ECHOCARDIOGRAPHY

ECHOCARDIOGRAPHY

HARVEY FEIGENBAUM, M.D.

Distinguished Professor of Medicine
Director of Hemodynamic Laboratories
Indiana University School of Medicine
Senior Research Associate
Krannert Institute of Cardiology
Indianapolis, Indiana

3rd Edition

LEA & FEBIGER

Philadelphia   1981

Cover: Echograms are from a patient with bi-atrial tumors and were obtained during a visit to the People's Republic of China.

Library of Congress Cataloging in Publication Data

Feigenbaum, Harvey.
  Echocardiography.

  Includes index.
  1. Ultrasonic cardiography. I. Title. [DNLM:
1. Echocardiography. WG141.5.E2 F298e]
RC683.5.U5F44   1980   616.1′207544   80-20682
ISBN 0-8121-0758-6

Published in Great Britain by Henry Kimpton Publishers, London

PRINTED IN THE UNITED STATES OF AMERICA

Print Number 6 5 4 3 2 1

To my wife, Phyllis,
who endured many lonely hours
while this book was being written

Preface

The tremendous growth of echocardiography in the past eight years is reflected by the relative sizes of the first, second, and third editions of this book. One of the most difficult tasks was trying to provide comprehensive coverage of the field without making this edition too large and cumbersome. Many changes in echocardiography had to be included. Probably the major advance has been the expanded use of two-dimensional echocardiography. This relatively new ultrasonic technique represents a sizable portion of this edition and accounts for the increase in its size.

The status of echocardiography has also changed significantly in the past four years—this diagnostic technique is now an integral part of clinical cardiology. To reflect this change in status, I have reorganized the book. Individual parts of the echocardiogram, such as valves and chambers, are not discussed as isolated entities in separate chapters. Instead the book is organized to demonstrate the relationship between echocardiography and clinical cardiology. After discussing instrumentation and the technical aspects of the echocardiographic examination, I primarily attempt to show how echocardiography can help in many potential cardiologic problems. Various echocardiographic techniques are critically reviewed, with discussion of both advantages and disadvantages as well as projected future developments in the field.

This book may serve multiple purposes. Because an extensive list of references follows each chapter, this book can serve as a reference source. With more than 700 illustrations, this book functions as an atlas as well. A fairly detailed description of instrumentation and the echocardiographic examination is included for those actively involved in echocardiography. However, as in previous editions, most technical information is limited to specific chapters or sections so that physicians not intimately involved in echocardiography can read this book without the burden of excessive technical detail.

I have attempted to preserve the continuity, cohesiveness, and readability of previous editions. Since the chapters are interrelated, considerable overlap and repetition occur throughout the text. Many illustrations appear more than once for the reader's convenience.

Although this book has one author, it in no way represents the work of one individual. The text, again, is primarily the product of the echocardiographic laboratories at the Indiana University School of Medicine. Ned Weyman, Betty Corya, and Jim Dillon have been primarily responsible for the investigative activities and daily operation of these laboratories. Without their efforts this book would not have been possible. I also wish to thank Randy Caldwell for many of the pediatric echocardiograms. I am particularly indebted to the technical assistance provided by Jane Marshall, Debbie Green, and Licia Mueller. Not only did they perform many of the echocardiographic examinations illustrated here, but they also considerably assisted in the preparation of this text. Thanks again go to Phil Wilson for his outstanding artwork and to Joe Demma for the photographic reproductions. And last, I wish to express special gratitude to my secretary, Cheryl Childress. Not only did she type the entire manuscript, but she also did most of the artwork for this edition.

Indianapolis, Indiana   HARVEY FEIGENBAUM

Contents

Instrumentation

The early evolution of echocardiography was primarily a result of clinicians developing a variety of applications for the M-mode echocardiographic technique. During this time there were relatively minor changes in instrumentation. Probably the only major advance was the use of strip-chart recorders rather than Polaroid film.

Over the past four to five years, however, with the advent of cross-sectional or two-dimensional echocardiography, dramatic changes in instrumentation have occurred. These changes have revolutionized the clinical uses of echocardiography and have expanded the overall value of this diagnostic tool. At the same time these developments have forced echocardiographers to acquire more knowledge of the instrumentation involved in this diagnostic examination. Since much of the future growth of echocardiography will be directly related to developments in instrumentation, it is becoming increasingly important for the echocardiographer to fully understand how the instruments produce the necessary clinical information.

Since an extensive description of the physics and engineering of echocardiography is beyond the scope of this text, I have attempted to simplify an otherwise extremely complicated subject. Some of the references provide more detailed information for readers who wish to delve more deeply into the principles of ultrasonic instrumentation.[1-4]

PHYSICAL PROPERTIES OF ULTRASOUND

By definition, ultrasound is sound having a frequency greater than 20,000 cycles per second,[2] that is, the sound is above the audible range. Actually, frequencies in the range of millions of cycles per second are used for medical diagnostic purposes. The principal advantages of high frequency sound or ultrasound as a diagnostic tool are: (1) ultrasound can be directed in a beam, (2) it obeys the laws of reflection and refraction, and (3) it is reflected by objects of small size. The principal disadvantage of ultrasound is that it propagates poorly through a gaseous medium. It is virtually impossible for ultrasound to pass to or from a gaseous medium such as air. As a result, the ultrasound-producing element or transducer must have airless contact with the body during the examination of a patient. In addition, it is difficult to examine parts of the body that contain air.

When discussing any type of sound one must understand the following terms: cycle, wavelength, velocity, and frequency.[3,5] Figure 1–1 demonstrates that a sound wave is a series of compressions and rarefactions. Such changes are frequently depicted as a sine wave with the peak of the hill representing the pressure maximum and the nadir of the valley the pressure minimum. The combination of one compression and one rarefaction represents one cycle, and the distance between the onset or peak compression of one cycle to the next is the wavelength. The velocity represents the speed at which sound waves travel through a particular medium. The frequency is the number of cycles in a given time. In other words, the velocity is equal to the frequency times the wavelength ($v = f \times \lambda$). Thus frequency and wavelength are inversely related; the higher the fre-

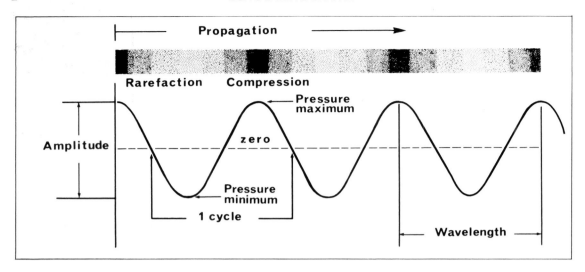

Fig. 1–1.   A soundwave is a series of compressions and rarefactions. The combination of one compression and one rarefaction represents one cycle. The distance between the onset (peak compression) of one cycle to the next is the wavelength.

quency, the shorter the wavelength. The velocity at which sound travels through a medium depends on the density and elastic properties of that medium. For example, sound travels faster through a dense medium, such as a solid, than it does through a less dense substance such as water. Velocity also depends on temperature. However, since body temperature is relatively constant within a fairly narrow range, changes in temperature are usually not an important factor in medical diagnostic work. The velocity of sound is fairly constant for human soft tissue, being approximately 1,540 meters per second.[6] There is a significant difference in the velocity if the sound passes through a solid structure such as bone.

How sound travels through a medium is frequently referred to as the acoustic impedance of that medium.[7] By definition, acoustic impedance is the density of the medium times the velocity that sound travels through that medium. For practical purposes, one may think of acoustic impedance in terms of the density of the medium. As a sound wave travels through a homogeneous medium, it essentially continues in a straight line. When the beam reaches an interface between two media with different acoustic impedances, it undergoes reflection and refraction. Figure

1–2 demonstrates the principles of reflection and refraction. As the sound wave travels through a relatively homogeneous medium (medium #1, Fig. 1–2), it is propagated essentially in a straight line. When it reaches an interface with a medium of different acoustic impedance or density (medium #2, Fig. 1–2), part of the beam is refracted and part is reflected. Almost all diagnostic ultrasound methods are based on the principle that ultrasound is reflected by an interface between media of different acoustic imped-

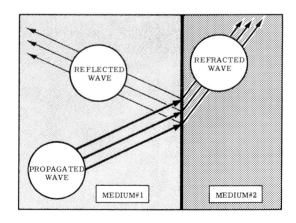

Fig. 1–2.   Ultrasound is reflected and refracted by an interface between two media of different acoustic impedance.

ances. The amount of sound that is reflected
depends on the degree of difference between the two media, i.e., the greater the
acoustic mismatch, the greater the amount of
sound reflected. For example, more sound is
reflected from an interface between gaseous
and solid media than from a liquid-solid
interface. In addition, the amount of ultrasound that is reflected depends on how
the ultrasonic beam strikes the interface and
the angle of incidence (Fig. 1–3). The closer
the angle of incidence is to 90°, the greater
the amount of reflected ultrasound.

When discussing ultrasonic echoes it is
important to distinguish between specular
echoes and scattered echoes (Fig. 1–4).
Specular echoes are produced by objects that
are fairly large with respect to the
wavelength and present a relatively smooth
surface to the ultrasonic beam. These objects
regularly reflect the ultrasonic energy and
are very angle dependent. The angles of the
echoes are predicted by the spatial orientation and the shape of the reflecting object or
interface. To date, echocardiography has
been principally concerned with specular
echoes originating from cardiac valves and
walls.

With increasing use of cross-sectional or
two-dimensional echocardiography as well
as increasing interest in examining the
myocardium, there is a greater need for understanding scattered echoes. Such echoes
originate from relatively small objects with
irregular surfaces. The resultant echoes are
reflected in multiple directions. Only a small

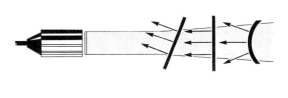

SPECULAR ECHOES

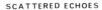

SCATTERED ECHOES

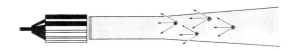

Fig. 1–4. Specular echoes originate from relatively large, strongly reflective, regularly shaped objects with smooth surfaces and are relatively intense
and angle dependent. Scattered echoes originate from
small, weakly reflective, irregularly shaped objects
and are less angle dependent and less intense.

percentage of the ultrasonic energy returns
to the transducer. However small, some energy does return to the transducer from scattered echoes. With specular echoes, if the
angle is improper, virtually none of the ultrasonic energy returns to the transducer.
Thus, although scattered echoes are difficult
to record, they are everpresent, are not angle
dependent, and are important for visualizing
objects essentially parallel to the ultrasonic
beam, such as the lateral or medial walls of
the left ventricle. With higher gain settings,
higher frequency transducers, and better
signal-to-noise ratio of instruments,
echocardiography will be increasingly concerned with recording scattered echoes.

Whether or not the ultrasound is reflected
by an interface also depends on the relative
sizes of the mismatched media and the
wavelength. If a solid object is submerged in
water, whether the ultrasound is reflected
from that object depends on the size of the
solid object with respect to the wavelength
of the ultrasound. The total thickness presented to the ultrasonic beam must be at least
one fourth the wavelength of the ultrasound.
Ultrasound having a higher frequency or a
shorter wavelength can reflect sound from
smaller objects. Thus a higher frequency ultrasonic beam has greater resolving power,
which is the ability to visualize objects or

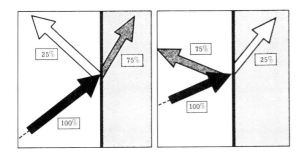

Fig. 1–3. The amount of ultrasound reflected or
refracted depends on the angle at which the ultrasonic
beam hits the interface between different media. As
the angle of incidence approaches 90°, a higher percentage of the ultrasound is reflected.

interfaces that are close to each other.[8] Echocardiography commonly utilizes ultrasound with a frequency of approximately 2,000,000 cycles per second or 2 megaHertz (mHz). (Hertz or Hz is another term for cycles per second.) Sound with a frequency of 2 mHz permits the recording of distinct echoes from interfaces that are approximately 1 mm apart. Since very high-frequency ultrasound is reflected by many small interfaces, a large percentage of the ultrasonic energy is reflected by these interfaces and less energy is available to penetrate deeply into the body. Thus penetration of the ultrasonic beam decreases as frequency increases.[1] Sonic absorption and scattering, which occurs even in a homogeneous medium, also determine how well ultrasound penetrates.[9] Again, ultrasound with higher frequencies has greater absorption and scattering, and thus poorer penetration. Naturally, the less homogeneous the medium, the more difficult it is for the ultrasound to penetrate, since reflection and refraction are important factors in diminishing the intensity of the beam as it travels through any nonhomogeneous medium.

The loss of ultrasound as it traverses a medium is known as attenuation, which is a combination of absorption and scattering. A term used to express the amount of absorption and attenuation of ultrasound in tissue is the "half-value layer,"[6] or "half-power distance."[4] These terms refer to the distance that ultrasound will travel in a particular tissue before its energy or amplitude is attenuated to half its original value. Table 1–1 gives the half-power distances for tissues and substances important in echocardiography. These values obviously depend on

the frequency, and those listed in Table 1–1 are for a frequency of 2 mHz. As noted in this table, ultrasound can travel 380 cm in water before its power decreases to half its original value. The loss of power when ultrasound travels through blood, although considerably greater, is still relatively low considering the distances involved in echocardiography. As expected, the attenuation is greater for soft tissue and even higher for muscle. Thus it is not surprising that a thick muscular chest wall would offer a significant obstacle to the transmission of ultrasound. Nonmuscular soft tissue such as fat has a longer half-power distance than muscle and is not quite as attenuating. The half-power distance for bone is still less than for muscle, which documents why bone is such a barrier to ultrasound. Cartilage is not listed, but its attenuating properties are clearly less than those of bone. Air and lung have extremely short half-power distances and represent severe obstacles to the transmission of ultrasound.

The absorption or attenuation of ultrasound need not always be uniform throughout the recording.[11] A localized object that reflects or attenuates sound may impede the transmission of ultrasound only in that area. Such an object may produce an "acoustic shadow." Since little ultrasonic energy passes through this particular object, structures distant to or behind the "shadowing" object may not be recorded echographically. Acoustic shadowing is an important parameter in other areas of diagnostic ultrasound, especially in examinations of the abdomen or breast. This phenomenon occurs in echocardiography when examining dense structures such as prosthetic valves or calcifications.

TRANSDUCERS AND THE PRODUCTION OF ULTRASOUND BEAMS

The use of ultrasound became practical with the development of piezoelectric transducers.[10] Piezoelectric means "pressure-electric." Piezoelectric substances change shape under the influence of an electrical field;[3] quartz was one of the first elements noted to have this property. If one impresses an electrical current through a quartz crystal

Table 1–1. Half-power Distances for Tissues and Substances Important in Echocardiography

Material	Half-power Distance (CM)
Water	380
Blood	15
Soft tissue except muscle	5 to 1
Muscle	1 to 0.6
Bone	0.7 to 0.2
Air	0.08
Lung	0.05

(Fig. 1–5), the shape of the crystal varies with the polarity. As the crystal expands and contracts it produces compressions and rarefactions or sound waves. The reverse is also true; when the crystal is struck by a sound wave, it produces an electrical impulse. Such a piezoelectric element is the primary component of an ultrasonic transducer. Commercial transducers use ceramics, such as barium titanate or lead zirconate titanate, as the piezoelectric element. Figure 1–6 is a diagram of the essential components of a transducer showing the piezoelectric element with electrodes connected to an electrical source on both sides. Behind the piezoelectric element is some backing material, which absorbs sound energy directed backward and improves the shape of the forward energy.

Recent transducer design has made the thickness of the piezoelectric element one fourth the inherent wavelength of the transmitted frequency. Designing the transducer in this fashion has apparently improved significantly the efficiency and sensitivity of the transducer. Thus "quarter wavelength" transducers are becoming the standard of the industry.

Because of the recent advances in instrumentation, the nature of the ultrasonic beam generated by the transducer must be understood. If one used a single small-element transducer, the ultrasonic waves would radiate from that transducer much as

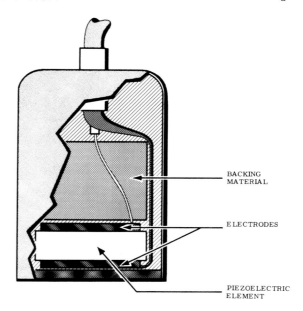

Fig. 1–6. The essential components of an ultrasonic transducer.

would the ripples created by a pebble dropped into water (Fig. 1–7). If one were to use a series of multiple small elements to produce the ultrasonic beam, then the individual curved waves or "ripples" would combine to form a linear wave front moving perpendicularly from the linearly arranged elements. Thus, by using multiple small elements that fire simultaneously, a unidirectional ultrasonic beam can be generated. If a single large element is used, a common procedure in echocardiography, an infinite number of small elements would essentially result. The individual wave fronts form a compact linear wave front that moves perpendicularly away from the face of the transducer (Fig. 1–7).

The principal sound waves produced by a transducer are longitudinal waves. These waves, which occur primarily in fluid, move parallel to the direction of the propagation of the sound waves. Other waves, such as sheer waves, move perpendicular to the propagation; however, these primarily occur in such solids as bone and play a relatively minor role in echocardiography. A more important secondary wave front presents the problem of "side lobes." As noted in Figure 1–7, the ultrasonic beam is comprised of multiple,

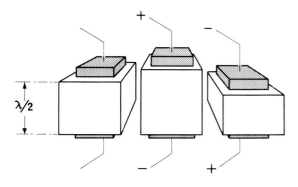

Fig. 1–5. Sketch of a crystal that has piezoelectric properties. The crystal changes shape as the surrounding electrical field is reversed. The wavelength (λ) of the emitted ultrasound is a function of the size of the crystal.

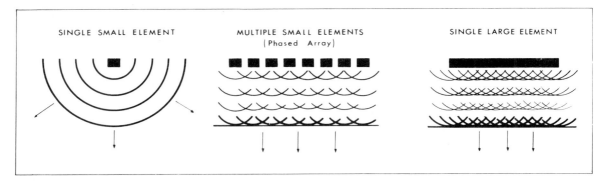

Fig. 1–7. Diagram demonstrating how longitudinal ultrasonic wave fronts are produced. The ultrasonic wavelets travel in a circular fashion from a single, small element. With either multiple element or single large element transducer, the circular wavelets combine to produce a longitudinal wave front directed away from the face of the transducer.

circular wavelets that originate from each element, especially from the edges, and move in directions different from those of the principal longitudinal wave. This problem is greatest with a single small element and is least prominent with a single large element. Partially because of the increased number of edges, an ultrasonic beam generated by multiple small elements will have more extraneous ultrasonic beams or side lobes than one formed from a single large element. These side lobes can produce artifactual information and will be discussed later in this chapter.

The series of longitudinal waves comprise the ultrasonic beam. As the beam propagates, it remains essentially parallel for a given distance and then begins to diverge (Fig. 1–8). That part of the beam closest to

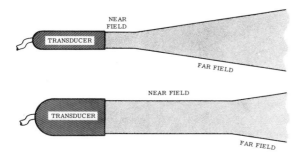

Fig. 1–8. Diagram demonstrating the influence of transducer size on the ultrasonic beam. The near field is much shorter and divergence considerably greater when the transducer is smaller.

the transducer and parallel to it is known as the near field or Fresnel zone. When the beam begins to diverge, it is called the far field or Fraunhofer zone. The diagnostic use of ultrasound works best when the objects being examined are located in the near field because the beam is more parallel, the reflecting interfaces are more perpendicular to the transducer, and thus the returning echoes are of greater intensity. One can detect many interfaces in the far field, although this becomes progressively more difficult the farther one goes into the far field.

The length of the near field (l) is a function of the radius of the transducer (r) and the wavelength (λ) and has been calculated as equal to the square of the radius divided by the wavelength ($l = \frac{r^2}{\lambda}$).[12] Thus, to lengthen the near field one would either decrease the wavelength or increase the size of the transducer. Figure 1–8 illustrates the effect of transducer size and Figure 1–9 the effect of frequency on the length of the near field. Doubling the size of the transducer quadruples the near field (Fig. 1–8). With a 12-mm diameter transducer, a 2.25-mHz transducer has a near field of 5.26 cm (Fig. 1–9). A 3.5-mHz transducer with a 12-mm diameter has a near field of 8.2 cm. Increasing the frequency to 5 mHz increases the near field to 11.6 cm (Fig. 1–9).

One can decrease the amount of diversion in the far field by using a focused transducer; such focusing is done by placing an acoustic

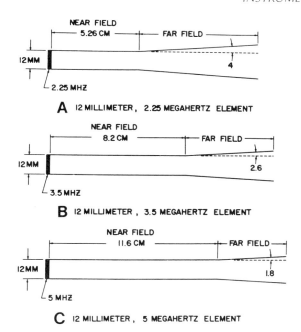

Fig. 1–9. The effect of transducer frequency on the near field. Higher frequency transducers have much longer near fields.

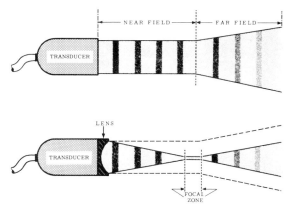

Fig. 1–10. Diagrams of the ultrasonic beam emitted by an unfocused, A, and a focused, B, transducer.

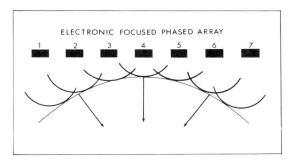

Fig. 1–11. Diagram demonstrating how a phased array transducer can focus the ultrasonic beam. By appropriate timing of the individual elements, the leading edges of the wavelets can produce a concentrically curved wave front so that the resultant ultrasonic beam focuses at a given point from the transducer.

lens on the surface of the transducer or by altering the curvature of the transducer itself. Using a lens with a concave surface or a transducer with a concave face, the ultrasonic beam is brought to a narrow zone at a predetermined distance from the transducer (Fig. 1–10). Narrowing the ultrasonic beam increases its intensity at the focal zone where the beam is narrowest and decreases the amount of divergence of the sound in the far field.

It is also possible to focus the ultrasonic beam electronically. By using a transducer made up of multiple small elements, the wave front can be shaped according to the timing of the individual elements. Figure 1–11 shows a transducer made up of multiple small elements that are individually fired so that the ultrasonic beam is curved. By firing the outside elements, 1 and 7, first, then elements 2 and 6, 3 and 5, and 4, one can shape the ultrasonic beam so that it converges much as the beam would converge when an acoustic lens is used. The curve can be varied according to when the individual elements are fired, and thus the location of the

focal zone can be changed. One can have a fixed-focus electronic beam or one can change the focal zone rapidly and generate a dynamically focused ultrasonic beam.[8,13,17] Such a transducer, which consists of multiple small elements fired individually in a controlled manner (in order to manipulate the ultrasonic beam), is known as a phased array transducer.

When discussing the ultrasonic beam it should be recognized that the beam is three-dimensional and not two-dimensional. Figure 1–12 illustrates the three-dimensional nature of the ultrasonic beam. When a transducer with a single, circular crystal is used, the beam is cylindrical in nature and

SINGLE CRYSTAL

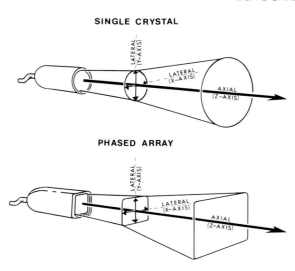

PHASED ARRAY

Fig. 1–12.   Three-dimensional presentation of the ultrasonic beam from a circular single-crystal transducer and from a phased array transducer demonstrating the various beam axes.

circular in cross-section. An ultrasonic beam generated by a phased array transducer made up of multiple, rectangular-shaped small elements produces an ultrasonic beam with a rectangular cross-section. The dimensions of the ultrasonic beam have been divided into axial (i.e., parallel to the direction of the ultrasonic beam) and lateral (i.e., perpendicular) to the ultrasonic beam. (Occasionally, axial is referred to as "linear" or "longitudinal" and lateral as "azimuthal."[5] In this text, the more common terms axial and lateral will be used.) Because of the three-dimensional nature of the beam, the lateral dimension has been subdivided into y axis (vertical dimension) and x axis (horizontal dimension). With a single, circular crystal the x and y axes are equal; with a phased array rectangular beam, however, the x and y axes are frequently dissimilar.[15] Acoustic focusing using a lens or shaping of the ultrasonic element will change the x and y axes equally (Fig. 1–13A). Electronic focusing utilizing the phased array principle and a transducer with multiple, rectangular-shaped elements will decrease the x axis without influencing the y axis (Fig. 1–13, B and C).[18] A dynamically focused beam will have a long focal zone (Fig. 1–13C).[16] If the phased array elements were circles or a

A

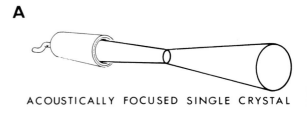

ACOUSTICALLY FOCUSED SINGLE CRYSTAL

B

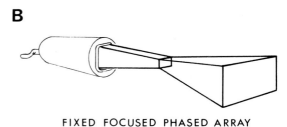

FIXED FOCUSED PHASED ARRAY

C

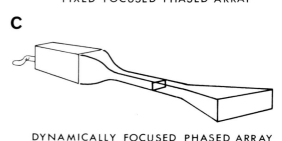

DYNAMICALLY FOCUSED PHASED ARRAY

Fig. 1–13.   Diagram demonstrating the ultrasonic beams emitted by A, an acoustically focused single-crystal transducer, B, a fixed-focused phased array transducer, and C, a dynamically focused phased array transducer.

series of rings rather than a series of long, thin elements, then electronic focusing would decrease the y as well as the x axis. Such a phased array system is known as annular phased array[19] and is available for some forms of ultrasonic imaging.[20] Since annular phased array is not currently used in echocardiography, it will be discussed later in this chapter in the section on future developments.

The ultrasonic beam is not absolute. The beam is greater in amplitude or intensity in the center, with decreasing intensity toward the edges of the beam (Fig. 1–14). Thus one must recognize the relative nature of beam width or sound intensity profile. When the shape of the ultrasonic beam is diagrammed, one usually draws the edge of the beam to the half-value limit of the beam plot. Figure 1–15 shows a transaxial beam plot and illus-

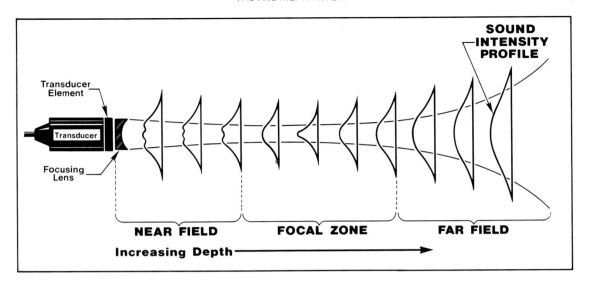

Fig. 1–14. The sound intensity profile of an acoustically focused transducer.

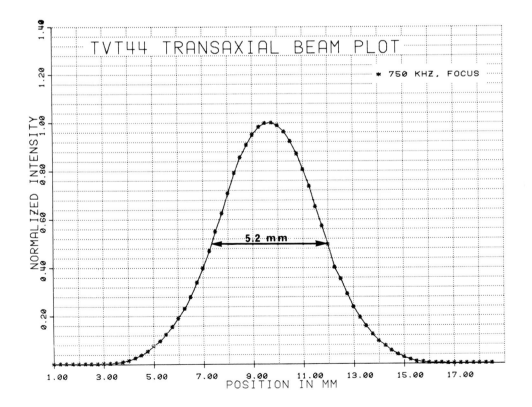

Fig. 1–15. Transaxial beam plot. The beam width or lateral resolution is a function of the intensity of the ultrasonic beam. The beam width is commonly measured at the half-intensity level.

trates the relative nature of the beam width. The beam at its peak intensity may only be 1 mm wide. However, the beam width at its weakest intensity is more than 12 mm wide. It is customary to measure the beam width at its half amplitude or intensity. In this particular example the beam width of this ultrasonic beam would be 5.2 mm. It should be apparent that if one used a higher gain setting on the echograph, the weaker portion of the ultrasonic beam would be recorded and the beam width would be larger. Conversely, if one used a low-gain setting and only the most intense portion of the ultrasonic beam were recorded, then the beam width would be narrowed. Understanding beam width is important since it is the cause for many potential artifacts in echocardiography.

PRINCIPLES OF M-MODE AND TWO-DIMENSIONAL ECHOCARDIOGRAPHY

The instrument used to create an image using ultrasound is known as an echograph. Figure 1–16 shows a block diagram of an echograph. The essential components include the transducer, which is in contact with the tissue being examined and which both sends and receives the ultrasound. The transmitter regulates the sending of the ultrasound by the transducer by way of a timer that controls the duration and frequency of the ultrasonic pulses emitted by the transducer. The transducer converts the returning echoes to electrical impulses, which then go to the receiver and the signal amplifier. The

returning echoes or impulses are processed so that they can be displayed on the cathode ray tube or oscilloscope.

Figure 1–17 demonstrates how one may use ultrasound to obtain an image of an object. Such acoustic imaging, sometimes called "echo ranging," depends primarily on the property of reflection together with pulsing of the ultrasonic beam.[21] The electric energy is intermittently fed into the transducer so that the piezoelectric element sends out ultrasound for brief periods of time. The duration of each ultrasonic impulse may be as short as one microsecond and influences the shape of the ultrasonic pulse. Following the emission or burst of ultrasound, the transducer becomes a receiver waiting to record any reflected ultrasound waves or echoes. Following a relatively long period of time, another burst of ultrasound is emitted and the cycle is repeated. The rate with which the bursts of ultrasonic energy are emitted is the pulse repetition rate or pulse repetition frequency of the echograph. Commercial diagnostic echographs have repetition rates between 200 to 5,000 per second. M-mode echographs have repetition rates of approximately 1,000 to 2,000 per second, whereas cross-sectional instruments have repetition rates between 3,000[22] and 5,000 per second. Many standard M-mode echographs have approximately 1½-microsecond bursts of ultrasound with a repetition rate of 1,000 per second. Thus the transducer functions as a receiver nearly 99 percent of the time. The commercial diagnostic echographs are extremely sensitive receivers and can detect a signal even when less than one percent of the ultrasonic energy is reflected.

In Figure 1–17, a transducer is placed on the side of a beaker of water and sends out short bursts of ultrasound at a given frequency. These bursts of ultrasound travel through the homogeneous water and are reflected by the interface between the water and the far side of the beaker. The reflected ultrasound or echo then retraces its original path and strikes the transducer, which is now functioning as a receiver. An electrical signal is created as the sound hits the piezoelectric element and is registered on the oscilloscope of the echograph. If one knows the velocity

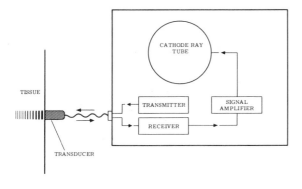

Fig. 1–16.   Block diagram of the components of an ultrasonic echograph.

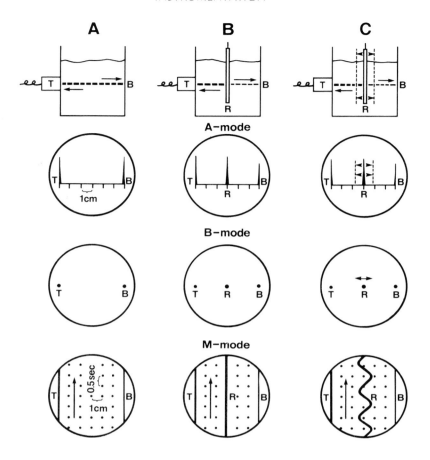

Fig. 1–17. Diagrams illustrating the principles of acoustic imaging using pulsed, reflected ultrasound (see text for details). T = transducer; B = beaker; R = rod. (From Feigenbaum, H. and Zaky, A.: Use of diagnostic ultrasound in clinical cardiology. J. Indiana State Med. Assoc., 59:140, 1966.

of sound traveling through the medium being examined as well as the time it takes for the ultrasound to leave the transducer, strike the interface, and return as an echo, then calculating the distance of the reflecting interface from the transducer is simple. By calibrating the echograph for the velocity of sound of the medium being examined, the conversion of time to distance may be done automatically. Thus, instead of indicating how long it takes for a burst of ultrasound to leave the transducer and to return as an echo, the electrical signal generated by the returning echo is actually displayed on the oscilloscope of the echograph at a certain distance from the transducer. In this particular example (Fig. 1–17A), the reflecting interface or the side of the beaker (B) is indicated as

being 6.0 cm away from the transducer. A built-in electrical artifact (T) is used to indicate the position of the transducer.

If a rod (R, Fig. 1–17B) is placed in the center of the beaker, the ultrasound strikes the rod first. Since the rod is closer to the transducer than to the far side of the beaker, the echo reflected from this interface reaches the transducer earlier than it would from the far side of the beaker. The shorter time is converted to a shorter distance, and the echo from the rod is displayed on the oscilloscope as being only 3.0 cm from the transducer. Some ultrasonic energy will continue to move past the rod, strike the far side of the beaker, and return to the transducer as it did when the rod was absent. Thus on the oscilloscope the echo from the rod is indicated as being 3.0 cm from the transducer and the echo from the far side of the beaker is 6.0 cm from the transducer.

If the rod is moving, its distance from the transducer is constantly changing (Fig. 1–17C). When the first burst of ultrasonic energy hits the rod, it may be 4.0 cm from the transducer. The next burst may be 3.0 cm away, and the next 2.0 cm away. Thus the oscilloscope shows that the position of the rod with respect to the transducer is constantly changing. How well this motion is visualized depends in part on the repetition rate or sampling rate of the echograph. With a repetition rate of approximately 1,000 per second, this echo motion is almost continuous.

If the interface from which the echo is derived is constantly moving (Fig. 1–17C), then the echo position will change constantly with reference to the transducer. The echo signal will move back and forth on the face of the oscilloscope. The motion could be recorded by filming or videotaping the oscilloscopic image. Another technique for displaying echo motion utilizes intensity modulation. This type of modification converts the amplitude of the echo to intensity; the signal is converted from a spike (Fig. 1–17, A-mode) to a dot (Fig. 1–17, B-mode). Within limits, the taller the echo, the brighter the dot. This presentation is known as B-mode, the B standing for brightness. Having converted the signal to a dot, one now has another dimension available for the recording. Since the heart is a moving object, one can record the motion by introducing time as the second dimension. For example, if the tracing is swept from bottom to top, as in the bottom diagram of Figure 1–17C, a wavy line will be inscribed if the rod or interface is moving. If the object is stationary (bottom tracing, Fig. 1–17B), a straight line will be inscribed. For calibration one may use a grid or a series of dots that are 1 cm apart in one axis and 0.5 sec apart in the other. Since all interfaces of the heart constantly move, this type of display has been the backbone of echocardiography.

The term adopted for this type of echo presentation is "M-mode;" M stands for motion. "Time motion" or TM is another name

given to this presentation. The standard display that presents the echo as a spike is known as "A-mode;" the A indicates the amplitude of the echo. The M-mode presentation may be recorded by taking a Polaroid photograph of the cathode ray tube. Such a photograph would be a time exposure as the intensity-modulated dots sweep from bottom to top or left to right across the oscilloscope. Most early commercial echographs had the oscilloscopic image sweep from bottom to top for the convenience of the A-mode presentation and Polaroid photography.

Since an electrocardiographic tracing is usually displayed on the oscilloscope, and since the electrocardiogram is read from left to right rather than from bottom to top, one usually displays the echocardiogram as moving from left to right. Some echocardiographers record the M-mode tracing on continuous 35-mm film.[24,25] However, most echocardiographers currently use strip-chart recorders to display their M-mode tracings. The advantages of strip-chart recordings are that the film does not need to be developed after the examination is performed, and the display does not need to be magnified for interpretation. The introduction of strip-chart recorders has greatly facilitated the M-mode examination and has been an important factor in the growth of echocardiography.

Figure 1–18 shows how the echocardiographic system can record an M-mode tracing of the heart. In this particular examination the ultrasonic beam is directed at the heart in the vicinity of the left ventricular cavity. A small portion of the right ventricular cavity is also intersected by the ultrasonic beam. The actual M-mode recording was made on a strip-chart recorder. As would be expected, the chest wall structures are not moving with cardiac motion and are exhibited as a series of straight lines. The echoes from the anterior right ventricular wall (ARV) are not visualized clearly and are comprised of a fuzzy band of echoes that are thicker in systole than in diastole. The relatively echo-free space between the right ventricular echo (ARV) and the right side of the interventricular septum (RS) is a segment of the right ventricular cavity tran-

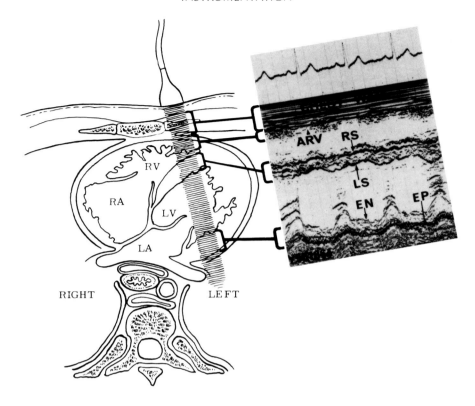

Fig. 1–18.   Diagram and echocardiogram illustrating how echocardiography can obtain an "ice-pick" or one-dimensional view of the heart through the right and left ventricles. ARV = anterior right ventricular wall; RS = right septum; LS = left septum; EN = posterior left ventricular endocardium; EP = posterior left ventricular epicardium; RA = right atrium; RV = right ventricle; LV = left ventricle; LA = left atrium.

sected by the ultrasonic beam. The interventricular septum (RS and LS) is represented by the band of echoes running through the middle of the tracing. The left side of the septum (LS) moves downward in systole and upward in diastole. The next major group of echoes originate from the posterior left ventricular wall with the endocardial (EN) echo having a greater amplitude during systole than the epicardial (EP) echo. The space between the two ventricular wall echoes represents the myocardium. The relatively echo-free space between the left side of the septum (LS) and the posterior left ventricular endocardium (EN) is the cavity of the left ventricle. Within the cavity, echoes from the mitral valve apparatus are visible occasionally.

If the spatial orientation of the transducer is tracked electronically, one could obtain a spatially oriented M-mode examination.

Such an examination has been used in Japan.[26,27] Spatial tracking of the ultrasonic beam is more commonly used to create a spatially oriented B-mode or cross-sectional examination. Figure 1–19 diagrams how a spatially oriented B-mode scan can provide a cross-sectional or two-dimensional image of an object. When the ultrasonic transducer is close to the top of the beaker, it traverses the circular object at the point at which the walls are relatively close together (Fig. 1–19A). As the transducer moves toward the bottom of the beaker, the beam transects the center of the circular object (Fig. 1–19B). Now the two B-mode echoes from the walls are farther apart and in the center of the oscilloscope. Moving the transducer closer to the bottom of the beaker causes the ultrasonic beam to again traverse the object at the point at which the walls are closer together (Fig. 1–19C). The oscilloscope shows two B-mode dots

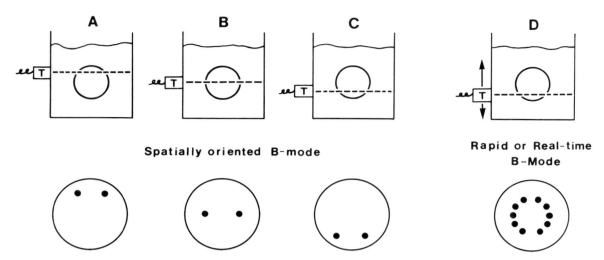

Fig. 1–19. Diagrams demonstrating how a spatially oriented B-mode scan can produce a two-dimensional image.

closer together and nearer the bottom of the transducer. In combination, these dots reveal the shape and size of the object being examined (Fig. 1–19D). If the object is motionless, one may take as much time as desired to move or scan the ultrasonic beam across the object. If the object is moving, however, then one should move the ultrasonic beam as rapidly as possible. A rapid B-mode scan is also known as a "real-time" scan. A real-time B-mode scan of the heart is commonly called "cross-sectional" or "two-dimensional" echocardiography.

Unfortunately, the terminology for real-time B-mode scanning of the heart is confusing. The most popular terms are "cross-sectional" or "two-dimensional" echocardiography, or just "real-time" echocardiography. However, many other terms have been used in the literature. One of the first investigators called the technique "ultrasonic cinematography."[28] This particular technique used a mirror system on a rotating ultrasonic transducer in a water tank. Similar techniques have been proposed.[29] Other terms that have been used include "cine ultrasound cardiography,"[30] "ultrasonic tomography,"[31] "ultrasonocardiotomography,"[32] "cardiac ultrasonography,"[33] and "ultrasonic cardiokymography."[26] Although the term two-dimensional echocardiography is most popular, I prefer cross-sectional

echocardiography because the examination does in fact produce cross-sectional images of the heart. One must not forget that M-mode echocardiography is also two-dimensional since time is plotted against distance. Despite this argument, most echocardiographers prefer the term two-dimensional echocardiography, which has been formally adopted by the American Society of Echocardiography. In keeping with this effort to standardize terminology, I will use the term two-dimensional echocardiography in this text and occasionally cross-sectional echocardiography.

There are various ways in which ultrasonic scans can be obtained. Figure 1–20 demonstrates some types of scans available in medical diagnostic work. Figure 1–19 exemplifies a linear scan. Although linear scans of the heart are being done, sector scans are more popular. The principal advantage of a sector scan is that it functions better within the confines of the limited echocardiographic window that is frequently available for examining the heart.

Figure 1–21 compares the standard M-mode echocardiographic examination with a real-time two-dimensional sector scan. The object in question is a sphere or ball moving as a pendulum within a beaker of water. When utilizing the M-mode examination (Fig. 1–21A), the oscilloscope shows a

TYPES OF SCANS

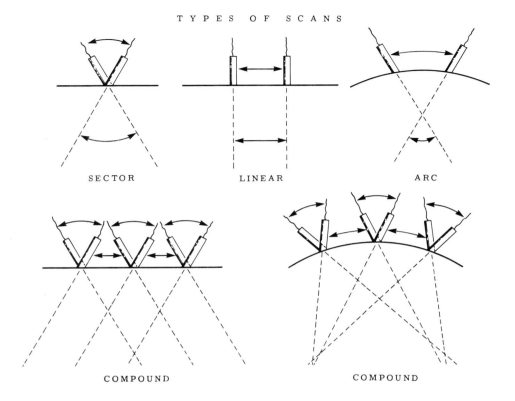

Fig. 1–20.   Various types of scanning maneuvers.

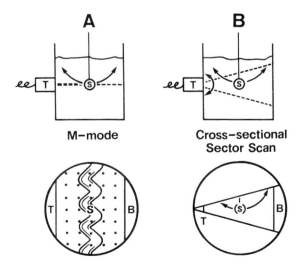

Fig. 1–21. Diagram comparing M-mode and cross-sectional sector scan of a spherical object moving as a pendulum in a beaker of water. (From Feigenbaum, H.: Echocardiography. *In* Heart Diseases. Edited by E. Braunwald. Philadelphia, W.B. Saunders Co., 1980.)

series of wavy lines principally from the leading and trailing edges of the sphere. Because of the beam width one might see multiple secondary, less intense echoes from the leading and trailing edges. The M-mode examination gives an excellent evaluation of the diameter of the object and the amount of motion in the axial direction. The examiner would have no appreciation of motion in the lateral direction (perpendicular to the ultrasonic beam), and he would not understand the shape of the object being examined. From the M-mode examination, one could say that there was an object approximately 1 cm in diameter moving approximately 1 cm in the axial direction.

With a cross-sectional scan the examiner would now appreciate that the object was spherical in nature. One might not be able to see the entire circle of the object because part of the walls might be parallel to the ultrasonic beam. However, it would be obvious that the object was spherical and not rectangular. In addition, one could appreciate that the object was moving in an arc rather than in a straight line. Thus the two-dimensional examination would provide the added information of lateral motion and shape.

Table 1–2 compares M-mode and two-dimensional echocardiography. For obtaining axial dimensions or axial motion, M-mode echocardiography is excellent. The sampling rate is approximately 1,000 per second, which provides an outstanding recording of axial motion. The processing of M-mode echoes is such that the axial resolution is usually better than with two-dimensional echocardiography. This factor plus the convenience of a strip-chart recorder make M-mode echocardiography particularly useful for axial dimensions. Since there are many important echocardiographic applications that depend on axial motion and axial dimensions, it is highly unlikely that M-mode echocardiography will be replaced in the near future. However, there are situations whereby it is necessary to know lateral dimensions, lateral motion, and the shape of the object. With M-mode echocardiography, it is very difficult, if not impossible, to obtain this information. Because of the spatial orientation inherent in two-dimensional echocardiography, this technique can determine lateral dimensions, lateral motion, and shape. Thus the two examinations are truly complementary. There are many situations whereby the rapid sampling rate, the recording of time on a strip-chart recorder, and the rapidity with which interpretations and measurements can be made, make the M-mode examination preferable. At other times the spatial orientation inherent in

two-dimensional echocardiography is required to fill in missing or vital data. This complementary relationship between M-mode and two-dimensional echocardiography and their relative advantages and disadvantages are emphasized throughout the text.

Real-time two-dimensional echocardiography is still an evolving field. Many commercial instruments are available, each with its advantages and disadvantages. There are basically two types of real-time scanners, mechanical and electronic (Fig. 1–22). Mechanical scanners move the ultrasonic beam by way of an electric motor, whereas electronic systems steer the ultrasonic beam electronically. The mechanical systems may use a probe with an oscillating transducer whereby the active element rocks through a given angle.[22,23,32,34–36] This angle may vary from 0° to 60°. A commonly used angle is 30°; 60° is probably the upper limit by which this system can function unless used with a water bath.[37] It must be remembered that the oscillating transducer must start and stop at the end of each excursion. As a result, the trans-

Table 1–2. Comparison Between M-Mode and Two-Dimensional Echocardiography

	M-Mode	2-D
Axial dimension	Excellent	Good
Axial motion	Excellent	Good
Lateral dimensions	Impossible	Good
Lateral motion	Poor	Good
Shape	Poor	Good

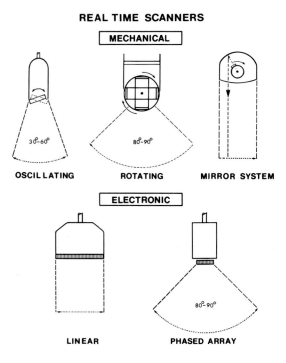

Fig. 1–22. Various types of real-time scanners.

ducer moves a little slower at the beginning and end of each sweep; thus the ultrasonic lines may not be distributed evenly. With oscillating transducers, the probes are usually placed directly on the chest, and there is some physical vibration of the transducer. The vibrations are not as troublesome as initially contemplated, but when the scan angle is greater than 45° they may become excessive. Although the vibratory sensation produced by the oscillating transducer is a nuisance, it is possible that the mechanical irritation of the chest could potentially benefit the ultrasonic examination. Several echocardiographers believe that the mechanical vibrating system, especially the narrow angle system, frequently obtains usable echocardiograms in patients in whom other systems were unsuccessful. The reason is unclear. Possible explanations include the high line density of the narrow-angle scan, the direct contact of the transducer with the chest, and the excellent maneuverability of the probe. An intriguing factor as yet unsubstantiated is whether the mechanical vibrations on the chest could in any way alter the acoustic properties of the chest wall. The chest becomes reddened and hyperemic in some individuals examined with an oscillating probe. Whatever the proper explanation, some echocardiographers feel that with a narrow-angle, oscillating probe, fewer technically unsatisfactory cross-sectional studies result.

A mechanical rotating transducer uses a series of active elements, usually three or four, mounted in a wheel located in a plastic housing filled with a liquid. Such a device has the advantage of providing a wider scan angle than can be provided by the oscillating transducer. The ultrasonic lines are also laid down uniformly since the sweeping of the transducer is constant. In addition, since the transducer is housed in plastic and the elements are not rocking back and forth, no appreciable vibration is noted by the patient. The disadvantage of such a transducer is that because it must transmit the ultrasonic beam through the plastic housing, potential reverberation artifacts are introduced, and there is slight attenuation of the ultrasonic beam by the plastic. In addition, there is the added expense of multiple transducer elements.

Another mechanical system that has not played much of a role in echocardiography utilizes a mirror system.[28,29] By rotating the transducer and reflecting the beam off of a parabolic mirror, one essentially obtains a linear scan. Such a system has been used for abdominal scanning but is not popular in echocardiography.

There are two basic electronic real-time scanners. The first such scanner utilized a series of small elements that were fired sequentially (Fig. 1–23). The sequential firing of the transducers essentially moved the ultrasonic beam linearly.[38–41] This device, known as a multi-element linear array transducer, was probably the first commercially available, practical, real-time cardiac scanner and was responsible for much of the enthusiasm for cross-sectional echocardiography. There have been many improvements in this instrument. The beam can be improved by electronic focusing and by firing multiple elements for each ultrasonic line of information. Real-time linear array scanners are now popular in abdominal ultrasound examinations. For cardiac examinations, however, these scanners have the principal disadvantage of requiring a fairly large

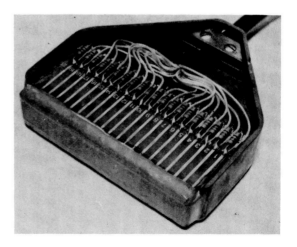

Fig. 1–23. Multi-element linear array transducer that provides an electronic scan of the heart. This particular probe consists of twenty piezoelectric elements. (From Bom, N.N., et al.: Multi-scan echocardiography. I, Technical description. Circulation, 48:1066, 1973.)

acoustic window. The large probe must overlie ribs and cannot be angled easily in the plane of the scan axis.

The most popular electronic real-time scanners utilize the phased array principle.[13,14,17,18] This type of scanner uses a multi-element transducer to create a single ultrasonic beam, the direction of which can be altered by controlling the timing when each element is fired. As noted in Figure 1–11, a multi-element transducer has the capability of electronic focusing by firing the individual elements so that a curved or focused wave front is formed. A similar technique can be used to change the direction of the angle of the wave front with a phased array system (Fig. 1–24). In this example, the ultrasonic wave front created by the multi-element, phased array transducer can be directed at a given angle and direction by firing each element individually, that is, elements one, two, three, four, and so on. Thus the leading edge of the wave front from the first transducer is farther away from the face of the probe than is that part of the wave front contributed by firing the seventh element. The resultant ultrasonic beam moves perpendicularly to the wave front. Changing the sequence of the firing of each element alters the direction of the wave front. Thus, by using a computer or microprocessor to control the firing of each element, it is possible to rapidly and randomly control the direction of the ultrasonic beam.

Table 1–3 compares some of the features of mechanical and phased array real-time sector scanners. Since the ultrasonic beam is

Table 1–3. Comparison of Mechanical and Phased Array Real-Time Sector Scanners

Features	Mechanical	Phased Array
Simultaneous M-mode and 2–D echo	No	Yes
Sequential M-mode and 2–D echo	Yes	Yes
Dual M-mode echo	No	Yes
Simultaneous 2–D and Doppler	No	Yes
Sequential 2–D and Doppler	Yes	Yes
Small acoustic window for wide-angle scan	No	Yes*
Can be electronically focused in lateral (y) axis	No	Yes
Compatible with ring or annular phased array transducer technology	Yes	No
Minimal side lobe artifacts	Yes	No
Easily compatible with transducers 5 mHz or above	Yes	No
Portable	Yes	±
Relatively inexpensive	Yes	No

*Size of phased array transducer depends on whether it is dynamically focused and on the frequency used.

electronically controlled with the phased array system, the direction of each line of information can be randomly distributed throughout the scan. By time sharing or alternating the lines of information between a one-dimensional M-mode examination and a two-dimensional cross-sectional examination, it is possible to obtain both examinations simultaneously. One merely directs an electronically generated cursor line through the desired portion of the cross-sectional examination for the appropriate M-mode examination. One can even electronically move the cursor throughout the scan to obtain an M-mode scan of the area. The mechanical system must move the beam in a designated fashion, either oscillating back and forth or rotating in one direction. Such a system does not have random access to the ultrasonic beam, and thus simultaneous, high-quality M-mode and two-dimensional examinations are not feasible. A crude low line density M-mode study is possible with a mechanical scan, but the quality of the

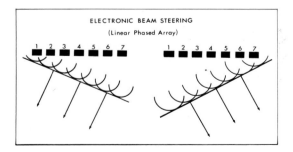

Fig. 1–24. Principles of electronic beam steering using linear phased array. By controlling the firing of the individual elements, the direction or the angle of wave front can be altered.

M-mode study does not compare with one derived from a phased array scanner. It is conceivable that once data are in digital form and can be manipulated by a computer, then simultaneous M-mode and two-dimensional examinations using a mechanical system might be possible in the future. At present, however, simultaneous M-mode and two-dimensional studies are done best with a phased aray scanning system.

Sequential M-mode and two-dimensional echocardiograms are of course possible with either mechanical or phased array systems. The mechanical system merely stops moving the transducer, and one automatically obtains a standard M-mode examination. A cursor again may indicate exactly where the transducer stops. The transducer usually stops in the center of the scan, although one may be able to direct the transducer at a different angle for the M-mode study.

Because of the random feature of electronic sector scanning, two simultaneous M-modes (or dual M-mode echo) are possible using this electronic approach. Figure 1–25 illustrates how two electronic cursors can be displayed on a two-dimensional study. Figure 1–26 shows the resultant simultaneous, dual M-mode examinations. Cursor 1 is passing through the level of the mitral valve and cursor 2 through the aortic

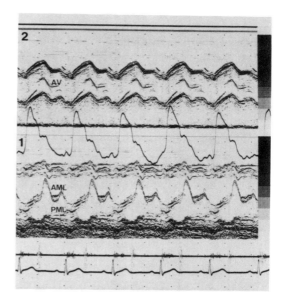

Fig. 1–26. Dual simultaneous M-mode echocardiograms using the phased array sector scanner illustrated in Figure 1–25. (From Machii, K.: Atlas of Cross-sectional Echocardiography. Tokyo, Toshiba Corp., 1978.)

valve. This feature is not available with the mechanical systems.

Obtaining simultaneous two-dimensional and Doppler echocardiograms would again require phased array technology because of the random access available with electronic steering. Sequential Doppler and two-dimensional recordings could of course be obtained with either technique. If a practical instrument is developed whereby the Doppler signal is displayed directly on the two-dimensional image, then phased array two-dimensional scanning will probably be required.

An important factor in scanning the heart is the size of the aperture or the face of the probe from which the scan is generated. With a phased array system, the limiting factor is the size of the transducer. With a mechanical system, the limiting factor is the arc through which the transducer moves. With a narrow-angle oscillating transducer, the arc is fairly small. For a 30-degree scan the transducer only arcs 15 degrees in either direction and the resultant aperture is small. As the angle increases, the size of the aper-

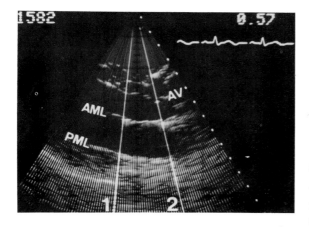

Fig. 1–25. Photograph demonstrating the capability of phased array sector scanner to obtain two simultaneous M-mode echocardiograms. (From Machii, K.: Atlas of Cross-sectional Echocardiography. Tokyo, Toshiba Corp., 1978.)

ture increases. With a rotating mechanical system, the aperture is even larger since the transducer elements must traverse a certain distance rather than pivot on one spot as with an oscillating system. The size of the phased array transducer depends on whether or not the system is electronically focused and on the frequency of the transducer. Unfocused or fixed-focus electronic sector scanners have a relatively small aperture with the face of the transducer being about 1 cm². Dynamically focused phased array transducers have traditionally been significantly larger than even mechanical systems. Newer focused transducers are being introduced that are smaller partially because of a higher frequency (3.0 to 3.5 mHz). Phased array transducers using frequencies higher than 3.5 mHz require a smaller aperture but are technically difficult to manufacture.

As already discussed, phased array systems have the advantage of electronically focusing the beam, either at some fixed distance or dynamically to give a relatively long focal zone (see Fig. 1–13C). Electronic focusing not only permits shaping of the beam, but one can also focus the received echoes by controlling the timing in a manner opposite from that used in creating the focused beam. Thus phased array systems can focus the beam in the y axis by focusing the transmitted beam and the returning echoes.

Current mechanical sector scanners do not have electronic focusing. However, there is interest in using annular array transducers that can electronically focus the beam not only in the y axis but in the x as well. If this feature is perfected, mechanical systems would have the capability of using such electronically focused transducers. It would be extremely difficult, if not impossible, for current phased array systems to use annular phased array transducers because of the complexity in electronically steering an annular array beam. Moving the annular array transducer mechanically would be far easier.

Side lobes have been briefly discussed and will be discussed in more detail later. This potential artifact presents more of a problem for phased array systems than it does with mechanical scanners.

There are obvious advantages to using higher frequency transducers. The most immediate need for such high-frequency systems is in examinations of small children or infants. The resolution is significantly better and, as already noted, so is the beam shape with high-frequency transducers. Because of the manner in which phasing is accomplished to steer the ultrasonic beam, creating phased array transducers in excess of 3.5 mHz is extremely difficult. Thus, if one needs transducers with higher frequencies, the mechanical system can probably provide this capability more readily.

The computer or microprocessor necessary for controlling the sequence of firing of phased array systems adds to the physical bulk of the system. As a result, it is frequently necessary for part of the recording system to be on a separate cart or else the total system is rather cumbersome. Thus, although some smaller, more portable phased array systems are being introduced, they still tend to be large and to have some limitations on portability. Since microprocessors are becoming smaller, this problem may be only temporary.

Probably the most portable echocardiographic instrument currently available is a small, hand-held multi-element cross-sectional system (Fig. 1–27).[44,45] This instrument is basically a small linear electronic scanner similar to that depicted in Figure 1–23. Equipped with a small television monitor screen, the device is intended to be used as an on-line, bedside diagnostic tool. The instrument's principal advantage is its portability and ease of use. The disadvantages include all of those present in any linear scanner in addition to the very small image and the relatively poor resolution.

Excessive electronic hardware and the technology required in manufacturing the components of phased array transducers render phased array systems more expensive than mechanical systems. Again, the difference in cost between mechanical and phased array systems may be temporary. Microprocessors and computers are decreasing in cost fairly dramatically. In addition, many mechanical systems are becoming more sophisticated, especially as they begin using multiple transducers. Thus it is conceivable

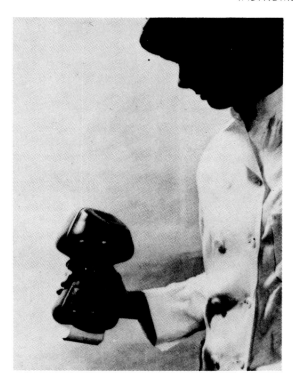

Fig. 1–27. Handheld multi-element linear scanner. (From Ligtvoet, C., et al.: Real-time ultrasonic imaging with a hand-held scanner. I. Technical description. Ultrasound Med. Biol., 4:91, 1978.)

that the difference in cost between the two systems may gradually decrease.

A somewhat minor factor is the size and weight of the transducer cable. Because of the complex nature of the phased array transducer, many more wires are required in the transducer cable. Thus the cable is heavier and the transducer more difficult to torque than in a mechanical system.

There are several relatively minor disadvantages to the electronic and mechanical sector scanners. A minor disadvantage of the phased array system is that the ultrasonic beam varies somewhat with the angle. The beam profile is not exactly the same with the beam perpendicular to the face of the transducer as when it is 45° from the center. To what extent this difference alters the image has not been demonstrated. A minor disadvantage of the mechanical system is that the transducer is constantly moving and is therefore in a slightly different location when it

sends and receives a given burst of ultrasound. The angle of the transducer changes slightly when the returning echoes hit the transducer. The importance of this difference is probably minor and does not significantly alter the image.

VARIABLES INVOLVED IN REAL-TIME SECTOR SCANNING

In order to understand the nature of real-time sector scanning, one must appreciate the variables involved in obtaining such images. One must remember that we are creating images with a relatively slow-moving modality—sound. Although two-dimensional echocardiograms have a similarity to angiograms or to photographs, one does not use fast-moving energy sources such as X rays or light to obtain these images. The speed of sound is considerably slower. Thus the limiting factor is the speed of sound in soft tissue and compromises must be made when generating a real-time two-dimensional image.

The variables and compromises to be considered are the depth of the examination desired, the line density, the pulse repetition frequency, the angle of the sweep, and the sweep or frame rate. Because the terms sweep, field, and frame are frequently used interchangeably, they can be confusing. A sweep indicates the movement of the ultrasonic beam through the desired angle. Field and frame usually refer to the television system on which most of these recordings are made. Television is made up of fields, each of which is one sixtieth of a second. Two fields are interlaced; the lines are laid down between each other to improve line density. Two interlaced 1/60-second "fields" produce one 1/30-second "frame." Thus, if the sector scanner is sweeping at a rate of 60 times per second, then each sweep is comparable to a single field, and two sweeps can be interlaced to produce one television frame. The frame rate therefore would be 30 per second, whereas the field or sweep rate would be 60 per second.

Table 1–4 presents some examples of how these variables interact in creating a real-time cross-sectional image. If the examination is to include 20 cm of depth, then each

Table 1–4. Variables in Real-Time Sector Scanning

Variables	Possible Combinations			
Depth of Examination (cm)	20	20	20	10
Time for each ultrasonic line (total distance traveled by ultrasound divided by velocity of sound plus fly-back time)	(40 cm or 0.4 m ÷ 1540 m/sec = 0.26 msec + 0.02 msec fly-back time = 0.28 msec)	(40 cm or 0.4 m ÷ 1540 m/sec = 0.26 msec + 0.02 msec fly-back time = 0.28 msec)	(40 cm or 0.4 m ÷ 1540 m/sec = 0.26 msec + 0.02 msec fly-back time = 0.28 msec)	(20 cm or 0.2 m ÷ 1540 m/sec = 0.13 msec + 0.02 msec fly-back time = 0.14 msec)
Sweep Rate (sweeps per second)	60	60	30	60
Time for each sweep (msec)	17	17	34	17
Lines per sweep time/sweep ÷ time/line	60 17 msec ÷ 0.28 msec	60 17 msec ÷ 0.28 msec	120 34 msec ÷ 0.28 msec	120 17 msec ÷ 0.14 msec
Pulse Repetition Frequency (pulses/sec) lines/sweep × sweeps/sec)	3600 60 × 60	3600 60 × 60	3600 120 × 60	7200 120 × 60
Angle	30°	90°	90°	90°
Line Density (lines/degree) lines/sweep–angle	2 60–30°	0.67 60–90°	1.33 120–90°	1.33 120–90°

ultrasonic line must travel 40 cm as the impulse leaves the transducer and returns as an echo. Since the velocity of ultrasound is 1,540 M/sec, it would take 0.28 msec for each ultrasonic line when one includes 0.02 msec for fly-back time. If the sweep rate is 60 per second, then 17 msec are available for each sweep of the ultrasonic beam. The lines per sweep are determined by the time available for one sweep and the time necessary for each ultrasonic line to be generated. In this particular case, one would have approximately 60 lines of ultrasonic information available for every sweep of the beam. The pulse repetition frequency that would be necessary to generate the necessary lines per sweep and the sweeps per second would be 3,600 pulses per second, a result obtained by multiplying the sweep rate by the lines per sweep. If one desires a 30° scan angle, there would be two lines per degree available for line density. If all variables remain constant, except for the scan angle, which is increased from 30° to 90° (Table 1–4, Column 2), only the line density changes. It would move from two lines per degree with a 30° scan to 0.67 lines per degree using a 90° examination. Thus there would be a significant degradation of line density and image quality.

Some loss in line density could be recovered by decreasing the sweep rate (Table 1–4, column 3). By sweeping the ultrasonic beam 30 rather than 60 times per second, the time for each sweep would double, the lines per sweep would double, and the line density would be 1.33 lines per degree or twice that when recording at a rate of 60 sweeps per second. The line density could also be improved by decreasing the depth of the examination (Table 1–4, column 4). If one were satisfied with examining only 10 cm of depth, he could again have twice the number of lines per sweep available and a line density of 1.33 lines per degree. Thus, multiple combinations could be utilized depending on the desired information and on the compromises one is willing to make.

Figure 1–28 shows a two-dimensional image using a 30° mechanical sector scanner. The principal disadvantage of such a scan is that only a small portion of the heart is visualized, making it difficult to become oriented to the area of examination. This difficulty is particularly troublesome when using a still picture of a single field or frame. As a result, the remainder of the heart frequently must be artistically rendered in order to orient the viewer to the portion of the heart being

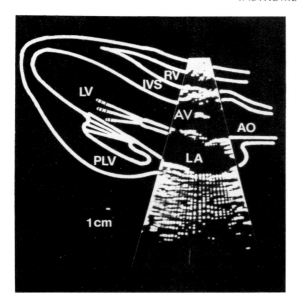

Fig. 1–28. A thirty-degree sector image of the aortic valve (AV) and left atrium (LA). AO = aorta; RV = right ventricle; IVS = interventricular septum; LV = left ventricle; PLV = posterior left ventricular wall.

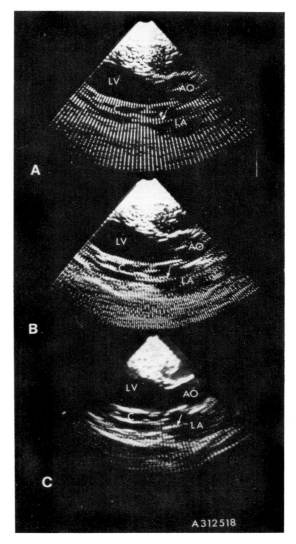

Fig. 1–29. Illustration demonstrating how line density in *A* can be improved by interlacing, *B*, and by the use of television persistence, *C*. LV = left ventricle; AO = aorta; LA = left atrium; C = chordae.

examined. This problem is less severe for the person performing the examination since he or she can move the transducer sufficiently to be better oriented. The principal advantages of a 30° scanner are that it gives high line density, utilizes a fairly small aperture, and has versatility in angulation of the transducer.

Figure 1–29 shows a wide-angle examination of the heart. Figure 1–29A shows a single 1/60-sec sweep with an 82° scan angle. The wide-angle image of the heart immediately enhances the viewer's orientation as it provides sufficient anatomic information. Thus wide-angle sector scanning has many advantages, particularly with still frames. As predicted in Table 1–4, column 2, the major sacrifice with the wide-angle scan is the loss of line density, which basically degrades the quality of the image. Sixty lines of information are spread over 82° rather than over 30°, as in Figure 1–28. Figure 1–29B shows one effort at solving the problem in line density. In this case two sweeps or fields are interlaced to fill in the gaps created by the wider angle. The line density is doubled and the image quality improved. However,

one must recognize that the two sweeps or fields were 1/60 sec apart, and the cardiac structures move slightly in that time. Thus careful examination of Figure 1–29B shows irregularities in the walls and valves owing to motion artifact of this interlaced picture.

Figure 1–29C shows a more common effort at improving the image quality of wide-angle sector scans. This illustration was obtained from a television monitor rather than from an x–y oscilloscope or cathode ray tube.

The gaps in the image seen in Figure 1–29A are filled in by the persistence present in the television camera. This picture was obtained by directing a television camera at the oscilloscopic image and recording the image on videotape. The persistence inherent in television cameras fills in the missing information. Although the image in Figure 1–29C represents one 1/60-sec sweep, the history of the previous sweeps is also visible owing to the television-induced persistence. Unfortunately, a television camera introduces artifact and some degradation of the image; newer instruments are replacing the camera by way of digital scan converters or by direct ultrasonic recording on videotape.

Another reason why Figure 1–29C has a more pleasing quality is the fact that it is

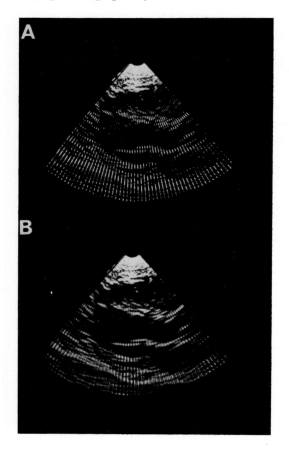

Fig. 1–30. Illustration demonstrating how the image quality and apparent line density can be improved by electronic "jitter." The spaces between the lines in A are partially eliminated by rapidly oscillating the image and taking a time photograph, B.

slightly smaller than Figures 1–29A and B. The smaller image again tends to minimize the gaps. Figure 1–30 shows another way in which the quality of the image can be improved. Figure 1–30A shows a 1/60-sec wide-angle sweep with many gaps between the ultrasonic lines. By rapidly oscillating the image electronically and by using a time-delayed photograph of that image, one can partially eliminate the gaps (Fig. 1–30B). The motion artifact inherent in interlacing is not present. Figure 1–30B is not only more pleasing to the eye, but the elimination of the black gaps between the ultrasonic lines also enhances whatever gray scale may be present in the system. For example, the echoes in the vicinity of the posterior left ventricular wall are more distinct using the processed echo in Figure 1–30B.

One can anticipate that computer processing of the images will play an increasingly important role in improving image quality. Figure 1–31 shows an example of an early computer system designed to improve the quality of the images. The pictures in Figure 1–31 represent computer-processed images that originally resembled those in Figures 1–29A and 1–30A. The gaps were eliminated by introducing multiple interlaced lines that were statistically predicted by means of a computer. As a result, a smooth, lineless image is produced with theoretically little artifact being introduced.

SIGNAL PROCESSING

When the ultrasonic energy returns as an echo and strikes the piezoelectric element of the transducer, an electrical impulse is created and transmitted back to the echograph. This impulse is in the form of a radio frequency or RF signal. The RF presentation is seen on the oscilloscope as a burst of signals rising above and below the baseline on the oscilloscope (Fig. 1–32A). A better method of presenting this information is by video display. With this method the RF signal is processed so that merely the envelope or the outline of the upper half of an electric signal is presented on the face of the oscilloscope (Fig. 1–32B). The most common display used in all routine echographs, video display may be further modified by accen-

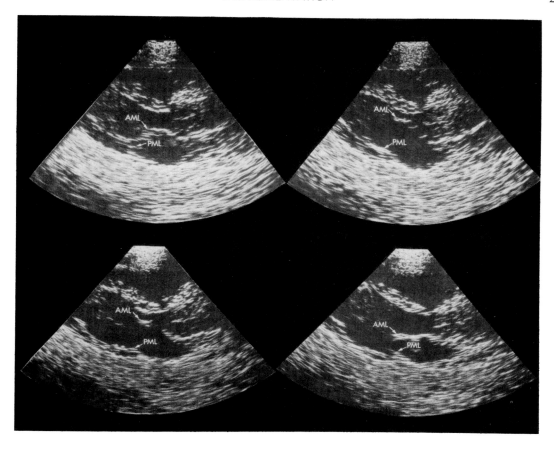

Fig. 1–31.   Computer-enhanced two-dimensional echocardiogram. The original images were similar to those in Figures 1–29A and 1–30A.

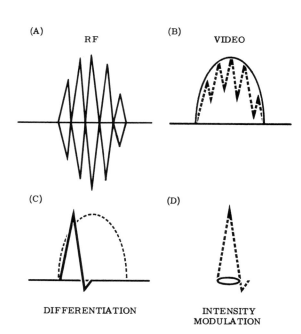

Fig. 1–32.   Ways of processing the returning ultrasonic echo. *A* represents the RF or radio frequency type of echo display. The video display in *B* represents the average height of the upper half of the RF signal. The differentiation in *C* is obtained by taking the first derivative of the video display. Intensity modulation in *D* represents the conversion of signal amplitude to intensity and changing the signal from a spike to a dot.

tuating the leading edge of the echo. This modification is accomplished by taking the first derivative of the video signal (Fig. 1–32C), which converts the echo to a thinner signal. There is also a small negative echo following the initial spike. This negative signal, in association with DC restoration, further accentuates the leading edge of the signal. This type of differentiation, sometimes called "fast-time constant" or "leading-edge enhancement," helps to accentuate individual echoes and to differentiate echoes that are closer together. Thus this display has the effect of enhancing the resolution of the total system and has been exceptionally useful in echocardiography, since individual echoes are frequently close together.

Figure 1–33 shows some of the effects of using differentiation in the signal processing. In a system with differentiation, the

amplitude of the signal in A-mode merely becomes taller and not wider as the gain is increased. In the B-mode presentation the dot or spot becomes brighter but not larger. In systems without differentiation, an increase in the gain not only produces an increase in amplitude of the A-mode, but the base or width of the spike also increases. This increase in the width of the echo is reflected in the B-mode presentation as well. Thus the width of the signals are gain dependent in systems that have minimal or no differentiation and are less gain dependent in echographs that are highly differentiated.

A concept that is becoming increasingly important with advances in instrumentation is that of dynamic range. The diagram in Figure 1–34 attempts to display the concept of dynamic range. In essence, the dynamic range is the range of useful ultrasonic signals that can be recorded and is usually expressed in decibels (db) as a ratio between the largest and smallest signals measured at the point of input to the display. As indicated in Figure 1–34, the dynamic range does not include all available signals. Some signals represent noise and some represent undesired echoes that are eliminated using reject control. There are also signals beyond the saturation level of the recording system. Since a large dynamic range is desirable, one strives to keep the noise level and undesired echoes requiring reject control to a minimum.

The recording of all available signals is limited by the cathode ray tube's ability to record these echoes. For example, there is

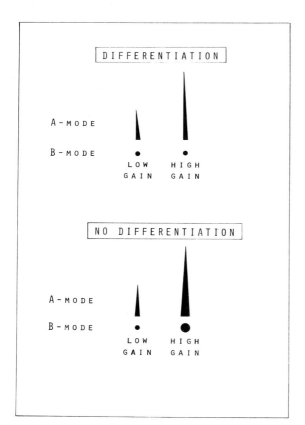

Fig. 1–33.   The effect of gain on differentiated and nondifferentiated echoes. Echoes with no differentiation have a much greater increase in width and gain.

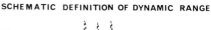
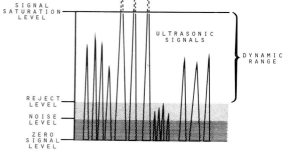

Fig. 1–34.   Schematic definition of dynamic range.

usually about 100 db of ultrasonic information, but the cathode ray tube can only record about 30 db. As a result, many weak echoes were eliminated in early echocardiographs. The M-mode systems were principally concerned with recording specular echoes originating from valves and leading edges of heart walls. As a result, the systems were adjusted to merely record the very strong, dominant specular echoes. As interest in two-dimensional echocardiography increases, so does concern over weaker echoes, especially those arising from the myocardium. These echoes are primarily scattered and are very weak compared with the specular valvular echoes.

One method for recording all ultrasonic information, both strong specular echoes and weak echoes, or, in other words, a method for increasing the dynamic range of the system, utilizes logarithmic compression. Figure 1–35 attempts to explain the logarithmic compression system. An input dynamic range of 100 db, which has a 100,000 to 1 input signal range, is beyond the capability of the cathode ray tube. Thus the 100-db range is logarithmically compressed to a 30-db range with a 32 to 1 output signal range. Every 3.3 db on the input is mapped into 1 db on the output. Needless to say, this description oversimplifies a fairly complicated means of signal processing. There are many different ways of accomplishing the same effect.

A wide dynamic range is necessary for recording gray scale. Gray scale indicates the ability of a display to record both bright and weak echoes in varying shades of gray. The number of gray scale levels is a measure of the dynamic range. Early echocardiographs had very little gray scale since the primary interest was locating specular echoes and mapping their motion. Now there is considerably more interest in judging the brightness of echoes as well as their location and motion. As a result, gray scale and dynamic range are becoming increasingly important. Figure 1–36B shows a two-dimensional image with gray scale, and Figure 1–36A has minimal or no gray scale. One can more readily appreciate the differences in brightness in recordings that have gray scales. The echocardiogram in Figure 1–36B uses digital processing, which helps to enhance or accentuate the gray scale. The recording of gray scale has proved immensely important in other medical applications of ultrasound,

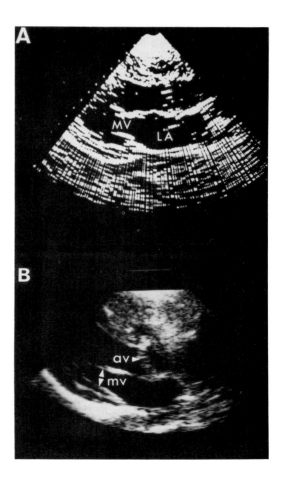

Fig. 1–36. Two-dimensional echocardiograms without, *A*, and with, *B*, gray scale.

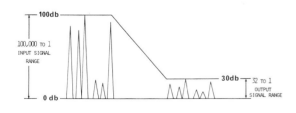

(EVERY 3.3db ON THE INPUT IS MAPPED INTO 1db ON THE OUTPUT)

Fig. 1–35. Logarithmic dynamic range compression: linear scheme. This diagram demonstrates how 100 db of ultrasonic information can be compressed to a 30-db output using logarithmic compression.

especially in abdominal scanning. One would anticipate that gray scale will become equally important in cardiac imaging.

Gray scale has also been important in the strip-chart recorders used to record M-mode echocardiographs. Figure 1–37 attempts to illustrate how the presence of gray scale on a strip-chart recorder can enhance axial resolution. With gray scale (Fig. 1–37A), the center of the signal is more intense than are the edges. Without gray scale the entire signal is of equal intensity, and if the edges touch, then the two echoes "bleed" into each other and appear as one. Standard oscilloscopes and strip-chart recorders have gray scale although some have more than others. Photographic film also has varying degrees of gray scale. Standard storage oscilloscopes have no gray scale. As a result, new, more expensive gray-scale storage oscilloscopes are necessary if one is to use storage mode. Another way of losing gray scale is to process

or digitize a signal electronically with an insufficient number of gray scales. There are strip-chart recorders that electronically manipulate the signals to improve the recording of the phonocardiogram and pulse tracings. Unfortunately, the gray scale recording of the echocardiograms may suffer, and one may lose the inherent resolution of the system.

ECHOCARDIOGRAPHIC CONTROLS

There are a variety of controls that modify the echocardiogram on all commercial echocardiographs. These controls can greatly influence the echo display and, as will be demonstrated, are vitally important in the recording of specific cardiac echoes. First, since ultrasound is attenuated and decreases in intensity as it travels through the body, some mechanism for enhancing the distant echoes is necessary. All commercial echocardiographs have a circuit for suppressing near-field echoes and for enhancing far-field echoes. Such a device appears under many names, including "time-gain-compensation" (TCG), "depth compensa-

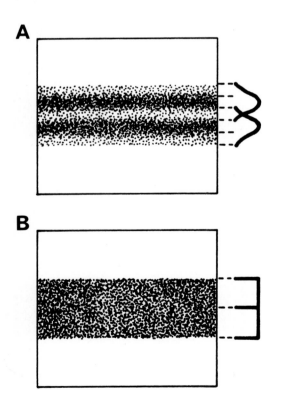

Fig. 1–37. Diagrams demonstrating how a recording of gray scale, A, can distinguish between two close echo-producing objects, whereas without gray scale, B, the two objects blend into one large signal.

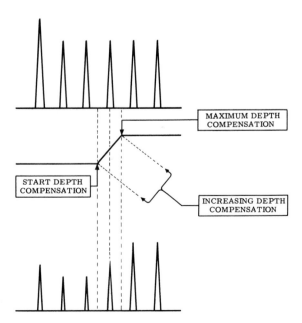

Fig. 1–38. Diagram illustrating how depth compensation reduces the amplitude of the near field echoes and enhances those originating from interfaces in the far field.

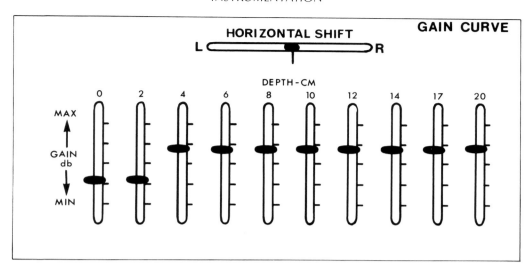

Fig. 1–39.   Illustration of depth compensation control whereby each lever controls the gain of a given segment of the echocardiogram.

tion," or "electronic distance compensation." A representation of the compensating wave form is frequently displayed as a break in the base line with a variable slope (Fig. 1–38). Both the beginning of this compensating mechanism, or "ramp," and the slope of the ramp may be varied. All echoes to the left of the ramp are suppressed (Fig. 1–38). The ramp itself represents increasing depth compensation. Maximal depth compensation is reached at the plateau to the right of the ramp. Figure 1–38 shows how this form of depth compensation is used to suppress near-field echoes and to relatively enhance far-field echoes. The exact way in which this depth compensation mechanism is used varies in several commercial echocardiographs. Near-field gain may be altered by a control called "near-gain." On other instruments there may be a control that increases or reduces the ramp on the depth compensation and thus influences the near-field echoes. Several commercial echocardiographs have a variable depth-compensation control that consists of a series of levers that alter the relative gain throughout the entire tracing (Fig. 1–39). Figure 1–40 demonstrates how the depth compensation can be varied with this system.

The depth-compensation control is undoubtedly the most confusing and frequently the most difficult to use for the

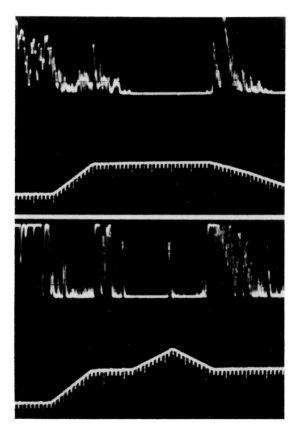

Fig. 1–40.   Echocardiograms demonstrating how the multiple depth compensation controls in Figure 1–39 can influence the gain. In the lower recording the gain has been increased at eight centimeters and helps to bring out an echo that is not visible in the above tracing.

echocardiographer. One can distort the recording by varying this particular control. If one remembers that the purpose of this device is to compensate for the loss of ultrasonic energy or attenuation as the beam enters the body, then one better understands how the control should be used. The general purpose is to enhance the far echoes and to suppress the near echoes. Where one places the ramp depends in part on that portion of the recording to be suppressed or enhanced. This topic will be discussed further in the chapter on the echocardiographic examination.

Because of the confusion involved in depth compensation, an automatic depth-compensation control has been introduced in some newer echocardiographs.[46] The depth compensation is controlled electronically, and there is no manual manipulation.

Most echocardiographs have sensitivity or gain controls that merely increase or amplify the height or intensity of the echoes as they are received. As mentioned previously, some echocardiographs permit one to selectively control the near field, that area to the left of the depth compensation ramp, as well as the overall gain of the entire display. Turning up a gain control increases the amplitude and number of echoes recorded. Some commercial instruments use an attenuator whereby an increase in that control actually reduces the number of echoes displayed. The damping control present on some instruments functions in a manner similar to an attenuator in that the higher the control the fewer the echoes; however, the

"damping" control essentially regulates the ringing of the transducer and influences the amount of ultrasonic energy entering the body rather than modifies the received signals. Damping may also enhance the resolution by decreasing the amount of ringing of the element and the size of the pulse.

The gain of the instrument can be rapidly switched between high and low settings in order to enhance the recording of certain strong echoes.[47] This "switch gain" technique eliminates some of the changes in damping or gain frequently made to record such structures as the pericardium or anterior right ventricular wall.

Whether one uses a gain, attenuator, or damping control, he or she essentially uniformly increases or decreases the number of echoes being displayed (Fig. 1–41). On the other hand, the reject control (Fig. 1–42) selectively eliminates the recording of echoes according to the reject level. This control essentially varies the threshold necessary for an echo to be displayed; those echoes below the threshold necessary for display are totally eliminated. Figure 1–42 shows how elevating the threshold by increasing the reject control eliminates the recording of weaker echoes.

FACTORS INFLUENCING RESOLUTION

Resolution or resolving power is the ability to distinguish or identify two objects that are close together. If two objects are a millimeter apart and one can identify both objects as distinctly separate entities, then the system has a 1-mm resolution. If the objects

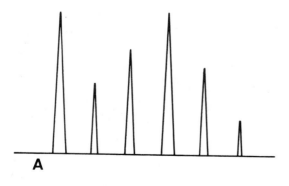
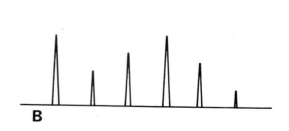

Fig. 1–41. Effect of damping or overall gain control. A decrease in gain or an increase in damping, B, will uniformly lower the amplitude of all echoes.

need to be two millimeters apart before they can be identified as distinct entities, then the system has 2-mm resolution. Multiple factors affect resolution.

The frequency or wavelength of the ultrasonic beam is one of the important determinants in axial resolution. To identify or record small objects, one needs a small wavelength. In addition, the manner in which the returning echo signal is processed influences the axial resolution. Figure 1–43 shows echoes in both the A-mode and the

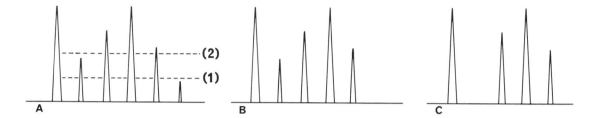

Fig. 1–42. Diagram showing the effects of reject control. By elevating the reject control to level 1, the smallest echo in A is eliminated, B. Elevating the reject control to level 2, the next smallest echo which is below this threshold is also eliminated, C. The remaining echoes retain their full amplitude.

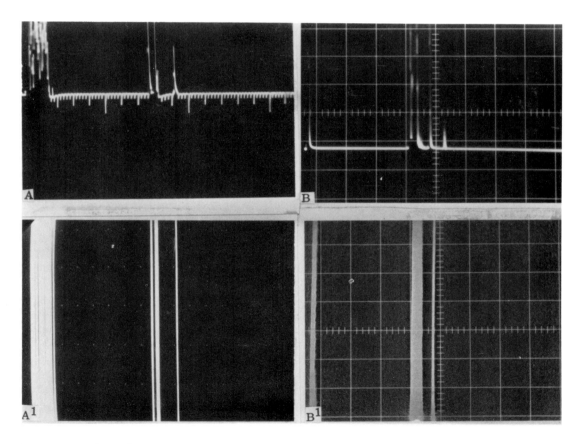

Fig. 1–43. Echocardiograms illustrating variations in resolving power of two different echographs. In the A-mode presentation, both systems demonstrate two strong echoes close together and a weaker third echo slightly farther away from the transducer, A and B. With the M-mode presentation, the system in A' again shows three separate echoes. However, in B' the initial two echoes, which are close together, fuse into one broad echo, and one cannot clearly identify two separate echo-producing structures.

M-mode recorded on two echocardiographic systems from the same test block. In the A-mode presentation (A and B), both systems record two strong echoes that are close together and a third, weaker echo farther away from the transducer. In the M-mode recording (A′ and B′), one can again distinguish all three echoes with the left-hand system (A′), but on the right (B′) the two echoes that are close together now appear as one broad, thick echo. One cannot determine how many echo-producing interfaces are present in this thick echo. Thus the echocardiographic system on the left has better resolution than that on the right. The reasons for the poor resolution with the right-hand system are, first, the echocardiograph did not differentiate the returning echoes so that the signals or echoes were not as narrow initially. Second, the M-mode recording on the right was taken with a nongray-scale storage oscilloscope. Without gray scale the individual echo was either all black or all white.

Ideally, the ultrasonic beam should be extremely narrow so that one can obtain a true "ice-pick" view of the heart. Unfortunately, as already described, the beam has a finite width and tends to widen further or to diverge as it enters the body. The amount of divergence is a function of frequency and size of the transducer. Efforts at decreasing the size of the beam width have already been discussed. In keeping with the principles of the ultrasonic beam, Figure 1–44 shows the interplay between the size of the beam, its relative intensity, and the relative acoustic properties of the reflecting object. The intensity of the ultrasonic beam obviously varies; the center of the beam is more intense than are the edges (Fig. 1–44). If the center of the ultrasonic beam (dark area) intersects a strong reflecting object (black dots) or a weak reflecting object (gray dots), one records an echo from both objects with the stronger reflecting object transmitting a stronger signal. On the other hand, if these objects are being intersected by the edges of the ultrasonic beam (light area), then only the stronger reflecting objects (black dots) may produce a signal. Less ultrasonic energy at the edge of the beam may be insufficient to produce an echo from a weaker object (gray dots). In

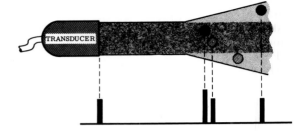

Fig. 1–44. Diagram illustrating the interrelationship between the intensity of the ultrasonic beam and the acoustic impedance of objects being examined. The center of the beam has a greater intensity *(dark area)* than do the edges of the beam *(light area)*. Whether or not an echo is produced and with what amplitude it is recorded depends on the relationship between the intensity of the beam and the acoustic mismatch of the object being examined. Objects with high acoustic impedance *(black dots)* will produce echoes even at the edges of the ultrasonic beam. Weak echo-producing objects *(gray dots)* only produce echoes of reduced amplitude in the center of the beam.

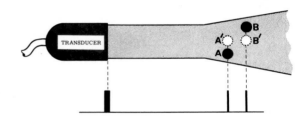

Fig. 1–45. Diagram illustrating how beam width can distort interpretation of the returning echoes. Objects A and B are essentially side by side; although object B is farther away from the transducer than object A, they are not directly behind each other. Because of the width of the ultrasonic beam, both objects are recorded simultaneously. The resulting echoes suggest that the two objects are directly behind each other (A′ and B′) rather than side by side.

addition, the returning echo from the strong object (black dots) will be weaker when intersected by the edge of the beam than when intersected by the center of the beam.

Figure 1–45 shows some of the distortion that can be produced by the width of the ultrasonic beam. This illustration shows how two point objects (A and B) that are primarily side by side appear as if one is behind the other (A′ and B′) if both are in the path of the ultrasonic beam. The distortion produced by the beam width has led to many confusing

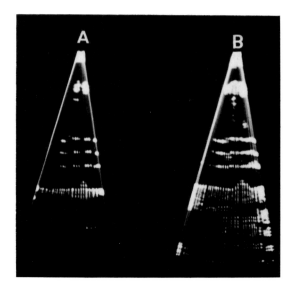

Fig. 1–46.   Effect of gain on lateral resolution of a two-dimensional sector scan, A. With an increase in gain, the individual echoes from the wires in the water tank blend into continuous horizontal lines, B. One cannot identify the individual wires. Gain does not significantly alter axial resolution in this echocardiograph.

echocardiograms and is an important factor that must be kept in mind when interpreting echocardiograms.[48]

Beam width artifacts in M-mode echocardiography can produce confusing echoes and hence misinterpretations because echoes seem to appear in certain areas where they actually do not exist. With two-dimensional echocardiography, beam width artifact is probably even more important because it actually distorts the basic image. Probably the most important point with regard to beam width in two-dimensional echocardiography is that it is the primary determining factor of lateral resolution. Figure 1–46 illustrates an attempt to determine lateral resolution using a two-dimensional scanner. The test object is a series of small wires in a tank of water. In Figure 1–46A one can clearly identify 12 reflecting objects that are a certain distance apart. Although this system was adjusted for the best possible resolution, it is clear that the lateral resolution is not nearly as good as the axial resolu-

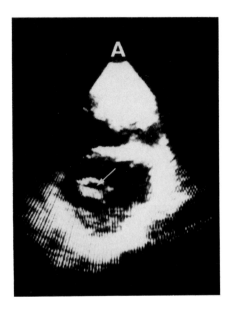
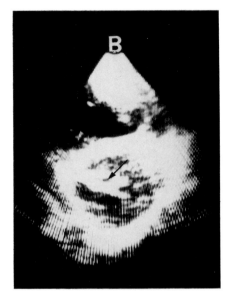

Fig. 1–47.   Two-dimensional echocardiograms illustrating how lateral and axial resolution is impaired by an increase in gain. The mitral valve orifice (arrows) is much smaller with an increase in gain, B.

tion. Although the wires were equal in all directions, one records a series of lines rather than small dots. Thus the axial resolution is inherently better than the lateral resolution in virtually all cross-sectional systems. Figure 1–46B demonstrates that the lateral resolution is also dependent on the gain. As one increases the gain, the lines become wider, and one can no longer even distinguish that there are 12 individual wires being examined. As predicted from Figure 1–44, as one increases the gain more of the available ultrasonic beam is recorded, the beam width increases, and lateral resolution decreases. Thus, in order to enhance lateral resolution, one should attempt to use a minimum amount of gain.[49] Figure 1–47 shows a clinical example of how gain setting can drastically alter lateral resolution. In this record-

ing of a stenotic mitral valve, one can identify two different mitral valve orifices with two different gain settings. With a low gain setting (Fig. 1–47A), one sees an orifice (white arrow) that is significantly larger than when the gain is increased (Fig. 1–47B, black arrow). It should be noted that this particular echocardiograph had both gain-sensitive axial and lateral resolution. The echoes became fatter as well as wider with an increase in gain. The echocardiographic system demonstrated in Figure 1–46 showed gain-sensitive lateral resolution, but because of more differentiation of the echo signals, the axial resolution did not change appreciably with an increase in gain.

Figure 1–48 demonstrates how the beam width is important in the basic configuration of the two-dimensional image. If one scans a series of objects that represent small dots, the beam width displays these dots as a series of lines depending on the size of the beam. A nonfocused ultrasonic beam gives a series of increasingly longer lines (Fig. 1–48A). Focusing the ultrasonic beam improves the situation and diminishes the size of the lines so that they more appropriately reproduce the actual objects, which would appear as a series of dots (Fig. 1–48B).

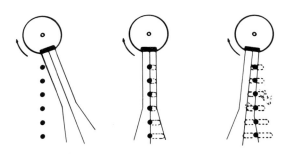

A   POINT SPREAD FUNCTION PRODUCED BY A NON-FOCUSED BEAM OF ULTRASONIC ENERGY

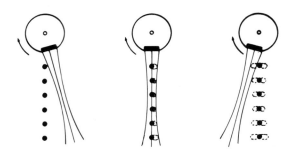

B   POINT SPREAD FUNCTION PRODUCED BY A FOCUSED BEAM OF ULTRASONIC ENERGY

Fig. 1–48. Diagrams demonstrating how beam width distorts the image with a two-dimensional sector scan, A, and how a focused beam can reduce the distortion, B. The true image should be a series of dots; beam width, however, distorts the image into a series of lines.

POTENTIAL ARTIFACTS

Side Lobes

Side lobes were recognized relatively recently as potential artifacts that must be considered with the newer ultrasonic instruments. These extraneous beams of ultrasound are generated from the edges of the individual transducer elements and are not in the direction of the main ultrasonic beam. Although all transducers generate side lobes, the problem is significantly greater with phased array transducers.

Figure 1–49 illustrates how side lobes can produce artifactual information. If the main ultrasonic beam is directed at the object in question (Fig. 1–49A) then an echo from that object is displayed on the oscilloscope. However, if the main ultrasonic beam is directed away from the object (Fig. 1–49B), then no echoes are generated by the main beam. However, the side lobe may be hitting the object and producing echoes from it. These echoes again hit the transducer and the echocardiograph displays the resultant echoes as though they were generated by the main beam. The echocardiographic system does not know the location of the side lobes. All returning signals are interpreted as if they originated from the main beam. Thus an echo of probably weaker intensity is recorded on the oscilloscope in the direction of the main beam. In fact, no such echo exists at this location. If the beam is oscillating rapidly, as in Figure 1–49C, then the multiple artifactual echoes produced by the side lobes are displayed as a curved line at the same level as the true object.

It should be emphasized that the side lobes are considerably weaker than the main beam, thus the returning echoes are clearly weaker than the dominant, real echoes. In fact, many side lobe echoes are not actually seen because they are overshadowed by true echoes in the same vicinity. Side lobes usually become evident when they do not conflict with real echoes. For example, in Figure. 1–50 the very large, relatively echo-free left atrium provides an opportunity for the side lobes to be displayed within the cavity of the left atrium. If the left atrium had been of normal size, then the side lobe would be

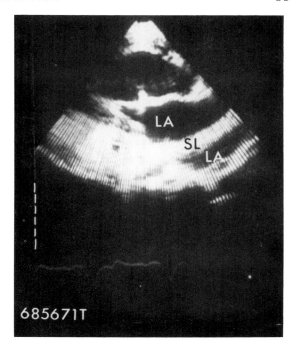

Fig. 1–50. Two-dimensional echocardiogram demonstrating a side lobe (SL) within a dilated left atrium (LA).

masked by the echoes from the posterior left atrial wall and lung. Another prerequisite for a dominant side lobe artifact is that the artifactual echoes must originate from a fairly strong reflecting surface. The atrioventricular groove and the fibrous skeleton of the heart represent good sources for side lobe echoes. If these artifactual echoes are not recognized, one can easily see how misinterpretations could occur. In Figure 1–50 considerable confusion could arise concerning the size of the left atrium or whether the left atrium is divided into two sections. Lesser degrees of side lobe artifact can merely increase the general noise level of the system and thus decrease the dynamic range. One may need to increase the reject level or to decrease the gain to eliminate some of these artifacts, but in so doing one decreases the dynamic range.

Reverberations

Reverberations are another important potential artifact. Figure 1–51 illustrates the principle of reverberations. The ultrasonic

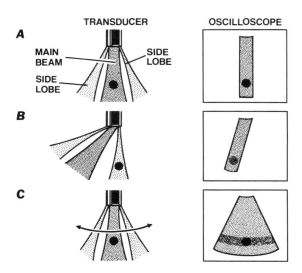

Fig. 1–49. Diagram demonstrating the principle of how side lobes produce artifacts on two-dimensional echocardiograms (see text for details).

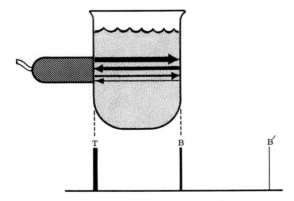

Fig. 1–51.   Diagram of the origin of reverberations. The ultrasonic beam leaves the transducer, strikes the side of the beaker, and returns to the transducer. The returning ultrasound produces echo B. Some ultrasound is also reflected by the transducer and returns to the side of the beaker. Returning to the transducer a second time, it produces a weaker echo, B'. Echo B' is a reverberation and gives the false impression of a second interface twice as far from the transducer as the side of the beaker.

beam travels through the homogeneous water, strikes the opposite side of the beaker, returns to the transducer, and the echocardiograph displays a signal or echo at point B. However, it is still possible that the near side of the beaker or the transducer may function as another reflecting surface and that the ultrasonic beam will retrace itself, hit the far side of the beaker again, and then return to the transducer. This added distance traveled by the same burst of ultrasound produces another signal (B') at twice the distance from the transducer as does the original echo (B). The second echo or reverberation may be weaker than the original echo. If the echo is moving, the amplitude of motion may be twice as great as that of the original echo. This type of echo is an artifact known as a reverberation; reverberations can be troublesome if not understood. Such artifacts may not only result from the ultrasonic beam

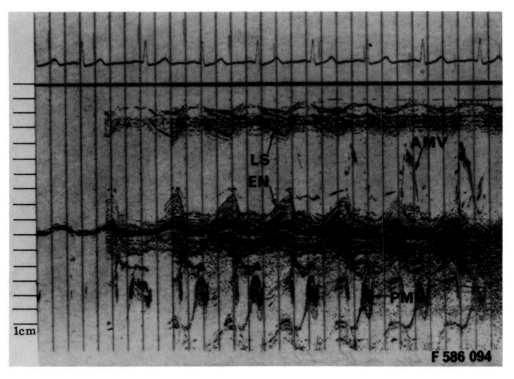

Fig. 1–52.   An M-mode echocardiogram demonstrating a reverberation. The left septal (LS) and posterior endocardial (EN) echoes are clearly identified as is the faint echo from the anterior mitral leaflet (AMV). Below the borders of the heart one can again see signals that have cardiac motion. This motion would suggest that the echoes originate from the mitral valve. Although their exact origin is unclear, the signals probably represent reverberations from echoes originating from the posterior mitral valve leaflet (PMV') The pattern of motion is correct, and the amplitude is much greater. Thus reverberations can be seen from structures that do not produce primary echoes on the echocardiogram.

reflecting from the transducer, but they may originate from some other echo-producing structures within the heart or chest. Thus it is not entirely predictable how the reverberations may be displayed. Fortunately, most important reverberations are recorded behind the usual cardiac recordings.

Figure 1–52 shows a reverberation behind the left ventricle; the desired echoes from the heart are primarily from the left ventricular cavity, which is bordered by the left side of the septum (LS) and the posterior left ventricular endocardium (EN). An echo from the anterior mitral valve leaflet (AMV) is seen toward the right-hand portion of the recording. In addition, there is a moving echo behind the posterior left ventricular wall. The motion of this echo is clearly from the mitral valve; however, there is nothing on the original recording that entirely resembles this extra posterior mitral valve echo. This posterior echo is clearly a reverberation and most likely originates from the posterior mitral leaflet; it is thus labeled PMV'. As can be noted, the amplitude of motion is greater than it was for the original posterior mitral valve echo. In fact, the primary posterior mitral valve leaflet is not well recorded within the actual left ventricular cavity. This illustration demonstrates how confusing reverberations can be and how one must be careful not to attempt a diagnosis based on echoes that appear outside the true cardiac border.

Unfortunately, the reverberations may occur within the cardiac recording and their origin may not be obvious.[50] Such reverberations may be particularly troublesome. Some of the new instruments, especially those that use plastic housing, have introduced new potential reverberations, many of which may appear within the cardiac echoes. Figure 1–53 illustrates artifacts within the cardiac image owing to reverberations. Figure 1–53A demonstrates two such artifacts. There is a small bright dot that oscillates in real time (Fig. 1–53A-1). There is a second long echo in the center of the left ventricular cavity (Fig. 1–53A-2). By readjusting the angle of the transducer (Fig. 1–53B), these artifacts can be eliminated. Whenever one sees confusing unidentifiable echoes, the

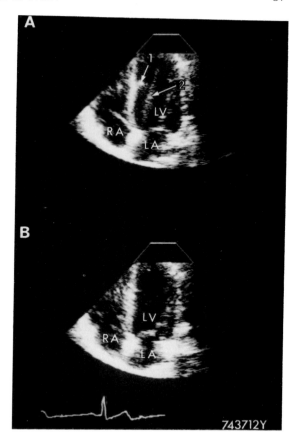

Fig. 1–53. Reverberations in a two-dimensional echocardiogram. A, Reverberation 1 oscillated in real time. Reverberation 2 probably originates from the plastic that surrounds the transducer. B, Both reverberation artifacts could be eliminated by readjusting the angle of the transducer.

possibility that they represent reverberation must be considered.

Television Artifact

A relatively minor potential artifact occurs with the use of television cameras in two-dimensional imaging. Because of the persistence of such cameras, the history or ghosts of echoes may be present on individual frames long after the true echo has disappeared. For example, in Figure 1–54 one notes echoes from an aortic valve vegetation (VEG) in diastole. Although in systole the vegetation is actually in the aorta and out of the field of vision, one still sees a "ghost echo" from the vegetation in the left ventricular outflow tract (arrow). The vegetation

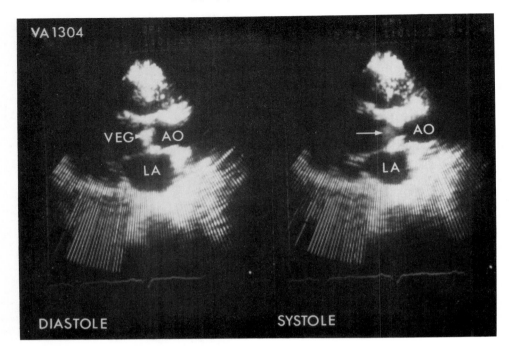

Fig. 1–54. Two-dimensional echocardiogram demonstrating an artifact produced by television persistence. The apparent vegetation faintly visible in systole *(arrow)* does not exist; it is merely a persistence artifact from an earlier diastolic frame.

does not in fact exist at that location in systole. The faint "ghost echo" is merely a persistence artifact of the television system. With the use of digital scan converters or direct ultrasonic recording instead of television cameras, the persistence artifact should be eliminated.

DOPPLER ECHOCARDIOGRAPHY

Doppler ultrasound uses a different principle by which to obtain information from the cardiovascular system. The usual Doppler technique utilizes a continuous ultrasonic beam rather than a pulsed beam.[51,52] When this beam hits a moving target, which might be either a valve leaflet, wall, or flowing blood, there is a change in the frequency of the returning ultrasonic signal. This change in frequency is known as the "Doppler shift" and is proportional to the velocity of the moving target. The frequency of the Doppler signal, which represents the difference between the outgoing and the returning ultrasonic frequencies, is usually within the audible range so that it comes back as an audible sound. The frequency of this audible sound is proportional to the velocity of motion of the object being examined. For example, if the ultrasonic beam is directed at a moving column of blood, then the Doppler sound is recorded within the audible range and is proportional to the velocity of motion of the blood. The velocity of the blood can be actually calculated provided that one knows the angle between the sound beam and the moving target.[52] The results of such a Doppler examination can be obtained by listening to the signals with a stethoscope, earphone, or loud speaker. One may also graphically display this audible sound in a variety of ways. An ideal graphic display has not been devised. The lack of such a display is one of the reasons why Doppler echocardiography has developed so slowly.

Most clinical data on Doppler ultrasound are based on experience with peripheral vessels.[53-55] Peripheral arteries and veins have been studied extensively, and such examinations have proved clinically useful in many situations.[56,57] Several investigators have used continuous-wave Doppler ultrasound to examine the heart and great vessels.[58,59] Much of the early work used this technique to obtain signals from the heart walls and valves.[60,61] Later, investigators began observing the blood flow in the aorta by placing the ultrasonic transducer in the suprasternal notch and by directing the beam at the arch, descending aorta, and ascending aorta.[62-67] This technique has been used to record the velocity of blood flow in the aorta and, it is hoped, to determine cardiac output. One of the problems associated with this technique is that the angle of the ultrasonic beam with respect to the column of blood is obviously critical; in addition, the velocity within the aorta varies, and the blood flow is slower near the edge of the aorta than it is in the center of the vessel.

Directional continuous-wave Doppler ultrasound can also reveal clinically useful information. This particular technique can provide information concerning aortic regurgitation.[69,70] A certain amount of backward flow during diastole is apparently normal; however, if this backward flow is excessive, it is indicative, if not diagnostic, of aortic regurgitation. This technique has not been widely popular, but it could be a useful means of not only detecting aortic regurgitation, but even of quantitating the degree of regurgitation. Variations in the pattern of aortic blood flow in patients with hypertrophic subaortic stenosis have also been noted using this Doppler examination.[71]

Probably one of the most promising developments in the use of Doppler ultrasound has been the introduction of pulsed Doppler echocardiography.[72-77] By using a pulsed system similar to that of echo ranging or routine echocardiography, one can now not only obtain a Doppler signal, but one can also record the various cardiac structures as routinely performed with echocardiography. A group of investigators in Seattle has been instrumental in developing such a pulsed Doppler or Doppler echocardiographic system.[75,78] Figure 1-55 shows one of their diagrams demonstrating how the system works. The ultrasonic transducer not only provides for echo ranging and the location of various cardiac structures, but it also samples a cer-

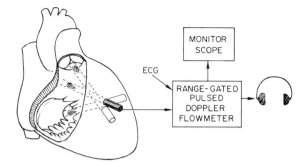

Fig. 1–55. Diagram demonstrating the principle of Doppler echocardiography. This system permits one to obtain the Doppler signal from a gated sample (*stippled tear drops*) within the heart. The returning signal is within the audible range of sound and can be heard with earphones. (From Johnson, S.L., et al.: Doppler echocardiography: the localization of cardiac murmurs. Circulation, *48*:810, 1973.)

tain area within the heart for the Doppler signal. Their initial system had an audible output, and the examiner listened for the frequencies and intensity of the returning sound.

Although many diagnoses depend on an interpretation of the audible Doppler signal, there is increasing effort toward using a graphic display for interpretation of the examination. One system of displaying the Doppler signal is the use of a "time-interval histogram."[76,79,80] By using multiple zero-crossing techniques to analyze the frequencies of the returning sound, such a technique plots the frequencies of the sound against time. The direction of the flow is also indicated on the tracing; flow toward the transducer is plotted above the baseline and flow away from the transducer below the baseline. Figure 1–56 demonstrates how time-interval histograms can identify "laminar flow" and "turbulent flow." If the sampling volume is recording an area of laminar blood flow, all returning frequencies are relatively homogenous and the dots being plotted are close together. The recording would indicate that all the blood being sampled is moving in the same direction and at approximately the same frequencies. If the sampling volume is in an area of turbulent or disturbed flow, then a different time-interval histogram pattern is recorded. There will be

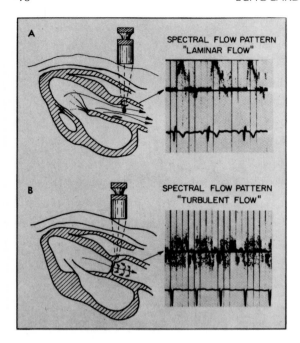

Fig. 1–56. Illustration demonstrating the principle of how a time interval histogram can distinguish "laminar flow" from "turbulent flow." With the Doppler sample in an area of laminar or normal flow, all dots that comprise the time interval histogram are close together since all velocities at a given instant are relatively equal, A. With turbulent or disturbed flow, B, there are multiple velocities and directions of flow, and thus the Doppler signals are scattered above and below the baseline. (From Baker, D.W., Rubenstein, S.A. and Lorch, G.S.: Pulsed Doppler echocardiography: principles and applications. Am. J. Med., 63:69, 1977.)

however, to date, they are still under clinical evaluation.

Figure 1–57 is a Doppler echocardiographic recording of a patient with rheumatic mitral regurgitation. The M-mode echocardiogram is seen in the upper half of the recording. The site of the sample volume is indicated by a line on the M-mode tracing. The time-interval histogram is in the lower half of the recording. During systole the mitral regurgitation jet generates a turbulent signal with multiple frequencies, most of which are moving away from the transducer (arrow).

Thus far Doppler echocardiography has not enjoyed the popularity of M-mode or two-dimensional echocardiography. The reasons for this slower development are many. There is still some question concern-

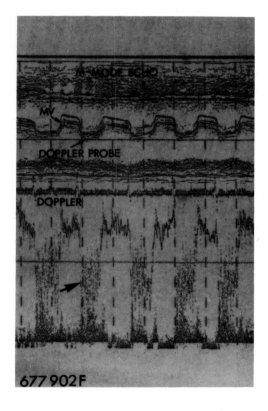

Fig. 1–57. Doppler echocardiogram of a patient with rheumatic mitral regurgitation. The Doppler probe is placed on the atrial side of the mitral valve. Turbulent blood flow moving away from the transducer is visible in systole (arrow). (From Feigenbaum, H.: Echocardiography. In Heart Disease. Edited by E. Braunwald. Philadelphia, W.B. Saunders Co., 1980.)

multiple Doppler signals of differing frequencies and directions. Thus on the time-interval histogram one sees multiple dots displayed indicating variations in both frequency and direction. As one might expect, the ability to distinguish laminar from turbulent flow is one of the principal diagnostic uses of this Doppler echocardiographic system.[81,82]

One must recognize that the time-interval histogram is not a true spectral analysis of the sound profile. Other investigators use a true spectral analysis.[83,84] Unfortunately, such systems require time and usually are performed as an off-line evaluation of the recording and not in real time.[84] Rapid spectrum analyzers are becoming available;

ing the interpretation and significance of the returning Doppler signal.[85] The different limitations and potential artifacts inherent in the Doppler approach are at times difficult to overcome. For example, the Doppler signal is highly sensitive to any change in angulation. Attempts at recording a true velocity of blood flow have been frustrating to date. Although many investigators have obtained reliable information, the angulation is even more critical with Doppler approaches than with either M-mode or two-dimensional cardiac imaging. There are significant limitations with the current graphic recordings of the Doppler signal.[79,86] Another limitation of pulsed Doppler echocardiography is that the depth of the examination is limited by the available frequency. With the frequency in the range of 3.0 to 3.5 mHz, it is difficult to examine structures beyond 10 cm away from the transducer. Frequencies above this level have poor penetrating power in adults. Although the use of Doppler echocardiography has been slow in developing, it is definitely increasing; discussion of many Doppler echocardiographic techniques are included throughout this book.

FUTURE DEVELOPMENTS IN INSTRUMENTATION

There is every reason to expect continued, rapid development of echocardiographic instrumentation. There will undoubtedly be changes in transducer design and technology. Use of both higher and lower frequency transducers can be anticipated. The advantage of higher frequency transducers is fairly obvious. The beam characteristics are improved, and both axial and lateral resolution are increased with higher frequency transducers.[87] Penetration of the ultrasound is still a problem. There remain significant numbers of individuals from whom satisfactory echocardiograms cannot be obtained. Higher frequency transducers will not overcome the problem of penetration. This limitation of echocardiography can possibly be overcome by the use of lower frequency transducers. Naturally, lower frequency transducers produce poorer beam characteristics for axial and lateral resolution. However, it is possible to use computer pro-

cessing to reconstitute some of the lost resolution, making it possible to use low-frequency transducers for better penetration.

One can expect increased interest in the use of multiple ring transducers and phased annular array transducers.[19] Figure 1–58 demonstrates how such transducer design can improve the ultrasonic beam. With a coaxial or two-element ring transducer, the center transducer functions as a sender of ultrasound and the outer ring as the receiver. Echoes that originate from objects in the center of the beam (solid dots) strike the receiving transducer simultaneously since they are equidistant from the outer ring. Objects that are not in the center of the ultrasonic beam (open dots) and are not equidistant from the receiving transducer produce echoes that strike the outer or receiving transducer at different times. Because of the nonsimultaneous registration of these echoes, they are suppressed and virtually eliminated. Thus a ring transducer only registers those echoes originating from objects within the center of the beam. The effective beam width is significantly reduced. The disadvantage of this approach is that some echoes are lost, and the overall sensitivity is reduced.

The phased annular array transducer functions on the same principle as the phased

COAXIAL OR TWO-ELEMENT RING TRANSDUCER

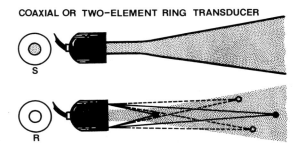

PHASED ANNULAR ARRAY TRANSDUCER

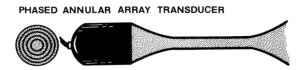

Fig. 1–58. Diagram demonstrating the principles of ring and phased annular array transducers (see text for details).

linear array transducer (see Fig. 1–11). The firing of the individual ring elements is controlled in order to focus the beam. Such electronic focusing can be done dynamically to produce a long focal zone. The obvious advantage of the annular array over the linear array transducer is that the focusing is done in both the x and y axes. Annular or circular phased array transducers have been used for ultrasonic imaging of organs other than the heart.[20] Thus their superior beam characteristics are well recognized. It is conceivable that such transducers could be adapted to current mechanical two-dimensional systems.

Preliminary work already exists that attempts to create three-dimensional echocardiographic images.[88–91] A variety of different approaches have been suggested. The principal added information necessary for such a display is the spatial orientation of the two-dimensional probe. Once that information is introduced into the system, reconstruction of two-dimensional images into three-dimensional images is possible. There are many technical details and problems to be overcome before three-dimensional echocardiography becomes a practical clinical tool.

One should certainly anticipate further developments in the field of Doppler echocardiography. Combining Doppler with two-dimensional echocardiography is already being contemplated[92] and such an instrument is commercially available.[93] Figure 1–59 shows how one system combines two-dimensional and Doppler echocardiography. One advantage of combining these two systems is that the two-dimensional examination can be used to determine the angle of the Doppler probe. It is hoped that better quantitative information is forthcoming that combines the spatial information from two-dimensional echocardiography and the velocity information from the Doppler examination.

Another interesting development with regard to Doppler echocardiography is the use of multiple sampling gates in the ultrasonic array with display of the Doppler information directly on the echocardiographic image. Doppler imaging of peripheral vessels

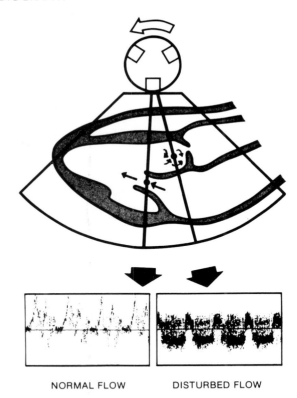

Fig. 1–59. Diagram demonstrating how Doppler echocardiography can be combined with two-dimensional echocardiography.

has been available for many years.[94,95] Figure 1–60 shows the use of multiple-gated Doppler and M-mode echocardiography.[97,98,98a] The velocities are coded according to color and are plotted on the M-mode tracing. This rather dramatic display shows the blood flow pattern within the heart directly on the M-mode recording. One can anticipate that with further development a similar type of display will be shown on a two-dimensional cardiac image. Such a display certainly should improve the utility of the Doppler echocardiographic examination and should enhance our ability to gain useful information from cardiac blood flow.

Color encoding of the image can occur either in the M-mode or two-dimensional mode.[99] Figure 1–61 shows how gray scale can be displayed in color rather than in shades of black and white. This approach has the advantage of enhancing the appreciation of gray scale. Whether or not the added cost

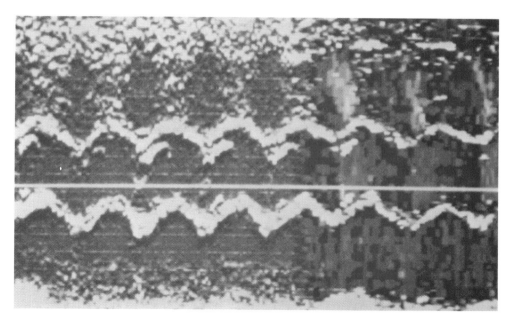

Fig. 1–60. A combined M-mode and Doppler recording whereby the Doppler signal is superimposed on the M-mode tracing. The direction and velocity of the Doppler signal are displayed in varying colors. This particular recording shows the right ventricular outflow tract (RVOT) and aorta. (From Brandestini, M.A., Eyer, M.K., and Stevenson, J.G.: M/Q-mode echocardiography. The synthesis of conventional echo with digital multigate Doppler. *In* Echocardiography. Edited by C.T. Lancee. The Hague, Martinus Nijhoff, 1979.)

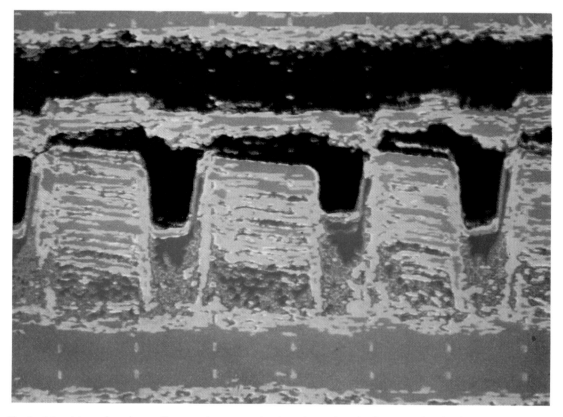

Fig. 1–61. M-mode echocardiogram demonstrating how intensity of echoes can be displayed in color rather than in gray scale. (From Flinn, G.S.: Color encoded display of M mode echocardiograms. J. Clin. Ultrasound, 4:339, 1976.)

of color is warranted remains to be verified by further investigations.

A new area of echocardiographic investigation involves tissue parameter identification.[100-103] This topic is discussed in more detail, especially in the chapter on coronary artery disease and the detection of ischemic myocardium. To some degree, tissue parameter identification has already been accomplished in that we are able to distinguish calcified or fibrotic tissue. A calcified mitral annulus and calcified valves are readily identified on echocardiograms. Echocardiographers have also noted the clinical appearance of scarred myocardium.[104] Investigations into tissue parameter identification utilize a great deal of sophisticated computer analysis of the individual echoes. In addition, as one attempts to identify myocardial echoes, one can anticipate greater interest in recording scattered echoes from the myocardium. Figure 1–62 shows an effort to identify the ischemic myocardium using computer processing of the two-dimensional information.[104a] This particular study used only three grades of gray scale. The echocardiographic demonstration of the ischemic area is noted by the bright group of echoes (arrow), the pathologic specimen is shown in the lower half of the photograph, and the ischemic area is stained dark. The use of ultrasound for gaining further insight into the identity of the tissues being examined has tremendous potential, and one can expect significant growth in this area.

There are a variety of ultrasonic parameters being utilized in attempts to identify various tissues. Some work has utilized transmission ultrasound and has measured the attenuation of the ultrasound as it passes through the tissue.[105,106] Various tissue changes, especially ischemia or scarring, clearly cause changes in the attenuation characteristics of that particular tissue possibly because of the increase in collagen content.[107,108] Measuring attenuation obviously has the disadvantage of requiring through transmission ultrasound, which is not commercially available. In addition, the clinical use of such an approach would have significant limitations.

Other investigation has been looking at

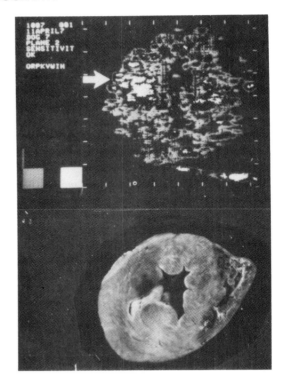

Fig. 1–62. Experimental technique using ultrasound to identify infarcted myocardium. An area of early infarction (arrow) is detected by white echoes. The lower panel represents a corresponding Thyoflavin S fluorescence image in which the perfusion defect appears black with some adjacent mottling. (From Gramiak, R., et al.: Ultrasonic imaging of experimental myocardial infarcts. In Echocardiography. Edited by C.T. Lancee. The Hague, Martinus Nijhoff, 1979.)

changes in the reflected echoes or "backscatter."[109,110] There has been considerable work already done with regard to looking at the amplitude of the returning echoes in tissue identification of eye pathology. Similar approaches are being used to examine returning echoes from different myocardial tissues. Many of these changes are quite subtle and require computer analysis to note the variations. Preliminary success with laboratory specimens suggests that this work will not only continue but that a clinically useful technique for identifying many pathologic histologic changes will be developed.

Computers will undoubtedly play an increasing role in all echocardiography. Many computers and microprocessors are already involved in electronic steering and shaping of the ultrasonic beam with phased array systems. As more echocardiographs become digital the electronic processing will play a bigger role in enhancement of the images. It is anticipated that computers will play an even bigger role in the analysis of the echocardiographic information. Computers are already widespread in this field and used for analyzing M-mode data. Two-dimensional echocardiographic images are analyzed by minicomputers and microprocessors. The major problem with using computers for analysis is entering the echocardiographic data into the system so that they can be handled electronically. Most systems require manual drawing of the various echoes.[111,112] Considerable work is being done to devise computers that can identify the pertinent echoes so that they can be entered into the system for analysis without requiring manual tracing.[113,114] In view of the voluminous amount of information on an echocardiogram, it is not surprising that this can represent a formidable problem.

BIOLOGIC EFFECTS OF ULTRASOUND

One of the principal reasons for the popularity of and interest in echocardiography is that the examination apparently poses no hazard to the patient.[115] In contrast to the usual invasive techniques that require catheterization and angiography, the risk to the patient is virtually negligible. At times, even the avoidance of routine roentgenography is an advantage of ultrasound. This is one of the reasons for the widespread use of ultrasound in examining the pregnant uterus. Ultrasonic examinations of all parts of the body, including such sensitive tissues as a pregnant uterus and the eye, have been performed on thousands of patients all over the world without report of a single untoward reaction. However, the question of safety of this external energy source must still be constantly reviewed since there are obvious biologic effects of ultrasound.[116-118]

When discussing the safety or biologic effects of diagnostic ultrasound, it is necessary to understand some of the terms used. Any biologic effect of ultrasound depends on the energy in question. The amount of acoustic energy (capacity to do work or to produce a biologic effect) is measured in joules.[119] A joule is the amount of heart generated by the energy in question, in this case, ultrasound. A joule is equal to 0.239 calories. A calorie is the amount of heat energy required to raise the temperature of 1 gm of water 1°C. Acoustic power is the amount of acoustic energy per unit time. For example, the power is one watt (1 W) if one joule of energy is produced per second. A milliwatt (mW) is 0.001 W and the kilowatt (kW) is 1000 W. The biologic effects of ultrasound are usually discussed in terms of power, and the units of power are in the milliwatt range.[119]

Another term used to describe the amount of energy used in diagnostic ultrasound is intensity. Intensity may also be called "power density," and is the concentration of power within an area usually expressed as watts per meter squared (W/m^2) or in milliwatts per centimeter squared (mW/cm^2). As previously discussed in this chapter, ultrasonic intensity varies spatially within the ultrasonic beam. For example, if one uses a continuous-wave ultrasonic beam, the average intensity, frequently called the spatial average (SA) intensity, is obtained by dividing the total power emitted by the transducer by the surface area of the face of the transducer. If the power output of the transducer were 2.0 mW and the radiating surface of the transducer were 1.0 cm^2, then the spatial average intensity would be 2.0 mW/cm^2. Since the shape and amplitude of the ultrasonic beam varies (see Fig. 1–14), so does the intensity of the ultrasonic energy. Thus the peak or spatial peak (SP) intensity varies at different locations within the ultrasonic beam. As expected, the SP intensity is greater in the center of the beam than at the periphery. The peak or spatial peak intensity can be measured by using a small thermocouple temperature sensor to detect minuscule rises in temperature in certain areas of the sound field. One may also measure intensity by using a second tiny receiving piezoelectric transducer and noting the resultant voltage changes within the beam.

Evaluating the intensity of the ultrasonic beam with a pulsed system is more complicated. The intensity of the ultrasound now varies not only with the spatial pattern of the beam, but it also varies according to the temporal pattern of the pulsing. In order to make the necessary calculations, one must know the pulse repetition frequency or pulse repetition rate. The duration of the pulse must also be known. For M-mode echocardiography a pulse repetition rate of 1,000 per second and a pulse duration of 1.5 μsec is fairly common. In order to calculate the energy from a pulsed ultrasonic beam, one must know the duty factor, which represents that fraction of time during which the transducer emits ultrasound. If the pulse duration is 1.5 μsec and the pulse repetition rate is 1,000 per second, then the pulse repetition period, i.e., the time between the onset of each pulse, would be 1,000 μsec or 1 msec. Thus the duty factor would be 1.5 divided by 1,000 or 0.0015 (0.15%). The duty factor must be known to calculate power or intensity of pulsed ultrasonic systems. The average power of a pulsed echocardiograph would be the peak power multiplied by the duty factor. For example, if the peak power were about 10 W and the duty factor were 0.0015, then the average power would be 0.015 W or 15 mW.

When discussing intensity for pulsed mode systems, one must talk not only about spatial average (SA) intensity and spatial peak (SP) intensity, but also about temporal average (TA) intensity and temporal peak (TP) intensity.[119] The spatial average, temporal average (SATA) intensity is obtained by measuring the average power of a transducer and dividing it by the surface area of the transducer. This measure, frequently quoted by manufacturers, is the lowest of the various intensities measured with a pulsed system. The spatial average, temporal peak (SATP) intensity is the spatial average value of intensity during a given pulse and is calculated by taking the spatial average, temporal peak (SATP) intensity and dividing it by the duty factor. This calculation allows for the fact that the transducer is transmitting pulsed and not continuous ultrasound. One can of course calculate the intensity by using the spatial peak intensity and the temporal average intensity, which would result in a measurement that indicates the intensity in the center of the beam rather than at the edges. There is a spatial peak (SP)/spatial average (SA) factor. This factor divides the measured peak intensities in the center of the ultrasonic beam by the average intensities over the entire ultrasonic beam. The spatial peak intensity is usually two to three times greater than the spatial average intensity. The highest possible intensity within a pulsed ultrasonic beam would be calculated using the spatial peak and temporal peak measurements. The spatial peak, temporal peak (SPTP) intensity would be calculated by multiplying the spatial average intensity by the SP/SA factor and then dividing it by the duty factor. For example, if one had a pulsed ultrasonic system with a spatial average, temporal average intensity of 3 mW/cm^2, with a duty factor of 0.001 and an SP/SA factor of 3, then the SATA intensity would be 3 mW/cm^2, SATP intensity 3,000 mW/cm^2 or 3 W/cm^2, SPTA intensity 9 mW/cm^2, and SPTP intensity 9,000 mW/cm^2 or 9 W/cm^2.

Commercial ultrasonic instrument companies offer various pulsed ultrasonic devices that have SPTA intensities in the range of 0.001 to 200 mW/cm^2.[120] Thus far, using ultrasound in a frequency of 0.5 to 10 mHz has revealed no significant biologic effect in the many tissues exposed to SPTA intensities below 100 mW/cm^2. In addition, using an ultrasonic exposure time of less than 500 sec and more than 1 sec has demonstrated no side effects, even with higher intensities when the product of the intensity and exposure time is less than 50 joules per cm^2.

One of the biologic effects of ultrasound is the production of heat, which is a principal goal of ultrasonic therapy. With the pulsed ultrasound used in echocardiography, it is extremely unlikely that the duty factor is long enough for any heat to be generated within the body.[121] The evidence available at present indicates that the brief pulses of ultrasound used in echocardiography are not likely to cause any cumulative damage.[122–124] The pulse repetition rate of two-dimensional echocardiography is higher; hence the duty factor is higher. However, the beam is constantly moving so that, except for the skin surface, the heart actually receives less ultrasonic energy. Even the higher average intensities used with continuous ultrasound, such as continuous-wave Doppler, probably are too low to produce any heat in in vivo tissues.[121]

Another physical effect of ultrasound is cavitation.[125] This effect is apparently produced by gaseous cavitations formed during the negative phase of the sound wave cycle. Unfortunately, there are no accurately sensitive techniques for detecting cavitation in vivo. However, it is highly unlikely that such an effect could occur in blood or soft tissue because of the relatively high viscosity of these substances.

There are a variety of other physical forces that might be produced by ultrasonic energy, including oscillatory, sheer, and Oseen forces, radiation, pressure, Venoulli effect, and microstreaming. All these effects have been demonstrated in vitro, but few are fully understood. No evidence of any of these physical effects has been demonstrated in any experimental animal, let alone in any patients. Many investigators have attempted to study the safety of ultrasonic procedures in a variety of laboratory settings. Despite numerous approaches, virtually no consistent biologic effects have been demonstrated using ultrasound at diagnostic power levels. There have been a few reports that some change might occur at the chromosomal level that affects fetal behavior and movement.[126–128] These observations obviously caused considerable concern for people using Doppler devices in obstetrics. However, several investigators have had difficulty duplicating these studies. Thus there are still no confirmed reports of deleterious effects produced by ultrasound in experimental animals, using the dosage parameters of current clinical applications.[121]

Research is continuing in this area. However, all findings thus far indicate that diagnostic ultrasound, particularly that used in echocardiography, is an extremely safe tool with no known deleterious effects. A reassuring factor is that a large percentage of all ultrasonic energy used in echocardiography is absorbed by the chest wall. It is estimated that probably a small percentage of the ultrasonic energy leaving the transducer ever enters the heart. In addition, the blood pool and cardiac structures should not be very

sensitive to the effects of ultrasound. Thus we probably have a wide margin of safety.

REFERENCES

1. Wells, P.N.T.: Biomedical Ultrasonics. London, Academic Press, 1977.
2. Kossoff, G.: Diagnostic applications of ultrasound in cardiology. Australas Radiol., 10:101, 1966.
3. Wells, P.N.T.: Absorption and dispersion of ultrasound in biological tissue. Ultrasound Med. Biol., 1:369, 1975.
4. Wells, P.N.T.: Physics: An Introduction to Echocardiography. Edited by G. Leech and G. Sutton. London, Medi-Cine Ltd., 1978.
5. Eggleton, R.C.: Interim AIUM Standard Nomenclature. Reflections, 4:275, 1978.
6. Goldman, D.E. and Jueter, T.F.: Tabular data of the velocity and absorption of high-frequency sound in mammalian tissues. J. Acoust. Soc. Am., 28:35, 1956.
7. Gregg, E.C. and Palogallo, G.L.: Acoustic impedance of tissue. Invest. Radiol., 4:357, 1969.
8. Reid, J.: A review of some basic limitations in ultrasonic diagnosis. In Diagnostic Ultrasound. Edited by C.C. Grossman, J.H. Holmes, C. Joyner, and E.W. Purnell. Proceedings of the First International Conference, University of Pittsburgh, 1965. New York, Plenum Press, 1966.
9. Fry, W.J.: Mechanism of acoustic absorption in tissue. J. Acoust. Soc. Am., 24:412, 1952.
10. Mason, W.P.: Piezoelectric crystals and their application to ultrasonics. New York, Van Nostrand, 1950.
11. Goss, S.A., Frizzell, L.A., and Dunn, F.: Ultrasonic absorption and attenuation in mammalian tissues. Ultrasound Med. Biol., 5:181, 1979.
12. Hertz, C.H.: Ultrasonic engineering in heart diagnosis. Am. J. Cardiol., 19:6, 1967.
13. Morgan, C.L., Trought, W.S., Clark, W.M., VonRamm, O.T., and Thurstone, F.L.: Principles and applications of a dynamically focused phased array real time ultrasound system. J. Clin. Ultrasound, 6:385, 1978.
14. VonRamm, O.T. and Thurstone, F.L.: Thaumascan: design considerations and performance characteristics. In Ultrasound in Medicine. Edited by D. White. New York, Plenum Press, 1975.
15. Eggleton, R.C. and Johnston, K.W.: Real-time mechanical scanning system compared with array techniques. I.E.E.E. Proc. Sonics Ultrasonics, Catalog No. 74–CH 0896–1, p. 16, 1974.
16. Vogel, J., Bom, N., Ridder, J., and Lancee, C.: Transducer design considerations in dynamic focusing. Ultrasound Med. Biol., 5:187, 1979.
17. Kisslo, J.A., VonRamm, O.T., Thurstone, F.L.: Dynamic cardiac imaging using a focused, phased-array ultrasound system. Am. J. Med., 63:61, 1977.
18. VonRamm, O.T. and Thurstone, F.L.: Cardiac imaging using a phased array ultrasound system. Circulation, 53:258, 1976.
19. Melton, H.E., Jr., and Thurstone, F.L.: Annular array design and logarithmic processing for ultrasonic imaging. Ultrasound Med. Biol., 4:1, 1978.
20. Kossoff, G., Garrett, W.J., Dadd, M.J., Paoloni, H.J., and Wilcken, D.E.L.: Cross-sectional visu-

alization of the normal heart by the UI OCTOSON. J. Clin. Ultrasound, 6:3, 1978.

21. Feigenbaum, H. and Zaky, A.: Use of diagnostic ultrasound in clinical cardiology. J. Indiana State Med. Assoc., 59:140, 1966.

22. Griffith, J.M. and Henry, W.L.: A sector scanner for real time two-dimensional echocardiography. Circulation, 49:1147, 1974.

23. Eggleton, R.C., Feigenbaum, H., Johnston, K.W., Weyman, A.E., Dillon, J.C., and Chang, S.: Visualization of cardiac dynamics with real-time B-mode ultrasonic scanner. In Ultrasound in Medicine. Edited by D. White. New York, Plenum Press, 1975.

24. Gramiak, R. and Shah, P.M.: Cardiac ultrasonography: a review of current applications. Radiol. Clin. North Am., 9:469, 1971.

25. Gramiak, R. and Shah, P.M.: Echocardiography. J.A.M.A., 229:1099, 1974.

26. Nagayama, T., Nakamura, S., Hayakawa, K., and Komo, Y.: Ultrasonic cardiokymogram. Acta Med. U. Kagoshima, 4:229, 1962.

27. Matsumoto, M., Matsuo, H., Ohara, T., and Abe, H.: Use of kymo-two-dimensional echocardiography for the diagnosis of aortic root dissection and mycotic aneurysm of the aortic root. Ultrasound Med. Biol., 3:153, 1977.

28. Asberg, A.: Ultrasonic cinematography of the living heart. Ultrasonics, 6:113, 1967.

29. Hertz, C.H. and Lundstrom, K.: A fast ultrasonic scanning system for heart investigation. 3rd International Conference on Medical Physics. Gotenburg, Sweden. August 1972.

30. Gramiak, R., Waag, R., and Simon, W.: Cine ultrasound cardiography. Radiology, 107:175, 1973.

31. Kratochwil, A., Jantsch, C., Mosslacher, H., Slany, J., and Wenger, R.: Ultrasonic tomography of the heart. Ultrasound Med. Biol., 1:275, 1974.

32. Ebina, T., Oka, S., Tanaka, M., Kosaka, S., Terasawa, Y., Unno, K., Kikuchi, D., and Uchida, R.: The ultrasono-tomography of the heart and great vessels in living human subjects by means of the ultrasonic reflection technique. Jpn. Heart J., 8:331, 1967.

33. King, D.L.: Cardiac ultrasonography: cross-sectional ultrasonic imaging of the heart. Circulation, 47:843, 1973.

34. Griffith, J.M., Henry, W.L., and Epstein, S.E.: Real time two-dimensional echocardiography. Circulation (Suppl. IV), 48:124, 1973. (Abstract)

35. Eggleton, R.C.: Ultrasonic visualization of the dynamic geometry of the heart. Second World Congress on Ultrasonics in Medicine. Excerpta Medica, June, 1973.

36. Kambe, T., Nishimura, K., Hibi, N., Sakakibara, T., Kato, T., Fukui, Y., Arakawa, T., Tatematsu, H., Miwa, A., Tada, H., and Sakamoto, N.: Clinical application of high speed B mode echocardiography. J. Clin. Ultrasound, 5:202, 1977.

37. Nishimura, K., Hibi, N., Kato, T., Fukui, Y., Arakawa, T., Tatematsu, H., Miwa, A., Tada, H., Kambe, T., Nakagawa, K., and Takemura, Y.: Real-time observation of cardiac movement and structures in congenital and acquired heart diseases employing high-speed ultrasonocardiotomography. Am. Heart J., 92:340, 1976.

38. Bom, N., Lancee, C.T., Honkoop, J., and Hugenholtz, P.C.: Ultrasonic viewer for cross-sectional analyses of moving cardiac structures. Biomed. Eng., 6:500, 1971.

39. Bom, N., Lancee, C.T., VanZwieten, G., Kloster, F.E., and Roelandt, J.: Multi-scan echocardiography. I. Technical description. Circulation, 48:1066, 1973.

40. Yoshikawa, J., Owaki, T., Kato, H., Yanagihara, K., Suzuki, T., Takagi, Y., and Okumachi, R.: Electroscan echocardiography: application to the cardiac diagnosis. J. Cardiography, 7:33, 1977.

41. Pedersen, J.F. and Northeved, A.: An ultrasonic multitransducer scanner for real-time heart imaging. J. Clin. Ultrasound, 5:11, 1977.

42. Reference deleted.

43. Reference deleted.

44. Ligtvoet, C., Rijsterborgh, H., Kappen, L., and Bom, N.: Real-time ultrasonic imaging with a hand-held scanner. I. Technical description. Ultrasound Med. Biol., 4:91, 1978.

45. Roelandt, J., Wladimiroff, J.W., and Baars, A.M.: Ultrasonic real time imaging with a hand-held scanner. Ultrasound Med. Biol., 4:93, 1978.

46. Roelandt, J., Lima, L., Hajar, H.A., Walsh, W., and Kloster, F.E.: Clinical Experience with an automatic echocardiograph. CVP, 7:27, 1979.

47. Griffith, J.M. and Henry, W.L.: Switched gain: a technique for simplifying ultrasonic measurement of cardiac wall thickness. I.E.E.E. Trans. Biomed. Eng., 22:337, 1975.

48. Roelandt, J., VanDorp, W.G., Bom, N., Laird, J.D., and Hugenholtz, P.G.: Resolution problems in echocardiography: a source of interpretation errors. Am. J. Cardiol., 37:256, 1976.

49. Martin, R.P., Rakowski, H., Kleiman, J.H., Beaver, W., London, E., and Popp, R.L.: Reliability and reproducibility of two-dimensional echocardiographic measurements of the stenotic mitral valve orifice area. Am. J. Cardiol., 43:56, 1979.

50. Yeh, E.: Reverberations in echocardiograms. J. Clin. Ultrasound, 5:84, 1977.

51. Kalmanson, D., Veyrat, C., Derai, C., Savier, C.H., Berkman, M., and Chiche, P.: Non-invasive technique for diagnosing atrial septal defect and assessing shunt volume using directional Doppler ultrasound. Correlations with phasic flow velocity patterns of the shunt. Br. Heart J., 34:981, 1972.

52. Rushmer, R.F., Baker, D.W., and Stegall, H.F.: Transcutaneous Doppler flow detection as a nondestructive technique. J. Appl. Physiol., 21:554, 1966.

53. Lavenson, G.S., Rich, N.M., and Baugh, J.H.: Value of ultrasonic flow detection in the management of peripheral vascular disease. Am. J. Surg., 120:522, 1970.

54. Sigel, B., Popley, G.L., Boland, J.P., Wagner, D.K., and Mopp, E. McD.: Augmentation of flow sounds in the ultrasonic detection of venous abnormalities. Invest. Radiol., 2:256, 1967.

55. Strandness, D.E., McCutcheon, E.P., and Rushmer, R.F.: Application of a transcutaneous Doppler flow meter in evaluation of occlusive arterial disease. Surg. Gynecol. Obstet., 122:1039, 1966.

56. Fronek, A., Coel, M., and Bernstein, E.F.: Quantitative ultrasonographic studies of lower extremity flow velocities in health and disease. Circulation, 53:957, 1976.

57. Johnston, K.W., Maruzzo, B.X., and Cobbold, R.S.C.: Doppler methods for quantitative measurement and location of peripheral arterial occlusive disease by analysis of the blood flow velocity wave form. Ultrasound Med. Biol., 4:209, 1978.

58. Yoshida, T., et al.: Analysis of heart motion with

ultrasonic Doppler method and its clinical application. Am. Heart J., 61:61, 1961.

59. Yoshida, T., et al.: Study of examining the heart with ultrasonics. III. Kinds of Doppler beats. IV. Clinical applications. Jpn. Circ. J., 20:228, 1956.

60. Kostis, J.B., Fleischmann, D., and Bellet, S.: Use of the ultrasonic Doppler method for the timing of valvular movement. Circulation, 40:197, 1969.

61. Kostis, J.B., Mavrogeorgis, E., Slater, A., and Bellet, S.: Use of a range gated, pulsed ultrasonic Doppler technique for continuous measurement of velocity of the posterior heart wall. Chest, 62:597, 1972.

62. Huntsman, L.L., Gams, E., Johnson, C.C., and Fairbanks, E.: Transcutaneous determination of aortic blood flow velocities in man. Am. Heart J., 89:605, 1975.

63. Light, L.H.: Transcutaneous observation of blood velocity in the ascending aorta in man. Biol. Cardiol., 26:214, 1969.

64. Light, L.H., Gross, G., and Hansen, P.L.: Noninvasive measurement of blood velocity in the major thoracic vessels. Proc. R. Soc. Med., 67:142, 1974.

65. Sequeira, R.F., Light, L.H., Gross, G., and Raftery, E.B.: Transcutaneous aortovelography: a quantitative evaluation. Br. Heart J., 38:443, 1976.

66. Buchtal, A., Hanson, G.C., and Peisach, A.R.: Transcutaneous aortovelography: potentially useful technique in management of critically ill patients. Br. Heart J., 38:451, 1976.

67. Huntsman, L.L., Gams, E., Johnson, C.C., and Fairbanks, E.: Transcutaneous determination of aortic blood flow velocities in man. Am. Heart J., 89:605, 1975.

68. Reference deleted.

69. Boughner, D.R.: Assessment of aortic insufficiency by transcutaneous Doppler ultrasound. Circulation, 52:874, 1975.

70. Thompson, P.D., Mennel, R.G., MacVaugh, H., and Joyner, C.R.: The evaluation of aortic insufficiency in humans with a transcutaneous Doppler velocity probe. Ann. Intern. Med., 72:781, 1970.

71. Joyner, C.R., Jr., Harrison, F.S., Jr., and Gruber, J.W.: Diagnosis of hypertrophic subaortic stenosis with a Doppler velocity flow detector. Ann. Intern. Med., 74:692, 1971.

72. Baker, D.W.V. and Johnson, S.L.: Doppler echocardiography. In Cardiac Ultrasound. Edited by R. Gramiak, et al. St. Louis, C.V. Mosby Co., 1973.

73. Baker, D.W.: Pulsed ultrasonic Doppler bloodflow sensing. I.E.E.E. Trans. Sonics Ultrasonics, SU-17, No. 3, July 1970.

74. Kalmanson, D., Veyrat, C., Bouchareine, F., and Degroote, A.: Non-invasive recording of mitral valve flow velocity patterns using pulsed Doppler echocardiography. Application to diagnosis and evaluation of mitral valve disease. Br. Heart J., 39:517, 1977.

75. Ward, J.M., Baker, D.W., Rubenstein, S.A., and Johnson, S.L.: Detection of aortic insufficiency by pulsed Doppler echocardiography. J. Clin. Ultrasound, 5:5, 1977.

76. Baker, D.W., Rubenstein, S.A., and Lorch, G.S.: Pulsed Doppler echocardiography: principles and applications. Am. J. Med., 63:69, 1977.

77. Schwartz, M.D. and DeCristofaro, D.: Review and evaluation of range-gated, pulsed, echo-Doppler. J. Clin. Eng., 3:153, 1978.

78. Johnson, S.L., Baker, D.W., Lute, R.A., and Dodge, H.T.: Doppler echocardiography: the localization of cardiac murmurs. Circulation, 48:810, 1973.

79. Goldberg, S.J., Areias, J.C., Spitaels, S.E.C., and deVilleneuve, V.H.: Echo Doppler detection of pulmonary stenosis by time-interval histogram analysis. J. Clin. Ultrasound, 7:183, 1979.

80. Lorch, G., Rubenstein, S., Baker, D., Dooley, T., and Dodge, H.: Doppler echocardiography. Use of a graphical display system. Circulation, 56:576, 1977.

81. Stevenson, J.G., Kawabori, I., Dooley, T., and Guntheroth, W.G.: Diagnosis of ventricular septal defect by pulsed Doppler echocardiography. Circulation, 58:322, 1978.

82. Stevenson, J.G., Kawabori, I., and Guntheroth, W.G.: Differentiation of ventricular septal defects from mitral regurgitation by pulsed Doppler echocardiography. Circulation, 56:14, 1977.

83. Bommer, W.J., Miller, L.R., Mason, D.T., and DeMaria, A.N.: Enhancement of pulsed Doppler echocardiography in the evaluation of aortic valve disease by the development of computerized spectral frequency analysis. Circulation (Suppl. II), 58:187, 1978. (Abstract)

84. Holen, J. and Simonsen, S.: Determination of pressure gradient in mitral stenosis with Doppler echocardiography. Br. Heart J., 41:529, 1979.

85. Atkinson, P.: A fundamental interpretation of ultrasonic Doppler velocimeters. Ultrasound Med. Biol., 2:107, 1976.

86. Goldberg, S.J., Areias, J.C., Spitaels, S.E.C., and deVilleneuve, V.H.: Use of time interval histographic output from echo-Doppler to detect left-to-right atrial shunts. Circulation, 58:147, 1978.

87. Cooperberg, P.L., Robertson, W.D., Fry, P., and Sweeney, V.: High resolution real time ultrasound of the carotid bifurcation. J. Clin. Ultrasound, 7:13, 1979.

88. Nixon, J.V. and Saffer, S.I.: Three-dimensional echocardiography. Circulation (Suppl. II), 58:157, 1978. (Abstract)

89. Brinkley, J.F., Moritz, W.E., and Baker, D.W.: Ultrasonic three-dimensional imaging and volume from a series of arbitrary sector scans. Ultrasound Med. Biol., 4:317, 1978.

90. Smith, R.P.: A technique for generating three-dimensional images from ultrasonography. J. Clin. Ultrasound, 4:49, 1976.

91. Matsumoto, M., Matsuo, H., Kitabatake, A., Inque, M., Hamanaka, Y., Tamura, S., Tanaka, K., and Abe, H.: Three-dimensional echocardiograms and two-dimensional echocardiographic images at desired planes by a computerized system. Ultrasound Med. Biol., 3:163, 1977.

92. Griffith, J.M. and Henry, W.L.: An ultrasound system for combined cardiac imaging and Doppler blood flow measurement in man. Circulation, 57:925, 1978.

93. Miyatake, K., Kinoshita, N., Nagata, S., Beppu, S., Park, Y–D., Sakakibara, H., and Nimura, Y.: Intracardiac flow pattern in mitral regurgitation studied with combined use of the ultrasonic pulsed Doppler technique and cross-sectional echocardiography. Am. J. Cardiol., 45:155, 1980.

94. Green, P.S., et al.: A real-time ultrasonic imaging system for carotid arteriography. Ultrasound Med. Biol., 3:129, 1977.

95. Bournat, J.P., Peronneau, P., and Herment, A.:

Yes-No ultrasonic Doppler method of detection for vascular imaging. Ultrasound Med. Biol., 3:105, 1977.

96. Reference deleted.

97. Stevenson, G., Brandestini, M., Weiler, T., Howard, A., and Eyer, M.: Digital multigate Doppler with color echo and Doppler display-diagnosis of atrial and ventricular septal defects. Circulation (Suppl. II), 60:800, 1979. (Abstract)

98. Brandestini, M., Howard, A., Eyer, M., Stevenson, J., and Weiler, T.: Visualization of intracardiac defects by M/Q-mode echo/Doppler ultrasound. Circulation (Suppl. II), 60:13, 1979. (Abstract)

98a. Brandestini, M.A., Eyer, M.K., and Stevenson, J.G.: M/Q-mode echocardiography. The synthesis of conventional echo with digital multigate Doppler. In Echocardiography. Edited by C.T. Lancee. The Hague, Martinus Nijhoff, 1979.

99. Flinn, G.S.: Color encoded display of M-mode echocardiograms. J. Clin. Ultrasound, 4:339, 1976.

100. Linzer, M.: The ultrasonic tissue characterization seminar: an assessment. J. Clin. Ultrasound, 4:97, 1976.

101. Mimbs, J.W., O'Donnell, M., Bauwens, D., Miller, J.G., and Sobel, B.E.: Characterization of the evolution of myocardial infarction by ultrasonic backscatter. Circulation (Suppl. II), 60:17, 1979. (Abstract)

102. Dines, K.A., Weyman, A.E., Franklin, T.D., Jr., Cuddeback, J.K., Sanghvi, N.T., Avery, K.S., Baird, A.I., and Fry, F.J.: Quantitation of changes in myocardial fiber bundle spacing with acute infarction, using pulse-echo ultrasound signals. Circulation (Suppl. II), 60:17, 1979. (Abstract)

103. Bauwens, D., O'Donnell, M., Miller, J.G., and Mimbs, J.W.: Detection of acute myocardial ischemia in vivo with quantitative ultrasonic backscatter. Circulation (suppl. II), 60:17, 1979. (Abstract)

104. Rasmussen, S., Corya, B.C., Feigenbaum, H., and Knoebel, S.B.: Detection of myocardial scar tissue by M-mode echocardiography. Circulation, 57:230, 1978.

104a. Gramiak, R., Waag, R.C., Schenk, E.A., Lee, P.P.K., Thompson, K., and Macintosh, H.P.: Ultrasonic imaging of experimental myocardial infarcts. In Echocardiography. Edited by C.T. Lancee. The Hague, Martinus Nijhoff, 1979.

105. Mimbs, J.W., Yuhas, D.E., Miller, J.G., Weiss, A.N., and Sobel, B.E.: Detection of myocardial infarction in vitro based on altered attenuation of ultrasound. Circ. Res., 41:192, 1977.

106. Mimbs, J.W., O'Donnell, M., Miller, J.G., and Sobel, B.E.: Changes in ultrasonic attenuation indicative of early myocardial ischemic injury. Am. J. Physiol., 236:H340, 1979.

107. O'Brien, W.D.: The relationships between collagen and ultrasonic attenuation and velocity in tissue. In Proceedings: Ultrasonics International '77. Guilford, England, IPC Science and Technology Press, 1977.

108. O'Donnell, M., Mimbs, J.W., Sobel, B.E., and Miller, J.G.: Collagen as a determinant of ultrasonic attenuation in myocardial infarcts. In Ultrasound in Medicine. Vol. 4. Edited by D. White. New York, Plenum Press, 1978.

109. Sigelmann, R.S. and Reid, J.M.: Analysis and measurement of ultrasound and backscattering from an ensemble of scatterers excited by sine wave bursts. J. Acoust. Soc. Am., 53:1351, 1973.

110. Greenleaf, J.F., Johnson, S.A., and Lent, A.H.: Measurement of spatial distribution of refractive index in tissues by ultrasonic computer assisted tomography. Ultrasound Med. Biol., 3:327, 1978.

111. Soffer, S.I., Nixon, J.V., and Mishelvich, D.J.: Simple method for computer-aided analysis of echocardiograms. Am. J. Cardiol., 38:34, 1976.

112. Chen, W. and Gibson, D.: Relation of isovolumic relaxation to left ventricular wall movement in man. Br. Heart J., 42:51, 1979.

113. Hestenes, J.D., Meerbaum, S., Wyatt, H.L., and Corday, E.: Echo tracking in ultrasound images of the left ventricle of dogs with induced ischemia. Circulation (Suppl. II), 60:145, 1979. (Abstract)

114. Skorton, D.J., McNary, C.A., Child, J.S., and Shah, P.M.: Computerized image processing in cross-sectional echocardiography. Am. J. Cardiol., 45:403, 1980. (Abstract)

115. Woodward, B. and Warwick, R.: How safe is diagnostic sonar? Br. J. Radiol., 43:719, 1970.

116. Veluchamy, V.: Medical ultrasound and its biological effects. J. Clin. Eng., 3:162, 1978.

117. Erdmann, W.A., Johnson, L.K., and Baird, A.I.: Ultrasonic toxicity study. Ultrasound Med. Biol., 3:351, 1978.

118. Galperin-Lemaitre, H.: Safety threshold of ultrasound in medical use? Am. Heart J., 94:260, 1977.

119. Who's afraid of a hundred milliwatts per square centimeter (10 mW/cm², SPTA)? Prepared by the American Institute of Ultrasound in Medicine Bioeffects Committee. American Institute of Ultrasound in Medicine, 1979.

120. Nyborg, W.L., Buxbaum, C., Carson, P.L., Carstensen, E.L., O'Brien, W.D., Jr., Rooney, J.A., Stratmeyer, M.E., and Taylor, K.J.W.: Should there be upper limits to intensities for diagnostic ultrasound equipment? A panel discussion. Reflections, 4:293, 1978.

121. Taylor, K.J.W.: Current status of toxicity investigation. J. Clin. Ultrasound, 2:149, 1974.

122. Edler, I., Gustafson, A., Karlefors, T., and Christensson, B.: Ultrasound cardiography. Acta Med. Scand. (Suppl). 370:68, 1961.

123. Huter, T.F., Ballantine, H.T., Jr., and Coller, W.C.: Production of lesions in the central venous system with focused ultrasound: a study of dosage factors. J. Acoust. Soc. Am., 28:192, 1956.

124. Lehmann, J.: The biophysical basis of biological ultrasonic reactions with special reference to ultrasonic therapy. Arch. Phys. Med. Rehabil., 34:139, 1953.

125. Flynn, H.G.: Physics of acoustic cavitation in liquids. In Physical Acoustics. Edited by W.P. Mason. New York, Academic Press, 1964.

126. Macintosh, I.C.C. and Davey, D.A.: Relationship between intensity of ultrasound and induction of chromosome aberrations. Br. J. Radiol., 45:320, 1972.

127. Murai, N., Hoshi, K., and Nakamura, T.: Effects of diagnostic ultrasound irradiated during fetal state on development of orienting behavior and reflex ontogeny in rats. Tohoku J. Exp. Med., 47:640, 1976.

128. David, H., Weaver, J.B., and Pearson, J.F.: Doppler ultrasound and fetal activity. Br. Med. J., 2:62, 1975.

CHAPTER 2

The Echocardiographic Examination

The ability to obtain a high-quality echocardiographic recording is probably the most important factor in determining how useful an echocardiographic examination will be. No matter how expertly one interprets echocardiograms, there is no possible way of obtaining useful information from an inadequate tracing. The technical details involved in getting a high-quality echocardiogram are somewhat unique to this particular type of examination. Unfortunately, examinations must be customized for each patient. One cannot place the transducer in routine positions over the chest as one does electrocardiographic leads and hope that the recording will be comparable from one patient to another. The examination is considered adequate when the echocardiographer performing the study records what he recognizes and feels is necessary for that individual patient. Thus the echocardiographic examination has become a highly sophisticated technique that requires experience, skill, and an understanding of the requirements for an adequate echocardiogram.

SELECTION OF TRANSDUCERS

The type of transducer used depends on the patient being examined. In adult echocardiography, a 2.0- or 2.25-megaHertz (mHz) transducer is most often used. This particular frequency represents a good compromise between penetration and resolution. As mentioned in Chapter 1, penetration is the ability of ultrasound to enter the body and to record structures located far from the transducer. Resolution represents the ability to identify two different objects or interfaces that might be close together. High-fre-

quency transducers emit ultrasound with small wavelengths having excellent resolution but poor penetration. Low-frequency transducers are the reverse; they have good penetration but poor resolution. Some newer echocardiographs, with better signal to noise ratios, permit the use of 3.0 to 5.0 mHz transducers in adults. However, there are some adult patients with extremely thick chest walls in whom even a 2.25-mHz transducer may not have sufficient penetration. Occasionally, a lower frequency transducer may be helpful in such an individual. In his early studies, Edler noted that a 1.0-mHz transducer was sometimes necessary in certain patients.[1] We have noted that by using a 1.6-mHz transducer, one frequently records cardiac echoes from a chest otherwise difficult to examine with a routine 2.25-mHz transducer.

In infants and young children, the problem of penetration is significantly less. These patients rarely have ossified ribs, and the amount of tissue through which the ultrasonic beam passes before entering the heart is small. In addition, since the cardiac structures are close to the transducer, the near-field structures are extremely important. In these patients a higher frequency transducer is usually preferable. A transducer with a frequency of 3.5 or 5.0 mHz is most useful. Some examiners have even used a 7.0-mHz transducer, although one with a frequency of 5.0 mHz is probably sufficient even for premature infants.

The size of the transducer is another important factor. The diameter of the crystal influences the shape of the ultrasonic beam (see Chapter 1). A larger transducer has a longer near field and thus a more parallel, relatively narrow beam because the diverging far field occurs farther from the transducer. On the other hand, a large transducer is difficult to angulate and when one tries to tilt a ¾-inch or a 1-inch transducer, much of the surface is lifted from the chest, resulting in lost contact. Hence the size of the transducer again represents a compromise between multiple factors. For routine adult echocardiography, a ½-inch transducer seems most useful. Occasionally, there is an adult patient who has depressed intercostal spaces, making it impossible to place a ½-inch transducer within such an interspace and still maintain good contact. In such individuals a ¼-inch transducer might be necessary. One must remember, however, that when a ¼-inch transducer is used in an adult patient, the excessive divergence inherent in small transducers is a problem and there is more beam-width distortion.

In barrel-chested individuals, especially those who require a frequency lower than 2.25 mHz, a larger transducer, such as a ¾-inch transducer, might be useful. Because the cardiac structures lie so far from the transducer, the angles through which the transducer is tilted are small. In addition, the large diameter of the crystal face also permits a larger surface for recording the returning echoes.

In young children and infants, a ¼-inch transducer is usually preferred. Because the heart lies so close to the transducer, the angles through which the transducer is tilted may be quite steep in many cases. The length of the near field is not as critical since the heart is close to the transducer, and the higher frequency ultrasound used in these patients has an inherently narrower beam width. Thus the most common transducer used in pediatric echocardiography is a ¼-inch transducer with a frequency of either 3.5 or 5.0 mHz.

Many echocardiographic transducers are focused or collimated. This effect is usually accomplished by an acoustical concave lens on the surface of the transducer. There is also a way to focus the transducer internally so that the face of the transducer remains flat. Although this alteration of the transducer is probably useful, it has not proved to be as major a factor as originally believed. It is usually difficult to determine whether or not a transducer is focused at 5, 7, or 10 cm. One possible reason for the inability to detect significant differences among the various focused transducers is that the state of the art may not be sufficient to give good standardization of this particular maneuver. In any case, the focusing aspect of the transducer is probably not as important as the size and frequency of the transducer.

One must also recognize that the manufacturing of a transducer is an art as well as a science. Probably no two transducers are identical. Since the crystal or ceramic used varies somewhat, the sensitivity of a given transducer should probably be checked periodically and certainly immediately when first received from the manufacturer.

There are differences in transducer shape and design for M-mode and two-dimensional echocardiography. However, the discussions thus far with regard to frequency and size of the transducers are valid for both techniques. The two-dimensional transducers, whether mechanical or electronic, are more complicated and usually larger than a simpler M-mode transducer. The shapes of the transducers vary considerably. As a general rule, the face or aperture of the transducer should be as small as possible to maximize maneuverability of the transducer and to permit access to the intercostal spaces. The transducer design should allow adequate examination from the various positions used in echocardiography.

POSITION OF THE PATIENT

Although most echocardiographic examinations are performed with the patient in the supine position, varying the position of the patient may enhance the recording of echoes from certain portions of the heart. The patient may be examined on his left or right side, or in varying degrees of the upright position. A commonly used position is to have the patient lie on his left side with or without elevating the head of the bed. This particular position utilizes gravity, bringing more of the heart to the left of the sternum and facilitating the recording of certain intracardiac echoes, especially the interventricular septum. Usually the patient is only tilted to the left side at approximately a 30° angle; however, it is sometimes beneficial to have the patient lie entirely on his left side. Unfortunately, this left-lateral position may also distort some of the cardiac dimensions, especially the right ventricle. Thus the patient is usually examined in the supine position initially; if this is difficult, the patient is then turned to the left-lateral position. The patient may be examined in the upright position, especially when looking for mitral valve prolapse. When examining infants, it is frequently advisable to examine the patient while in his mother's arms to minimize apprehension and excessive motion. There has even been a recent attempt to examine the patient in the prone position in order to maximize the effect of gravity in bringing the heart close to the chest wall. This technique requires using a table with a hole in it, which presents obvious technical difficulties. Another possible position is sitting up and leaning forward, which may be helpful in the difficult patient.

PLACEMENT OF THE TRANSDUCER

As stated in Chapter 1, sound travels poorly through a gaseous medium such as air. It is not possible for ultrasound to traverse any significant amount of lung tissue and still obtain adequate echoes from the heart. Acoustic mismatch between bone and soft tissue is great. If one tries to direct the ultrasonic beam through bone, almost all ultrasonic energy is reflected or absorbed. Thus an echocardiographic examination is impractical if the transducer is placed over the sternum or ribs. This problem may not be as great in infants or young children since the ribs and the sternum may not be calcified. However, with adults one is limited in performing the echocardiographic examination with respect to transducer placement. The usual echocardiographic "window" lies between the second to fifth intercostal spaces and within 3 to 4 cm to the left of the left sternal border (Fig. 2–1). The transducer may be held in the left hand; some examiners find it more comfortable to use the right hand (Fig. 2–2). With the heavier two-

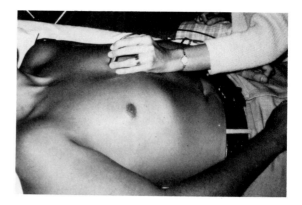

Fig. 2–1. M-mode transducer held with the left hand and positioned along the left sternal border. (From Chang, S.: M-mode Echocardiographic Techniques and Pattern Recognition. Philadelphia, Lea & Febiger, 1976.)

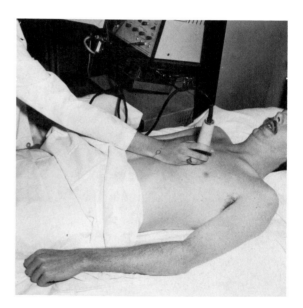

Fig. 2–2. Two-dimensional transducer held with the right hand along the left sternal border.

dimensional transducers it is somewhat easier to carry the weight of the transducer with the fingers of the right hand rather than with the thumb of the left. One can usually examine the heart from at least two or sometimes three interspaces along the left sternal border. In many adult patients, the second interspace has lung overlying the heart, making it a difficult location for the echocardiographic examination. In some adults with low-lying diaphragms even the third or fourth interspace might render examination extremely difficult because of overlying lung. On the other hand, in children the higher interspaces are usually available for the echocardiographic examination, and in young infants the transducer can probably be placed directly over the sternum and the ribs if necessary.[3]

Although the examination from the left sternal border is the most important transducer position for echocardiography, the other available transducer positions are gaining in importance. Because of the increasing use of different transducer positions, the American Society of Echocardiography (A.S.E.) has attempted to standardize the nomenclature used for these various locations.[3a] Figure 2–3 diagrammatically demonstrates the various positions where transducers can be placed for both M-mode or two-dimensional studies. The usual left sternal border examination, as depicted in Figures 2–1 and 2–2, is called "parasternal." When the term is used alone, it is assumed that a left parasternal location is indicated. This area is bounded superiorly by the left clavi-cle, medially by the sternum, and inferiorly by the apical region. The right parasternal area would have the similar landmarks on the right side of the chest. When the transducer is located over the apex impulse, this transducer location is referred to as "apical." The apical location is always left-sided, except in the rare patient with a right-sided apex. The transducer may also be placed below the sternum and the beam directed at the heart from that position. This transducer location is referred to as "subcostal." (Another term used in the literature is "subxiphoid.") A "suprasternal" examination refers to the transducer placement in the suprasternal notch. Thus the four basic transducer locations are the parasternal, apical, subcostal, and suprasternal.

Figure 2–4 illustrates the examination with the transducer placed over the cardiac apex. Although the patient in this figure is being examined in the supine position, it is generally preferred that the patient lie in the left lateral position for the apical examination. This transducer position is a relatively old technique, originally described for recording motion from the mitral ring annulus.[4] It was next used primarily for examining the prosthetic mitral valve. With the

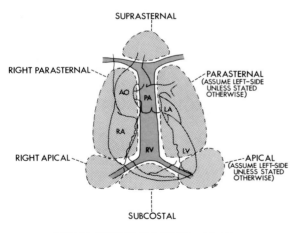

NOMENCLATURE FOR TRANSDUCER LOCATION

Fig. 2–3. Diagram demonstrating the various transducer locations for echocardiography. AO = aorta; PA = pulmonary artery; LA = left atrium; RA = right atrium; RV = right ventricle; LV = left ventricle. (From Henry, W.L., et al.: Report of the American Society of Echocardiography Committee on Nomenclature and Standards in Two-dimensional Echocardiography. Circulation, in press.)

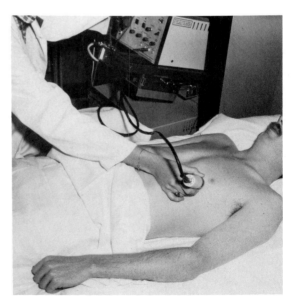

Fig. 2–4. Echocardiographic examination from the cardiac apex.

advent of two-dimensional echocardiography, the apical window is becoming an extremely important transducer position.[5]

An increasingly important echocardiographic examination places the transducer in the subcostal or subxiphoid area (Fig. 2–5).[6,7] This particular technique has been extremely helpful in obtaining echocardiographic information in patients who otherwise were extremely difficult to examine because of a barrel chest. This approach is especially suited to patients with emphysema and low diaphrams. If the patient has a high diaphragm owing to abdominal distention, obesity, or ascites, then this approach may be unsatisfactory since the heart will be far from the transducer. The subcostal examination also permits the examination of slightly different areas of the heart. For example, this approach has been useful in the M-mode examination of the ischemic left ventricle and the right ventricular free wall.[8-10] Examining the heart from the subcostal position is proving to be even more important with the advent of two-dimensional echocardiography. In patients with congenital heart disease, especially in the newborn and young infant, the subcostal examination is extremely useful in studying various structures

not readily seen with the transducer in other positions.[11,12]

The transducer can also be placed in the suprasternal notch (Fig. 2–6).[13] This particular approach examines the aorta, right pulmonary artery, and left atrium (Fig. 2–7). This technique has renewed interest in two-dimensional echocardiography. The two-dimensional examination from this position permits the examination of the arch of the aorta and the descending aorta.[14,15] It also provides the opportunity to examine the right pulmonary artery and the left atrium from a different perspective.[16,17] The suprasternal approach is also a technique commonly used for Doppler studies that record the velocity of blood flow within the thoracic aorta.[18,19]

At present, the principal transducer positions include the parasternal, apical, subcostal, and suprasternal locations. However, there are several other positions described in the literature with specific applications. Examinations with the transducer to the right of the sternum have been attempted, especially in looking at the right atrium and interatrial septum,[20,21,21a] and even at the ascending aorta.[22] In addition, as expected, the right sternal border examination is help-

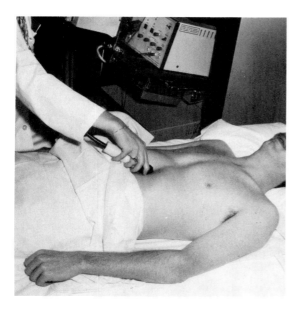

Fig. 2–5. Ultrasonic transducer in the subxiphoid or subcostal position.

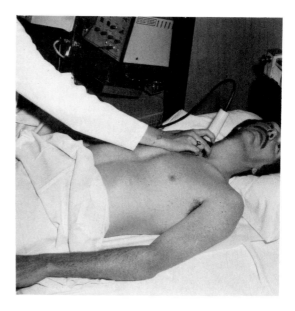

Fig. 2–6. Echocardiographic transducer in the suprasternal position.

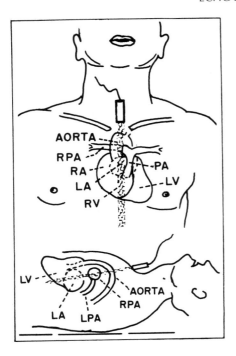

Fig. 2–7. The transverse aorta, the right pulmonary artery (RPA), and the left atrium (LA) as recorded with the transducer placed in the suprasternal notch. (From Goldberg, B.B.: Suprasternal ultrasonography. J.A.M.A., 215:245, 1971.)

ful in patients with dextrocardia. The right parasternal examination may be useful in examining the right ventricle and interventricular septum in some patients. The right supraclavicular fossa is also occasionally used for the echocardiographic examination. Thus far the only application suggested for this approach is to examine the prosthetic aortic valve (see Chapter 6). There is even a report of placing the transducer posterior to the heart in patients with left pleural effusion.[23]

Irrespective of where the transducer is placed, it must have airless contact with the skin. Usually an ultrasonic gel is used as a coupling medium. Occasionally it may be difficult to maintain transducer contact with the skin because of depressed intercostal spaces. In these cases a smaller transducer that better fits between the interspaces is preferable. Some of the larger two-dimensional transducers can be a problem in maintaining good contact with the skin.

Some older two-dimensional scanners use water baths with a thin membrane between the transducer and the skin. The rotating mechanical sector scanners use a fluid-filled plastic housing that separates the patient from the transducer. The plastic offers some attenuation to the ultrasonic beam and also represents a potential source of reverberations. Fortunately, these problems are relatively minor and rotating mechanical scanners have been quite useful.

There has been recent interest in obtaining two simultaneous M-mode echocardiograms.[24,25] For example, it may be of value to obtain simultaneous recordings of mitral and tricuspid valves. Such an examination may involve the use of two M-mode transducers located on the surface of the chest. With phased array two-dimensional transducers it is possible to obtain simultaneous dual echocardiograms (see Chapter 1). Thus only one transducer need be used.

Although echocardiography is considered a noninvasive cardiologic examination, the transducer can be made very small and placed in the body through the use of a catheter. One technique involves placing a small M-mode transducer at the end of an esophageal catheter (Fig. 2–8).[26–29] The transducer is swallowed and the heart is examined through the esophageal wall. The principal advantage of this approach is that it

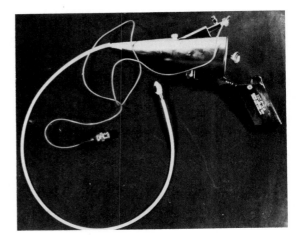

Fig. 2–8. Transducer and catheter used for esophageal echocardiography. The direction of the transducer can be altered by a control in the handle.

avoids the problem inherent in obtaining a satisfactory echocardiogram through the chest wall. There is the occasional patient in whom satisfactory echocardiograms are difficult if not impossible to obtain. The esophageal approach may provide the necessary information. The esophageal echocardiogram has also been used to follow patients during cardiac surgery.[27] This technique thus permits monitoring of left ventricular dimensions during the procedure. The disadvantages of esophageal echocardiography is the semi-invasive nature of the technique. The transducer must be swallowed with some discomfort and inconvenience. In addition, manipulation of the transducer is somewhat limited and may cause esophageal discomfort. There have also been attempts to obtain two-dimensional echocardiograms using the esophageal technique.[28,30]

One may also record the echocardiogram with the transducer placed directly on the epicardial surface of the heart. This approach is primarily limited to laboratory animals;[31] however, there have been some reports of using such an examination intraoperatively to judge the efficacy of cardiac surgery.[32]

SETTING THE CONTROLS ON THE ECHOCARDIOGRAPH

The echocardiographic examination is usually begun with the oscilloscope in the A-mode presentation, which is useful in setting up the echocardiographic controls and especially the depth compensation or TGC. This control is unique to diagnostic ultrasound and is frequently confusing. As stated in Chapter 1, this control essentially compensates for the loss of ultrasonic energy as the beam enters the body. The principal purpose of this control is to suppress those echoes close to the transducer and to increase the intensity of those farther away. Different instruments have a variety of electronic devices for accomplishing this goal. As noted in the previous chapter, some of the newer echocardiographs have a series of levers that permit one to vary the gain control at several distances from the transducer. A more commonly used technique employs an electronic ramp that gradually rises on the

baseline of the A-mode presentation (Fig. 2–9). Those echoes on the left side of the record, on the lower portion of the ramp, are suppressed, whereas those on the right side, on the upper plateau of the ramp, are enhanced. Those echoes in the middle of the slope are either enhanced or suppressed depending on their location.

There is no strict rule as to exactly where the depth compensation ramp should be placed or what the angle of the slope should be. One must merely remember the purpose of this control. If there are a great many confusing echoes in the near field, then the ramp should be placed beyond those near-field echoes so they can be suppressed. If on the other hand one is looking for a weak echo in the far field, then one must be certain that the echo lies to the right of the ramp so that it can

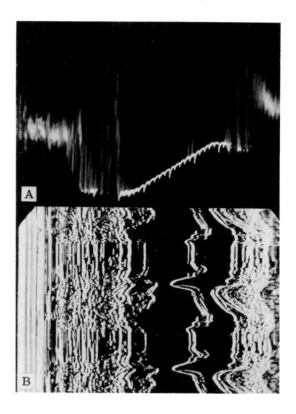

Fig. 2–9. A-mode and M-mode echocardiograms illustrating the use of the depth compensation control when examining the left ventricle. The depth compensation ramp is set to start on the right of the interventricular septum. The rate of rise of the ramp is maximal. All echoes from the posterior left ventricular wall are to the right of the ramp.

be enhanced. For any given individual one may be unable to predict exactly where the ramp should be placed. For example, in some patients the interventricular septum may be best seen if the septal echoes are on the left side of the ramp in the area of the suppressed echoes. On the other hand, interventricular septal echoes frequently may be difficult to record and it is best to adjust the ramp so that the interventricular septal echoes are to the right of the depth compensation ramp and thus enhanced. Another possible way of using the depth compensation ramp is to make a gradual slope throughout the entire tracing. The echocardiographic systems that use automatic depth compensation essentially utilize a gradual slope. The exact location of the depth compensation is not entirely critical since the other controls can help modify or correct the echocardiographic recording. As a matter of practice, the depth compensation is not usually changed during the echocardiographic examination once it is set for an individual patient.

Figure 2–10 illustrates the effect of the reject control. This electronic device essentially eliminates the weaker echoes. Remaining echoes are recorded at full intensity. This illustration shows that when the reject is off (reject 0), there may be so many echoes that those in which one might be interested, for example, the left septal echo (LS), may not be visible. Even with the reject set at 1, so many echoes may come from the left ventricular cavity that the border-forming echoes may be indistinct. On the other hand, with excessive reject (reject 4) the weaker echoes from the left side of the septum (LS) and the posterior left ventricular endocardium (EN) may be eliminated, resulting in an unsatisfactory recording. In this particular illustration, reject 2 probably provides the best-quality tracing, although reject 1 or 3 is also satisfactory.

Damping, gain, or attenuation controls essentially function in a similar manner. By increasing the setting, these controls uniformly influence the number of echoes. As a damping or attenuation setting increases, the number of echoes decrease. The difference between the damping control and an attenuator is that the attenuator works on the received signal similar to the gain control, whereas damping influences the amount of ultrasonic energy entering the body. Figure 2–11 shows the effect of damping on an echocardiographic recording. Similar examples could be given using gain or attenuation controls. This illustration shows that with a damping setting of 4 or 5, much echocardiographic information remains unrecorded.

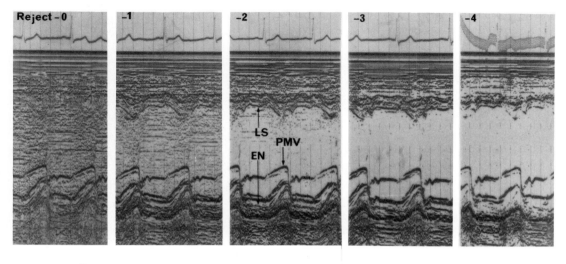

Fig. 2–10.   Illustration of the effect of the reject control. Note changes in the echocardiographic recording as the amount of reject control is increased. LS = left septum; PMV = posterior mitral valve leaflet; EN = posterior left ventricular endocardium. (From Chang, S.: M-mode Echocardiographic Techniques and Pattern Recognition. Philadelphia, Lea & Febiger, 1976.)

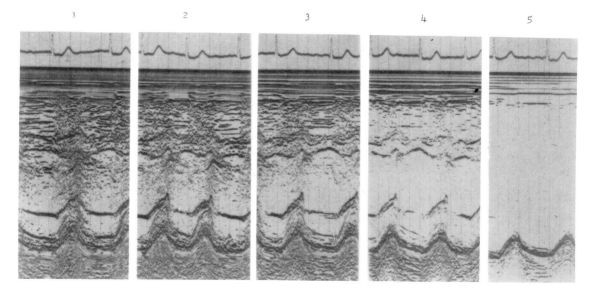

Fig. 2–11. Effect of increasing the damping control on the echocardiograph. (From Chang, S.: M-mode Echocardiographic Techniques and Pattern Recognition. Philadelphia, Lea & Febiger, 1976.)

When the damping setting is 4 or 5, one only sees a strong epicardial echo and virtually no other cardiac structures. Damping settings of 1, 2, or 3 would all be satisfactory for recording the available echocardiographic information. There may be excessive echoes with a damping setting of 1.

As a general rule, one should attempt to use minimum reject and minimum gain controls. The reject control obviously eliminates echoes, many of which are noise and of no clinical value. However, one does not know whether or not some of the eliminated echoes represent true information. As the signal-to-noise ratio improves with newer instrumentation, it is hoped that minimal or no reject will be necessary so that all available information can be utilized. The gain control should be at a minimum to enhance the lateral resolution and beam characteristics of the system. Again, this problem is a function of signal-to-noise. If the signal is too weak, one must increase the gain to see the desired echoes. It is hoped that as instrumentation improves the signal may be sufficiently strong to permit the use of relatively low gain settings.

Most commercial echocardiographs have a control for selectively influencing the echoes in the near field. In some instruments the control is called "near gain." In others the near gain is controlled by changing the left side of the depth compensation ramp. In most cases this near-field gain is related to the depth compensation control. Figure 2–12 shows the effect of a near-gain control. The depth compensation ramp is set so that the septal echoes (LS) are on the right side of the depth compensation ramp and thus are not influenced by the near-gain control. Only the chest wall echoes and the right ventricular (RV) cavity echoes are influenced by this particular gain. In the left photograph, one completely eliminates the chest wall echoes and the right ventricular echoes by reducing the near gain. When the near gain is high, one cannot appreciate the relatively echo-free right ventricular cavity as seen in the illustration on the right. One usually tries to obtain a recording similar to the middle tracing in which the chest wall echoes and the right ventricular cavity are not totally obscured by excessive echoes. Unfortunately, one cannot always set the gain and depth compensation appropriately for such a recording, and one may have to change the

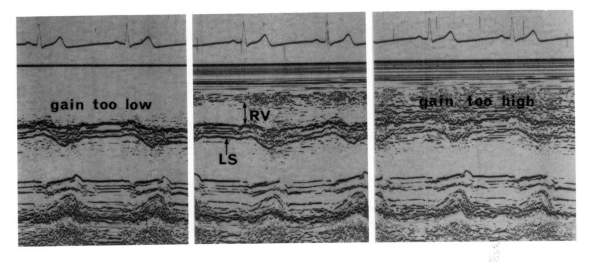

Fig. 2–12.   Echocardiogram showing the effect of altering the near gain. With deficient gain the chest wall and right ventricular echoes can be obliterated *(left)*. With excessive gain, all echoes of the right ventricular cavity can be obscured *(right)*. RV = right ventricle; LS = left septum. (From Chang, S.: M-mode Echocardiographic Techniques and Pattern Recognition. Philadelphia, Lea & Febiger, 1976.)

overall gain or damping settings to achieve proper identification of the right ventricular cavity.

Although the discussion on echocardiographic controls is illustrated by M-mode recordings, these same controls influence the two-dimensional examination identically. Some of the two-dimensional devices have additional controls that alter the character of the echoes, making them fatter or thinner as desired. One may also select a linear or logarithmic display of the echoes, depending on how much dynamic compression is desired. The brightness and contrast knobs on the television monitor are additional controls that can be utilized for picture enhancement.

M-MODE EXAMINATION

Because M-mode echocardiography is still more commonly used than the two-dimensional approach, I will first discuss the M-mode examination. In addition, explaining the M-mode examination sometimes makes it easier to explain the manipulation of the transducer and the controls with a single ultrasonic beam. As will be discussed in the section on the two-dimensional examination, the multiple planes available for examining the heart have complicated

this newer examination. It is possible, however, that with increasing use of two-dimensional echocardiography and with newer instruments that can obtain high-quality two-dimensional and M-mode recordings, the more logical approach would be to perform and discuss the two-dimensional examination prior to the M-mode technique. One can anticipate that many M-mode studies will be done as part of or in conjunction with two-dimensional examinations.

While performing any echocardiographic examination, the examiner must constantly identify the cardiac echoes so that he knows the location of the ultrasonic beam. With M-mode echocardiography, he must have a preconceived idea of the pattern of specific cardiac echoes before he can obtain a recognizable or useful echocardiogram. In short, the first step in learning how to obtain an echocardiogram is knowing what an echocardiogram looks like.

With the M-mode transducer placed along the left sternal border in approximately the third or fourth intercostal space, one can sweep the ultrasonic beam in a sector between the apex (Fig. 2–13, position 1), and the base of the heart (Fig. 2–13, position 4). When the transducer is pointed toward the apex of the heart (Figs. 2–13 and 2–14, posi-

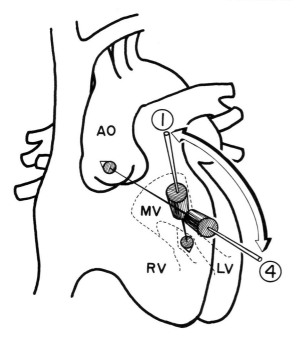

Fig. 2–13. The manner in which a parasternal M-mode examination scans the heart from the apex to the base. AO = aorta; MV = mitral valve; RV = right ventricle; LV = left ventricle. (From Feigenbaum, H.: Clinical applications of echocardiography. Prog. Cardiovasc. Dis., *14*:531, 1972.)

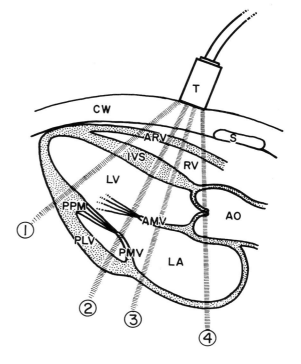

Fig. 2–14. A cross-section of the heart showing the structures through which the ultrasonic beam passes as it is directed from the apex toward the base of the heart. CW = chest wall; T = transducer; S = sternum; ARV = anterior right ventricular wall; RV = right ventricular cavity; IVS = interventricular septum; LV = left ventricle; PPM = posterior papillary muscle; PLV = posterior left ventricular wall; AMV = anterior mitral valve leaflet; PMV = posterior mitral valve leaflet; AO = aorta; LA = left atrium. (From Feigenbaum, H.: Clinical applications of echocardiography. Prog. Cardiovasc. Dis., *14*:531, 1972.)

tion 1), the ultrasonic beam traverses the left ventricular cavity (LV) at the level of the posterior papillary muscle (PPM) and passes through a small portion of the right ventricular cavity (RV). Tilting the transducer superiorly and medially (Fig. 2–14, position 2) causes the ultrasonic beam to travese the left ventricular chamber at the level of the edges of the mitral valve leaflets (AMV and PMV) or the chordae. The beam again passes through a small portion of the right ventricle. By directing the transducer more superiorly and medially (Fig. 2–14, position 3), one records more of the anterior mitral valve leaflet (AMV), and the beam may traverse part of the left atrial cavity (LA). Continuing to tilt the transducer further superiorly and medially (position 4) permits the beam to go through the root of the aorta (AO), the aortic valve leaflets, and the body of the left atrium (LA).

Figure 2–15 is a diagrammatic representation of the echocardiographic recording as the transducer is directed from the apex to the base of the heart. The areas between the dotted lines correspond to the direction of the transducer in Figures 2–13 and 2–14. An electrocardiogram helps to identify systole and diastole. Beginning on the left side of Figure 2–15 (area 1), one initially records the chest wall echoes and then the anterior right ventricular wall (ARV). The right ventricular cavity may or may not be recorded as an echo-free space depending on the individual patient and the setting of the controls. The next structure is the interventricular septum with the right side of the septum (RS) frequently indicated as a double or triple line, while the left side of the septum (LS) is recorded as a single echo. Posterior to the left ventricular cavity, frequently but not always,

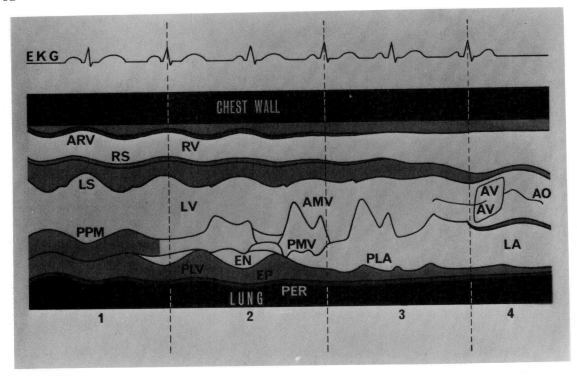

Fig. 2–15.   Diagrammatic presentation of the M-mode echocardiogram as the transducer is directed from the apex *(position 1)* to the base of the heart *(position 4)*. The areas between the dotted lines correspond to the transducer position as depicted in Figure 2–14. LS = left septum; RS = right septum; EN = endocardium of the left ventricle; EP = epicardium of the left ventricle; PER = pericardium; PLA = posterior left atrial wall. For explanation of other symbols see Figure 2–14. (From Feigenbaum, H.: Clinical applications of echocardiography. Prog. Cardiovasc. Dis., *14*:531, 1972.)

is a mass of echoes originating from the posterior papillary muscle (PPM). Located further posteriorly is part of the posterior left ventricular wall (PLV). The dark echoes behind the entire heart originate from the lung.

In transducer position 2 (Figs. 2–13 and 2–15), the principal change in the echocardiogram is that one records parts of the mitral valve apparatus within the left ventricular cavity (LV). These echoes are either chordae or the edges of the leaflets (AMV and PMV). In this position, one also goes through more of the body of the left ventricle, particularly in the posterior left ventricular endocardium (EN). As one tilts the transducer slightly superiorly and medially, the anterior (AMV) and posterior (PMV) mitral valve leaflets can be recorded. Tilting the transducer even further (Figs. 2–14 and 2–15, position 3) causes the posterior leaflet to drop out, and one only records the anterior mitral valve.

The posterior left ventricular wall (PLV), which was moving anterior to or toward the chest wall with ventricular systole, now changes into the posterior left atrial wall (PLA), which moves posteriorly or away from the chest wall during ventricular systole. Directing the transducer toward the base of the heart (Figs. 2–14 and 2–15, position 4) changes the interventricular septum into the anterior wall of the aortic root,[33] and the anterior mitral valve becomes the posterior wall of the aortic root, which is also the anterior wall of the left atrium.[34] Between the two aortic walls one can frequently record two or more leaflets of the aortic valve (AV).[35] These leaflets separate and form a boxlike structure during systole, coming together as a single line in diastole. The left atrial cavity (LA) lies behind the aorta (AO).[34]

The type of echocardiogram depicted in Figure 2–15 is called an "M-mode" scan because echo motion is recorded and the transducer is moved. In this case the transducer remains in one spot on the chest and is tilted in a sector, and hence this scan is called a "sector scan." Figure 2–16 is an actual M-mode section scan. Many of the structures illustrated in Figure 2–15 can be recognized in Figure 2–16. In positions 1 and 2, the right ventricular cavity is not visible. This cavity, frequently only a potential cavity, can be visualized only when the gain is turned down to record fewer echoes in the near field, close to the transducer. In position 1, the papillary muscle is recorded as a mass of somewhat ill-defined echoes approximately 2 to 3 cm from the left side of the interventricular septum. In position 2, one begins to see echoes with a pattern of motion characteristic of mitral valve leaflets within the left ventricular cavity (LV). This pattern is best noted by a sharp spike on the echoes in early diastole.

The anterior leaflet has a spike that moves anteriorly, and the posterior leaflet has a spike that moves posteriorly. In addition, this transducer position provides the best view of the posterior left ventricular wall with a clearly defined endocardial echo behind the posterior leaflet. As demonstrated later, this is the echocardiogram that provides the most information concerning the left ventricle. In position 3, one records a good anterior mitral valve echo, but the posterior leaflet is not seen. With the ultrasonic beam in this direction, the posterior left ventricular wall begins to change into the left atrial wall. In position 4, one records the aorta (AO) and the body of the left atrium (LA). One can see the echoes from the aortic valve leaflets (AV) in the last two cardiac cycles of the echocardiogram. These leaflets appear as thin echoes that form a box-like configuration during ventricular systole.

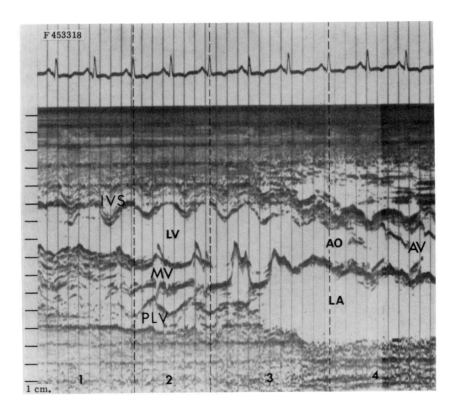

Fig. 2–16. M-mode echocardiographic scan of the heart. The areas between the dotted lines correspond to those in Figure 2–15. IVS = interventricular septum; LV = left ventricular cavity; MV = mitral valve; PLV = posterior left ventricular wall; AV = aortic valve; AO = aorta; LA = left atrium. (From Feigenbaum, H.: Clinical applications of echocardiography. Prog. Cardiovasc. Dis., *14*:531, 1972.)

When an M-mode sector scan is performed between the root of the aorta and the left ventricular apex near the papillary muscles, the transducer does not pass through a single plane. To record the root of the aorta and the aortic valve, one directs the transducer superiorly and medially (Fig. 2–17). As the mitral valve is recorded, the beam is directed almost directly posterior. The left ventricular examination requires a more lateral as well as inferior direction of the transducer.

The tricuspid and pulmonary valves can also be recorded echocardiographically. The tricuspid valve is medial to the aortic and mitral valves, and the pulmonary valve is lateral to the aortic valve and almost directly anterior to the mitral valve. Figure 2–18 shows the relationship between the cardiac valves and the left ventricular apex from the frontal view. Usually only one leaflet of both the pulmonary and the tricuspid valves are recorded echocardiographically. Figure 2–19 shows an M-mode scan from the aortic valve (AV) to the anterior tricuspid valve

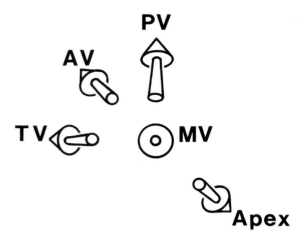

Fig. 2–18. Relationship between the cardiac valves and the left ventricular apex in the frontal projection.

leaflet (ATV). This tricuspid leaflet resembles the anterior leaflet of the mitral valve. Figure 2–20 is an M-mode scan that demonstrates the posterior leaflet of the pulmonary valve (PV) and shows its relationship to the aortic valve (AV). The similarity between the two semilunar valves is apparent on this recording.

It is possible to record echoes from the interatrial septum. This structure can be recorded with the transducer placed either along the left or right sternal borders. Figure 2–21 shows an examination of the tricuspid valve, right atrium, interatrial septum, and left atrium with the transducer placed along the right sternal border. Contrast echoes that help to identify that structure are seen on both sides of the interatrial septum.

A recently described technique notes the identity of the descending thoracic aorta posterior to the heart.[15] Figure 2–22 shows an M-mode scan with the area of the descending aorta lying behind the junction of the left ventricule and left atrium.

When obtaining an M-mode echocardiogram one frequently begins by identifying and recording the mitral valve. It is sometimes useful to feel for a slight left ventricular lift along the left sternal border. If one can feel such a lift, the transducer should be placed directly over the heave or slightly to the left and inferior to it. If no heaves can be palpated, begin by placing the transducer 1

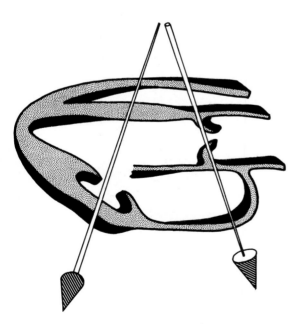

Fig. 2–17. Diagram demonstrating that the left ventricular outflow tract and the cardiac apex are not in the same plane. When examining the base of the heart in the vicinity of the aortic valve, the ultrasonic transducer is directed medially and superiorly. As the angle of the transducer is tilted toward the cardiac apex, the direction changes inferiorly and laterally.

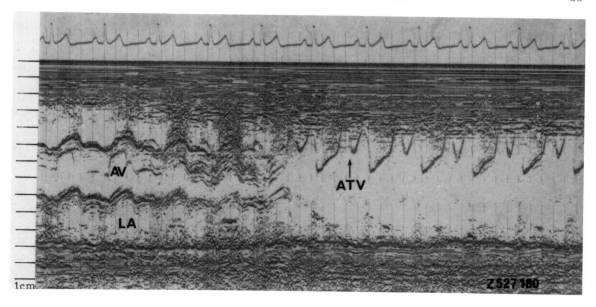

Fig. 2–19. M-mode echocardiographic scan from the aortic valve to the anterior tricuspid valve leaflet (ATV). The echo resembles that of the anterior mitral valve leaflet. AV = aortic valve; LA = left atrium.

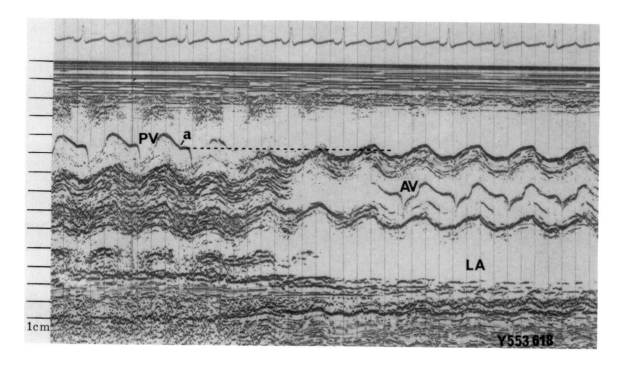

Fig. 2–20. M-mode echocardiographic scan showing the relationship of the pulmonary valve (PV) to the aortic valve (AV). LA = left atrium. (From Chang, S.: M-mode Echocardiographic Techniques and Pattern Recognition. Philadelphia, Lea & Febiger, 1976.)

to 2 cm from the left sternal border in the fourth intercostal space, pointing it almost directly posteriorly. If one does not record the mitral echo, the sound beam should be directed superiorly and medially until the characteristic "snapping" motion of the an-

terior leaflet is recognized. Once the mitral valve is located, one may zero in on the strongest echo by clockwise rotation in tiny circles with any necessary shifting of the transducer upward, downward, or laterally. The pattern of motion inscribed by the struc-

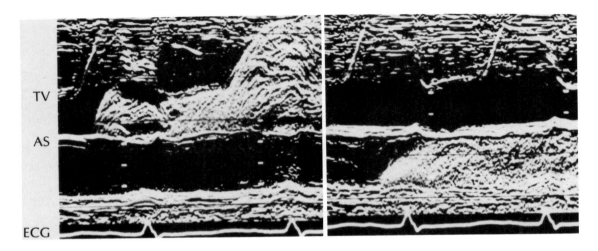

Fig. 2–21. M-mode echocardiographic scan of the tricuspid valve (TV) and atrial septum (AS) with the transducer along the right sternal border. Contrast injections are made in the right atrium (left tracing) and in the left atrium (right tracing). (From Nanda, N.C. and Gramiak, R.: Clinical Echocardiography. St. Louis, C.V. Mosby Co., 1978.)

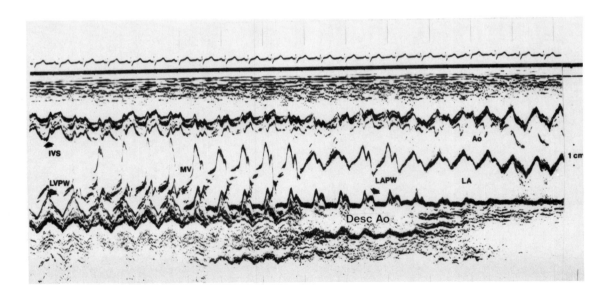

Fig. 2–22. M-mode echocardiographic scan from the left ventricle to the aorta showing the descending aorta posterior to the junction of the left ventricle and left atrium. IVS = interventricular septum; LVPW = left ventricular posterior wall; MV = mitral valve; LAPW = left atrial posterior wall; AO = aorta; LA = left atrium. (From Mintz, G.S., et al.: Two-dimensional echocardiographic recognition of the descending thoracic aorta. Am. J. Cardiol., 44:232, 1979.)

ture is quite distinctive and easily recognized even by the beginner in echocardiography.

Having located the anterior leaflet of the mitral valve, one has an excellent landmark for finding all other cardiac structures. To record the posterior left ventricular wall (PLV) and interventricular septum (IVS) (Fig. 2–16), gradually angle the sound beam inferiorly from the mitral valve position so that it assumes a more anteroposterior position. Continue to tilt the transducer in this general direction until a strong echo from the posterior left ventricular epicardium (EP) and pericardium (PER) (Fig. 2–15) is recorded. Continue to slowly rotate the transducer clockwise until the right and left sides of the interventricular septum come into view. If the septum still is not visible, shift the transducer a little to the left or toward the sternum and angle slightly laterally. Another maneuver might be to move the transducer slightly upward and to angle it somewhat laterally and inferiorly. If the septum is still not easily visible, roll the patient onto his left side and repeat the procedure, beginning

with the mitral valve. Turning the patient on his left side often throws the heart out from under the sternum and brings the septum into its proper place (Fig. 2–23).

To identify the posterior left ventricular wall, the operator must record an echo from the endocardium (EN) (Fig. 2–15), one of the more difficult echoes to record. This is a critical structure for many echocardiographic applications. The posterior left ventricular epicardial and pericardial echoes are easily recorded from many different positions; these echoes come from relatively smooth interfaces with large acoustic mismatches. Although the posterior left ventricular epicardial echo is easily recorded, many other echoes from the heart have similar patterns of motion. As a result, confusion can arise concerning the identity of the posterior left ventricular wall, unless one records the endocardial as well as the epicardial echoes. As a fairly posterior structure, the endocardium lies in the far field. In addition, it may be trabeculated, making it difficult to find a single echo from that structure. Frequently the best endocardial echo may be seen im-

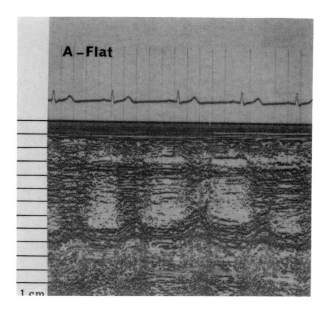
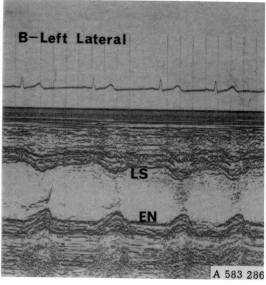

Fig. 2–23. Echocardiogram showing how echoes from the interventricular septum can be enhanced by moving the patient to the left lateral position. LS = left septum; EN = posterior left ventricular endocardium. (From Chang, S.: M-mode Echocardiographic Techniques and Pattern Recognition. Philadelphia, Lea & Febiger, 1976.)

mediately behind the posterior mitral leaflet (PMV) (Fig. 2–15) or behind the chordae tendineae attached to the posterior leaflet.

To record both sides of the left ventricular cavity, continue to maneuver the transducer laterally and slightly inferiorly until the two sides of the interventricular septum as well as the full left ventricular wall are visualized simultaneously. This transducer position is usually at that point where the amplitude of the anterior mitral leaflet is no longer greatest (Fig. 2–15, position 2). One may frequently see some mitral valve motion, but it is usually considerably damped and may actually represent the chordae.

A common error when examining the left ventricle with M-mode echocardiography is to direct the ultrasonic beam too medially. Medial orientation of the ultrasonic beam is due to the frequent presence of lung tissue overlying the lateral portion of the heart and,

to avoid this tissue, one automatically directs the beam medially. Medial orientation of the ultrasonic beam can frequently be detected by noting that the mitral valve is almost directly on top of the posterior left ventricular wall (Fig. 2–24B). One frequently sees an increased atrial component to the posterior ventricular wall motion, and both the interventricular septum and the posterior left ventricular wall have multiple echoes that confuse the identification of endocardial and epicardial structures. Another confusing point is a relatively echo-free space behind the posterior left ventricular wall that can be misinterpreted as pericardial effusion. The possible source of this echo-free space is the coronary sinus. The medial orientation of the ultrasonic beam is also partially due to pointing the transducer medially when examining the aorta and not correctly angling the beam toward the left ventricle. In any case, the

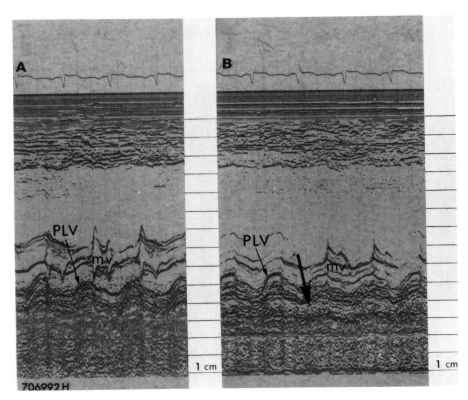

Fig. 2–24. M-mode echocardiograms demonstrating the common error of directing the ultrasonic beam too medially. A proper examination of the left ventricle is noted in *A*. In *B* the transducer is purposely directed medially, and one records distorted posterior left ventricular wall echoes (PLV). The mitral valve (MV) is very close to the posterior wall echoes, an atrial component to the wall motion is increased, and a relative echo-free space *(arrow)* appears behind the left ventricular wall echoes.

medial angulation of the transducer when examining the left ventricle can produce many erroneous measurements.

To record the echoes from the base of the heart, it may be necessary to place the transducer one interspace above the best location for the mitral valve. One should aim the transducer medially and superiorly away from the mitral valve until the anterior leaflet of the mitral valve smooths out in appearance and becomes the posterior wall of the aortic root (Figs. 2–15 and 2–16, position 4). In addition, the interventricular septum becomes the anterior wall of the aortic root.[33] Both aortic walls move parallel to each other and have a characteristic echocardiographic appearance. Posterior to the aorta is the left atrium (LA),[34] and the left atrial wall (LAW) either moves minimally or has a small posterior motion during ventricular systole.[36]

Having located the aortic root, one may or may not immediately record the leaflets of the aortic valve (AV) (Fig. 2–15). If the leaflets are not readily visible, minor changes in transducer angulation may be necessary. The adjustment necessary to record the aortic leaflets is frequently obtained by trial and error; there is no consistent angulation that will bring out the leaflets.

The tricuspid valve is not easily recorded; however, it is found best by first locating the aortic outflow tract. After identifying these structures, tipping the transducer medially and inferiorly frequently locates the anterior leaflet of the tricuspid valve (TV) (Fig. 2–19). The tricuspid valve appears the same as the anterior leaflet of the mitral valve; often it seems to be originating from the anterior root of the aorta. The location of the tricuspid valve is much closer to the chest wall than is the anterior mitral leaflet. The tricuspid valve is recorded much more easily in patients with dilated right ventricles than in patients with normal ones.

The pulmonary valve echo may also be recorded best by first locating the aortic outflow tract and the aortic valve. Having identified the aortic valve, one tilts the transducer laterally and superiorly to find the posterior leaflet of the pulmonary valve (Fig. 2–20).[37,38] As indicated in Figure 2–18, one may also go directly superiorly from the mi-

tral valve echo. The pulmonary valve echo is difficult to record, especially in normal patients. It is more readily visible when the pulmonary artery is dilated. Under these circumstances one can usually feel a lift above the right ventricular outflow tract or above the pulmonary artery. Frequently, one may place the transducer above that lift and find the pulmonary valve much more easily.[39]

It should be emphasized that the echocardiographic technique just described pertains to the parasternal approach and is primarily applicable to adults and older children. In infants and young children, one may direct the transducer in ways not available to echocardiographers who examine adults. In these young patients, the transducer may be placed directly above the valve in question, whether or not the sternum or rib overlies this valve since the chest cage is not ossified at this age and permits penetration of the sound beam.[3]

It should be apparent from this discussion that the direction of the transducer is critical in obtaining an adequate echocardiographic recording. How the ultrasonic beam strikes the cardiac structures is the most important factor in determining whether one will be able to record identifiable echoes. Although the controls also influence the recording, they are not as important and are more easily learned than is the manipulation of the transducer.

Effect of Transducer Location on the M-mode Echocardiogram

Transducer location obviously influences the appearance of the echocardiogram; however, only recently have echocardiographers called attention to this fact. The effect of transducer position is more dramatically demonstrated when one uses a condensed or compressed M-mode scan.[40] Such a scan is performed with the strip-chart recorder moving at a slow speed, usually 10 mm/sec. Figure 2–25 shows such a scan in a normal individual. The ultrasonic beam is directed from the left ventricular apex toward the aorta in the usual manner. Cardiac echoes such as those originating from the left septum (LS), posterior left ventricular endocardium (EN), aorta (AO), and left atrium (LA) can be appreciated. This particular recording was obtained with the transducer placed at approximately the fourth intercostal space. The transducer was equidistant from the interventricular septum and the anterior wall of the aorta since both structures are located at about the same level in this tracing. Figure 2–26 is another M-mode scan of the same patient, only with the transducer placed at a lower interspace. The tracing is altered in that the aorta (AO) is now farther from the transducer, and the anterior wall of the aorta is definitely more posterior than is the left side of the septum (LS). In addition, the left septal (LS) and posterior left ventricular endocardial echoes at the vicinity of the apex are closer together than in Figure 2–25. In fact, the left septal echoes in the vicinity of the mitral valve are not as distinct in Figure 2–26 as they were when the transducer was somewhat higher (Fig. 2–25).

Figure 2–27 shows another recording from the same patient with the transducer located in the third intercostal space. Now the transducer is much nearer the aorta, as demonstrated by the close proximity of the aorta to the chest wall echoes. The anterior wall of the aorta is now closer to the transducer than

is the left side of the septum (LS). Even the echoes from the posterior left ventricular endocardium (EN) are farther from the transducer than are the posterior left atrial echoes (LA). In most normal adults one cannot record echoes from this high interspace because it is frequently obscured by lung tissue; however, Figure 2–27 shows the differences one can obtain if the transducer is placed in such a relatively high position.

Unfortunately, one cannot entirely rely on the interspace as to whether the tracing will be high, low, or in a midposition. The relationship of the heart to the chest varies from one individual to another. A mid-examination may be in the third, fourth, or fifth interspace depending on the location of the diaphragm and on the orientation of the heart. It is important for the person interpreting the echocardiogram to have some idea of the location of the transducer. Condensed M-mode scans such as those in Figures 2–25, 2–26, and 2–27 can be helpful in identifying the location of the transducer by enabling one to evaluate the relationship of the aorta to the interventricular septum. Another possible way of identifying transducer location is to note the direction of the transducer

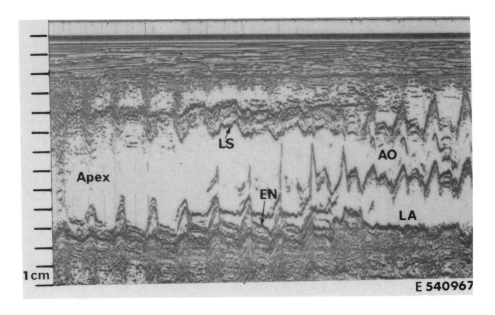

Fig. 2–25.   Condensed M-mode scan from the apex to the base of the transducer in a midposition. The anterior wall of the aorta and the interventricular septal echoes are approximately equidistant from the transducer. LS = left septum; AO = aorta; EN = posterior left ventricular endocardium; LA = left atrium.

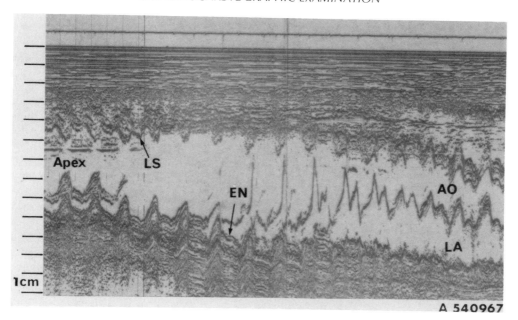

Fig. 2–26.   Condensed M-mode scan of the patient in Figure 2–25, with the transducer placed at a lower interspace. The echoes of the left septum (LS) are now closer to the transducer than is the anterior wall of the aorta. The distance between the left septal and posterior left ventricular endocardial (EN) echoes is less at the apex than at the vicinity of the mitral valve. LA = left atrium; AO = aorta.

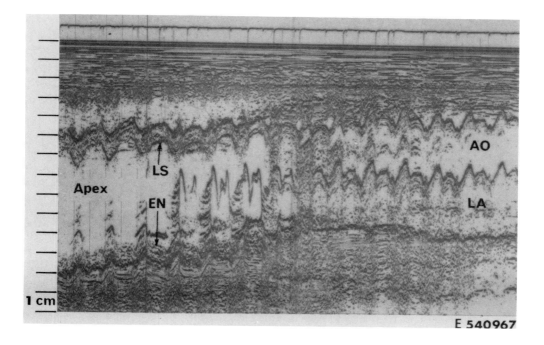

Fig. 2–27.   Condensed M-mode scan of the patient in Figures 2–25 and 2–26 with the transducer placed at a higher interspace. The anterior wall of the aorta is now closer to the transducer than are the septal echoes. LS = left septum; EN = posterior left ventricular endocardium; AO = aorta; LA = left atrium.

when recording the mitral valve. In the mid-position the transducer is perpendicular to the chest when examining this valve.[41] When placed at a higher or lower interspace, the transducer must be directed superiorly or inferiorly to record the mitral valve echoes.

Subcostal M-mode Examination. Figure 2–5 shows how the transducer is placed in the subcostal or subxiphoid area. The patient is supine and the transducer is usually placed slightly to the right of the patient's midline. The transducer is then directed toward the patient's throat and left shoulder. It is best if the patient is elevated slightly at 20° to 30° to relax the abdominal muscles. The examination works best on patients who have low diaphragms, such as those with emphysema. Held inspiration may also assist the subcostal study. In patients with high diaphragms or abdominal distention because of obesity or ascites, the subcostal examination can be extremely difficult.

Figure 2–28 diagrammatically shows how the ultrasonic beam traverses the heart from the subcostal direction. When the transducer is directed superiorly, it passes through the right ventricle, tricuspid valve, aorta, and pulmonary artery. Tilting the transducer toward the left directs the ultrasonic beam through the midportion of the interventricular septum and through the posterior-lateral wall of the left ventricle. Figure 2–29 shows a condensed or compressed M-mode scan with the transducer in the subcostal area. The distinguishing feature of the subcostal examination is the large mass of tissue located between the transducer and the cardiac echoes. The distance between the chest wall and the right ventricular cavity is considerably greater in Figure 2–29 than in Figure 2–27, which is a parasternal examination. The echoes from the left ventricle are similar with the subcostal approach. One can identify the left septal echoes (LS) and the echoes from the posterior left ventricular endocardium (EN) (Fig. 2–29). Near the apex, the distance between these two echoes decreases. Frequently the mitral valve echoes (MV) are not well seen using the subcostal approach. However, the tricuspid valve echoes (TV) are frequently readily seen with this examination. The aorta and

aortic valve echoes may be difficult to record from the subcostal position and may be quite indistinct as noted on this particular tracing. A better subcostal study of the aorta is seen in Figure 2–30. This examination is from a patient who had a catheter in the pulmonary artery. Note that the echo-producing catheter (C) is both anterior and posterior to the aorta, showing that the anterior space above the aorta represents the right ventricular cav-

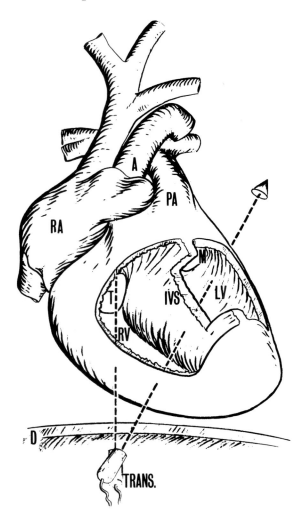

Fig. 2–28. Diagram demonstrating the cardiac structures intersected by the ultrasonic beam with the transducer in the subcostal area. RA = right atrium; A = aorta; PA = pulmonary artery; RV = right ventricle; T = tricuspid orifice; IVS = interventricular septum; M = mitral orifice; LV = left ventricular wall. (From Chang, S. and Feigenbaum, H.: Subxiphoid echocardiography. J. Clin. Ultrasound, 1:114, 1973.)

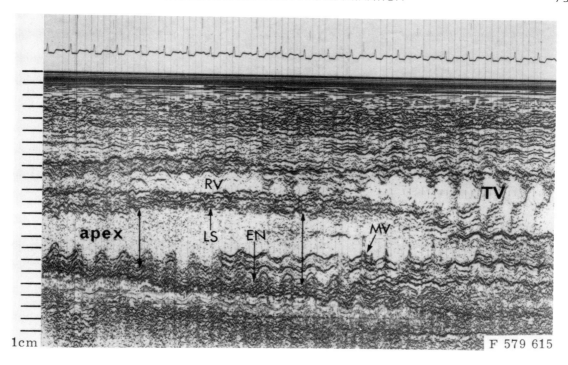

Fig. 2–29.   Condensed M-mode echocardiographic scan from the apex to the base of the heart with the transducer in the subcostal area. RV = right ventricle; LS = left septum; EN = posterior ventricular endocardium; MV = mitral valve; TV = tricuspid valve. (From Chang, S.: M-mode Echocardiographic Techniques and Pattern Recognition. Philadelphia, Lea & Febiger, 1976.)

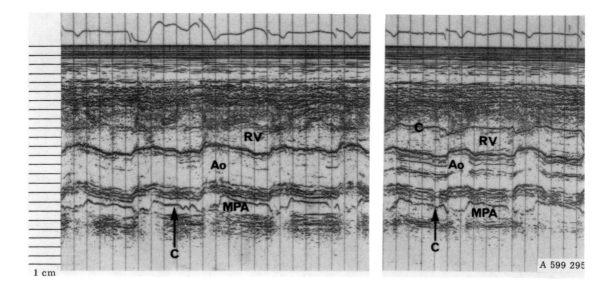

Fig. 2–30.   Subcostal M-mode echocardiogram with the catheter in the pulmonary artery, proving that the echo-free space behind the aorta is the pulmonary artery and not the left atrium. RV = right ventricle; AO = aorta; MPA = main pulmonary artery; C = catheter. (From Chang, S., Feigenbaum, H., and Dillon, J.C.: Subxiphoid echocardiography: a Review. Chest, 68:233, 1975.)

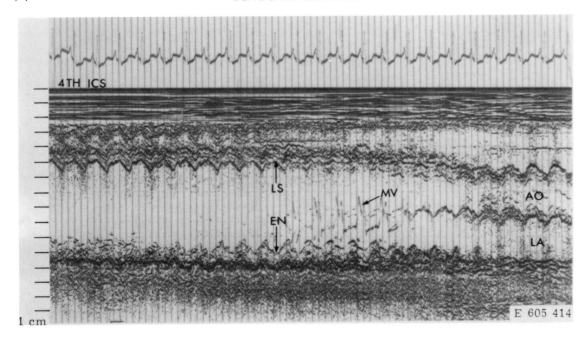

Fig. 2–31. M-mode echocardiographic scan with the transducer placed in the fourth intercostal space. LS = left septum; EN = posterior left ventricular endocardium; MV = mitral valve; AO = aorta; LA = left atrium. (From Chang, S.: M-mode Echocardiographic Techniques and Pattern Recognition. Philadelphia, Lea & Febiger, 1976.)

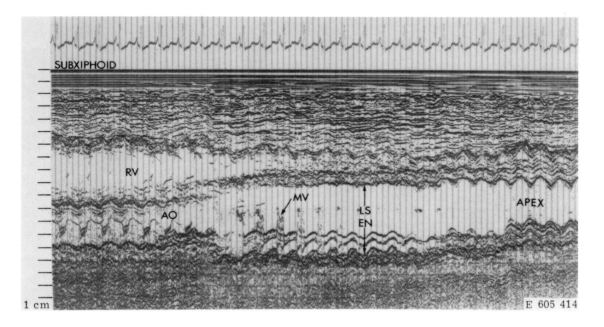

Fig. 2–32. M-mode scan of the patient in Figure 2–31 with the transducer placed in the subcostal area. RV = right ventricle; AO = aorta; MV = mitral valve; LS = left septum; EN = posterior left ventricular endocardium. (From Chang, S.: M-mode Echocardiographic Techniques and Pattern Recognition. Philadelphia, Lea & Febiger, 1976.)

ity and that the posterior space is part of the pulmonary artery.[7]

Figures 2–31 and 2–32 compare an echocardiographic study done on the same patient from both the left sternal border in the fourth intercostal space (Fig. 2–31) and from the subcostal area (Fig. 2–32). Some of the major differences are seen in the echoes originating from the base of the heart. The left atrial cavity is not seen in this subcostal examination. On the other hand, the right ventricular outflow tract is well seen with some faint echoes from the tricuspid valve (Fig. 2–32). In both recordings, one can see echoes from the aortic valve within the aorta (AO); however, the two views of the aortic valve are not entirely similar. As discussed later in the chapter on the left ventricle, the standard echocardiographic dimension between the left septum (LS) and the posterior ventricular endocardium (EN) is similar in the two examinations. Even though the septal motion may not be identical in the two tracings, the dimensions of both are approximately 6 cm in this particular patient. Thus one of the uses of the subcostal examination is obtaining a measurement of the left ventricle, especially in those patients who are technically difficult to examine with other approaches.

M-mode Examination from Other Transducer Locations. As indicated earlier in this chapter, it is possible to obtain useful echocardiographic information with the transducer placed at several locations. In addition to the parasternal and subcostal approaches, one can obtain echoes by placing the transducer in the suprasternal notch,[13] the right supraclavicular fossa,[42] the apex,[4] and the right sternal border.[20-22] These locations are additional to the multiple areas over the chest available to the pediatric echocardiographer examining the young infant.[3]

The suprasternal examination is done preferably with a small transducer having a relatively short handle. Some investigators are using a special right-angle transducer that fits this part of the body conveniently. One can put a pillow under the shoulders and allow the head to fall back slightly; however, this maneuver occasionally tenses the neck muscles and makes the examination even

more difficult. Usually, just turning the patient's head to one side sufficiently permits an adequate suprasternal examination.

Thus far, the right supraclavicular fossa has been used only to examine the ball or disc-type prosthetic aortic valve.[42] The transducer is placed in the supraclavicular fossa and directed toward the heart so that the ultrasonic beam is aligned parallel to the ascending aorta. With M-mode echocardiography the cardiac apex is used primarily for examining prosthetic valves. Both the aortic and mitral prosthetic valves can be seen with the transducer at the apex. An apical study is performed by feeling for the point of maximal impulse and by placing the transducer directly above it, then tilting the transducer to record the necessary structures.

Labeling the M-mode Echocardiogram

A variety of labels have been given to the M-mode echocardiographic recording, most of which refer to the M-mode tracings of the cardiac valves. Since the first recognized structure was the anterior leaflet of the mitral valve, this echo was the first to be labeled. Figure 2–33 is an M-mode examination of a

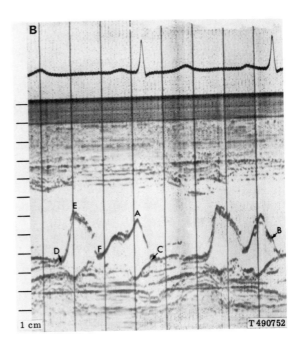

Fig. 2–33. Labeling of the mitral valve M-mode echocardiogram.

normal mitral valve. The various peaks and valleys of the anterior mitral leaflet are labeled. The end of systole, immediately prior to the opening of the valve, is designated D. As the anterior leaflet opens, it peaks at E. The nadir of the initial diastolic closing is labeled F. There may or may not be another upward motion of the mitral leaflet in mid-diastole, depending on the length of diastole. This interval is not given any specific label. In atrial systole, blood is propelled through the mitral orifice, and the mitral leaflets are re-opened. The peak of this phase of mitral valve motion is indicated as A. The valve begins to close with atrial relaxation. Ventricular systole begins during the downslope of the mitral leaflet and may produce a slight interruption in closure at B. Complete closure occurs following the onset of ventricular systole at C. During systole there is a gradual upward motion of the leaflet until the onset of mitral valve opening again occurs at D. The posterior mitral leaflet is a virtual mirror image of the anterior leaflet, except that the amplitude of motion is usually less. Specific letters are not assigned to the posterior leaflet, although occasionally those given to the anterior leaflet are used, with the addition of a prime. Thus there might be E', F', A', and so on. The slope between the E and F points is not necessarily straight, and occasionally an F_o is indicated where there is a break in the diastolic E to F slope.

Specific labels are not assigned to the aortic valve. However, labeling similar to that for the mitral valve is given to the tricuspid and pulmonary valves. Figure 2–34 shows the tricuspid valve echocardiogram with the appropriate labels. The tricuspid valve is similar in appearance to the mitral valve and the labels are also similar.

Figure 2–35 shows the labels commonly given to the pulmonary valve.[39] The letters essentially correspond to those used for the mitral valve. For example, the downward motion, labeled a, follows atrial contraction and coincides with the A wave of the mitral valve. The b point represents the onset of ventricular systole. With ejection of blood through the pulmonary valve, the leaflet opens to its maximum downward position

noted at c. During systole, the leaflet moves gradually anteriorly to point d, at which time closure begins. Closure is completed at point e. The configuration of diastole varies. The point immediately prior to the next A wave is the f point. There may be an early diastolic upward motion after the point designated e. In adults it is unusual to record any more than the posterior leaflet of the pulmonary valve (Fig. 2–35). In children or in patients with unusually large pulmonary arteries, one may also record an anterior leaflet. In fact, one can rarely record the entire excursion of the pulmonary valve throughout the cardiac cycle in adults. One more likely sees the diastolic and early systolic components of the pulmonary valve, as in Figure 2–35B. One usually can identify the e to f interval, the a dip, and the b to c opening.

TWO-DIMENSIONAL EXAMINATION

One initially expects the two-dimensional echocardiographic examination to be simpler than the M-mode examination. The spatial orientation inherent in the two-dimensional technique more readily identifies the cardiac anatomy and should theoretically enhance the ease with which the study is performed. It is true that for the neophyte in echocardiography, the two-dimensional examination enables an easier appreciation of that portion of the heart being examined. The two-dimensional recording resembles the correct anatomic configuration of the heart and is not a series of wiggles and waves as is the M-mode echocardiogram. Actually, the two-dimensional examination is more complicated than the M-mode examination. Instead of examining the heart with a single ultrasonic beam or "ice-pick" view, one is studying the heart using slices or planes. Thus one must not only recognize the direction of the ultrasonic beam, but also the plane through which the beam is being directed. Another point of confusion is that because our understanding of cardiac anatomy is preconditioned by our experience with radiography and angiography, we are accustomed to looking at cardiac silhouettes. Two-dimensional echocardiography has a superficial resemblance to angiography, but the ultrasonic technique records tomograms

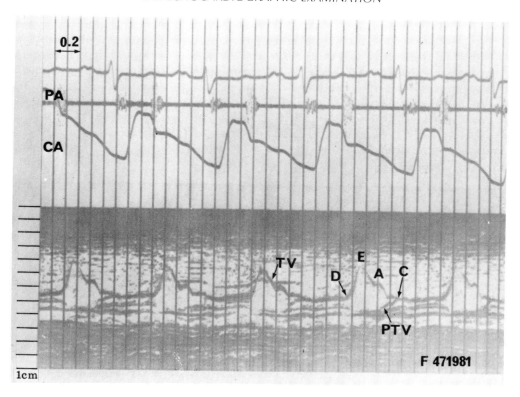

Fig. 2–34.   Labeling of the tricuspid valve M-mode echocardiogram. PA = phonocardiogram in pulmonary area; CA = carotid artery pulse; TV = anterior tricuspid valve leaflet; PTV = posterior tricuspid valve leaflet. (From Chang, S.: M-mode Echocardiographic Techniques and Pattern Recognition. Philadelphia, Lea & Febiger, 1976.)

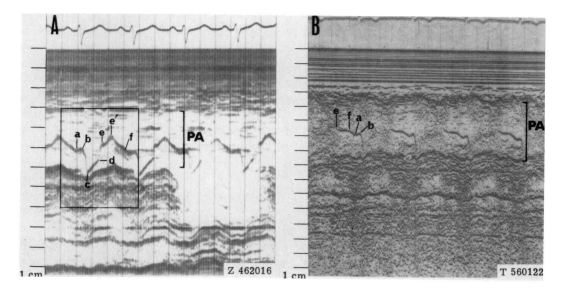

Fig. 2–35.   Labeling of the pulmonary valve echocardiogram. A shows a fairly complete M-mode recording of a posterior pulmonary valve leaflet. Usually only diastolic and early systolic motion can be detected, B. (From Weyman, A.E., Dillon, J.C., Feigenbaum, H., and Chang, S.: Echocardiographic patterns of pulmonic valve motion with pulmonary hypertension. Circulation, 50:905, 1974.)

or cross-sections and not silhouettes. Although some two-dimensional images resemble some angiocardiographic recordings, many views are available in two-dimensional echocardiography that are unavailable in angiography.

One can obtain an infinite number of slices through the heart using the two-dimensional echocardiographic technique.[43] The large number of such examinations has greatly increased the complexity of this technique. There is considerable confusion in the literature concerning terminology and orientation of the views that have been used by several investigators.[43,44] Attempts will be made to clarify the two-dimensional echocardiographic examination by first discussing this technique from a historic viewpoint and then by offering one possible approach to the many examinations described in the literature.

The initial efforts at using two-dimensional echocardiography were performed with the transducer placed along the left sternal border, as noted in Figure 2–2. With the transducer in this location, the plane through which the ultrasonic beam sweeps is

aligned parallel to the long axis of the heart or roughly to the long axis of the left ventricle (Fig. 2–36). With the transducer in this position, the heart is transected in a plane similar to the diagram depicted in Figure 2–37. This diagram is identical to that shown in Figure 2–14 when the M-mode examination was described. The principal difference is that now the ultrasonic beam is sweeping rapidly through the heart rather than remaining stationary or moving slowly as in Figure 2–14. The resultant recording from such an ultrasonic cross-sectional examination is a true anatomic slice through the heart in a plane parallel to the long axis of the heart. Figure 2–38 shows an actual two-dimensional recording obtained in this plane and an artist's sketch of an anatomic specimen sectioned in

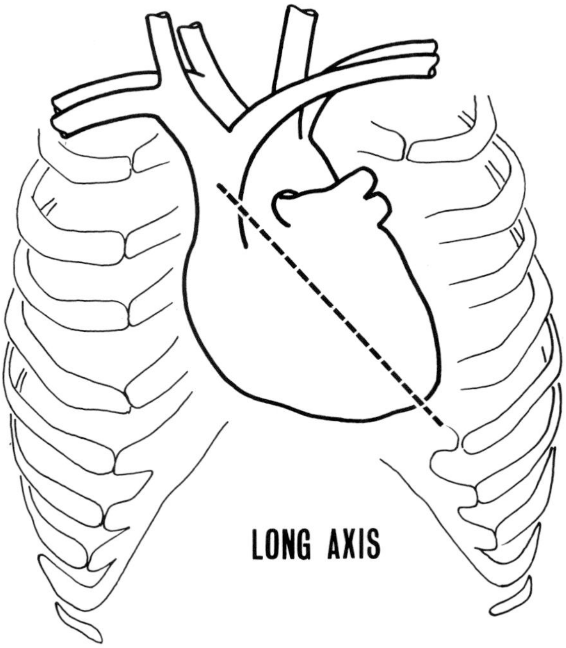

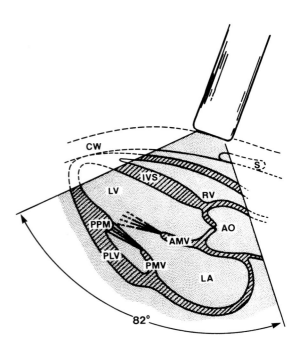

Fig. 2–37. Diagram of the heart similar to that shown in Figure 2–14 demonstrating how a two-dimensional sector scan can examine the heart parallel to the long axis. CW = chest wall; S = sternum; RV = right ventricle; AO = aorta; LA = left atrium; PMV = posterior mitral valve; AMV = anterior mitral valve; PLV = posterior left ventricular wall; PPM = posterior papillary muscle; LV = left ventricle; IVS = interventricular septum. (From Feigenbaum, H.: Echocardiography. In Heart Disease. Edited by E. Braunwald. Philadelphia, W.B. Saunders Co., 1980.)

LONG AXIS

Fig. 2–36.   Illustration of the long axis of the heart.

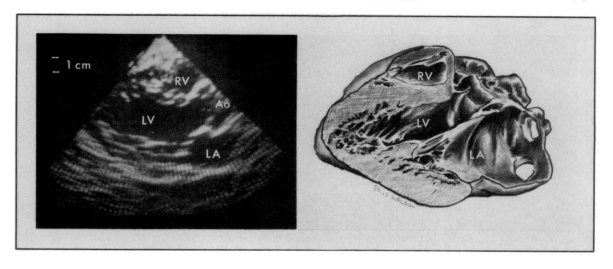

Fig. 2–38. Two-dimensional long-axis echocardiogram and a drawing of the corresponding anatomic specimen with the heart sliced through its long axis. RV = right ventricle; LV = left ventricle; AO = aorta; LA = left atrium. (From Rogers, E.W., Feigenbaum, H., and Weyman, A.E.: Echocardiography for quantitation of cardiac chambers. *In* Progress in Cardiology. Vol. 8. Edited by P.N. Yu and J.F. Goodwin. Philadelphia, Lea & Febiger, 1979.)

this manner. Such an examination provides a recording of much of the left ventricle, left atrium, root of the aorta, and a small portion of the right ventricular outflow tract.

It became readily apparent that one could turn the transducer so that the plane of the

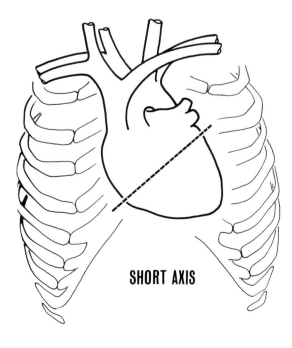

Fig. 2–39. Illustration of the short axis of the heart.

examination was perpendicular to the cardiac long axis. One would thus obtain a slice through the heart parallel to the short axis of the heart or the left ventricle (Fig. 2–39). Figure 2–40 shows some of the resultant cross-sectional pictures that are roughly parallel to the short axis of the left ventricle. Slicing the heart in this manner produced circular images of the left ventricle. An almost perfect circle or doughnut was obtained when slicing the left ventricle near the apex (Fig. 2–40–1). Directing the ultrasonic beam toward the base of the heart produces a slice at the level of the papillary muscles (Fig. 2–40–2). Tilting the transducer yet further to the base of the heart produces a two-dimensional slice of the left ventricle at the level of the mitral valve (Fig. 2–40–3). Figure 2–41 shows a two-dimensional echocardiogram parallel to the short axis of the left ventricle at the level of the papillary muscles, together with a drawing of the anatomic specimen. The left ventricular cavity is basically circular with indentations made by the papillary muscles. This section corresponds to Figure 2–40–2. Slicing the left ventricle in a short-axis plane at the level of the mitral valve produces a picture such as that seen within a circular left ventricle. Figure 2–42 corresponds to Figure 2–40–3.

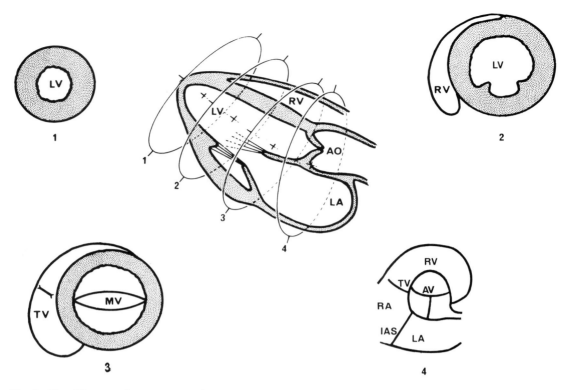

Fig. 2–40. Diagram demonstrating the various short-axis slices one can obtain through the heart. Short-axis echocardiogram 1 is at the level of the cardiac apex, echocardiogram 2 at the level of the papillary muscles, echocardiogram 3 at the mitral valve level, and echocardiogram 4 is through the base of the heart and the aorta. LV = left ventricle; RV = right ventricle; AO = aorta; LA = left atrium; MV = mitral valve; TV = tricuspid valve; RA = right atrium; IAS = interatrial septum; AV = anterior mitral valve. (From Feigenbaum, H.: Echocardiography. In Heart Disease. Edited by E. Braunwald. Philadelphia, W.B. Saunders Co., 1980.)

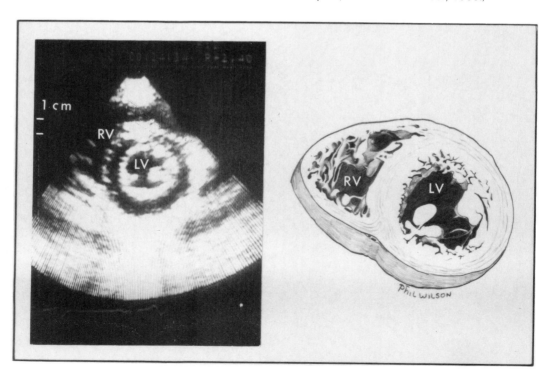

Fig. 2–41. Two-dimensional short-axis echocardiogram and corresponding anatomic specimen of the right ventricle (RV) and left ventricle (LV) at the level of the papillary muscles. (From Rogers, E.W., Feigenbaum, H., and Weyman, A.E.: Echocardiography for quantitation of cardiac chambers. In Progress in Cardiology. Vol. 8. Edited by P.N. Yu and J.F. Goodwin. Philadelphia, Lea & Febiger, 1979.)

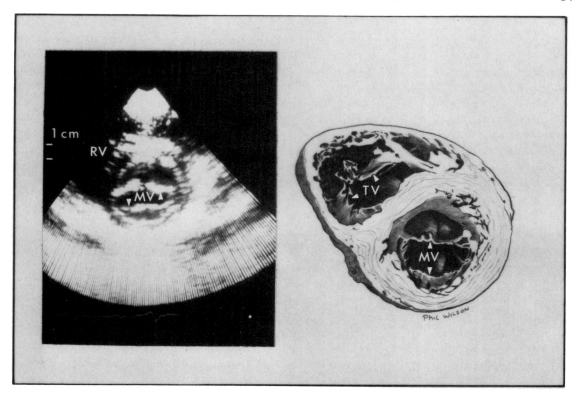

Fig. 2–42. Short-axis echocardiogram at the level of the mitral valve *(left)*. Diagram of the anatomic specimen *(right)*. MV = mitral valve; RV = right ventricle; TV = tricuspid valve. (From Rogers, E.W., Feigenbaum, H., and Weyman, A.E.: Echocardiography for quantitation of cardiac chambers. *In* Progress in Cardiology. Vol. 8. Edited by P.N. Yu and J.F. Goodwin. Philadelphia, Lea & Febiger, 1979.)

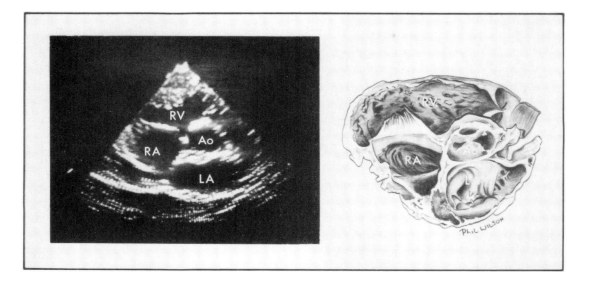

Fig. 2–43. Two-dimensional short-axis echocardiogram and drawing of the anatomic specimen at the base of the heart. RV = right ventricle; RA = right atrium; AO = aorta; LA = left atrium. (From Rogers, E.W., Feigenbaum, H., and Weyman, A.E.: Echocardiography for quantitation of cardiac chambers. *In* Progress in Cardiology. Vol. 8. Edited by P.N. Yu and J.F. Goodwin. Philadelphia, Lea & Febiger, 1979.)

Figure 2–43 shows the two-dimensional echocardiogram and anatomic drawing when the heart is sliced in a short-axis plane through the root of the aorta. Note the relatively circular aorta (AO) bounded on three sides by the right ventricle (RV), right atrium (RA), and left atrium (LA). Figure 2–43 corresponds to Figure 2–40–4.

The next development that dramatically changed the two-dimensional echocardiographic examination was the demonstration that the transducer could be placed at the cardiac apex, as noted in Figure 2–4, and the heart could be sectioned so that all four cardiac chambers were recorded. Figure 2–44 illustrates the anatomic specimen and a resulting two-dimensional echocardiogram when the heart is sliced in this plane. Needless to say, the four-chamber view or plane has become one of the basic examinations in two-dimensional echocardiography.

Shortly after the introduction of the four-chamber view of the heart, numerous other two-dimensional views were introduced into the literature. The American Society of Echocardiography has attempted to standardize and somewhat simplify the many two-dimensional examinations described.[3a] The Society felt that all views could be categorized into three orthogonal planes, as illustrated in Figure 2–45. These planes are the long-axis, short-axis, and four-chamber sections.

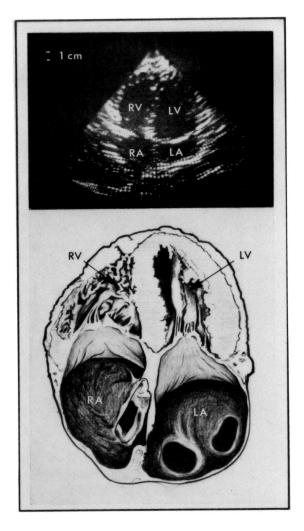

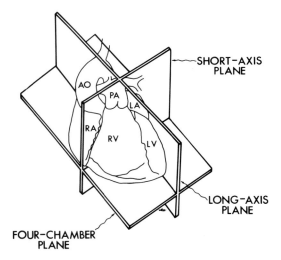

TWO–DIMENSIONAL ECHOCARDIOGRAPHIC IMAGING PLANES

Fig. 2–44. Two-dimensional echocardiogram and anatomic specimen of an apical four-chamber examination of the heart. RV = right ventricle; LV = left ventricle; RA = right atrium; LA = left atrium. (From Rogers, E.W., Feigenbaum, H., and Weyman, A.E.: Echocardiography for quantitation of cardiac chambers. *In* Progress in Cardiology. Vol. 8. Edited by P.N. Yu and J.F. Goodwin. Philadelphia, Lea & Febiger, 1979.)

Fig. 2–45. Diagram demonstrating the three orthogonal planes for two-dimensional echocardiographic imaging. AO = aorta; PA = pulmonary artery; LA = left atrium; RA = right atrium; RV = right ventricle; LV = left ventricle. (From Henry, W.L., et al.: Report of the American Society of Echocardiography Committee on Nomenclature and Standards in Two-dimensional Echocardiography. Circulation, in press.)

The long-axis plane is the imaging plane that transects the heart perpendicular to the dorsal and ventral surfaces of the body and parallel to the long axis of the heart. The plane transecting the heart perpendicular to the dorsal and ventral surfaces of the body, but perpendicular to the long axis of the heart, is defined as the short-axis plane. The plane that transects the heart approximately parallel to the dorsal and ventral surfaces of the body is referred to as the four-chamber plane.

These planes can be obtained from more than one transducer location. The long- and short-axis examinations with the transducer placed along the left sternal border have been discussed. Figure 2–46 shows how one could move the transducer toward the apex and examine the long axis from the apical approach. Theoretically, one might even be able to place the transducer in the suprasternal notch and obtain a long-axis study. (In actuality, the suprasternal examination can

rarely provide this type of information.) The short-axis and four-chamber planes can also be obtained with a subcostal transducer location. Thus the Society recommends that the two-dimensional examination be categorized according to three basic orthogonal planes and that the location of the transducer be identified.

The American Society of Echocardiography's approach to standardizing the two-dimensional echocardiogram is certainly a rational and useful step to correct some of the communication problems in the literature. The following discussion concerning the two-dimensional echocardiographic examination makes every attempt to stay within their suggested guidelines. However, as the Society recognizes, modifications must be introduced since the three orthogonal planes can vary according to the structure being examined. They recommend that any examination within 45° of a basic plane be identified with that plane. For example, an

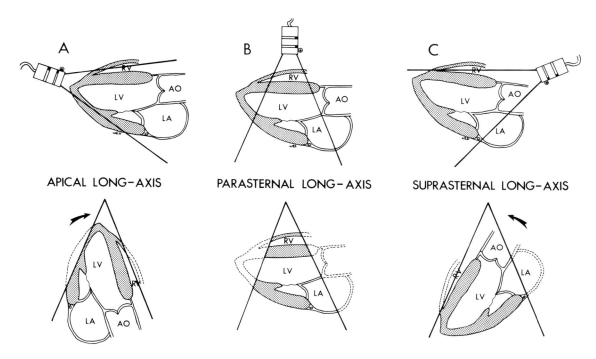

Fig. 2–46. Diagrams indicating how one can obtain a long-axis examination of the heart from the following transducer positions: *A*, apical, *B*, parasternal, and *C*, suprasternal. The suprasternal long-axis examination is more theoretical than actual since such an examination is difficult to obtain in most patients. RV = right ventricle; LV = left ventricle; LA = left atrium; AO = aorta. (From Henry, W.L., et al.: Report of the American Society of Echocardiography Committee on Nomenclature and Standards in Two-dimensional Echocardiography. Circulation, in press.)

examination that deviated 10° to 15° from the standard long axis would still be considered a long-axis examination of the heart. Thus there are multiple views within each examining plane. The modifications in angulation depend on the exact cardiac structure being examined.

Table 2–1 lists the various two-dimensional echocardiographic examinations categorized according to the location of the transducer, the plane of the examination, and the cardiac structure being examined. The parasternal transducer location is basically used for long- and short-axis examinations. Figure 2–47 shows the approximate transducer location for long- and short-axis studies of the root of the aorta. As with the

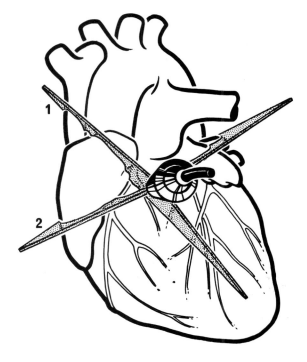

Fig. 2–47. Diagram demonstrating long-axis, *1*, and short-axis, *2*, sector scans of the root of the aorta. Note approximate transducer location.

Table 2–1. Two-dimensional Echocardiographic Examination

I. Parasternal approach
   A. Long-axis plane
      1. Root of aorta—aortic valve, left atrium, left ventricular outflow tract
      2. Body of left ventricle—mitral valve
      3. Left ventricular apex
      4. Right ventricular inflow tract—tricuspid valve
   B. Short-axis plane
      1. Root of the aorta—aortic valve, pulmonary valve, tricuspid valve, right ventricular outflow tract, left atrium, pulmonary artery, coronary arteries
      2. Left ventricle—mitral valve
      3. Left ventricle—papillary muscles
      4. Left ventricle—apex
II. Apical approach
   A. Four-chamber plane
      1. Four chamber
      2. Four chamber with aorta
   B. Long-axis plane
      1. Two chamber—left ventricle, left atrium
      2. Two chamber with aorta
III. Subcostal approach
   A. Four-chamber plane—all four chambers and both septa
   B. Short-axis plane
      1. Left ventricle
      2. Right ventricle
      3. Inferior vena cava
IV. Suprasternal approach
   A. Four-chamber plane
      1. Arch of aorta—descending aorta
   B. Long-axis plane
      1. Arch of aorta—pulmonary artery, left atrium

M-mode examination, the transducer is tilted slightly medially. The long-axis examination (Fig. 2–47, plane 1), provides a long-axis view of the aorta, aortic valve, left atrium, and left ventricular outflow tract (Fig. 2–48). Although the mitral valve may be seen in this examination, this valve is best examined in a slightly different plane. The aortic valve can be seen opening as two parallel echoes running near the walls of the aorta in systole (Fig. 2–48A). The leaflets close in diastole and one sees a dominant echo where the commissures meet. There may also be faint echoes from the body of the leaflets. These echoes are usually recorded only when the valve is thickened or when the patient is unusually easy to examine.

The short-axis view through the aorta and base of the heart (Fig. 2–47, plane 2), is approximately 90° to the long-axis aortic examination. This examination is comparable to that depicted in Figures 2–40 and 2–43. Figure 2–49 illustrates another echocardiogram comparable to that seen in Figure 2–43 and demonstrates the many cardiac

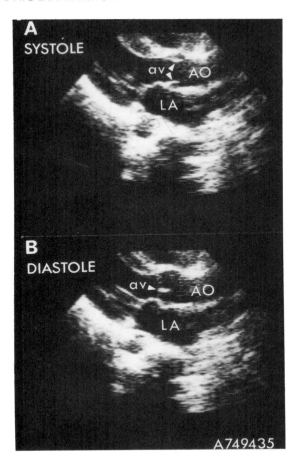

Fig. 2–48. Systolic, *A*, and diastolic, *B*, parasternal long-axis echocardiograms through the aorta (AO), aortic valve (av), and left atrium (LA).

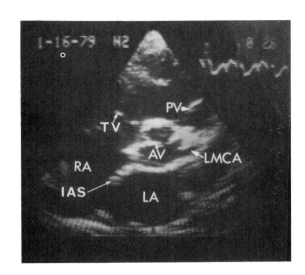

Fig. 2–49. Two-dimensional short-axis echocardiogram of the base of the heart demonstrating the aortic valve (AV) within the aorta, the pulmonary valve (PV), the tricuspid valve (TV), the right atrium (RA), the interatrial septum (IAS), the left atrium (LA), and the left main coronary artery (LMCA).

structures that can be seen with this two-dimensional short-axis view. Besides the aorta, left atrium, right atrium, and right ventricle, noted in Figure 2–43, Figure 2–49 also demonstrates the aortic valve (AV), pulmonary valve (PV), tricuspid valve (TV), interatrial septum (IAS), and left main coronary artery (LMCA).

Figure 2–50 is a short-axis examination of the aorta in a patient with well-defined aortic leaflets. The right (r), left (l), and noncoronary (n) cusps of the aortic leaflets in this patient can be readily identified in both diastole and systole.

Figure 2–51 demonstrates that with a slight change in angulation of the transducer, it is also possible to record the length of the

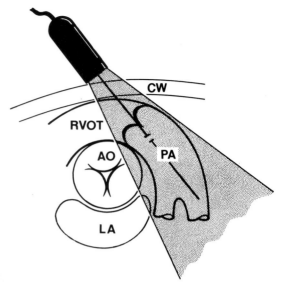

Fig. 2–51. Diagram demonstrating how the pulmonary artery (PA) can be visualized with a parasternal short-axis examination. CW = chest wall; RVOT = right ventricular outflow tract; AO = aorta; LA = left atrium.

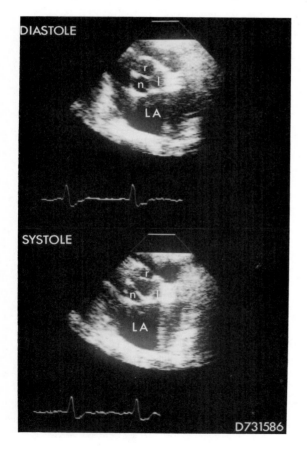

Fig. 2–50. Diastolic and systolic short-axis echocardiograms of the aortic valve showing right coronary (r), left coronary (l), and noncoronary (n) aortic valve leaflets. The patient had a low cardiac output; thus the aortic valve orifice is not circular in systole. LA = left atrium.

pulmonary artery to the point of its bifurcation. Figure 2–52 shows a diastolic and systolic short-axis examination through the base of the heart. During diastole (Fig. 2–52A), the pulmonary valve (PV) and proximal portion of the pulmonary artery (PA) is seen. With ventricular systole, the heart moves into a position that reveals the echo-free space from the pulmonary artery and its two major branches (Fig. 2–52B). These echocardiograms provide a good view of how the pulmonary artery curves around the aorta and bifurcates posteriorly.

The parasternal long-axis view of the body of the left ventricle is in a slightly different plane than that of the left ventricular outflow tract and aorta. The body of the left ventricle is best recorded using the transducer position shown in Figure 2–53, plane 1. The transducer is almost perpendicular to the surface of the chest and is at the same location as that used for the M-mode examination of the mitral valve. The resultant two-dimensional echocardiogram is comparable to that seen in Figure 2–38. This is the best view for recording the long axis of the mitral valve. Figure 2–54 shows three frames from

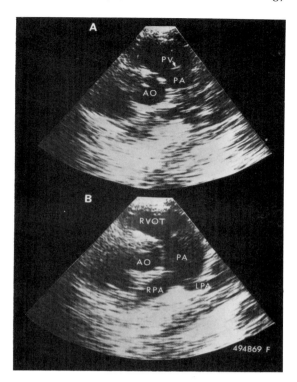

Fig. 2–52. Diastolic (A) and systolic (B) short-axis echocardiograms at the levels of the aorta and pulmonary artery. With systole, the pulmonary artery can be visualized and its two major branches seen. PV = pulmonary valve; PA = pulmonary artery; AO = aorta; RPA = right pulmonary artery; LPA = left pulmonary artery; RVOT = right ventricular outflow tract.

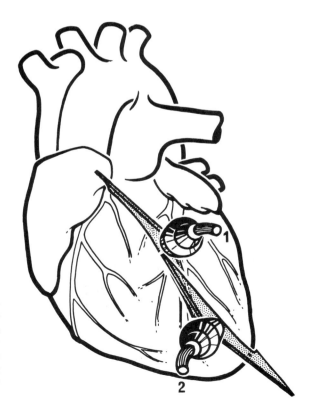

Fig. 2–53. Diagram demonstrating the transducer position and the direction of the ultrasonic beam for parasternal long-axis examinations of the left ventricle and mitral valve. Both the transducer location and the direction of the beam for examining the mitral valve and body of the left ventricle (position 1) are different than those for the apical portion of the left ventricle (position 2).

a two-dimensional study of the mitral valve with the valve in early diastole (Fig. 2–54A), mid-diastole (Fig. 2–54B), and systole (Fig. 2–54C). It is important to note that one rarely records the left ventricular apex with the transducer in this plane. Figure 2–55 shows a long-axis parasternal view through the body of the left ventricle and the mitral valve showing an "apparent apex." This rounded

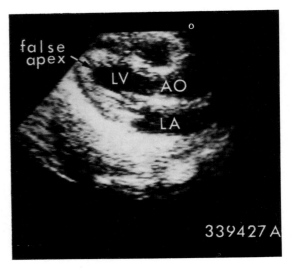

Fig. 2–55. Long-axis parasternal examination of the left ventricle showing a "false apex." The apparent apex probably originates from the medial wall of the left ventricle. LV = left ventricle; AO = aorta; LA = left atrium.

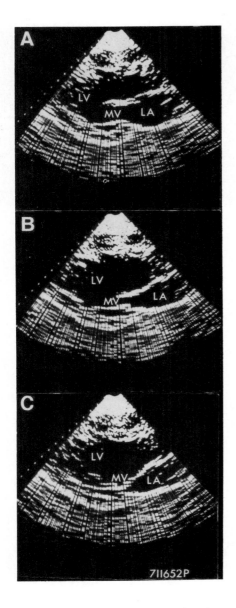

Fig. 2–54. Long-axis, parasternal echocardiograms of the mitral valve (MV), left ventricle (LV), and left atrium (LA) in early diastole, A, mid-diastole, B, and systole, C.

apical segment of the body of the left ventricle is probably a truncated view created by the ultrasonic beam transecting the medial wall of the left ventricle. To truly record the left ventricular apex, the transducer should be moved to a lower interspace and directed somewhat laterally (Fig. 2–53, plane 2). Figure 2–56 shows two long-axis parasternal views of the left ventricle. Figure 2–56A records the body of the left ventricle from a slightly lower position than that seen in Figure 2–54. The apex is recorded in Figure 2–56B by directing the transducer laterally as well as by moving it to a slightly lower interspace.[45,46] The fact that the left ventricular outflow tract, body, and apex are in slightly different echocardiographic planes is in keeping with what we have learned from the M-mode examination (see Fig. 2–17).

Figure 2–57 shows three transducer positions for short-axis examinations of the left ventricle. The interspace is the same for planes 1 and 2. One merely changes the angle of the transducer. Examining plane 3 requires moving the transducer to a lower interspace. Figure 2–58 shows the resultant short-axis left ventricular echocardiograms.

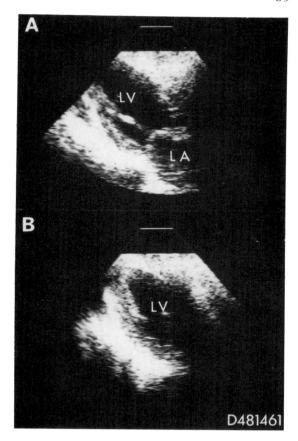

Fig. 2–56. Long-axis parasternal echocardiograms of the left ventricle through the body of the chamber, A, and over the left ventricular apex, B. LV = left ventricle; LA = left atrium.

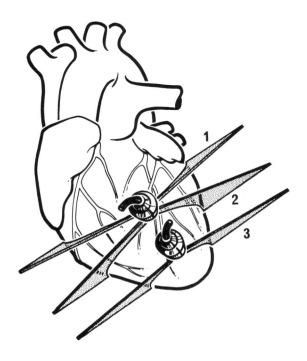

Fig. 2–57. Transducer positions for short-axis examinations of the left ventricle. Plane 1 passes through the mitral valve, plane 2 through the papillary muscles, and plane 3 through the left ventricular apex.

The first short-axis view (Fig. 2–58A) is at the level of the mitral valve and is produced by examining plane 1 in Figure 2–57. The mitral valve is visible within the circular left ventricular cavity. Transducer position 2 in Figure 2–57 produces an echocardiogram similar to that in Figure 2–58B at the level of the papillary muscles. The echoes from the papillary muscles can be seen indenting the cavity of the left ventricle. The short-axis examination resulting from examining plane 3 in Figure 2–57 is at the level of the cardiac apex and produces an echocardiogram similar to Figure 2–58C. Neither the mitral valve nor the papillary muscles are visible.

The short-axis left ventricular examination provides an opportunity for a short-axis study of the mitral valve. Figure 2–59A shows the mitral valve in its open position. Figure 2–59B illustrates a partially closed mitral

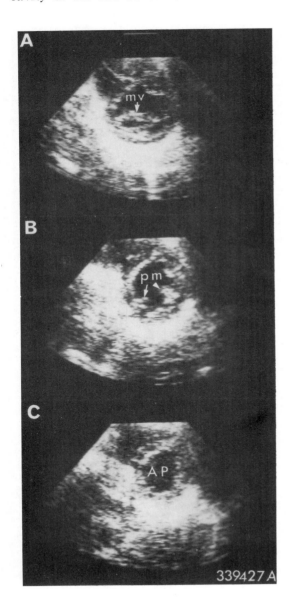

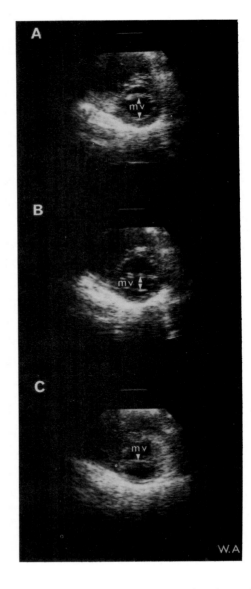

Fig. 2–58. Short-axis parasternal echocardio-grams at *A*, the mitral valve (mv), *B*, the papillary muscles (pm), and *C*, the left ventricular apex (AP).

Fig. 2–59. Short-axis parasternal echocardio-grams of the mitral valve (mv) in early diastole, *A*, mid-diastole, *B*, and systole, *C*.

valve, and a completely closed mitral valve is shown in Figure 2–59C. It should be remembered that the mitral valve and the mitral annulus are constantly moving in a superior-inferior direction so that recording the mitral valve throughout the cardiac cycle in one short-axis plane is not always easy. To best see the valve in diastole may require one plane, whereas mitral valve closure may be best recorded in a slightly different plane. The mitral valve and annulus move toward the apex with systole and in the reverse direction in diastole.

The right ventricle and tricuspid valve can also be recorded with the transducer in the parasternal position (Fig. 2–60). The plane of the examination does not exactly fit either the long or short axis. However, the plane is closer to that of the long axis rather than the short axis, and thus is categorized as a long-axis study. Figure 2–61 shows the right ventricular inflow tract and right atrium, by way of such a parasternal examination. This examination provides an opportunity to record the motion of the tricuspid valve. Figure 2–62 shows diastolic and systolic frames of the tricuspid valve in the long axis.

Figure 2–63 diagrammatically illustrates the two commonly used two-dimensional echocardiographic views with the transducer placed at the cardiac apex. Examination plane 1 demonstrates the apical four-chamber view of the heart. Figure 2–64A shows an example of a four-chamber apical echocardiogram. This view is similar to that in Figure 2–44. With slight angulation of the transducer, one can record the root of the aorta with the apical four-chamber view. Figure 2–65A demonstrates a four-chamber apical examination. By tilting the transducer slightly anteriorly, one can record the aorta (Fig. 2–65B).

It is possible to obtain an apical view of the long axis of the heart similar to that seen from the parasternal view. Such an examination would include portions of the right ventricle and the aorta. A more common examination is the so-called apical two-chamber view (Fig. 2–63, plane 2). This examination requires slight clockwise rotation of the trans-

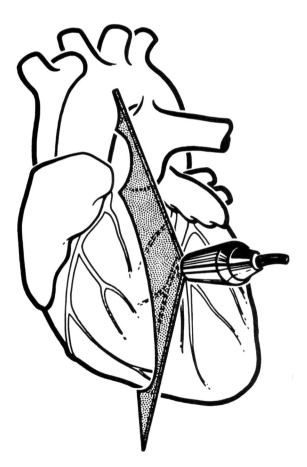

Fig. 2–60. Transducer position for a long-axis parasternal examination of the tricuspid valve, right atrium, and right ventricular inflow tract.

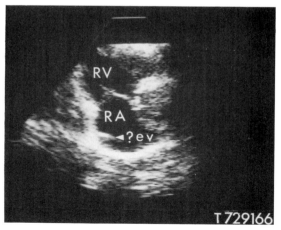

Fig. 2–61. Two-dimensional echocardiogram of the right atrium (RA) and right ventricular inflow tract (RV). EV = eustachian valve.

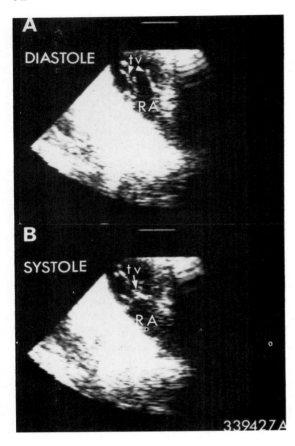

Fig. 2–62.   Diastolic, A, and systolic, B, long-axis echocardiograms of the tricuspid valve (TV). RA = right atrium.

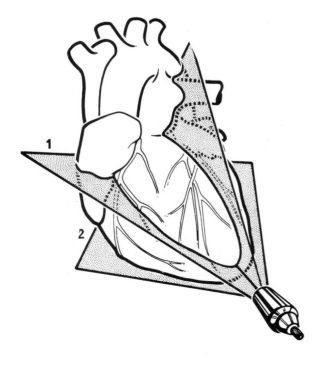

Fig. 2–63.   Transducer position and examining planes for apical, two-dimensional echocardiograms. Plane 1 passes through the four-chamber plane of the heart. Plane 2 represents the path of the ultrasonic beam for the two-chamber apical examination.

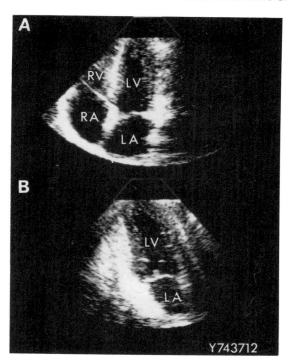

Fig. 2–64. Four-chamber, *A*, and two-chamber, *B*, apical two-dimensional echocardiograms. RV = right ventricle; LV = left ventricle; RA = right atrium; LA = left atrium.

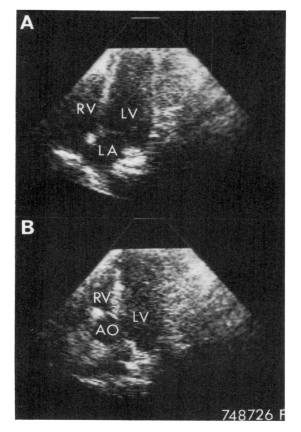

Fig. 2–65. Echocardiograms demonstrating how a small change in the angulation of the transducer can modify a four-chamber apical view, *A*, so that the aorta can be recorded from this position, *B*. RV = right ventricle; LV = left ventricle; LA = left atrium; AO = aorta.

ducer to completely avoid the right ventricle. Thus one only records the left ventricle and the left atrium (Fig. 2–64B). This view can be considered a slight modification of an apical long-axis view.

There is a slight difference between the apical two-chamber view and the parasternal long-axis view of the apex. Figure 2–66 attempts to demonstrate the subtle but at times real differences between these two examinations. The transducer position for the examination in Figure 2–66a is directly above the cardiac apex, and one sees the left ventricular apex and the entire posterior left ventricular wall. Much of the anterior wall of the left ventricle is not recorded. The apical two-chamber view is noted in Figure 2–66B. The transducer is now slightly below the apex and the beam is directed upward toward the heart. One now sees the entire posterior and anterior walls of the left ventricle as well as much of the left atrium. Since these two views are critical in examining the left

ventricle, a more detailed comparison of the two studies is given in the next chapter.

The subcostal transducer location produces examinations roughly in the four-chamber and short-axis planes. The ultrasonic plane indicated in Figure 2–67A is similar to examining plane 1 in Figure 2–63. The resultant subcostal four-chamber echocardiogram appears in Figure 2–68A. Figure 2–67B shows how the transducer can be rotated 90° to provide a subcostal short-axis examination of the heart.[44] Figure 2–68C demonstrates an approximate short-axis study through the left ventricle. The left ventricle is almost but not quite circular in this examination. The subcostal four-chamber view is particularly helpful in examining the interatrial and interventricular septum (Fig. 2–68B).[11,12] By directing the transducer in a slightly modified short-axis examination (Fig. 2–69A), one can obtain an excellent view of the right side of the heart (Fig. 2–70).[47] This study may be particularly help-

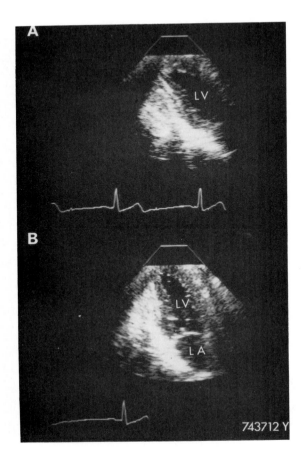

Fig. 2–66. Two-dimensional echocardiogram demonstrating the subtle difference between the long-axis parasternal study of the left ventricular apex, A, and an apical two-chamber echocardiogram, B. LV = left ventricle; LA = left atrium.

A   **B**

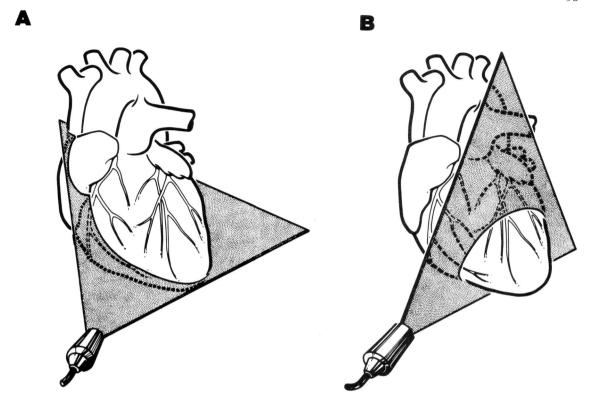

Fig. 2–67. Diagrams showing the transducer position and examining planes for a subcostal four-chamber examination, *A*, and a subcostal short-axis examination, *B*.

ful when looking at the right ventricular outflow tract in patients with congenital heart disease. The subcostal location also permits an opportunity to direct the ultrasonic beam through the inferior vena cava and hepatic vein (Fig. 2–69B). This examination is again a modified short-axis examination. Two-dimensional echocardiographic views of the inferior vena cava and hepatic veins are noted in Figure 2–71. One feature of this study is the collapse of the systemic veins with inspiration. Examination of the inferior vena cava can also be obtained with M-mode echocardiography.

The two examining planes with the transducer in the suprasternal notch are depicted in Figure 2–72. The ultrasonic view in Figure 2–72A is roughly equivalent to that of a four-chamber plane, and the view in Figure 2–72B is somewhat comparable to that of the long-axis plane. However, it is probably best to orient the ultrasonic beam with regard to

the arch of the aorta rather than to the heart since one does not record much of the heart with the transducer in this position, especially in the adult. In addition, the planes are different than with the transducer at the apex or subcostal region. Thus better terminology with regard to the examining planes from the suprasternal location would be *parallel* or *perpendicular* to the arch of the aorta. Figure 2–73 shows a suprasternal examination parallel to the arch of the aorta. Note the curved arch and descending aorta (DA)[14,15] as well as several branches of the aorta. One can frequently identify the innominate (I), the left carotid (LC), and the left subclavian (SC) arteries. A short-axis suprasternal examination of the arch of the aorta reveals a circular aorta, the pulmonary artery, and part of the left atrium (Fig. 2–74). Note also the bifurcation of the pulmonary artery.

There is a variety of less commonly used two-dimensional views of the heart. There

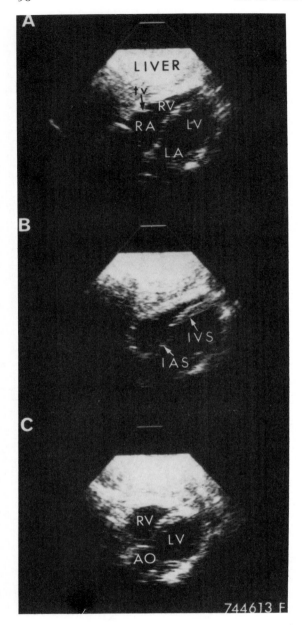

Fig. 2–68. Subcostal two-dimensional echocardiograms through the four-chamber plane, A, and
short-axis plane, C. With slight modification of the
four-chamber examination, the interventricular septum (IVS) and interatrial septum (IAS) can be well seen,
B. tv = tricuspid valve; RV = right ventricle;
RA = right atrium; LV = left ventricle; LA = left atrium; AO = aorta.

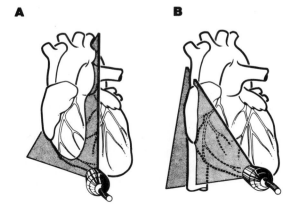

Fig. 2–69. Diagram demonstrating the examining
planes and transducer positions for the subcostal
examination of the right side of the heart, A, and the
inferior vena cava, B.

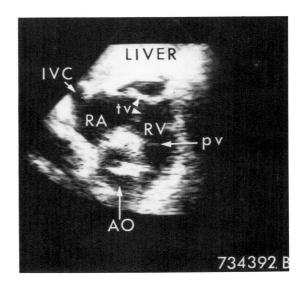

Fig. 2–70. Subcostal two-dimensional echocardiogram of the right side of the heart demonstrating the inferior vena cava (IVC), right atrium (RA), tricuspid valve (tv), right ventricle (RV), and pulmonary valve (pv). AO = aorta.

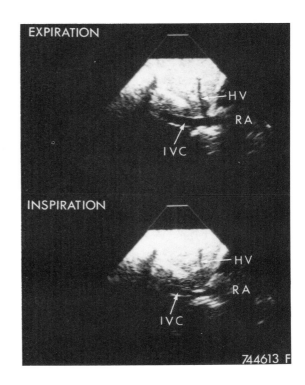

Fig. 2–71. Subcostal two-dimensional echocardiogram of the inferior vena cava (IVC) and hepatic veins (HV). The inferior vena cava decreases in size with inspiration. RA = right atrium.

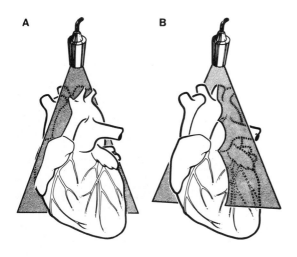

A   B

Fig. 2–72. Transducer position and examining plane for the suprasternal examination parallel to the arch of the aorta, *A*, and perpendicular to the arch of the aorta, *B*.

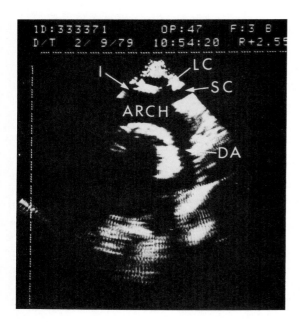

Fig. 2–73. Two-dimensional suprasternal echocardiogram parallel to the arch of the aorta. The innominate (I), left carotid (LC), and subclavian (SC) arteries can be seen originating from the aorta. DA = descending aorta.

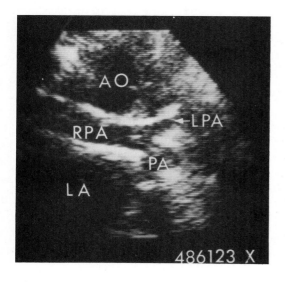

Fig. 2–74. Suprasternal echocardiogram perpendicular to the arch of the aorta demonstrating a circular aorta (AO) and a more horizontal right pulmonary artery (RPA). A somewhat distorted view of the main pulmonary artery (PA) and left pulmonary artery (LPA) are also visible. LA = left atrium.

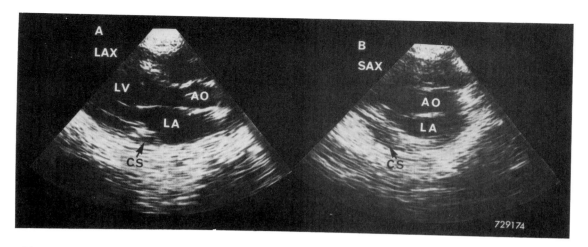

Fig. 2–75. Long-axis (LAX) and short-axis (SAX) parasternal two-dimensional echocardiograms demonstrating the coronary sinus (CS). LV = left ventricle; LA = left atrium; AO = aorta.

has been recent interest in examining the heart with the transducer placed along the right sternal border, which is called the right parasternal position. This view apparently offers an excellent opportunity for recording the interatrial septum.[21] The ultrasonic beam is almost perpendicular to the septum, thus allowing for good delineation of this structure.

Less frequently considered cardiac structures can also be seen in the various two-dimensional views already discussed. In the parasternal long-axis view of the left ventricle, it is possible to record an echo-free space in the coronary sinus (Fig. 2–75A). This structure is seen at the junction of the left ventricle and left atrium. It is important to note that this echo-free space moves along with the atrioventricular groove. The curved nature of the coronary sinus can be appreciated with a short-axis examination (Fig. 2–75B). Another echo-free space posterior to the heart originates from the descending aorta. Figure 2–76 illustrates the descending aorta as seen in a parasternal long-axis study. If one rotates the transducer so that the examining plane is parallel to the descending aorta, then two long parallel echoes can be recorded (Fig. 2–76B). Although the plane of the descending aorta closely approximates a true sagittal plane of the body, it would be considered part of a long-axis examination, according to the American Society of Echocardiography's recommendations.

Some investigators have described an echo originating from a prominent eusta-

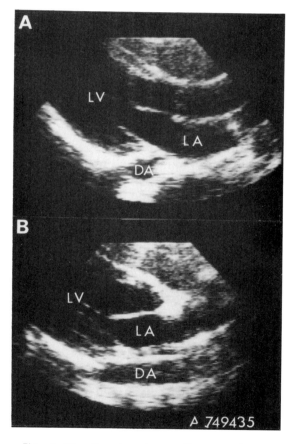

Fig. 2–76. Parasternal two-dimensional echocardiograms of the descending aorta. In the usual long-axis view of the left ventricle and left atrium, A, the descending aorta appears as a circular, echo-free space posterior to the left ventricular and left atrial walls. With a slight change in the angle of the beam rendering the examining plane parallel to the descending aorta, B, the length of the descending aorta can be recorded. LV = left ventricle; LA = left atrium; DA = descending aorta.

chian valve at the junction of the inferior vena cava and the right atrium.[48] Figure 2–61 demonstrates this structure in a parasternal long-axis view. The eustachian valve has also been noted in apical and subcostal four-chamber examinations. Since there has been little confirmation regarding the identity of the eustachian valve echo, it is indicated by a question mark in Figure 2–61.

The echocardiographic literature uses numerous terms for the same two-dimensional views. Long-axis examinations are also called "sagittal" or "longitudinal;" short-axis parasternal examinations are "horizontal," "transverse," or "cross-sectional;" and the apical four-chamber view is "frontal." To minimize confusion, these terms will not be used in this text in favor of following as closely as possible the terminology of the American Society of Echocardiography.

Orientation of Two-dimensional Images

The orientation of two-dimensional echocardiographic images may vary with different investigators. The first real-time, two-dimensional echocardiographic instrument was the multi-scan linear electronic scanner developed by a group in the Netherlands. Because of differences in instrumentation, the cardiac image was oriented so that the long-axis study was viewed as though the patient were standing (Fig. 2–77).[49,50] The base of the heart was at the top and the apex at the bottom. This orientation may have been partially prompted by the desire to make the echocardiogram similar to corresponding angiograms. Unfortunately, the short-axis examination is confusing with this approach. Since the transducer is always depicted on the left, the short-axis study is now viewed as though the patient were on his side, with the right side of the heart at the top and the left side at the bottom (Fig. 2–78). Although some early sector scanners also oriented their images in this way,[51,52] most echocardiographers placed the transducer at the top. Thus the studies were displayed as though the patient were supine and not standing upright, or lying on his side.

A few echocardiographers orient the parasternal long-axis views with the aorta on the left (Fig. 2–79B), as opposed to the usual

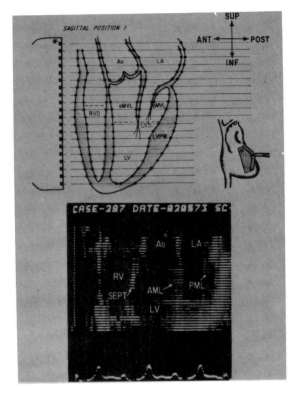

Fig. 2–77. Diagram and two-dimensional echocardiogram showing the parasternal long-axis orientation used with the multiscan echocardiograph. The heart is visualized as though the patient were in an upright position. AO = aorta; LA = left atrium; RV = right ventricle; SEPT = septum; AML = anterior mitral leaflet; PML = posterior mitral leaflet; LV = left ventricle. (From Sahn, D.J., et al.: Multiple crystal cross-sectional echocardiography in the diagnosis of cyanotic congenital heart disease. Circulation, 50:230, 1974.)

orientation (Fig. 2–79A). A more common left-right variation is to switch the left and right orientation of the apical four-chamber view (Fig. 2–80A and B).[43] Yet another variation is to invert the two-dimensional image, especially when using an apical or subcostal examination. Figure 2–80C shows an inverted four-chamber examination in which the position of the transducer is at the bottom of the illustration with the atria above the ventricles.

Because of the confusion in the literature, the American Society of Echocardiography has recommended the proper orientation of two-dimensional cardiac images. The Society suggests that all two-dimensional imag-

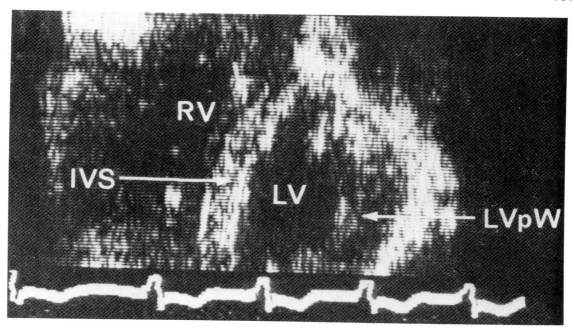

Fig. 2–78.   Short-axis orientation using the linear array multiscan system. Anterior position is on the left, and the right side of the patient is at the top. The echocardiogram is recorded as though the patient were lying on his left side. RV = right ventricle; LV = left ventricle; IVS = interventricular septum; LVpW = left ventricular posterior wall. (From Ligtvoet, C., et al.: A dynamically focused multiscan system. *In* Echocardiology. Edited by N. Bom. The Hague, Martinus Nijhoff, 1977.)

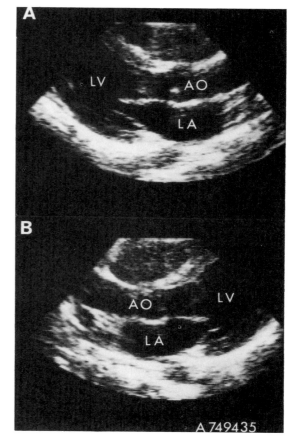

Fig. 2–79.   Parasternal long-axis examinations of the left ventricle (LV), aorta (AO), and left atrium (LA), using two different orientations. *A,* The cardiac apex is toward the left and the base of the heart toward the right. *B,* The reverse orientation.

ing transducers have an index mark that indicates the edge of the imaging plane, i.e., the direction in which the ultrasonic beam is angled (Fig. 2–81). The index mark should be located on the transducer to indicate the edge of the image to appear on the right side of the display. For example, in a parasternal long-axis examination the index mark should point in the direction of the aorta, making the aorta appear on the right side of the image

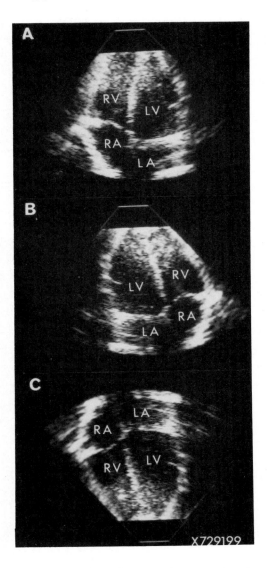

Fig. 2–80.   Echocardiograms demonstrating three orientations for apical four-chamber views. A, The four-chamber view used primarily in this text. B, Four-chamber view reversed. C, Inverted image of A. RA = right atrium; RV = right ventricle; LA = left atrium; LV = left ventricle.

display. In addition, the index mark should point either in the direction of the patient's head or to his left side. With this recommended transducer orientation, the long-axis parasternal view shows the aorta on the right, the short-axis parasternal view shows the left ventricle on the right, the apical four-chamber view shows the left ventricle on the right, and the subcostal four-chamber view shows the two ventricles on the right. The Society is leaving inversion of the image as a possible option (Fig. 2–80C). All of the two-dimensional examinations, excluding Figures 2–77, 2–78, 2–79B and 2–80B are in keeping with the recommended orientations of the Society. These standards are followed throughout this book.

CONTRAST ECHOCARDIOGRAPHY

The initial observation that the injection of indocyanine green dye though a cardiac catheter produces a cloud of echoes on the echocardiogram has proved to be a major development in the field.[53] The original use of this technique was to identify and verify the various cardiac structures being recorded echocardiographically.[53,54] More recently this technique has been used for diagnostic purposes.[55-62] It has been established that one need not use indocyanine green dye. The rapid injection through a catheter or needle of almost any liquid or gas produces a cloud of echoes. One may use saline solution, dextrose in water, the patient's own blood, or carbon dioxide gas for such injections.[63] Indocyanine green dye probably works somewhat better than the other substances because the surface tension permits the formation of smaller bubbles that stay in suspension for longer periods of time.[64] Carbon dioxide gives striking contrast effects but is more difficult and possibly more hazardous to use. Some investigations have used a variety of other substances to create microbubbles that can be injected and that produce a contrast effect.[64,65] One of the more promising substances is gelatin-coated microbubbles that are uniform in diameter, more reproducibly produce the contrast effect, and may possibly be made small enough to pass through the lungs.[65] Normally all echo-producing microbubbles are filtered by

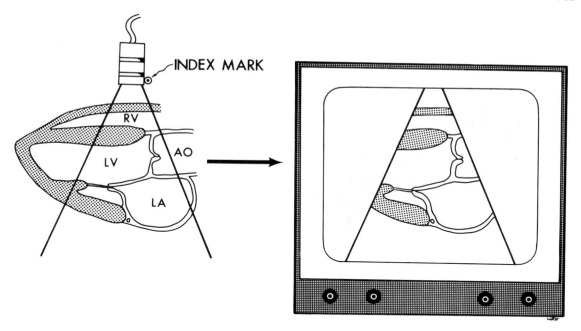

TRANSDUCER ORIENTATION   IMAGE DISPLAY

Fig. 2–81.   Illustration of the relation between transducer orientation (indicated by the direction of the index mark) and that of the resulting image on display. RV = right ventricle; LV = left ventricle; AO = aorta; LA = left atrium. (From Henry, W.L., et al.: Report of the American Society of Echocardiography Committee on Nomenclature and Standards in Two-dimensional Echocardiography. Circulation, in press.)

the pulmonary capillaries; however, injections made through an inflated balloon catheter in the "wedge" position produce contrast echoes on the left side of the heart.[63] Further experience is necessary to determine what risk, if any, is associated with this technique.

A technical detail that may aid in obtaining a good contrast effect from a peripheral venous injection is to have the patient pump the hand in which the injection is made during the injection. The muscular motion will aid the venous return. This maneuver may increase the concentration of contrast echoes recorded. Elevating the extremity may accomplish the same effect.

Figure 2–21 demonstrates the utility of intracardiac indocyanine green dye injections to help identify the origin of echoes. Similar intracardiac injections may also be used for diagnostic purposes similar to cineangiography.[57] Valvular regurgitation and intracardiac shunts can be detected with

this technique. The advantage is that angiographic dye or roentgenograms are not necessary. The disadvantage is that the examination is no longer noninvasive. Peripheral venous injections of indocyanine green dye or contrast can be made.[60] Figure 2–82 shows a peripheral venous injection in a normal individual. As the bolus of echo-producing bubbles reaches the right side of the heart, it is visible within the right ventricular outflow tract as a mass or cloud of echoes (arrow). One important feature of contrast echocardiography is that the tiny bubbles are too large to pass through a capillary bed. As a result, no contrast echoes are seen on the left side of the heart. If there is a right-to-left shunt whereby the blood can reach the left side of the heart without passing through a capillary bed, then one sees contrast echoes on the left side of the heart (Figure 2–83, arrow). As is readily apparent, this technique is extremely useful and sensitive for detecting right-to-left shunts.[60,66] This topic is dis-

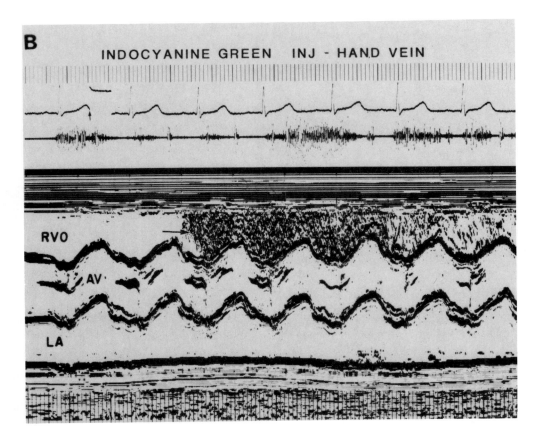

Fig. 2–82. A peripheral vein indocyanine green dye injection demonstrating the production of contrast echoes *(arrow)* in a patient with no evidence of an intracardiac shunt. The echoes appear in the right ventricular outflow tract (RVO) and not on the left side of the heart. AV = aortic valve; LA = left atrium. (From Seward, J.B., et al.: Peripheral venous contrast echocardiography. Am. J. Cardiol., 39:202, 1977.)

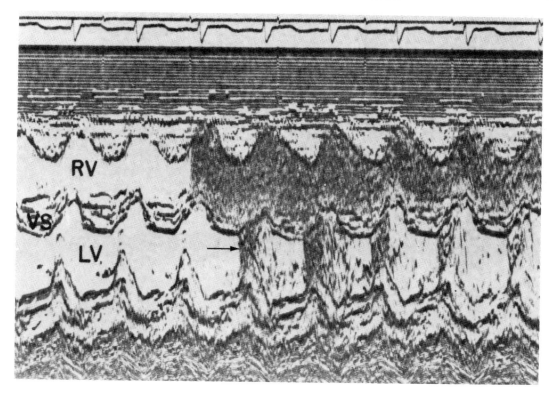

Fig. 2–83. Peripheral vein contrast echocardiographic study of a patient with a right-to-left shunt at the ventricular level. Contrast echoes are seen in the left ventricle (arrow) above the mitral valve. RV = right ventricle; VS = ventricular septum; LV = left ventricle. (From Seward, J.B., et al.: Echocardiographic contrast studies: initial experience. Mayo Clin. Proc., 50:163, 1975.)

cussed further in the chapter on congenital heart disease.

As with every aspect of echocardiography, potential artifacts must be appreciated when using contrast echocardiography. The echoes produced by the contrast material may be very intense depending on the particular patient and on the gain settings on the echocardiograph. As with all strong echoes, reverberations can be produced from the contrast echoes (Fig. 2–84).[60] The reverberation echoes appear within the left side of the heart and produce an artifactual right-to-left shunt. The artifactual nature of the left-sided contrast echoes in Figure 2–84 can be recognized by the fact that these echoes (arrows) are visible throughout the recording, even in the left atrium, and that they occur simultaneously with the real contrast echoes in the right ventricular outflow tract. This potential problem can be prevented or corrected by decreasing the gain control on the echocardiograph.

Contrast studies also can be done with two-dimensional echocardiography. Figure 2–85 demonstrates a short-axis two-dimensional examination through the base of the heart. The right atrium is echo-free during the control study (Fig. 2–85A). Following the peripheral injection of contrast, the echoes can be seen filling the right side of the heart (Fig. 2–85B, arrows). The two-dimensional examination has the advantage of noting the direction in which the bubbles pass as well as their spatial orientation. Unfortunately, because the contrast does not remain within the heart for long, the event is fleeting and diligent frame-by-frame analysis of the two-dimensional examination may be needed. M-mode contrast echocardiography, on the other hand, is much easier to analyze.

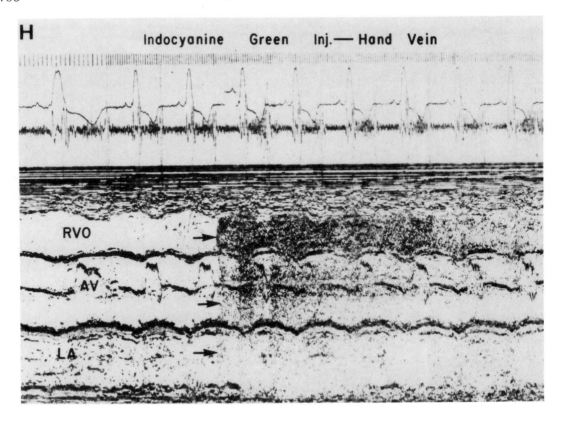

Fig. 2–84. Contrast echocardiogram demonstrating the artifacts that can occur with reverberations of the contrast echoes. The true contrast echoes are seen only in the right ventricular outflow tract *(arrow)*. The echoes seen within the aorta and left atrium *(arrows)* are artifacts due to reverberations from the contrast material in the right ventricle. RVO = right ventricular outflow tract; AV = aortic valve; LA = left atrium. (From Seward, J.B., et al.: Peripheral venous contrast echocardiography. Am. J. Cardiol., *39*:202, 1977.)

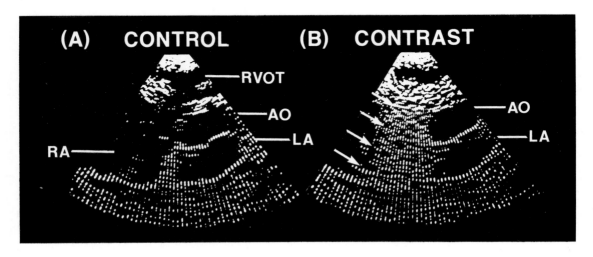

Fig. 2–85. Two-dimensional short-axis echocardiogram through the base of the heart before, *A*, and after, *B*, injection of indocyanine green dye in a peripheral vein. The contrast-producing echoes (arrows) are visible within the right atrium. RVOT = right ventricular outflow tract; AO = aorta; LA = left atrium; RA = right atrium. (From Weyman, A.E., et al.: Negative contrast echocardiography: a new method for detecting left-to-right shunt. Circulation, *59*:498, 1979.)

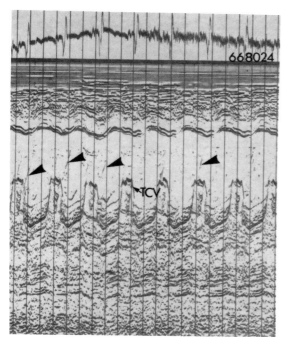

Fig. 2–86. Faint, mobile intracardiac echoes *(arrows)* passing through the right ventricle above the tricuspid valve (TCV) in a patient with chronic obstructive lung disease and heart failure.

Occasionally, one sees patients who spontaneously produce echoes similar to those produced by contrast echocardiography. Some of these echoes are actual contrast echoes since the patients may have an intravenous infusion at the time of the examination. However, Figure 2–86 shows a patient who has faint, mobile echoes (arrowheads) within the right side of the heart with no obvious cause. The patient merely had chronic obstructive lung disease and heart failure, and no adequate explanation for the origin of these echoes was ever determined. Similar echoes have been occasionally seen originating from prosthetic valves (see Chapter 6).

ECHOCARDIOGRAPHIC EXAMINATION WITH INTERVENTIONS

A variety of interventions to be used with the echocardiographic examination have been described. These include Valsalva maneuver[67-69] and isometric exercise.[70-74]

Studies have also been described that use infusions of water and salt overloading.[75] Various pharmacologic manipulations have been proposed.[76] Some of these studies attempt to manipulate afterload or preload with tourniquets and leg raising.[77] An intriguing noninvasive technique has been proposed for inducing premature ventricular systoles.[78,79] This maneuver involves an instrument that produces a mechanical thump above the cardiac apex, usually producing a timed ventricular systole. When done in conjunction with an echocardiogram, it is possible to note the post-extrasystolic effect on the echocardiogram.

The intervention that has recently generated much interest has been isotonic exercise.[71,74,79a,80-86] Because of the great interest in coronary artery disease and the necessity of bringing out the underlying pathology with stress-induced ischemia, several papers have described various ways of recording echocardiograms during exercise. The technical difficulties involved in performing echocardiograms during exercise are obvious. Any attempt at obtaining an echocardiogram during upright treadmill exercise would be fraught with extreme difficulty.[79a,85] Because the body moves up and down, such an echocardiographic examination is extremely impractical. Most techniques require some immobilization of the chest. Merely performing supine exercise is helpful in reducing the amount of chest motion during exercise.

Several investigators have noted that it is possible to obtain echocardiograms during supine exercise.[71,74,82,86] Most of these studies use a bicycle ergometer. Both M-mode and cross-sectional examinations have been performed during supine exercise. Figure 2–87 illustrates an M-mode examination of the left ventricle before and during supine bicycle exercise. The technical difficulties associated with the exercise tracing are readily apparent. However, it is possible to obtain some useful information, especially during expiration. Another exercise approach has the patient sit up on a stationary table and lean forward on his elbows to stabilize the chest.[71,85]

One benefit of the exercise echocardio-

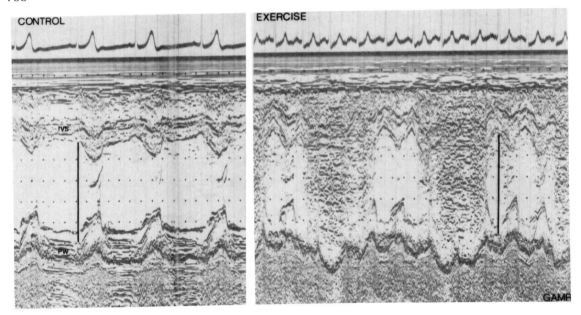

Fig. 2–87. Left ventricular M-mode echocardiogram before *(control)* and during *(exercise)* supine leg exercise. Despite marked interference from respiration, one can obtain left ventricular measurements during exercise. (From Corya, B.C. and Rasmussen, S.: Clinical usefulness of intervention echocardiography in evaluating regional and global left ventricular function. Cardiovascular Medicine [in press].)

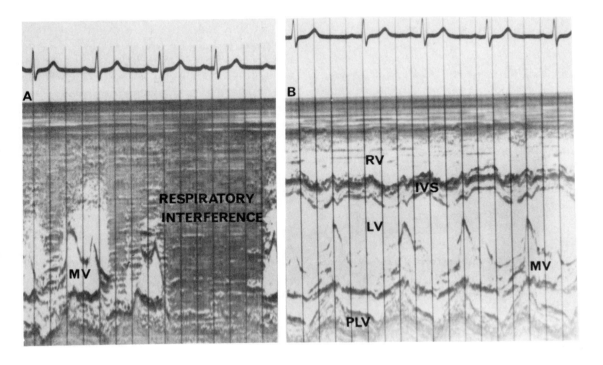

Fig. 2–88. M-mode echocardiogram showing interference that can occur with respiration, A. This interference can be avoided by moving the transducer to another interspace, B. MV = mitral valve; RV = right ventricle; IVS = interventricular septum; LV = left ventricle; PLV = posterior left ventricular wall. (From Chang, S.: M-mode Echocardiographic Techniques and Pattern Recognition. Philadelphia, Lea & Febiger, 1976.)

graphic studies is the examination of cardiac physiology under stress.[71,80,81,87-90] The possibility of obtaining satisfactory echocardiographic recordings on certain individuals is sufficiently great to permit such physiologic investigations. Unfortunately, the percentage of technically satisfactory recordings is still not high enough to warrant routine exercise examinations for diagnostic purposes. There will probably be at least 30 percent of the patients in whom satisfactory recordings cannot be obtained.[82] Some recent developments may reduce this percentage of unsatisfactory recordings. The use of the apical window for two-dimensional studies makes the incidence of satisfactory recordings higher.[82] In addition, two-dimensional echocardiography, because of the wider scan, is technically easier than the M-mode approach. Although further work in this area is necessary, the possibility of using echocardiography during various interventions, including exercise, seems real.

TECHNICAL DIFFICULTIES ASSOCIATED WITH THE ECHOCARDIOGRAPHIC EXAMINATION

One may face numerous technical problems when attempting an echocardiographic examination. Fortunately, solutions have been developed for many of these problems. For example, the subcostal examination has been an important development in examining patients with barrel chests and/or emphysema. The apical examination, especially when using two-dimensional echocardiography, has provided information on patients who were otherwise technically unsatisfactory. The use of a lower-frequency transducer with a larger diameter occasionally helps in the difficult, thick-walled individual. As noted in Figure 2–23, turning the patient on his side assists in recording the desired echoes. In addition to placing the patient in the left lateral position, the right lateral decubitus position is occasionally advantageous for recording certain echoes. For example, in patients who have large right ventricles, it is sometimes difficult to record adequate echoes from the relatively small left ventricle. Having the patient lie on the right side frequently brings out the left ven-

tricle so that it can be more easily recorded echocardiographically. Some difficult mitral valve echoes may be recorded if the patient is gradually raised to the sitting position, either by adding pillows or by raising the head of the bed.

Compensations may be necessary for some patients with peculiar body configurations. Tall, thin patients with vertical hearts have interventricular septa that lie in a plane almost parallel to the ultrasonic beam. These patients may need to be turned in an extremely lateral position. In addition, the plane of the transducer is almost vertical when scanning from aorta to apex. Obese patients, on the other hand, usually have horizontally positioned hearts. As a result, the transducer must be tilted medially to find the aorta and more laterally to record the posterior left ventricular wall. A scan from the base to the apex of the heart is almost horizontal. These variations in body type are even more important in two-dimensional echocardiography. A long-axis scan of a patient with a horizontal heart is definitely different from that of a patient with a vertical heart.

The lung is frequently a problem in obtaining satisfactory echocardiograms. Figure 2–88 shows a typical example of respiratory interference. When attempting to record a mitral valve echo, the tracing is obscured by frequent bands of echoes coming from respiratory interference. Figure 2–89 demonstrates the same problem with the two-dimensional echocardiogram. In Figure 2–89A, the lateral half of the left ventricle is obscured by echoes originating from lung tissue. One answer to this technical problem is to move the transducer to a lower interspace so that the lung does not overlie the heart, resulting in satisfactory tracings as exhibited in Figures 2–88B and 2–89B.

Great strides have been made in overcoming many technical problems involving the echocardiographic examination. However, our constant attempts to obtain more information from echocardiographic examinations only add to the complexity of the examination and introduce even more technical difficulties. Unfortunately, there still remain patients in whom satisfactory echocardio-

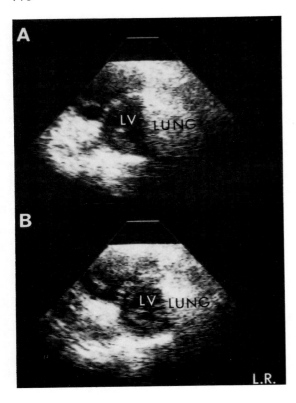

Fig. 2–89. *A*, Two-dimensional short axis echo-cardiogram showing the interference produced by lung tissue. *B*, This interference can be partially reduced by moving the transducer to a lower interspace. LV = left ventricle.

grams cannot be obtained, a phenomenon that represents one of the significant limitations of echocardiography.

PRINCIPLES OF ECHOCARDIOGRAPHIC MEASUREMENTS

Since the velocity of sound in human soft tissue is known, it is possible to calibrate echocardiographs so that quantitative measurements are possible. These measurements provide a quantitative aspect to echocardiography. Many of the measurements that have been introduced into the echocardiographic literature are discussed in detail in later chapters of this book. Normal values for some of the commonly used echocardiographic measurements are listed in the appendix. Although these measurements are popular, it is important to understand some basic principles behind making echocardiographic measurements.

One may make measurements on echocardiograms in a variety of ways. With respect to the A-mode or M-mode presentations, one should have an understanding of the concepts of "leading edges" and "trailing edges" of individual echoes. Each echo has a finite width. That edge of the echo closest to the transducer is the leading edge; the edge away from the transducer is the trailing edge (Fig. 2–90). When attempting to measure the distance between two objects, one can measure the distance between the trailing edge (TE) of the initial echo to the leading edge (LE) of the more distant echo. Such a measurement (TE-LE) is attractive since it corresponds visually to the space between the two objects. A large percentage of the echocardiographic measurements are made in this fashion. One of the problems with making measurements in this way is that the width of the individual echoes may vary from one instrument to another or may vary with the gain setting of the echocardiograph. If the instrument displays wide echoes, then the distance between the trailing edge of the first echo and the leading edge of the second echo (TE-LE) is less (Fig. 2–90B) than with an echocardiograph that displays thin echoes (Fig. 2–90A). With a system that records thick echoes, increasing the gain may aggravate the situation and make the TE-LE measurement even less (Fig. 2–90D). In those instruments that display thick echoes, the extra width displaces the trailing edge but not the leading edge. Thus the location of the leading edge is essentially identical, whether an instrument uses a thin or thick display. Therefore, measurements from leading edge to leading edge (LE-LE) are theoretically more accurate than those using the trailing edge of any echo. For this reason, the American Society of Echocardiography has recommended leading edge-to-leading edge M-mode measurements.[90a]

Despite this recommendation and the fact that leading edge measurements are theoretically more accurate, measurements between the trailing edge and leading edge continue to be used because of convenience and the fact that most echocardiographers use instruments that display thin echoes that are not gain dependent in the axial dimen-

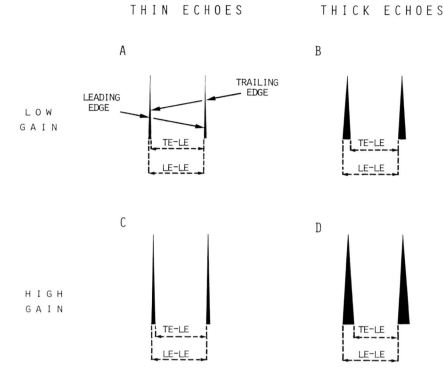

Fig. 2–90. Diagram demonstrating how echocardiographic measurements can differ whether one uses leading edge (LE) or trailing edge (TE) measurements. Echocardiographic measurements are commonly from leading edge to leading edge (LE–LE) or from trailing edge to leading edge (TE–LE). If the echocardiographic system has thin echoes (A and C), the gain makes little difference in either measurement. However, if the echocardiograph displays relatively thick echoes (B and D), then the trailing edge-to-leading edge measurement is significantly reduced with an increase in gain, D. The leading edge-to-leading edge measurement is uninfluenced by gain.

sion. One problem with the leading edge-to-leading edge standard is that finding the leading edge of the proximal echo, especially when buried among multiple echoes, is not easy. When using an echocardiograph that displays thin echoes, the width of the echo is not more than a millimeter. Thus the difference between trailing edge-to-leading edge measurements and leading edge-to-leading edge measurements is no more than a millimeter or two. In adults, such a difference is of questionable significance,[90b] whereas in children in whom the measurements are small, this difference may represent a significant percentage.

With two-dimensional echocardiography, echocardiographers measure the echo-free space between echoes, thus making measurements between trailing edge and lead-

ing edge as well as from the right lateral border to the left lateral border of an echo (Fig. 2–91). Since leading edge-to-leading edge measurements are meaningless with lateral and medial echoes, the M-mode ASE criteria have not been adopted for two-dimensional echocardiography. Any two-dimensional measurement that involves measuring area or lateral dimensions is clearly gain dependent because lateral resolution is gain dependent on all instruments. One way of overcoming this problem is to use the minimum gain setting necessary to display all required echoes. The better focused the beam, the less of a problem one has. The error may not be significant in judging a large chamber. A millimeter or two of difference may not represent a significant problem; however, when measuring a small

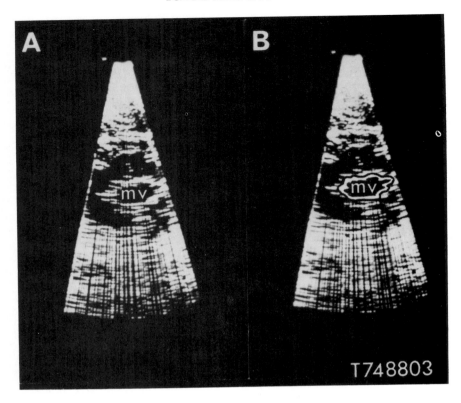

Fig. 2–91.   Two-dimensional echocardiograms demonstrating how area measurements can be obtained from two-dimensional examinations. As noted in *B*, the measurements are usually obtained from the trailing edge of the anterior echoes, the leading edge of the posterior echoes, and the inner aspects of the lateral and medial echoes. MV = mitral valve.

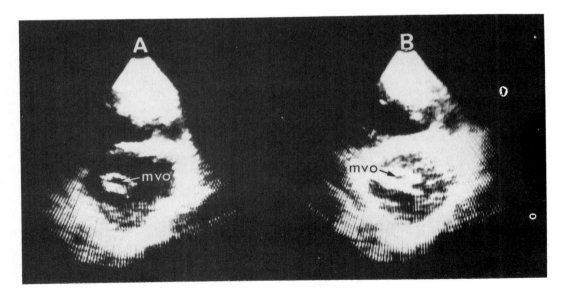

Fig. 2–92.   Echocardiograms demonstrating how the mitral valve orifice (mvo) can be significantly influenced by gain. The orifice is virtually eliminated with a high gain setting, *B*.

object, such as a mitral valve orifice (Fig. 2–92), an increase of a millimeter or two is significant. A basic rule is that since axial resolution is inherently better than lateral resolution, axial measurements are more accurate than lateral measurements.

From a technical point of view it is easier to make measurements on the M-mode echocardiogram than on the two-dimensional study. The convenience of displaying the recording on a strip-chart recorder is a great advantage of the M-mode technique. Other advantages are that most measurements can be made with simple calipers and calibration marks, the recording can be analyzed by merely unfolding the tracing, and a tracing that may have taken five minutes to record can be scanned, going back and forth at will, in one tenth of the time. One does not have this convenience when analyzing two-dimensional echocardiograms. First, if one has five minutes of recording on the videotape, it takes a minimum of five minutes to review the examination in real time. Any slow motion or frame-by-frame analysis only lengthens the analysis. Fortunately new videotape recorders are reducing this problem significantly. These recorders will permit analysis of the recording at twice normal speed. In addition video-disc attachments greatly facilitate slow motion and frame-by-frame analysis. The use of light pens and electronic calipers considerably aid in making measurements on two-dimensional recordings. Despite these technical advances it remains to be seen whether the quantitative analysis of two-dimensional echocardiography will approach the ease with which M-mode echocardiographic measurements can be made.

Another problem with analyzing two-dimensional echocardiograms is that there is significant dropout of echo information on any given frame.[91] Figure 2–93 shows diastolic and systolic short-axis views of the left ventricle. One can easily identify and trace the endocardial border of the left ventricle in systole (Fig. 2–93B). However, there is so much echo dropout in diastole (Fig. 2–93A) that one must estimate the location of the endocardium, especially in the medial and lateral walls.

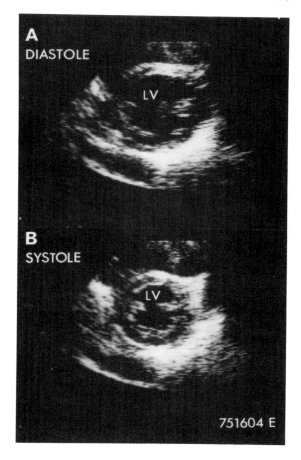

Fig. 2–93. Systolic and diastolic short-axis parasternal echocardiograms of the left ventricle at the level of the papillary muscles. A, In systole, one can identify the entire circumferences of the left ventricular walls and endocardium for possible measurement. B, In diastole, however, dropout of echoes is significant, especially in the medial and lateral walls, thus making measurement difficult.

Because the eye integrates a great deal of information in real time, it is highly unlikely to find one frame that looks as good as the image in real time. This problem is significant when trying to analyze information quantitatively or when trying to use a still picture to represent what is seen in real time. A partial solution to this problem may come with the advent of new videotape and videodisc recorders and electronic calipers so that the measurements can be made both on still frames and in real time.

To facilitate the analysis of two-dimensional tracings and to provide a hard copy recording, there have been efforts to put the frames on a strip-chart recorder. Thus far most instruments record one frame at a time, usually in real time. Unfortunately, it may take up to a minute for this recording to be put on the strip-chart recorder. Newer methods of analyzing the data using strip-chart recorders are undoubtedly forthcoming. It is hoped that less time will be required for the frames to be recorded on the strip chart and that multiple frames may be recorded both on-line and off-line. Many images are recorded according to electrocardiographic gating. One attractive feature is the use of a freeze frame whereby the frame is frozen until upgraded by the next frame at the same time in the cardiac cycle. One may even have multiple gates so that the frame changes more than once in the cycle. This strobe, freeze frame feature aids greatly in analyzing or recording structures which move rapidly or move in and out of the examining plane.

There is considerable interest in using computers to analyze the echocardiographic information. Thus far, most activity has concerned the analysis of the M-mode tracing. Current techniques use a sonic pen, light pen, bit pad or electronic calipers whereby one traces the portion of the echocardiogram desired in order to put information into the computer.[92,92a,93,93a] A popular technique is to trace the walls of the left ventricle and to have the computer analyze the dimensions and changes in dimensions. A similar approach can be used with any valvular or cardiac structure. Obviously, the data analyzed by the computer can be no better than the raw data entered. In addition, the human error involved in tracing influences the final results. One can anticipate an increased use of such computer analysis with two-dimensional echocardiographic data. It is hoped that it will be possible to have the computer identify and track the desired echoes to eliminate the necessity of manual tracing.[94,95]

The location of the transducer and the angle of the ultrasonic beam with respect to the heart can also influence echocardiographic measurements. Figures 2–25 and 2–26 demonstrate the distortion of the M-mode echocardiogram that can occur with varying the degree of the angle of the ultrasonic beam. For example, the distance between the left side of the interventricular septum (LS) and the posterior left ventricular endocardium (EN) is closer at the apex in Figure 2–25 than in Figure 2–26. The angle of the ultrasonic beam can also influence the amplitude inscribed by a moving echo. If the ultrasonic beam is parallel to the motion of a given echo, then the maximum amplitude is recorded (Fig. 2–94). However, if the ultrasonic beam is not parallel to the motion, then a lesser amplitude is inscribed on the M-mode echocardiographic tracing. The problems with angulation can usually be overcome by varying the location of the transducer on the chest. However, there are some patients in whom the echocardiographic window may be limited, so that multiple transducer positions may not be available. Fortunately, since the location of the ultrasonic beam is spatially registered with the two-dimensional examination, the limitations inherent in angulation are considerably less with this examination than with the M-mode technique. The spatial orientation of the two-dimensional probe is still not known, but this problem is far less serious than is the angulation of the beam in M-mode echocardiography.

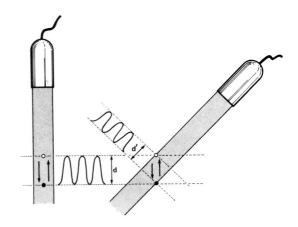

Fig. 2–94.   Diagram illustrating that the amplitude of motion of a moving echo depends on the angle of the ultrasonic beam with respect to that echo. The maximum amplitude of motion (d) is recorded when the beam is parallel to the direction of the moving echo. As the angle becomes less parallel, the amplitude of motion decreases (d').

Respiration is an important technical factor involved in recording echocardiograms. Not only does respiration completely wipe out a tracing at times (Fig. 2–87), but it alters the measurements because of possible displacement of the heart or because of actual changes in the hemodynamics incurred by respiration. One may also take advantage of the respiratory effect on the echocardiogram. Since an examination is frequently best obtained in expiration,[86] it may be advisable to have the patient stop breathing in expiration so that a satisfactory recording can be obtained. The reverse is true when using the subcostal approach. With inspiration the heart is brought closer to the transducer and frequently a better recording may result. Thus holding the breath with inspiration may occasionally improve the quality of the examination.

Other factors, such as position of the patient, age,[95a] training, and heart rate, may all influence echocardiographic measurements. These factors are discussed in more detail in later chapters. It is sufficient to say that one must be aware of the many factors and limitations that influence echocardiographic measurements.[96,97]

REFERENCES

1. Edler, I., Gustafson, A., Karlefors, T., and Christensson, B.: Ultrasound cardiography. Acta Med. Scand. (Suppl.), 370:68, 1961.
2. Reference deleted.
3. Solinger, R., Elbl, F., and Minhas, K.: Echocardiography in the normal neonate. Circulation, 47:108, 1973.
3a.Henry, W.L., et al.: Report of the American Society of Echocardiography Committee on Nomenclature and Standards in Two-dimensional Echocardiography. Circulation (in press).
4. Zaky, A., Grabhorn, L., and Feigenbaum, H.: Movement of the mitral ring: a study of ultrasound cardiography. Cardiovasc. Res., 1:121, 1967.
5. Silverman, N.H. and Schiller, N.B.: Apex echocardiography: a two-dimensional technique for evaluating congenital heart disease. Circulation, 57:503, 1978.
6. Chang, S. and Feigenbaum, H.: Subxiphoid echocardiography. J. Clin. Ultrasound, 1:14, 1973.
7. Chang, S., Feigenbaum, H., and Dillon, J.C.: Subxiphoid echocardiography: a review. Chest, 68:233, 1975.
8. Matsukubo, H., Furukawa, K., Watanabe, T., Asayama, J., Katsume, H., Kunishige, H., Endo, N., Matsuura, T., and Ijichi, H.: Echocardiographic measurement of right ventricular wall motion by subxiphoid echocardiography. J. Cardiogr., 6:15, 1976.
9. Matsukubo, H., Matsuura, T., Endo, N., Asayama, J., Watanabe, T., Furukawa, K., Kunishige, H., Katsume, H., and Ijichi, H.: Echocardiography measurement of right ventricular wall thickness. A new application of subxiphoid echocardiography. Circulation, 56:278, 1977.
10. Matsukubo, H., Furukawa, K., Watanabe, T., Asayama, J., Katsume, H., Kunishige, H., Endo, N., Matsuura, T., and Ijichi, H.: Echocardiographic measurement of right ventricular wall motion by subxiphoid echocardiography. J. Cardiogr., 6:15, 1976.
11. Lange, L.W., Sahn, D.J., Allen, H.D., and Goldberg, S.J.: Subxiphoid cross-sectional echocardiography in infants and children with congenital heart disease. Circulation, 59:513, 1979.
12. Bierman, F.Z. and Williams, R.G.: Subxiphoid two-dimensional imaging of the interatrial septum in infants and neonates with congenital heart disease. Circulation, 60:80, 1979.
13. Goldberg, B.B.: Suprasternal ultrasonography. J.A.M.A., 215:245, 1971.
14. Sahn, D.J., Goldberg, S.J., McDonald, G., and Allen, H.D.: Suprasternal notch real-time cross-sectional echocardiography for imaging the pulmonary artery, aortic arch, and descending aorta. Am. J. Cardiol., 39:266, 1977. (Abstract)
15. Seward, J.B. and Tajik, A.J.: Noninvasive visualization of the entire thoracic aorta: a new application of wide-angle two-dimensional sector echocardiographic technique. Am. J. Cardiol., 43:387, 1979. (Abstract)
16. Allen, H.D., Goldberg, S.J., Sahn, D.J., Ovitt, T.W., and Goldberg, B.B.: Suprasternal notch echocardiography: assessment of its clinical utility in pediatric cardiology. Circulation, 55:605, 1977.
17. Goldberg, S.J., Allen, H.D., and Sahn, D.J.: In Pediatric and Adolescent Echocardiography. Chicago, Year Book Medical Publishers, Inc., 1975.
18. Light, L.H.: Transcutaneous observation of blood velocity in the ascending aorta in man. Biol. Cardiol., 26:214, 1969.
19. Light, L.H., Gross, G., and Hansen, P.L.: Noninvasive measurement of blood velocity in the major thoracic vessels. Proc. R. Soc. Med., 67:142, 1974.
20. Gramiak, R. and Nanda, N.C.: Structure identification in echocardiography. In Cardiac Ultrasound. Edited by R. Gramiak and R. Waag. St. Louis, C.V. Mosby Co., 1975.
21. Tei, C., Tanaka, H., Kashima, T., Yoshimura, H., Minagoe, S., and Kanehisa, T.: Real-time cross-sectional echocardiographic evaluation of the interatrial septum by right atrium-interatrial septum-left atrium direction of ultrasound beam. Circulation, 60:539, 1979.
21a.Tei, C., Tanaka, H., Kashima, T., Nakao, S., Tahara, M., and Kanehisa, T.: Echocardiographic analysis of interatrial septal motion. Am. J. Cardiol., 44:472, 1979.
22. D'Cruz, I.A., Jain, D.P., Hirsch, L., Levinsky, R., Cohen, H.C., and Glick, G.: Echocardiographic diagnosis of dilatation of the ascending aorta using right parasternal scanning. Radiology, 129:465, 1978.
23. Parameswaran, R., Carr, V.F., Rao, A.V.R., and Goldberg, H.: The posterior thoracic approach in echocardiography. J. Clin. Ultrasound, 7:461, 1979.
24. Rothendler, J.A., King, D.L., and Green, W.M.:

Technique for dual transducer echocardiography. J. Clin. Ultrasound, 4:139, 1976.

25. Ito, M., Fujino, T., Kurata, E., Kanaya, S., Imanishi, S., Uasuda, H., Fujino, M., and Ueno, T.: Isometric contraction and relaxation times of the right ventricular overload measured by the bidirectional echocardiography. J. Cardiogr., 7:357, 1977.

26. Matsuzaki, M., Yorozu, T., Fukagawa, K., Anno, Y., Sasaki, T., Ishida, K., Kusukawa, R., Shimizu, M., Nomoto, R., Momona, E., Ikee, Y., and Tanikado, O.: Assessment of left ventricular wall motion: a new application of esophageal echocardiography. J. Cardiogr., 8:113, 1978.

27. Spotnitz, H.M., Maml, J.R., King, D.L., Pooley, R.W., Bowman, F.O., Jr., Bregman, D., Edie, R.N., Reemstsma, K., Korongrad, E., and Hoffman, B.F.: Outflow tract obstruction in tetralogy of Fallot. Intraoperative analysis by echocardiography. N.Y. State J. Med., 78:1100, 1978.

28. Hisanaga, K., Hisanaga, A., and Ichie, Y.: A new transesophageal real-time linear scanner and initial clinical results. Reflections, 4:203, 1978.

29. Frazin, L., Talano, J.V., Stephanides, L., Loeb, H.S., Kopel, L., and Gunnar, R.M.: Esophageal echocardiography. Circulation, 54:102, 1976.

30. Hisanaga, K., Hisanaga, A., and Ichie, Y.: A transesophageal ultrasound sector scanner for oblique scans. Circulation (Suppl. II), 60:245, 1979. (Abstract)

31. Kerber, R.E., Wilson, R.L., and Marcus, M.L.: An animal model for experimental echocardiographic studies. J. Clin. Ultrasound, 4:343, 1976.

32. Mary, D.A.S., Catchpole, L.A., and Ionescu, M.I.: Intraoperative echocardiographic studies of the mitral valve: assessment of commissurotomy and repair. J. Clin. Ultrasound, 4:349, 1976.

33. Gramiak, R. and Shah, P.M.: Echocardiography of the aortic root. Invest. Radiol., 3:356, 1968.

34. Hirata, T., Wolfe, S.B., Popp, R.L., Helmen, C.H., and Feigenbaum, H.: Estimation of left atrial size using ultrasound. Am. Heart J., 78:43, 1969.

35. Gramiak, R. and Shah, P.M.: Echocardiography of the normal and diseased aortic valve. Radiology, 96:1, 1970.

36. Winsberg, S. and Goldman, H.S.: Echo patterns of cardiac posterior wall. Invest. Radiol., 4:173, 1969.

37. Edler, I., Gustafson, A., Karlefors, T., and Christensson, B.: Ultrasound cardiography. Acta Med. Scand. (Suppl.), 370:68, 1961.

38. Gramiak, R., Nanda, N.C., and Shah, P.M.: Echocardiographic detection of pulmonary valve. Radiology, 102:153, 1972.

39. Weyman, A.E., Dillon, J.C., Feigenbaum, H., and Chang, S.: Echocardiographic patterns of pulmonic valve motion in pulmonic stenosis. Am. J. Cardiol., 34:644, 1974.

40. Chang, S., Feigenbaum, H., and Dillon, J.C.: Condensed M-mode echocardiographic scan of the symmetrical left ventricle. Chest, 68:93, 1975.

41. Popp, R.L., Filly, K., Brown, O.R., and Harrison, D.C.: Effect of transducer placement and echocardiographic measurement of left ventricular dimensions. Am. J. Cardiol., 35:537, 1975.

42. Gimenez, J.L., Winters, W.L., Jr., Davila, J.C., Connell, J., and Klein, K.S.: Dynamics of the Starr-Edwards ball valve prosthesis: a cinefluorographic and ultrasonic study in humans. Am. J. Med. Sci., 250:652, 1965.

43. Tajik, A.J., Seward, J.B., Hagler, D.J., Mair, D.D.,

and Lie, J.T.: Two-dimensional real-time ultrasonic imaging of the heart and great vessels: technique, image orientation, structure identification, and validation. Mayo Clin. Proc., 53:271, 1978.

44. Popp, R.L., Fowles, R., Coltart, J., and Martin, R.P.: Cardiac anatomy viewed systematically with two-dimensional echocardiography. Chest, 75:579, 1979.

45. Weyman, A.E., Peskoe, S.M., Williams, E.S., Dillon, J.C., and Feigenbaum, H.: Detection of left ventricular aneurysms by cross-sectional echocardiography. Circulation, 54:936, 1976.

46. Hickman, H.O., Weyman, A.E., Wann, L.S., Phillips, J.F., Dillon, J.C., Feigenbaum, H., and Marshall, J.: Cross-sectional echocardiography of the cardiac apex. Circulation (Suppl. III), 56:153, 1977. (Abstract)

47. Sahn, D.J., Sobol, R.G., and Allen, H.D.: Subxiphoid real-time cross-sectional echocardiography for imaging the right ventricle and right ventricular outflow tract. Am. J. Cardiol., 41:354, 1978. (Abstract)

48. Bommer, W.J., Kwan, O.L., Mason, D.T., DeMaria, A.N.: Indentification of prominent eustachian valves by M-mode and two-dimensional echocardiography: differentiation from right atrial masses. Am. J. Cardiol., 45:402, 1980. (Abstract)

49. Bom, N., Lancee, C.T., VanZwieten, G., Kloster, F.E., and Roelandt, J.: Multiscan echocardiography. I. Technical description. Circulation, 48:1066, 1973.

50. Bom, N., Hugenholtz, P.G., Kloster, F.E., Roelandt, J., Popp, R.L., Pridie, R.B., and Sahn, D.J.: Evaluation of structure recognition with the multiscan echocardiograph. A cooperative study in 580 patients. Ultrasound Med. Biol., 1:243, 1974.

51. Kisslo, J., VonRamm, O.T., and Thurstone, F.L.: Thaumascan: clinical cardiac imaging. J. Clin. Ultrasound, 2:237, 1974. (Abstract)

52. VonRamm, O.T. and Thurstone, F.L.: Cardiac imaging using a phased array ultrasound system. Circulation, 53:258, 1976.

53. Gramiak, R., Shah, P.M. and Kramer, D.H.: Ultrasound cardiography: contrast studies in anatomy and function. Radiology, 92:939, 1969.

54. Feigenbaum, H., Stone, J.M., Lee, D.A., Nasser, W.K., and Chang, S.: Identification of ultrasound echoes from the left ventricle using intracardiac injections of indocyanine green. Circulation, 41:615, 1970.

55. Duff, D.F. and Gutgesell, H.P.: The use of saline for ultrasonic detection of a right-to-left shunt in postoperative period. Am. J. Cardiol., 37:132, 1976. (Abstract)

56. Pieroni, D., Varghese, P.J., and Rowe, R.D.: Echocardiography to detect shunt and valvular incompetence in infants and children. Circulation (Suppl.), 48:81, 1973. (Abstract)

57. Seward, J.B., Tajik, A.J., Spangler, J.G., and Ritter, D.G.: Echocardiographic contrast studies: initial experience. Mayo Clin. Proc., 50:163, 1975.

58. Reference deleted.

59. Shub, C., Tajik, A.J., Seward, J.B., and Dines, D.E.: Detecting intrapulmonary right-to-left shunt with contrast echocardiography. Mayo Clin. Proc., 51:81, 1976.

60. Seward, J.B., Tajik, A.J., Hagler, D.J., and Ritter, D.G.: Peripheral venous contrast echocardiography. Am. J. Cardiol., 39:202, 1977.

61. Allen, H.D., Sahn, D.J., and Goldberg, S.J.: New serial contrast technique for assessment of left-to-right shunting patent ductus arteriosus in the neonate. Am. J. Cardiol., 41:288, 1978.

62. Weyman, A.E., Wann, L.S., Caldwell, R.L., Hurwitz, R.A., Dillon, J.C., and Feigenbaum, H.: Negative contrast echocardiography: a new method for detecting left-to-right shunts. Circulation, 59:498, 1979.

63. Reale, A.: Contrast echocardiography: transmission of echoes to the left heart across the pulmonary vascular bed. Am. J. Cardiol., 45:401, 1980. (Abstract)

64. Meltzer, R., Tickner, G., Sahines, T., and Popp, R.L.: The source of ultrasonic contrast effect. Circulation (Suppl. II), 60:795, 1979. (Abstract)

65. Bommer, W.J., Mason, D.T., and DeMaria, A.N.: Studies in contrast echocardiography: development of new agents with superior reproducibility and transmission through lungs. Circulation (Suppl. II), 60:17, 1979. (Abstract)

66. Valdes-Cruz, L.M., Pieroni, D.R., Roland, J-M.A., and Varghese, P.J.: Echocardiographic detection of intracardiac right-to-left shunts following peripheral vein injections. Circulation, 54:558, 1976.

67. Parisi, A.F., Harrington, B.S., Askenazi, J., Pratt, R.C., and McIntyre, K.M.: Echocardiographic evaluation of the Valsalva maneuver in healthy subjects and patients with and without heart failure. Circulation, 54:921, 1976.

68. Robertson, D., Stevens, R.M., Friesinger, G.C., and Oates, J.A.: The effect of the Valsalva maneuver on echocardiographic dimensions in man. Circulation, 55:596, 1977.

69. Yokoyama, H., Ishizawa, K., Okada, M., Matsumori, A., and Kawashita, K.: Alterations in left ventricular systolic time intervals induced by Valsalva maneuver: an echocardiographic-mechanocardiographic correlative study. J. Cardiogr., 7:49, 1977.

70. Laird, W.P., Fixler, D.E., and Huffines, F.D.: Cardiovascular response to isometric exercise in normal adolescents. Circulation, 59:651, 1979.

71. Crawford, M.H., White, D.H., and Amon, K.W.: Echocardiographic evaluation of left ventricular size and performance during handgrip and supine and upright bicycle exercise. Circulation, 59:1188, 1979.

72. Laird, W.P., Fixler, D.E., and Huffines, F.D.: Cardiovascular response to isometric exercise in normal adolescents. Circulation, 59:651, 1979.

73. DeMaria, A.N., Kwan, D.L., Bommer, W., Gandhi, H., and Mason, D.T.: Evaluation of left ventricular response to isometric exertion by two-dimensional echocardiography. Circulation (Suppl. II), 60:152, 1979. (Abstract)

74. Paulsen, W.J., Boughner, D.R., Friesen, A., and Persaud, J.A.: Ventricular response to isometric and isotonic exercise: echocardiographic assessment. Br. Heart J., 42:521, 1979.

75. Weyman, A.E., Luft, F.C., Bloch, R., Murray, R.H., Weinberger, M., and Marshall, J.: Echocardiographic assessment of left ventricular response to extremes of salt intake in normo-tensive man. Am. J. Cardiol., 41:403, 1978. (Abstract)

76. Gomes, J.A.C., Carambas, C.R., Moran, H.E., Dhatt, M.S., Calon, A.H., Caracta, A.R., and Damato, A.N.: The effect of isosorbide dinitrate on left ventricular size, wall stress and left ventricular function in chronic refractory heart failure. Am. J. Med., 65:794, 1978.

77. Masuya, K., Saga, T., Murakami, H., Matsui, S., Hara, S., Kin, T., Hiramaru, Y., Takegoshi, N., Murakami, E., and Maeda, M.: Echocardiographic measurement of change in preload after leg-raising and venous tourniquet of leg and estimation of left ventricular performance after change in preload. J. Cardiogr., 6:333, 1976.

78. Angoff, G.H., Wistran, D., Sloss, L.J., Markis, J.E., Come, P.C., Zoll, P.M., and Cohn, P.F.: Value of a noninvasively induced ventricular extrasystole during echocardiographic and phonocardiographic assessment of patients with idiopathic hypertrophic subaortic stenosis. Am. J. Cardiol., 42:919, 1978.

79. Cohn, P.F., Angoff, G.H., Zoll, P.M., Sloss, L.J., Markis, J.E., Graboys, T.B., Green, L.H., and Braunwald, E.: A new, noninvasive technique for inducing post-extrasystolic potentiation during echocardiography. Circulation, 56:598, 1977.

79a.Redwood, D.R., Henry, W.L., Goldstein, S., and Smith, E.R.: Design and function of a mechanical assembly for recording echocardiograms during upright exercise. Cardiovasc. Res., 9:145, 1975.

80. Weiss, J.L., Weisfeldt, M.L., Mason, S.J., Garrison, J.B., Livengood, S.V., and Fortuin, N.J.: Evidence of Frank-Starling effect in man during severe semisupine exercise. Circulation, 59:655, 1979.

81. Imataka, K., Kato, Y., Tomono, S., Ueda, S., Natsume, T., and Yazaki, Y.: Changes in left ventricular dimension during supine exercise assessed by continuous recordings of echocardiograms: an effect of beta-adrenergic blockade. J. Cardiogr., 8:729, 1978.

82. Wann, L.S., Faris, J.V., Childress, R.H., Dillon, J.C., Weyman, A.E., and Feigenbaum, H.: Exercise cross-sectional echocardiography in ischemic heart disease. Circulation, 60:1300, 1979.

83. Goldstein, R.E., Bennett, E.D., and Leech, G.L.: Effect of glyceryl trinitrate on echocardiographic left ventricular dimensions during exercise in the upright position. Br. Heart J., 42:245, 1979.

84. Sugishita, Y. and Koseki, S.: Dynamic exercise echocardiography. Circulation, 60:743, 1979.

85. Amon, K.W. and Crawford, M.H.: Upright exercise echocardiography. J. Clin. Ultrasound, 7:373, 1979.

86. Zwehl, W., Gueret, P., Meerbaum, S., Holt, D., and Corday, E.: Reproducibility of two-dimensional echocardiography during bicycle exercise. Am. J. Cardiol., 45:403, 1980. (Abstract)

87. Noda, H., Ogita, K., Amano, N., Koro, T., Ito, Y., Akaike, A., and Kogure, T.: Echocardiographic estimation of left ventricular responses to supine bicycle exercise: a study on normal subjects. J. Cardiogr., 8:237, 1978.

88. Ajisaka, R., Itoh, H., Niwa, A., Iiizumi, T., Fujiwara, H., Taniguchi, K., and Takeuchi, J.: Echocardiographic study of left and right ventricular functions during dynamic exercise by subxiphoid approach. J. Cardiogr., 8:737, 1978.

89. Stein, R.A., Michielli, D., Fox, E.L., and Krasnow, N.: Continuous ventricular dimensions in man during supine exercise and recovery. Am. J. Cardiol., 41:655, 1978.

90. Mason, S.J., Weiss, J.L., Weisfeldt, M.L., Garrison, J.B., and Fortuin, N.J.: Exercise echocardiography: detection of wall motion abnormalities during ischemia. Circulation, 59:50, 1979.

90a.Sahn, D.J., DeMaria, A., Kisslo, J., and Weyman, A.: Recommendations regarding quantitation in M-mode echocardiography: results of a survey of echocardiographic measurements. Circulation, 58:1072, 1978.

90b.Crawford, M.H., Grant, D., O'Rourke, R.A., Starling, M.R., and Grooves, B.M.: Accuracy and reproducibility of new M-mode echocardiographic recommendations for measuring left ventricular dimensions. Circulation, 61:137, 1980.

91. Beeder, C., Charuzi, Y., Meerbaum, S., Berman, D., Staniloff, H., Davidson, R., Corday, E., and Swan, H.J.C.: Cross-sectional echocardiography: Improved assessment of left ventricular function. Circulation (suppl. II), 60:26, 1979. (Abstract)

92. Saffer, S.I., Nixon, J.V., and Mishelevich, D.J.: Simple method for computer-aided analysis of echocardiograms. Am. J. Cardiol., 38:34, 1976.

92a.Johnson, M.D. and McSherry, D.: Rapid analysis of echocardiographic data and two-dimensional images with a mini-computer based system. Cardiovasc. Dis., 5:167, 1978.

93. Chen, W. and Gibson, D.: Relation of isovolumic relaxation to left ventricular wall movement in man. Br. Heart J., 42:51, 1979.

93a.Friedman, M.J., Sahn, D.J., Burris, H.A., Allen, H.D., and Goldberg, S.J.: Computerized echocardiographic analysis to detect abnormal systolic and diastolic left ventricular function in children with aortic stenosis. Am. J. Cardiol., 44:478, 1979.

94. Skorton, D.J., McNary, C.A., Child, J.S., and Shah, P.M.: Computerized image processing in cross-sectional echocardiography. Am. J. Cardiol., 45:403, 1980. (Abstract)

95. Hestenes, J.D., Meerbaum, S., Wyatt, H.L., and Corday, E.: Echo tracking in ultrasound images of the left ventricle of dogs with induced ischemia. Circulation (Suppl. II), 60:II–145, 1979.

95a.Gardin, J.M., Henry, W.L., Savage, D.D., Ware, J.H., Burn, C., and Borer, J.S.: Echocardiographic measurements in normal subjects: evaluation of an adult population without clinically apparent heart disease. J. Clin. Ultrasound, 7:439, 1979.

96. Kotler, M.N., Segal, B.L., Mintz, G., and Parry, W.R.: Pitfalls and limitations of M-mode echocardiography. Am. Heart J., 94:227, 1977.

97. Markiewicz, W., London, E., and Popp, R.L.: Effect of transducer placement on echocardiographic mitral valve motion. Am. Heart J., 95:555, 1978.

3

Echocardiographic Evaluation of Cardiac Chambers

LEFT VENTRICLE

Reports that echocardiography could be used to evaluate left ventricular function was probably more responsible for the rapid worldwide interest and growth in this field than was any other diagnostic application. The number of reports using echocardiography to examine the left ventricle has expanded a great deal. Because of the tremendous interest in ultrasound, we can safely assume that echocardiographic examination of the left ventricle must be of significant value. On the other hand, major limitations and considerable room for improvement remain in the various echocardiographic techniques thus far described. An even more distressing fact is that the literature is not always consistent. There are many contradictory articles concerning echocardiography's reliability in assessing the left ventricle. In addition, so many techniques are described that it is difficult to sort out those examinations that are of value and will continue to be so. Although the introduction of the two-dimensional echocardiographic examination of the left ventricle has enlarged the usefulness of this application, it has also added some confusion to the field. To minimize this confusion, I will separately discuss the M-mode and two-dimensional examinations of the left ventricle; however, much of the discussion of the M-mode examination is made in view of recent information on two-dimensional studies.

M-mode Examination

The diagram in Figure 3–1 shows a transverse section of the heart at approximately the level of the fourth intercostal space and demonstrates that the ultrasonic beam transects part of the right ventricle and interventricular septum as well as the posterior left ventricular wall. The corresponding echocardiogram is shown on the right. The borders of the left ventricle are the interventricular septum anteriorly and the posterior left ventricular wall posteriorly. The cavity of the chamber is bordered by the left side of the interventricular septum (LS) and the endocardial surface of the posterior left ventricular wall (EN). In order to make any measurements concerning the left ventricle, one must correctly identify the border-forming echoes. The learning process with regard to identifying the borders of the left ventricle was a result of a series of studies using indocyanine green contrast injections through a left ventricular catheter at the time of cardiac catheterization. These studies were necessary because confusing echoes are frequently present in the vicinity of the left ventricular posterior endocardium. Figure 3–2 shows a common situation whereby echoes from the mitral valve apparatus, most likely posterior chordae (PC), lie immediately anterior to the posterior left ventricular endocardium (EN). Without the benefit of the dye studies, it was difficult to determine whether the chordal echoes were

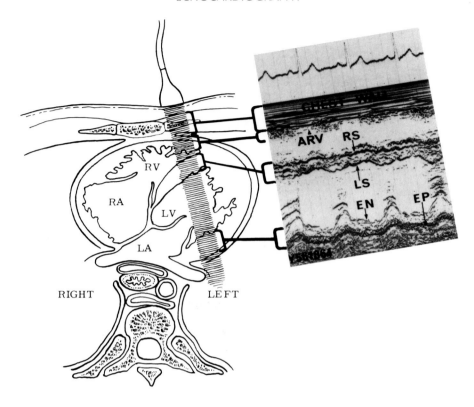

Fig. 3–1. Transverse section of the heart with corresponding echocardiogram showing the path of the ultrasonic beam during an M-mode examination of the left ventricle. ARV = anterior right ventricular wall; RS = right septum; LS = left septum; EN = left ventricular posterior endocardium; EP = left ventricular posterior epicardium. (From Feigenbaum, H., et al.: Ultrasound measurement of the left ventricle: a correlative study with echocardiography. Arch. Intern. Med., *129*:461, 1972.)

border forming or within the cavity of the ventricle. With more experience, it became possible to differentiate between chordal and endocardial echoes. As noted in Figure 3–2, the amplitude of motion of the true endocardial echo is greater than the amplitude of the chordal echoes. Thus a useful criterion in identifying the posterior left ventricular endocardial echo is that this echo is the one with the greatest amplitude of motion in the vicinity of the posterior left ventricular wall.

The left ventricular chamber can be examined from several directions. Figure 3–3 is a diagram showing the cardiac structures traversed by the ultrasonic beam as it is angled from the apex to the base of the heart. This diagram helps one appreciate the relationship between the left ventricle and other parts of the heart. The transducer direction in Figure 3–1 is the same as position 2 in

Figure 3–3. Figure 3–4 is a diagrammatic echocardiogram corresponding to Figure 3–3. As in Figure 3–1, the principal cardiac echoes recorded in position 2 of Figure 3–4 are the immobile chest wall echoes and those orginating from the anterior right ventricular wall (ARV), interventricular septum (RS and LS), and posterior left ventricular wall (PLV), comprised of the endocardium (EN) and the epicardium (EP). The mitral valve structures in Figure 3–4 can be seen faintly in the echocardiogram in Figure 3–1.

Figure 3–5 is an M-mode scan of the left ventricle in a normal subject. The left ventricular cavity (LV) is outlined by the left side of the interventricular septum (LS) and by the endocardial echo of the posterior left ventricular wall (EN). This particular scan is made with the ultrasonic beam initially directed toward the left ventricular apex and

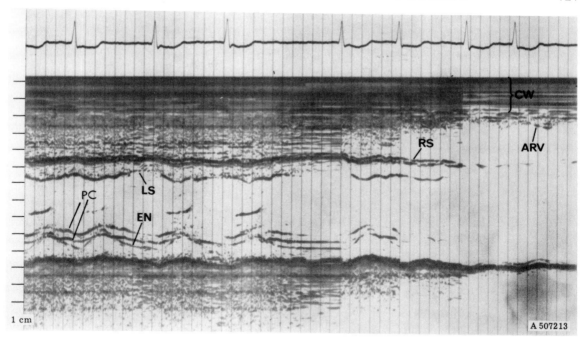

Fig. 3–2. M-mode echocardiogram showing the relationship between the posterior chordae (PC) and the posterior left ventricular endocardium (EN). CW = chest wall; ARV = anterior right ventricular wall; RS = right septum; LS = left septum.

Fig. 3–3. Diagram of the heart showing the cardiac structures traversed by the ultrasonic beam as the transducer scans the apex *(position 1)* to the base *(position 4)* of the heart. Standard examination of the left ventricle corresponds to *position 2*. CW = chest wall; T = transducer; S = sternum; ARV = anterior right ventricular wall; RV = right ventricle; IVS = interventricular septum; LV = left ventricle; AMV = anterior mitral valve; PPM = posterior papillary muscle; PLV = posterior left ventricular wall; PMV = posterior mitral valve; LA = left atrium; AO = aorta. (From Feigenbaum, H.: Clinical applications of echocardiography. Prog. Cardiovasc. Dis., *14*:531, 1972.)

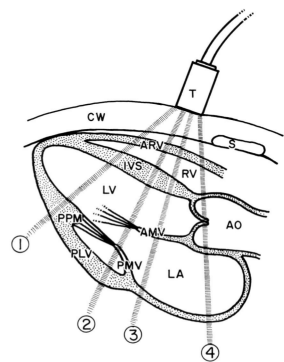

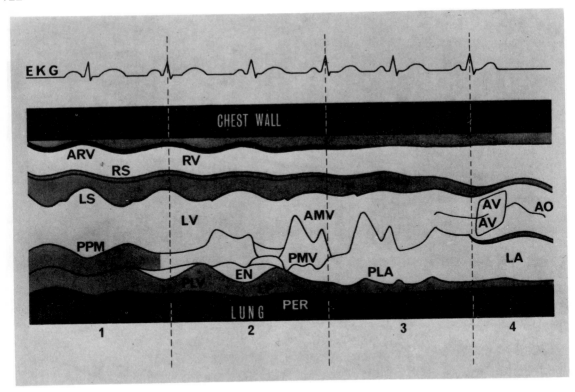

Fig. 3–4.   Diagram of an M-mode scan of the heart corresponding to the transducer position in Figure 3–3. The echocardiogram of the left ventricle is seen in *position 2*. PER = pericardium; PLA = posterior left atrial wall. For explanation of other symbols see Figures 3–1 and 3–3. (From Feigenbaum, H.: Clinical applications of echocardiography. Prog. Cardiovasc. Dis., *14*:531, 1972.)

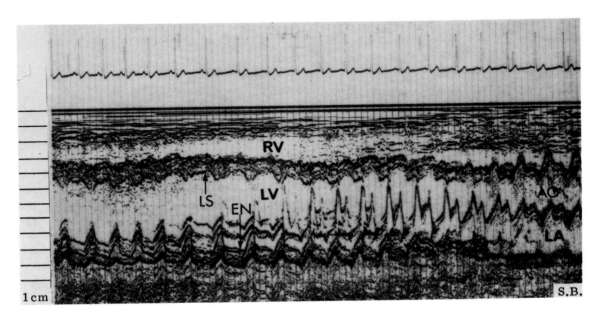

Fig. 3–5.   M-mode scan of the left ventricle (LV) in a normal subject. RV = right ventricle; LS = left septum; EN = posterior left ventricular endocardium; AO = aorta; LA = left atrium.

then gradually toward the base of the heart, which contains the aorta (AO) and left atrium (LA). During the course of the ultrasonic scan, the mitral valve appeared and then disappeared. Whether the mitral valve is being recorded reveals important information about the direction of the transducer. That one is examining the left ventricle near the ventricular apex on the left side of the tracing is confirmed by the fact that no mitral valve echoes are seen. As the ultrasonic beam approaches the left ventricular outflow tract, mitral valve echoes appear and then disappear as the aorta is recorded.

M-mode scanning has many advantages in helping to identify the left ventricular echoes. The left ventricular echocardiogram can be confusing when the beam is directed toward the apex, since the posterior papillary muscle (PPM) (Fig. 3–6) may be mistaken for the true left ventricular endocardial echoes. As the beam moves toward the left ventricular outflow tract, the true left ventricular endocardial echo (EN) becomes apparent, and the posterior papillary muscle (PPM) becomes continuous with the posterior chordal

(PC) echo. The chordal echo eventually attaches to the more apparent mitral valve echoes. The potential error in assuming a midventricular dimension when the beam is actually directed toward the papillary muscle can be significant if one attempts to measure left ventricular dimensions. The distance between the septal and posterior ventricular echoes is considerably less at the level of the papillary muscle than at the level of the chordae or mitral valve. In addition, the thickness of the left ventricular wall may be quite different at the level of the papillary muscle than at the level of the chordae or mitral valve. Thus it is important that the echocardiographer know exactly where the ultrasonic beam is directed by utilizing M-mode scanning and by clearly identifying the various mitral valve echoes.

Although M-mode echocardiograms can be obtained by way of two-dimensional echocardiographic equipment, thus far few recommend using two-dimensional orientation of the beam to record the M-mode left ventricular echocardiogram. One possible reason for this observation is that many two-

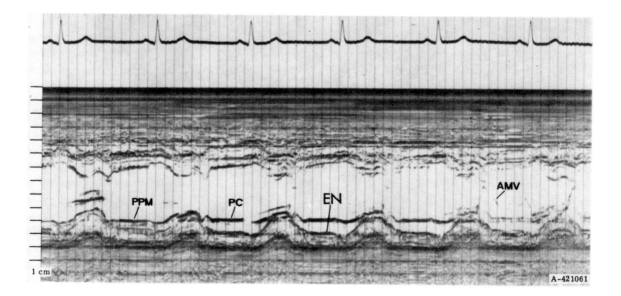

Fig. 3–6.   M-mode scan of the heart with the ultrasonic beam moving from the posterior papillary muscle (PPM) to the anterior mitral valve (AMV). This echocardiogram demonstrates how the posterior papillary muscle can be confused with the true left posterior ventricular wall. Proper identification of the posterior papillary muscle is made by scanning until the posterior papillary muscle becomes the posterior chordae (PC). If the left ventricle were measured in the vicinity of the posterior papillary muscle, the internal dimensions would be abnormally small and the posterior left ventricular wall abnormally thick. EN = posterior left ventricular endocardium.

dimensional echocardiographic instruments provide M-mode tracings that are inferior to the standard M-mode examination done with a single transducer and a standard M-mode instrument. As the M-mode examinations from two-dimensional instruments improve in quality, one can probably expect greater use of two-dimension information for orienting the M-mode examination.

Some common M-mode errors, such as not directing the ultrasonic beam through the center of the cavity of the left ventricle, should be overcome by using the two-dimensional study for initial orientation. For example, a common error is directing the ultrasonic beam too medially (Fig. 3–7). Such an error frequently occurs because of lung tissue overlying the lateral border of the left ventricle (Fig. 3–8). The echocardiographer thus directs the beam medially and

does not transect the center of the left ventricular cavity. The beam tangentially cuts across both the interventricular septum and the posterior left ventricular wall (Fig. 3–7). The echoes from the posterior left ventricular wall are distorted, and any measurements are usually inaccurate.

Two-dimensional echocardiography has also taught us that an M-mode scan of the left ventricle does not record equal amounts of the interventricular septum and the posterior left ventricular wall. Since the scan is done by tilting the transducer, the ultrasonic beam transects minimal amounts of tissue close to the transducer and considerably more amounts at the distal portion of the sweep. Thus, with a routine M-mode scan (as seen in Fig. 3–5), one may be examining 2 or 3 cm of the posterior left ventricular wall but only half that amount or less of the inter-

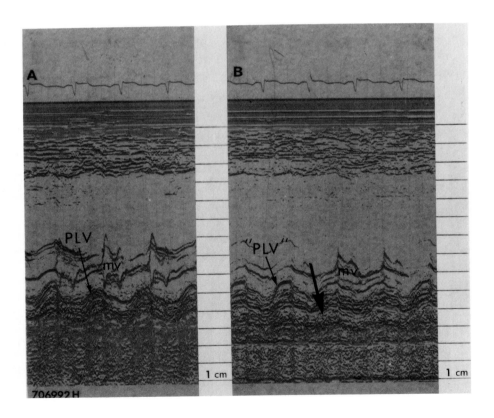

Fig. 3–7.   M-mode echocardiogram demonstrating the common error of directing the ultrasonic beam too medially. A, Proper examination of the left ventricle. B, The transducer is purposely directed medially, and one records distorted posterior left ventricular wall echoes (PLV). The mitral valve (mv) is very close to the posterior wall echoes, there is an increased atrial component to the wall motion, and a relatively echo-free space appears behind the left ventricular wall echoes (arrow).

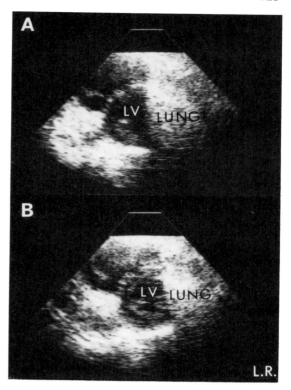

Fig. 3–8. Two-dimensional short-axis echocardiograms of the left ventricle showing how lung tissue can obscure the lateral border. Moving the transducer to a lower interspace will reduce lung interference, *B*.

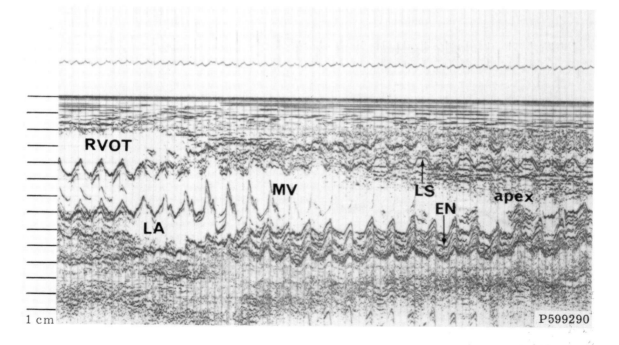

Fig. 3–9. M-mode scan of the normal heart with the transducer in a low intercostal space. Note again the difficulty in identifying the posterior left ventricular endocardium (EN) owing to chordal or mitral valve apparatus echoes that frequently lie immediately anterior to the endocardium. This patient also had multiple linear echoes below the left septum (LS) in the vicinity of the apex. RVOT = right ventricular outflow tract; LA = left atrium; MV = mitral valve.

ventricular septum. The M-mode tracing leads one to believe that there are equal amounts of both walls being recorded.

Figure 3–9 shows that not only are the posterior left ventricular endocardial (EN) echoes difficult to identify, but that the left septal (LS) echoes can also be troublesome. Again, the two posterior endocardial echoes (EN) are almost obscured by the dominant chordal or mitral valve apparatus echoes lying immediately anterior to it. In addition, the septal echoes may be obscured by a band or cloud of echoes within the left ventricular cavity. The exact origin of these echoes is not clear. It is possible that one is obtaining echoes from the sides of the cardiac walls because of beam width. These echoes may also be reverberations from the chest wall echoes. In any case, these linear, nonmoving echoes can be confusing in the identification of the true septal echoes, especially when the beam is directed toward the ventricular apex.

One criticism of the M-mode echocardiographic examination of the left ventricle is that it is limited to only a small area of the ventricle. It is possible to see more of the ventricle by moving the transducer to other positions. Figure 3–10 shows a tracing of the left ventricular apex when the transducer is placed in a lower interspace directly above the apex. In this patient with a relatively small ventricle, the interventricular septum and posterior left ventricular wall near the left ventricular apex are reasonably perpendicular to the ultrasonic beam, and both walls can therefore be adequately recorded. Unfortunately, the apex is frequently dilated or distorted by disease so that the beam may not be sufficiently parallel to the moving walls to record an adequate tracing. Thus, although the cardiac apex is visible with M-mode echocardiography, this is not a frequent examination and the apex is seen with far better reliability by way of two-dimensional echocardiography.

It is also possible to record the anterior wall of the left ventricle (ALV, Fig. 3–11) by sliding or moving the transducer laterally away from the portion of the right ventricle,

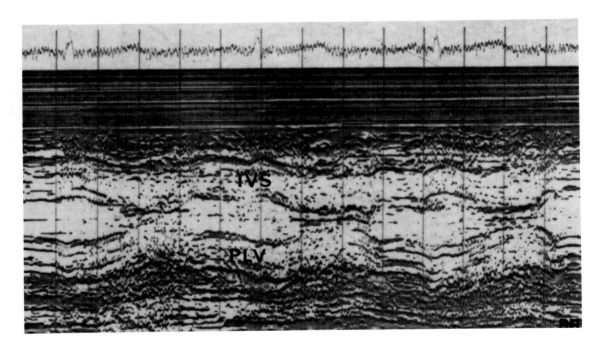

Fig. 3–10.   M-mode echocardiogram of the left ventricle with the transducer placed over the left ventricular apex. The interventricular septum (IVS) and posterior left ventricular wall (PLV) meet in systole, obliterating an already small left ventricular cavity. (From Corya, B.C.: Echocardiography in ischemic heart disease. Am. J. Med., 63:10, 1977.)

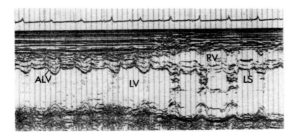

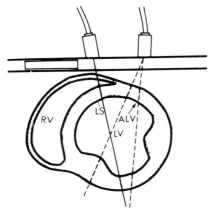

Fig. 3–11.   Echocardiogram and diagram demonstrating how the ultrasonic transducer can be moved laterally to record the anterior left ventricular wall (ALV). In the echocardiogram the transducer is actually moved from the level of the anterior left ventricular wall toward the right ventricle (RV) and interventricular septum (LS). LV = left ventricular cavity.

which overlies the left ventricle anteriorly.[1] As with the examination of the cardiac apex, this study is infrequently done. The lateral free wall of the left ventricle is often covered by some lung (Fig. 3–8) and recording it with an M-mode examination may be difficult. Nonetheless, investigators have demonstrated that multiple areas on the precordium are available for the M-mode ultrasonic examination of the left ventricle.

It is possible to examine the left ventricle with the transducer in the subxiphoid or subcostal position.[2–4] Figure 3–12 diagrammatically shows the direction of the ultrasonic beam during such an examination. With this approach the ultrasound traverses the medial portion of the interventricular septum and the posterior lateral wall of the left ventricular wall cavity. Figure 3–13 is a standard M-mode scan of the left ventricle with the transducer placed along the left

sternal border in the fourth intercostal space. The left septal (LS) and posterior endocardial (EN) echoes are identified. Figure 3–14 is a subcostal examination of the same patient. One can recognize that this recording was obtained with the subcostal approach by the much larger band of tissue between the skin surface and the cardiac echoes. The

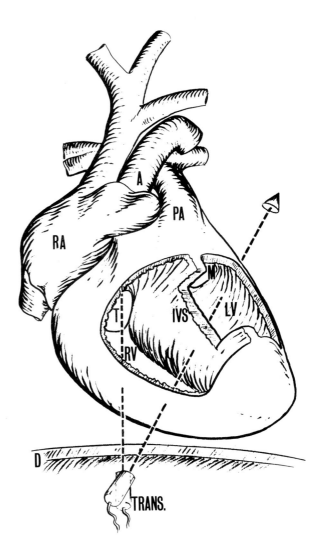

Fig. 3–12.   Diagram demonstrating the position of the transducer and the direction of the ultrasonic beam when examining the heart from the subcostal approach. A = aorta; RA = right atrium; PA = pulmonary artery; T = tricuspid valve orifice; RV = right ventricle; IVS = interventricular septum; LV = left ventricle; D = diaphragm. (From Chang, S. and Feigenbaum, H.: Subxiphoid echocardiography. J. Clin. Ultrasound, 1:14, 1973.)

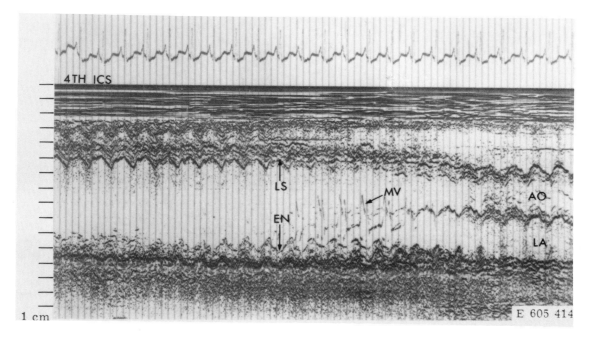

Fig. 3–13.   M-mode scan of the left ventricle with the transducer in the fourth intercostal space along the left sternal border. LS = left septum; EN = posterior left ventricular endocardium; MV = mitral valve; AO = aorta; LA = left atrium. (From Chang, S.: M-mode Echocardiographic Techniques and Pattern Recognition. Philadelphia, Lea & Febiger, 1976.)

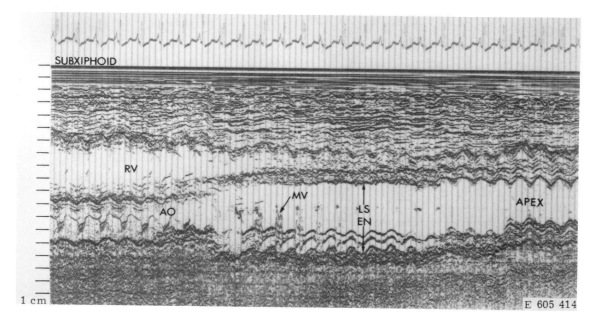

Fig. 3–14.   Left ventricular M-mode scan of the patient in Figure 3–13. The transducer is placed in a subcostal position. RV = right ventricle; AO = aorta; MV = mitral valve; LS = left septum; EN = posterior left ventricular endocardium. (From Chang, S.: M-mode Echocardiographic Techniques and Pattern Recognition. Philadelphia, Lea & Febiger, 1976.)

calibration is changed because the heart is farther from the transducer. The echoes toward the base of the heart include those from the right ventricle and aorta and appear markedly different from those obtained with the standard parasternal examination. However, the left ventricular examination is not grossly dissimilar in the two recordings. It is still possible to estimate the left ventricular dimensions and wall thicknesses.[2,4] Wall motion assessment can also be made using the subcostal approach. There are, however, some differences between the parasternal and subcostal approaches. In patients in whom the parasternal examination is difficult or impossible, the subcostal examination gives access to some information even though this information may not be completely comparable to that obtained in the routine type of study.[4]

M-mode Measurements

Numerous M-mode echocardiographic measurements of the left ventricle have been proposed. These measurements include cavity dimensions,[5-10] wall thickness,[11-17] and combinations thereof.[18,19] The echocardiographic measurements have also been combined with phonocardiographic[2] and pulse tracing recordings, or even intracardiac pressures.[21] A wide variety of calculations have been proposed, especially in view of the increasing use of computers. A new echocardiographic measurement to assess left ventricular function is proposed almost monthly in the cardiac literature.[22] Thus it would be virtually impossible to describe in detail all of the suggested echocardiographic measurements that relate to left ventricular performance. Only the more commonly used measurements are discussed in this text and many details must be obtained from reading the references in the literature. It cannot be emphasized too strongly that these measurements are all totally dependent on a high-quality echocardiographic recording of the left ventricle. It is totally useless and could be potentially dangerous to make sophisticated, complicated calculations on raw data that are of questionable value.

There are many articles in the literature concerning echocardiographic measurements of the left ventricular cavity. The observation that one could make a quantitative measurement between the interventricular septum and the posterior left ventricular wall was the impetus to much of the interest in echocardiography, especially with regard to its assessment of left ventricular performance. Figure 3–15 illustrates how one can make a measurement between the left side of the interventricular septum (LS) and the posterior left ventricular endocardium (EN). Measurements can be made during diastole (d) and systole (s). In Figure 3–15 the diastolic dimension is taken at the peak of the R wave and from the trailing edge of the left side of the interventricular septum (LS) to the leading edge of the posterior endocardial echo (EN). As discussed in the previous chapter, the width of the echoes may vary from one instrument to another and at times even with the gain used. Since the leading edge of echoes is less influenced by these factors, the American Society of Echocardiography (ASE) recommends that measurements be made from leading edge to leading edge.[23] Figure 3–16 diagrammatically demonstrates the ASE recommended method for obtaining left ventricular dimensions. The measurement is made from the leading edge of the septal and endocardial echoes, that is, the septal measurement is actually taken within the substance of the septum. In addition, the Society feels that the end of diastole is best indicated by the Q wave of the electrocardiogram rather than the R wave.[23] This recommendation is based on the fact that the electrocardiogram on the echocardiograms is frequently not of the highest quality, and the R wave may vary. In addition, there may be significant differences in the pediatric population.

Whether one uses the leading edge or trailing edge of the septal echo, and whether the measurement is made from the R wave or the Q wave probably makes relatively little difference in adult echocardiography. As shown in Figure 3–15, there is no significant difference between a Q- or an R-wave diastolic measurement, and the septal echo is probably no more than a millimeter in width. However, in Figure 3–17, which shows an echocardiogram of a young infant, one sees a

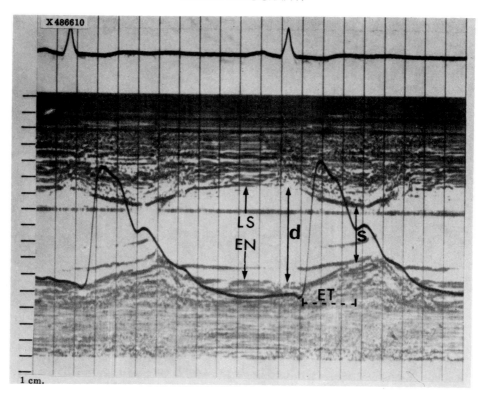

Fig. 3–15.   Simultaneous carotid pulse tracing and left ventricular echocardiogram recorded at 100 mm/sec. The peak upward motion of the posterior left ventricular endocardium (EN) occurs after the diastolic notch on the carotid pulse. LS = left septum; d = diastolic dimension; s = systolic dimension; ET = ejection time.

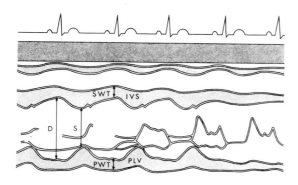

Fig. 3–16.   Diagram of the M-mode echocardiogram demonstrating the left ventricular measurements as recommended by the American Society of Echocardiography. D = left ventricular diastolic dimension; S = left ventricular systolic dimension; SWT = septal wall thickness; IVS = interventricular septum; PWT = posterior left ventricular wall thickness; PLV = posterior left ventricular wall.

marked downward motion of the posterior left ventricular wall shortly after the Q wave of the electrocardiogram. A measurement taken at the Q wave would significantly differ from one taken at the R wave during the rapid downward motion of the posterior ventricular wall. Such a difference would represent a sizable percent variation in this small chamber. A study examining the ASE criteria challenged the reliability of some of these criteria.[24] Although these standards are theoretically more accurate, whether or not they make a difference is still to be determined. Since most echocardiographers use instruments with relatively thin, highly differentiated echoes, echo width probably makes relatively little difference. Thus most of the literature still uses left ventricular measurements from the trailing edge of the

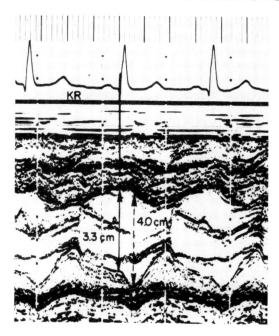

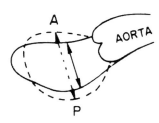

Fig. 3–17.   M-mode echocardiogram of an infant demonstrating the difference in left ventricular dimensions taken at the Q wave of the electrocardiogram and after the onset of ventricular systole. A = anterior; P = posterior. (From Meyer, R.A.: Pediatric Echocardiography. Philadelphia, Lea & Febiger, 1977.)

septum to the leading edge of the endocardium (Fig. 3–15). Since the R- and Q-wave measurements are relatively minor in most adult patients, most measurements in the literature are also derived from the R wave.

The location for making the end-systolic measurement varies among investigators. Many authors use the peak upward motion of the posterior left ventricular endocardium as the timing for end-systole. Others use the peak downward motion of the interventricular septum. One might initially assume that these two events occur simultaneously, but on closer inspection one notes that the peak downward motion of the septum occurs slightly before the maximum upward excursion of the endocardium (Fig. 3–15). The simultaneous carotid pulse tracing in Figure 3–15 shows that the peak upward motion of the posterior endocardium usually occurs after the dicrotic notch, or the second heart sound. Thus the peak downward motion of the interventricular septum more likely corresponds to end-systole than does the posterior endocardial echo. The American Society of Echocardiography therefore recommends

the peak downward motion of the septum as the location of end-systole; however, in many patients with abnormal septal motion, one may have to resort to the peak upward motion of the posterior endocardium.[23]

All investigators agree that the left ventricular dimensions should be obtained when the ultrasonic beam is directed at the chamber between the mitral valve echoes and the papillary muscle echoes (Fig. 3–16).[23] Some element of the mitral valve echoes, usually chordae, is present in such a recording. In the adult, it is unusual to record the best mitral valve echoes when making left ventricular measurements. At the mitral valve level the posterior ventricular wall is frequently not properly seen, and one may obtain a combination of left ventricular and left atrial echoes. The errors inherent in including the papillary muscle in the echocardiographic measurements have been described. There is some debate over whether the situation is different in pediatric echocardiography. Reasonably good mitral valve echoes are recorded in Figure 3–17 at the time when left ventricular dimensions are obtained. Many pediatric echocardiographers feel that the relationship of the mitral valve to the left ventricular cavity is different in the small hearts of neonates and infants and that frequently the best and most standardized left ventricular measurements are obtained when more mitral valve echoes are present in the recording.

After obtaining left ventricular cavity measurements, there are many ways in which these measurements can be used. They may be used merely as estimates of the size of the left ventricle.[7,8,10] With increasing usage many echocardiographers and nonechocardiographers are growing accustomed to echocardiographic left ventricular measurements, and there is less demand that echocardiographic numbers be converted to more commonly used angiographic terms, such as volumes or ejection fractions. In the early history of the echocardiographic examination of the left ventricle, many attempts were made to render the echocardiographic dimensions compatible with quantitative left ventricular angiography. Cardiologists were accustomed to speaking in terms of ventricular volumes and ejection fractions. Thus efforts were made to utilize the left ventricular dimensions to calculate ventricular volumes.[5,6,25–29]

The first attempt at comparing the echocardiographic measurements with angiography did demonstrate a correlation between the two techniques.[8] The correlation with left ventricular volumes was best when the echocardiographic dimensions were cubed. These correlations were made primarily to convince the medical community that some relationship existed between the echocardiographic measurements and the assessment of left ventricular size and function as judged by angiography. It was never anticipated that the dimensions would be used for actually measuring left ventricular volumes. It was apparent that one could not hope to measure a three-dimensional object with a single dimension unless that object were a sphere. The geometric shape of the left ventricular cavity is far more complicated than that of a sphere, and one should not expect to accurately measure volume with a single dimension. Nonetheless, the reasonably

good correlations between the left ventricular dimensions and the angiographic volumes prompted investigators to derive several approaches for estimating left ventricular volumes with a single M-mode measurement.[5,6,27,28] Their rationale was based on the fact that the left ventricle could be described as a prolate ellipse (Fig. 3–18), and that the two short axes (D1 and D2) are equal, the long axis is normally twice as long as the short axes, the echocardiographic left ventricular dimensions approximate the short axes, and the left ventricular wall contracts uniformly. Unfortunately, these assumptions are frequently erroneous,[28] and with more experience it appears that measuring left ventricular volumes using a single M-mode echocardiographic dimension is unreliable and fraught with sufficient error[30,31] to indicate that it should probably no longer be done except in special situations.[29,32,33] Recent evidence shows that even in a normal individual having no contraction abnormalities, the correlation between M-mode dimensions and ventricular volumes is too poor to be used clinically. Efforts at using multiple M-mode dimensions to calculate left ventricular volume have been described,[35] but are still in the investigative stages. These authors attempt to obtain a long-axis measurement by placing the transducer at the apex and by directing the beam toward the base of the heart.

Another attempt to use echocardiography to obtain measurements used by angiographers was the echocardiographic calcula-

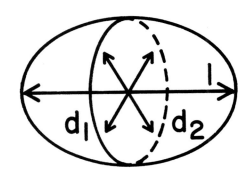

Fig. 3–18. Prolate ellipse demonstrating the long axis (1) and the two short diameters or short axes (d_1 and d_2).

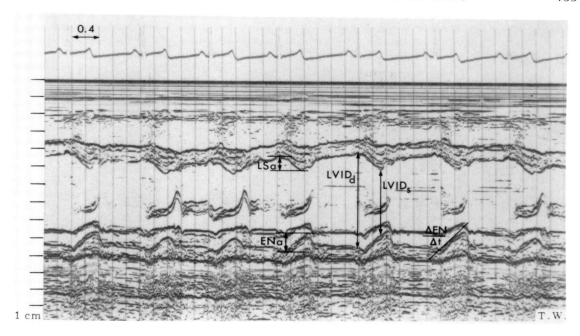

Fig. 3–19.   Left ventricular M-mode echocardiogram showing some of the measurements that can be obtained from such an examination. This recording also demonstrates some cyclical variations that may occur with respiration. LS_a = amplitude of motion of left septal echo; EN_a = amplitude of motion of posterior left ventricular endocardial echo; $LVID_d$ = diastolic left ventricular internal dimension; $LVID_s$ = systolic left ventricular internal dimension; $\Delta EN/\Delta t$ = rate of rise of posterior left ventricular endocardial echo.

tions of circumferential shortening.[9,36–41] The left ventricle can be described as a series of circles, and there is evidence that the rate of circumferential shortening is another way of describing the quality of ventricular contractions. Assuming that the left ventricular M-mode dimension (LVID, Fig. 3–19) is a diameter of this circle, one could calculate circumferential shortening. By obtaining a measurement of ejection time, one could then also measure a mean rate of circumferential shortening or mean Vcf.[42] Table 3–1 shows the rationale for calculating circumferential shortening of the left ventricle using M-mode left ventricular dimensions. Other proposed calculations include instantaneous Vcf or maximum Vcf.[42,43] The Vcf can also be "normalized" by dividing the diastolic diameter.[44] Circumferential shortening measurements are somewhat better than using the M-mode echocardiogram for calculating volumes since fewer assumptions are necessary. One does not have to estimate volume from a one-dimensional

measurement. However, the technique does assume that the short-axis cross-sectional configuration of the left ventricle is a circle and that the M-mode measurement is the diameter of that circle. This assumption is correct in most cases and is not a severe limitation. A more significant limitation is that this technique is not helpful in the overall assessment of left ventricular performance if regional wall abnormalities are present. The mean circumferential shortening of the portion of the left ventricle examined with routine M-mode studies may not necessarily be representative of the entire ventricle, which may have dyskinetic areas not visible on the M-mode study.

Fractional shortening of the left ventricle is similar to circumferential shortening except that one does not theoretically assume the measurement of circumferences.[19,45] The actual measurements and numbers are identical since the value π is cancelled in the calculation of circumferential shortening (Table 3–1). The term fractional shortening is more attractive because relatively few assumptions are made. One is merely calculating the percent shortening of the left ventricular dimension, and no assumptions are made concerning volumes or circumferences. There are inherent limitations to fractional shortening similar to those present in calculating ejection fraction or circumferential shortening in that one can only assess the areas of the ventricle examined by the ultrasonic beam. The only theoretic advantage of the term fractional shortening is that one at least does not assume knowledge of the entire ventricular function as one does when

Table 3–1.　Echocardiographic Measurements of Left Ventricular Performance

1. Posterior left ventricular wall velocity (cm/sec)

   a. Mean velocity $= \dfrac{ENa}{E.T.}$

   　　ENa = amplitude of motion of posterior left ventricular endocardium
   　　E.T. = ejection time

   b. Normalized velocity $= \dfrac{ENa}{LVIDd \times E.T.}$

   　　LVIDd = diastolic left ventricular internal dimension

2. Left ventricular ejection fraction (E.F.) (%)

   $$E.F. = \frac{LV\ diastolic\ volume - LV\ systolic\ volume}{LV\ diastolic\ volume}$$

   or

   $$E.F. = \frac{LV\ stroke\ volume}{LV\ diastolic\ volume}$$

3. Circumferential shortening of left ventricle (fraction)

   a. $\dfrac{Diastolic\ circumference - systolic\ circumference}{Diastolic\ circumference}$

   or

   $$\frac{\pi\ LVIDd - \pi\ LVIDs}{\pi\ LVIDd}$$

   or

   $$\frac{\pi\ (LVIDd - LVIDs)}{\pi\ LVIDd}$$

   or

   $$\frac{LVIDd - LVIDs}{LVIDd}$$

   b. Mean rate of circumferential shortening (mean Vcf) (circumferences/sec)

   $$mean\ Vcf = \frac{LVID - LVIDs}{LVIDd \times E.T.}$$

4. Fractional shortening of left ventricle (%)

   $$\frac{LVIDd - LVIDs}{LVIDd} \times 100$$

using the term ejection fraction. Thus, if one does use the M-mode left ventricular dimensions to assess overall ventricular function, the term fractional shortening probably has fewer objections, although no fewer limitations.

Another commonly used echocardiographic measurement is that of wall motion.[46,47] Wall motion may be measured in terms of total amplitude or rate of motion of the walls (Fig. 3–19). One may measure the total amplitude or excursion of the septal echo (LS_a) or of the posterior ventricular endocardial echo (EN_a). Mean velocity can be calculated by dividing the amplitude by the ejection time (Table 3–1). The measurement can then be "normalized" by dividing it by the diastolic dimension. The rate of motion of the posterior endocardium $\left(\dfrac{\Delta \ EN}{\Delta \ T} \right)$ may also be calculated. One way of measuring the rate change may be to merely draw a line through the rate of rise of the endocardial echo (Fig. 3–19). This slope can represent either the peak motion or the average motion, since the rate of rise is frequently a curve rather than a straight line.

More sophisticated assessments of wall motion and changes in cavity dimensions can be made with the use of computers.[48-51,51a] Using a sonic or light pen to trace the left ventricular echoes, one can more accurately assess changes in wall motion and rates of wall motion, as well as absolute and rate changes in cavity dimensions and wall thickening.[50,52] It is possible to obtain first derivatives of wall motion or changes in chamber dimensions. These observations need not be limited to systole. Increasing evidence indicates that the echocardiographic measurements of diastolic events have great clinical significance.[48,49,53-56] Computer analysis of left ventricular echoes also has the advantage of utilizing other parameters for calculations. For example, Figure 3–20 shows a simultaneous echocardiogram and apex cardiogram (ACG). By tracing both the left ventricular dimensions and the apex cardiogram, a computer can graphically display the changes in echocardiographic ventricular dimensions and apex echocardiographic motion.[57] Computer-drawn loops, such as those seen in Figure 3–21, provide a new way of assessing ventricular function. The timing provided by the apex cardiogram highlights the isovolumic

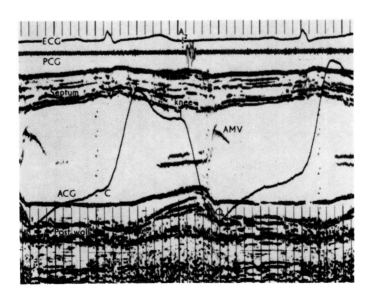

Fig. 3–20. Simultaneous M-mode left ventricular echocardiogram, apex cardiogram (ACG), phonocardiogram (PCG), and electrocardiogram (ECG). AMV = anterior mitral valve leaflet. (From Venco, A., Gibson, D.G., and Brown, D.J.: Relation between apex cardiogram and changes in left ventricular pressure and dimension. Br. Heart J., 39:117, 1977.)

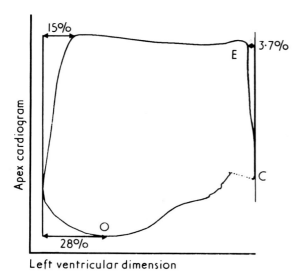

Fig. 3–21. A computer-derived plot comparing left ventricular echocardiographic dimensions against the apex cardiogram. C and E represent timing intervals on the mitral valve echocardiogram. O represents the O point on the apex cardiogram. (From Venco, A., Gibson, D.G., and Brown, D.J.: Relation between apex cardiogram and changes in left ventricular pressure and dimension. Br. Heart J., 39:117, 1977.)

periods and gives a good assessment of changes in ventricular dimensions during those critical times in the cardiac cycle.[49,57,58] One can also introduce timing of cardiac events by way of the mitral valve echocardiogram and thus further enhance the assessment of ventricular performance.[20,49] A computer greatly facilitates such relatively complex calculations. M-mode left ventricular dimensions may also be combined with intracardiac left ventricular pressures.[21,59–62] This combination of measurements has been used to calculate ventricular volume pressure loops, or compliance loops.[62] Such calculations have been useful in investigative studies concerning the properties of left ventricular performance in various disease states.

One of the most important measurements for which echocardiography is uniquely suited is that of wall thickness. Figure 3–22 illustrates how the posterior left ventricular wall thickness (PWT) and septal wall thickness (SWT) can be measured. These measurements can be obtained at any time throughout the cardiac cycle. Initially, the

measurements were taken at the R wave of the electrocardiogram (Fig. 3–22). With increased interest in wall thickness[58,64] and wall thickening,[52,65] there has been a variety of recommended measurements of posterior left ventricular wall thickness. The diastolic wall thickness measurements in Figure 3–22 are made at the R wave. Atrial contraction may produce significant thinning of the ventricular wall; therefore, some investigators measure diastolic wall thickness before atrial contraction. The most important observation is that in the normally functioning ventricle systolic thickness is clearly greater than diastolic thickness. With decreased ventricular function, the rate of thickening

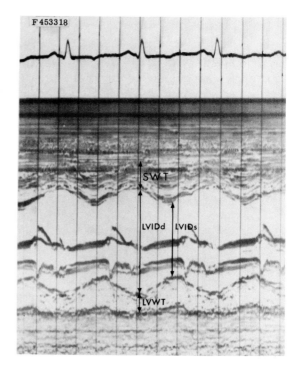

Fig. 3–22. M-mode echocardiogram of the left ventricle. The diastolic left ventricular internal dimension (LVID$_d$) is taken between the left side of the interventricular septum and the posterior left ventricular endocardium at end-diastole at the peak of the R wave of the electrocardiogram. The systolic left ventricular internal dimension (LVID$_s$) is taken at the peak downward motion of the interventricular septum. The diastolic thickness of the interventricular septum (SWT) and the posterior left ventricular wall (LVWT) are indicated. (From Feigenbaum, H.: Clinical applications of echocardiography. Prog. Cardiovasc. Dis., 14:531, 1972.)

decreases and on rare occasions, such as with ischemia, there may actually be thinning of the ventricular wall with systole.[52] Systolic thinning is usually seen in the interventricular septum, but it may occasionally occur in the posterior left ventricular wall. As with cavity dimensions, the wall thickness measurements should be taken from leading edge to leading edge according to ASE criteria (Fig. 3–16).[23] Such a leading edge-to-leading edge measurement is the usual technique for measuring the posterior ventricular wall. However, measurements of the interventricular septum are usually taken from the leading edge of the right septal echo to the trailing edge of the left septal echo (SWT, Fig. 3–22). Thus the septal thickness includes the widths of both right and left septal echoes, whereas the posterior ventricular wall measurement includes only the width of the endocardial echo and not the epicardial echo. A group of investigators who attempted to quantitate left ventricular wall thickness and left ventricular mass recommended that the thickness of the endocardial echoes be excluded from the measurement of both posterior wall thickness and interventricular septal wall thickness.[64] Interestingly, these same investigators found that their measurements correlated best with ventricular mass if the cavity dimensions included the thickness of the endocardial echoes.[64,66] Thus, despite the efforts of the American Society of Echocardiography to standardize M-mode dimensions, there is still considerable confusion in the literature regarding how to exactly obtain the measurements.

Having made measurements of left ventricular wall thickness and cavity dimensions, one can calculate ventricular mass.[67–69] Unfortunately, these calculations suffer partially from inaccuracies of the echocardiographic determinations of volume. The theory behind the calculation of mass is to estimate the volume of the epicardial surface of the ventricle and to subtract the volume of the cavity of the ventricle. The difference represents the volume of the left ventricular wall. One uses the specific gravity of cardiac muscle to convert the left ventricular wall volume into left ventricular mass.

The cavity and wall thickness measurements can also be combined to give a thickness-volume ratio[18,70,71] or vice versa.[72] These ratios attempt to estimate the relationship of hypertrophy to dilatation or even to predict systolic left ventricular pressure.[70,73,74] A ventricle with thick walls and small cavity dimensions would be in keeping with a ventricle that responds to a chronic pressure overload, whereas a ventricle whose wall thickness was relatively small compared to its cavity dimension might be responding to a chronic volume overload. The calculation of mass for both types of chambers might be relatively equal. The thickness-volume ratio has been used to determine the relative importance and severity of pressure and volume overload states.

Many factors may significantly influence the M-mode left ventricular dimensions. There are respiratory variations in the left ventricular measurements.[75,76] Careful examination of the echocardiogram in Figure 3–19 shows a slight variation in left ventricular dimensions during respiration in this normal individual. The left ventricular dimensions become slightly smaller during inspiration. This finding may be a result of normal physiologic factors owing to the effect of respiration on cardiac filling. Another possible explanation is that the heart moves slightly with respiration so that a somewhat different area of the ventricle is recorded during diastole versus systole. This is a possible factor in Figure 3–19 since one sees more of the mitral valve during inspiration than during expiration. Thus the ASE recommends that respiration should be indicated on the recording to help standardize the measurements with regard to the respiratory cycle.[23]

Two-dimensional echocardiography has helped to identify some factors that must be considered in the M-mode examination of the left ventricle. Slight rotation of the left ventricle during the cardiac cycle has been demonstrated.[53] The degree of rotation may vary in different cardiac conditions. Normally, a minimal counterclockwise rotation appears with ventricular systole. In patients with an atrial septal defect and a large right ventricular volume overload, there is an

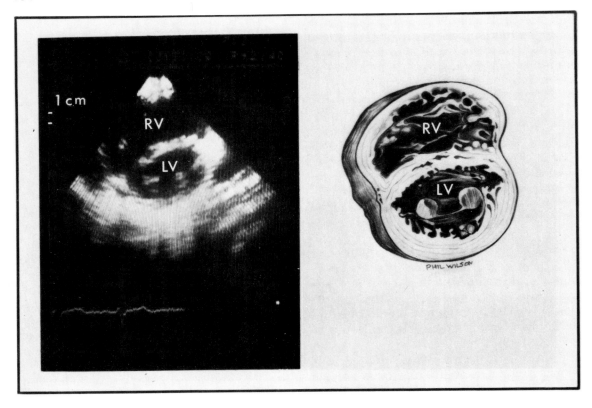

Fig. 3–23.   Short-axis echocardiogram through the right ventricle and left ventricle in a patient with an atrial septal defect. Note the dilated right ventricle (RV) and flattening of the interventricular septum. LV = left ventricle. (From Rogers, E.W., Feigenbaum, H., and Weyman, A.E.: Echocardiography for quantitation of cardiac chambers. *In* Progress in Cardiology. Vol. 8. Edited by P.N. Yu and J.F. Goodwin. Philadelphia, Lea & Febiger, 1979.)

exaggerated counterclockwise rotation of the ventricle.[53,77] Probably a more important limitation to the echocardiographic measurement, as learned from two-dimensional echocardiography, is that the shape of the left ventricle is not always circular in its short-axis plane. With aneurysmal dilatation of one of the walls one expects distortion of the overall shape. However, the shape may be altered when the right ventricle is markedly enlarged (Fig. 3–23).[77] With a right ventricular volume overload, this distortion is greatest in diastole. The effect on the left ventricular diastolic dimension varies depending on how the beam transects the abnormally shaped ventricle.

Anyone who has ever performed echocardiography is aware that technical difficulties may always be present in an examination of the left ventricle.[76] As a result, most patients are usually examined in the left lateral position. Although there are no gross differences in the left ventricular dimensions when the patient is moved from the supine to the left lateral positions, more careful measurements in recent studies have indicated that left ventricular dimensions may change with the position of the patient. These differences could influence serial studies of patients being followed for changes in left ventricular dimensions.[78,79] Thus it is possible that one may need to note the position of the patient when recording the left ventricular dimensions if comparison studies will be made at a later date. Some authors suggest that the location of the transducer should be marked on the chest and that the angle of the beam should be noted by an orthogonal reference system.[80]

In addition to all technical and theoretical

difficulties, one must always remember the human factor in making these measurements.[81] Even with the same examiner, reproducibility is not 100 percent. Thus all measurements must be made and interpreted with these variables in mind. For example, as a rule one should expect a difference of 2 to 3 mm in any adult left ventricular cavity measurement in order to be well within the margin of human error.

Mitral Valve Echocardiogram as a Reflector of Left Ventricular Function

Many studies have shown a relationship between the pattern of mitral valve motion and left ventricular function. Probably the oldest observation is that the mitral valve diastolic E to F slope is reduced in some ventricles. Although the exact mechanism for this reduced slope is not understood, it is thought to relate to the manner in which blood flows into the ventricle during diastole. A commonly accepted idea is that stiff or noncompliant ventricles fill relatively slowly, and thus the mitral valve does not close as rapidly as usual during early diastole. Another mitral valve observation that may indicate altered left ventricular function is the closure of the valve following atrial contraction. Normally the mitral valve begins to close with atrial relaxation and completes its closure with ventricular contraction. This closure is smooth and uninterrupted (Fig. 3–24A). In patients with abnormal ventricular performance, one may see an alteration in the mitral valve closure whereby the B point is interrupted immediately prior to ventricular contraction (Fig. 3–24B). This pattern is usually observed in patients with elevated left ventricular diastolic pressures and an elevated atrial component to the diastolic pressure.[82,83,84] Although the original investigators believed that this echocardiographic finding was specific for such an altered diastolic pressure, later studies showed that this correlation was not reliable.[85] In the original observation the interval between the A and C points was also measured. To correct for atrioventricular conduction, that echocardiographic measurement was subtracted from the echocardiographic PR interval.

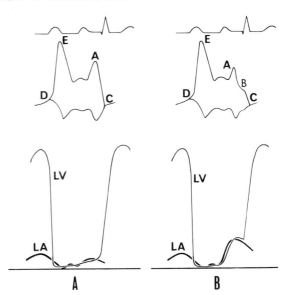

Fig. 3–24. Diagrams illustrating how the mitral valve echocardiogram may reflect changes in left ventricular diastolic pressure (see text for details).

Thus, a PR–AC measurement was proposed.[85] If the AC interval was prolonged disproportionate to the PR interval, that is, if the PR–AC measurement was short (less than 60 msec), then left ventricular function was considered abnormal with probable elevated left ventricular diastolic pressure. Unfortunately, with wider experience the PR–AC measurement proved to have many limitations. With a short PR interval, less than 150 msec, one may obtain an abnormally short PR–AC interval in patients who do not necessarily have an elevated diastolic pressure. In addition, the A to C interval is probably influenced also by the isovolumic contraction time as well as by the diastolic pressure. Thus the PR–AC interval does not correlate well with left ventricular diastolic pressure.[84,86] However, one can use this measurement and probably more reliably the presence of an abnormal mitral closure pattern, i.e., "B bump" or "notch" (Fig. 3–24B), to identify patients with probable abnormal ventricular function and an elevated left ventricular diastolic pressure. As with most echocardiographic techniques that measure altered hemodynamics, this sign is relatively insensitive. Patients can have abnormal ventricular function and elevated left ventricular diastolic pressure, especially below 20 mm Hg, with a normal mitral valve echocardiogram.

A more recent report on using the mitral valve echocardiogram to assess ventricular performance utilizes a measurement between the mitral valve E point and the left side of the interventricular septum.[87] In the original paper the investigators measured the maximum point of the mitral valve E point and the maximum downward motion of the interventricular septum.[87] These two points did not necessarily occur at the same time (Fig. 3–25–1). The mitral E point-septal separation (EPSS) correlated with the angiographic ejection fraction with an R value of 0.87.[87] The normal value was thought to be less than 5 mm and was found in only six of 160 patients with poor ejection fractions. However, almost all patients with abnormal ejection fractions had EPSS more than 5 mm. A modification of this technique was reported whereby one measured the distance between the E point and the septum at the E point (Fig. 3–25–2).[88] These authors also arrived at a good correlation with an R valve of 0.83 in 40 patients, all of whom had coronary artery disease. Another group of investigators found this technique useful even in the presence of left ventricular dilatation. There was concern that with a spherical configuration of the left ventricle this observation may not hold. In patients with dilated ventricles the EPSS continued to be fairly reliable.

Another study showed the measurement to be relatively insensitive even though it was specific for patients with coronary artery disease.[90] Correlating the EPSS with nuclear angiography in patients with acute and chronic coronary artery disease, these authors found that when the EPSS was abnormal, one could reliably predict an abnormally low ejection fraction. However, in a significant number of patients, the ejection fraction was reduced while the EPSS remained within normal limits.

This echocardiographic measurement will probably continue to be popular if for no other reason than it is easy to obtain. Undoubtedly, further research is necessary to judge the general reliability of this relatively simple measurement. Although simple, there is a reasonable rationale behind this measurement. As the left ventricle dilates, the septum moves anteriorly. As noted later, there is ample evidence that mitral valve motion is influenced by the amount of blood flowing through the mitral valve and that the excursion of the mitral valve at the E point correlates with the flow through that valve. Thus, with a decreased stroke volume one would anticipate a decreased amplitude of the mitral valve E point, and with left ventricular dilatation the septum should move anteriorly. With a decreased ejection fraction, which is stroke volume divided by diastolic volume, it is not unreasonable to expect an increase in the distance between the mitral valve E point and the interventricular septum. Despite the measurement's attractive simplicity and rationale, one must recognize its inherent limitations. If there is intrinsic valvular disease, such as mitral stenosis, then the excursion of the mitral valve is not a reliable indicator of flow through that orifice. In patients with aortic insufficiency, mitral valve flow is not an indicator of total left ventricular stroke volume, and one will not be able to provide an as-

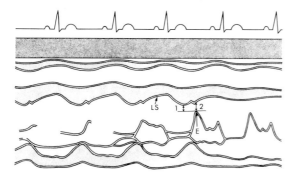

Fig. 3–25. Diagram of an M-mode echocardiogram demonstrating two ways of measuring the distance between the E point of the mitral valve and the left septal echo. E-point septal separation *number 1* represents the distance between the peak downward motion of the septum and the maximum upward excursion of the E point. E-point septal separation *number 2* represents the distance between the mitral valve and the septum at the time of the E point. LS = left side of the interventricular septum.

sessment of ejection fraction. In addition, with aortic regurgitation there probably is partial distortion of the excursion of the mitral valve by the regurgitant jet. Furthermore, the diastolic volume may be increased by segmented dilatation or aneurysm formation that may not produce anterior displacement of the system, and the EPSS may be normal with an angiographically reduced ejection fraction.

Some investigators have been looking at the peak opening[91] and peak closing[92] of the mitral valve as indicators of left ventricular function. In one study, the timing of peak motion of the mitral valve was measured.[91] In the other, the closing velocity (B–C slope) correlated with the velocity of blood ejected into the aorta.[92]

For many years, cardiology has used systolic time intervals to assess ventricular performance. Originally this noninvasive assessment of ventricular performance utilized the phonocardiogram, electrocardiogram, and carotid pulse tracings. By way of these measurements, one calculated left ventricular ejection time and pre-ejection period.[19] The M-mode echocardiogram that utilizes the aortic and mitral valves can also provide measurements of ejection time, pre-ejection period, and even isovolumic relaxation.[93] Several investigators have used these echocardiographic measurements to assess left ventricular performance.[94,95] For example, a "relaxation time index" was proposed as the time between the mininum left ventricular dimension and mitral valve opening.[95a] This interval is apparently prolonged with left ventricular hypertrophy. These measurements are often made through a combination of echocardiography, phonocardiography, and pulse tracings. The cardiac intervals can also be obtained from two simultaneous or dual M-mode echocardiograms of valves.[93,96,97]

Two-dimensional Examination

As described in the previous chapter, two-dimensional echocardiographic examinations of the left ventricle can be obtained with the transducer in three positions. Figure 3–26 diagrammatically shows how one can obtain long-axis parasternal views of the

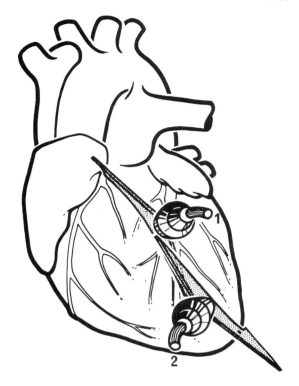

Fig. 3–26. Diagram demonstrating transducer positions and examining planes for parasternal, long-axis two-dimensional examinations of the left ventricle (see text for details).

left ventricle. Examining plane 1 records the body of the left ventricle and the mitral valve. Examining plane 2 transects the left ventricular apex.

One might expect that with a very wide scan angle, one might be able to examine the entire left ventricle with a long-axis parasternal study. Unfortunately, the basal and apical segments of the left ventricle are not in the same plane (Fig. 3–27). Several authors have recorded what they believed to be the left ventricular apex while recording the inflow and outflow tracts of the left ventricle. Figure 3–27A demonstrates such an examination with a "false apex." The echoes that form the pseudo apex are probably from the medial wall of the left ventricle. To record the true apex from the left sternal border, one must move the transducer to a lower interspace and then direct it somewhat laterally (Fig. 3–26, plane 2).[98,99]

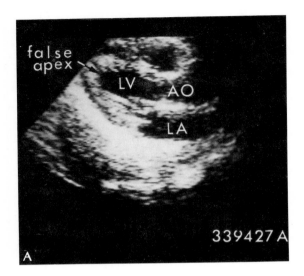

false
apex

LV   AO

LA

339427 A

A

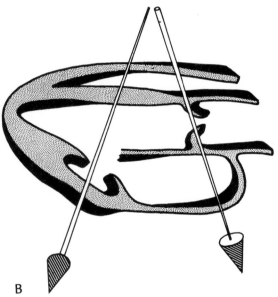

B

Fig. 3–27. Diagram demonstrating that the examining plane of the left ventricular outflow tract differs from that of the apical portion of the left ventricle. A. Long axis, parasternal echocardiogram of the left ventricle showing a "false apex." The apparent apex probably originates from the medial wall of the left ventricle. LV = left ventricle; AO = aorta; LA = left atrium.

Figure 3–28 demonstrates diastolic and systolic frames from a long-axis left ventricular examination through the body of the ventricle. This examination routinely records the posterior ventricular wall from the papillary muscles to the atrioventricular junction. At least the basal third to half of the interventricular septum is visible in this view. The visible amount of left ventricle depends on the distance between the transducer and the heart. When the heart is farther from the transducer, a larger portion of the sector angle transects the left ventricle. In Figure 3–28, one should note not only the change in location of the walls during systole and diastole, but also the increase in thickness of both the interventricular septum (IVS) and the posterior left ventricular wall (PLV) during systole. A diastolic and systolic frame of a long-axis parasternal apical view is shown in Figure 3–29. Again, note not only the decrease in size of the cavity, but also the increase in wall thickness during systole.

Figure 3–30 demonstrates diagrammatically how the left ventricle can be examined from the parasternal border with serial short-axis slices. The three most commonly used short-axis left ventricular echocardiograms are those at the levels of the mitral valve, papillary muscles, and cardiac apex. Figure 3–31 demonstrates a diastolic and systolic frame and examines the left ventricle in a short-axis plane at the level of the mitral valve. A similar examination at the papillary muscle level is shown in Figure 3–32. The apical short-axis study is illustrated in Figure 3–33. The examination illustrated in Figure 3–31 is identified by the echoes originating from the mitral valve within the recording. In Figure 3–32, the papillary muscles have fairly distinct echoes protruding into the left ventricular cavity. Indentations from the papillary muscles may or may not be seen at the level of the apex (Fig. 3–33). The differences between the three levels of examination are not always clear cut, as there may be some overlaps. For example, some authors introduce a fourth plane at the level of the chordae. One cannot be too dogmatic about the classification of short-axis slices because, with the motion of

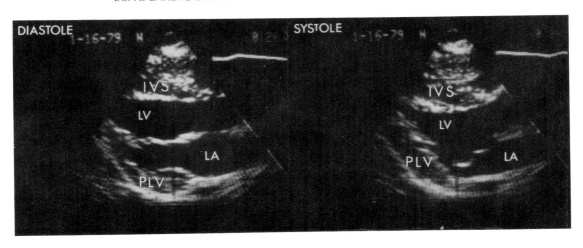

Fig. 3–28.   Diastolic and systolic parasternal examination of the body of the left ventricle (LV). IVS = interventricular septum; PLV = posterior left ventricular wall;LA = left atrium.

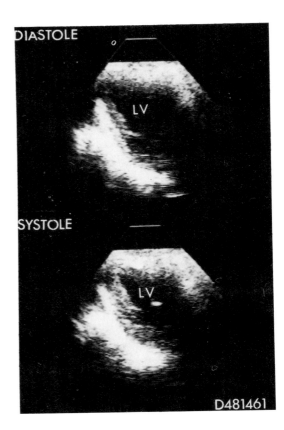

Fig. 3–29.   Diastolic and systolic parasternal examination of the left ventricle over the left ventricular apex. LV = left ventricle.

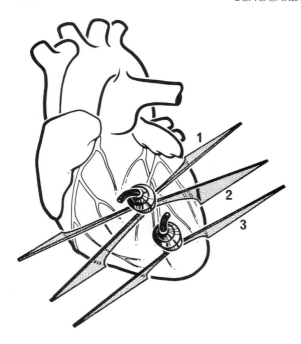

Fig. 3–30. Transducer positions and examining planes for short-axis, parasternal two-dimensional images of the left ventricle. Examining plane *1* passes through the mitral valve, plane *2* through the papillary muscles, and plane *3* through the cardiac apex.

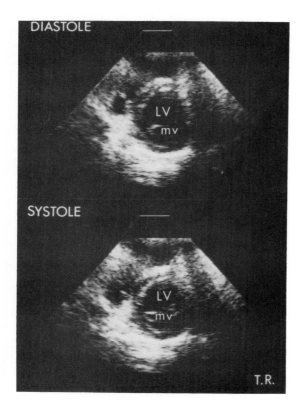

Fig. 3–31. Diastolic and systolic short-axis examinations of the left ventricle (LV) at the level of the mitral valve (mv).

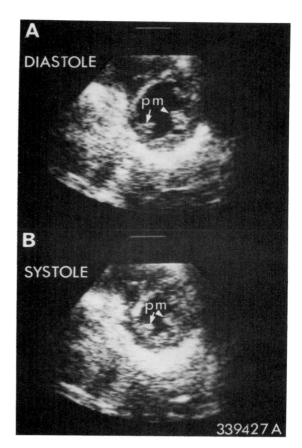

Fig. 3–32. Diastolic, *A*, and systolic, *B*, short-axis, two-dimensional echocardiograms of the left ventricle at the level of the papillary muscles (pm).

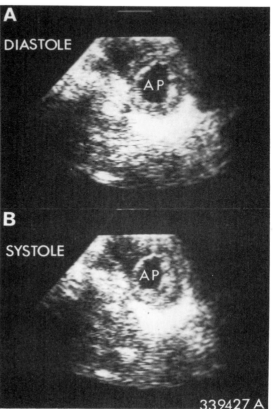

Fig. 3–33. Short-axis left ventricular echocardiograms in diastole, *A*, and systole, *B*, at the level of the left ventricular apex (AP).

the heart, an examination at the papillary muscle level may record papillary muscle in diastole but mitral valve in systole. Technically, it is important to be as parallel to the left ventricle as possible. The proper short-axis examination of the normal ventricle should produce an almost perfect circle. If one examines the left ventricle at an improper angle, then an oval-shaped chamber is recorded. Being aware of this potential problem is important since pathologic situations may produce abnormally shaped ventricles.

Figures 3–31, 3–32, and 3–33 also point out that it is not always possible to obtain complete echoes with the short-axis examination. Dropout of echoes, frequently along the lateral and medial walls, is common. The systolic frame usually has fewer dropouts than the diastolic image. A possible explanation for this phenomenon is that with systole, the left ventricular cavity becomes more irregularly shaped and produces more specular echoes from the endocardial surface. During diastole, the ventricular walls are smoother, with virtually no specular echoes originating from the medial and lateral walls. One must depend entirely on scattered echoes for visualizing these walls during diastole. As expected, frequent echo dropout is an important limitation when one attempts to make quantitative measurements. On the other hand, when the examination is viewed in real time, the dropout is not as troublesome because the eye integrates a large number of frames. Missing echoes in some frames are filled in by echoes in other frames.

Figure 3–34 diagrammatically shows how the heart can be examined with the transducer at the cardiac apex. The introduction of this technique has proved significant for a variety of reasons. Most important, this examination provides a new view of the heart that yields additional information. Second, the apex of the heart frequently offers an echocardiographic window that is more accessible in many patients. In barrel-chested patients, the lingula of the lung may lie between the chest wall and the heart along the left sternal border. The apex, on the other hand, lies closer to the chest wall and lung rarely overlies it. Thus satisfactory

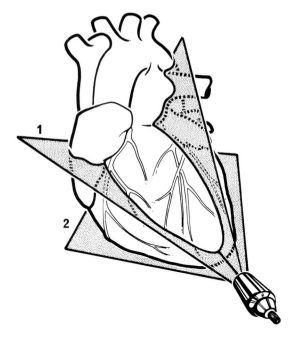

Fig. 3–34.   Diagram demonstrating the examining planes with the transducer placed at the cardiac apex. Examining plane *1* passes through the four-chamber plane; plane *2* is the location of the two-chamber apical examination.

examinations may be made with the transducer placed at the apex in patients in whom parasternal examinations are inadequate. Figure 3–35 shows a systolic and diastolic frame of an apical four-chamber examination (Fig. 3–34, plane 1). One can appreciate the change in size of the left ventricular cavity from systole to diastole and also the increase in wall thickness during diastole. Rotating the transducer 90° produces a left ventricular tomogram so that the right side of the heart is no longer recorded (Fig. 3–34, plane 2, and Fig. 3–36). Such an examination provides the apical two-chamber view of the heart that principally visualizes the left ventricle and left atrium. With minor angulation of the transducer, it is also possible to see the aorta. This plane has also been called the "right anterior oblique (RAO) equivalent." This terminology is used to acknowledge the similarity between this echocardiographic view and the right anterior oblique angiocardiogram. There are many important differences between an-

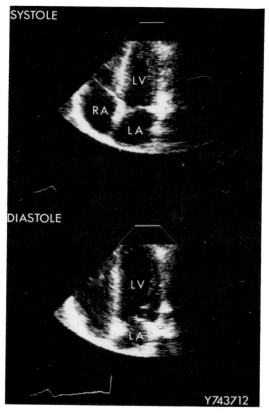

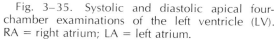

Fig. 3–35. Systolic and diastolic apical four-chamber examinations of the left ventricle (LV). RA = right atrium; LA = left atrium.

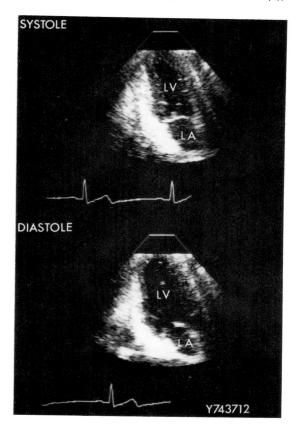

Fig. 3–36. Systolic and diastolic apical two-chamber examinations of the left ventricle (LV). LA = left atrium.

giography and echocardiography; to minimize the confusion, the term apical two-chamber view is used in this text instead of the RAO equivalent.

There is confusion and lack of uniformity concerning some of the two-dimensional views of the left ventricle. One point of confusion is comparing the long-axis parasternal examination of the left ventricular apex (Fig. 3–29) and the apical two-chamber view (Fig. 3–36). There are some similarities between the two examinations, but there are also some differences. Figure 3–37 attempts to compare the two examinations. The location of the transducer for the two studies is slightly different. For the parasternal apical view, the transducer is placed over the apex (Fig. 3–36, plane 2). The basal portion of the anterior left ventricular wall is not clearly visible, and the left ventricular outflow tract

is rarely seen. The tip of the left ventricular apex and the entire posterior left ventricular wall are visualized well.[98] The principal advantage of this examination is that the tip of the apex is always recorded, and one examines the anterior and posterior ventricular walls by using mostly the axial rather than the lateral aspects of the ultrasonic beam. Thus the full thickness of the posterior left ventricular wall is usually recorded (Figs. 3–29, 3–37A). The apical two-chamber view is obtained with the transducer position somewhat more inferiorly and laterally and is actually below the apex (Fig. 3–34, plane 2). The ultrasonic beam is directed up toward the apex rather than directly over it. Thus the principal difference between the long-axis parasternal apical view and the apical two-chamber view is the location of the transducer. With the apical two-chamber

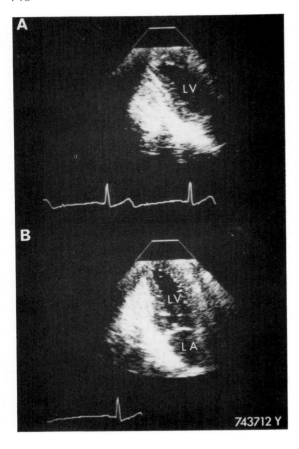

examination, one can more readily visualize the entire anterior wall of the left ventricle, including the left ventricular outflow tract (Figs. 3–36, 3–37B). One routinely obtains a more complete study of the entire ventricle with this examination than with the parasternal apical examination. Thus this examination has become popular for evaluating the left ventricle since it provides the one view that comes closest to visualizing the entire left ventricle with one single echocardiographic study. The disadvantage of this particular view is that the tip of the apex may not always be recorded with either the two- or four-chamber apical views. In addition, the anterior and posterior ventricular walls are evaluated primarily with the lateral resolution of the ultrasonic beam. As noted in Chapter 1, axial resolution is inherently superior to lateral resolution. Thus the thickness of the walls may not be as accurately recorded with the apical views as with the parasternal ones.

It is also possible to examine the left ventricle with the transducer in the subcostal position (Fig. 3–38). This examination is not applicable to all patients. If the diaphragm is reasonably high, then one will not obtain a good examination of the left ventricle. This approach is most useful in patients with low diaphragms, particularly those with em-

Fig. 3–37. Comparison of A, parasternal long-axis apical echocardiogram and B, apical two-chamber examination. LV = left ventricle; LA = left atrium.

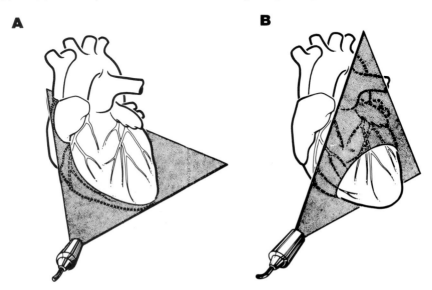

Fig. 3–38. Diagram illustrating transducer position and examining planes for A, subcostal four-chamber examination and B, subcostal short-axis examination.

physema. In addition, the subcostal examination is proving extremely important in pediatric echocardiography, especially in the newborn, the infant, and the young child. In Figure 3–39A, the subcostal examination is similar to a four-chamber apical view (Fig. 3–38A). Figure 3–38B is roughly equivalent to a short-axis left ventricular study.

Two-dimensional Measurements

Ever since it was known that echocardiography offered another opportunity for examining the left ventricle, there has been considerable interest in using this ultrasonic technique to measure left ventricular volumes. Efforts to use M-mode echocardiography for this purpose have been discussed. Despite numerous reports demonstrating a statistical relationship between M-mode echocardiographic measurements and corresponding angiographic volumes, there are many limitations. At best one can say that the M-mode echocardiographic measurements estimate left ventricular volumes in a limited number of clinical situations. M-mode echocardiography does not and probably never will actually measure left ventricular volume.

Two-dimensional echocardiography theoretically overcomes many problems inherent in using M-mode echocardiography to measure left ventricular volume. Whereas the M-mode examination is limited as to the amount of ventricle examined, the two-dimensional technique can visualize the entire left ventricle. In fact, with the multiple examinations now possible, two-dimensional echocardiography probably can examine the left ventricle more completely than can any other technique currently available, including angiography or radionuclide studies. Thus, as expected, numerous investigators have reported their efforts at using two-dimensional echocardiography for calculating left ventricular volumes[100–108] and left ventricular mass.[109,110] There has even been an attempt to reconstruct a three-dimensional display of left ventricular volume through two-dimensional echocardiography.[111]

Before discussing the various ways to calculate volumes in echocardiography, it is necessary to review how one can justify such measurements. Much effort with echocardiographic volume measurements has been based on previous experience with angiocardiography. The left ventricle has been compared with the geometric shape of a prolate ellipse. Considerable angiographic data justify such an assumption. If one describes the left ventricle as a prolate ellipse, then the volume can be calculated by knowing the length, or long axis, and the two minor axes (Fig. 3–40). These measurements can be obtained by directly measuring the length and the two minor axes either angiographically or echocardiographically. An alternate technique is to measure the long axis directly and to calculate the minor axes by measuring the area of the cavity in various projections or planes. This second technique is frequently

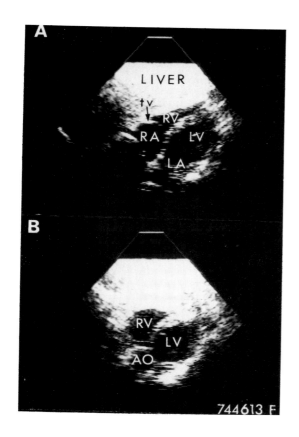

Fig. 3–39. A, Four-chamber and B, short-axis subcostal examinations of the left ventricle (LV). RV = right ventricle; RA = right atrium; AO = aorta; tv = tricuspid valve.

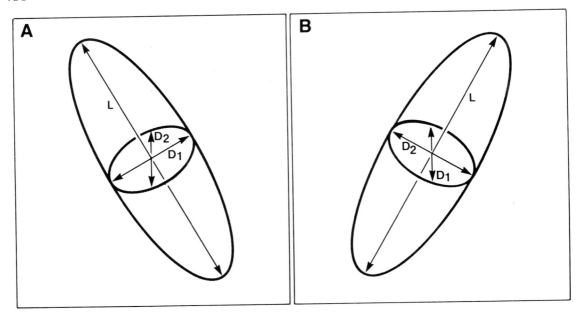

Fig. 3–40.   Two views of a prolate ellipse and its three axes. L = long axis; D_1 and D_2 = minor axes. (From Rogers, E.W., Feigenbaum, H., and Weyman, A.E.: Echocardiography for quantitation of cardiac chambers. *In* Progress in Cardiology. Vol. 8. Edited by P.N. Yu and J.F. Goodwin. Philadelphia, Lea & Febiger, 1979.)

called the "area-length method" for calculating the volume of a prolate ellipse. The long-axis measurements are usually obtained from apical views of the left ventricle, usually the two-chamber view. One could also obtain a long-axis dimension using the parasternal apical view from the tip of the apex to the atrioventricular junction. The minor axes could be directly measured from a short-axis examination at the level of the papillary muscles. An alternate technique would be to use the area-length method from the two- or four-chamber apical examination.[101] The mathematical formula for calculating the volume of a prolate ellipse is $4/3\ \pi \dfrac{L}{2} \times \dfrac{D_1}{2} \times \dfrac{D_2}{2}$, where L is the long-axis dimension and D_1 and D_2 are the short-axis dimensions (Fig. 3–40).

The principal difficulty with using the prolate ellipse model for the left ventricle is that the chamber frequently does not resemble a prolate ellipse. With any significant dyskinesis or aneurysmal dilatation, the geometric model is significantly distorted. Even the normal ventricle does not resemble a prolate ellipse in systole. As a result, many

investigators have been looking for techniques to calculate volumes that do not require the assumption of a geometric model. The technique that has proved most attractive is Simpson's rule. The basis for measuring volume by way of Simpson's rule is to divide the object into slices of known thickness. The volume of the object is then equal to the sum of the volumes of the slices. One need only know the surface area and the thickness of the slices in order to determine the volume. If the shape of the chamber being studied is quite regular, only a small number of slices are required to adequately define its volume. As the shape becomes more irregular, thinner slices are needed for accurate volume quantitation. If infinitely thin slices were obtainable, one could accurately measure the volume regardless of the shape of the object. In Figure 3–41, the left ventricle is represented as a prolate ellipse and is divided into slices that are circular discs. Summing the volume of the discs provides a measurement of left ventricular volume. Even with distortion of the shape of the left ventricle, such as with an aneurysm (Fig. 3–42), Simpson's rule permits a calculation

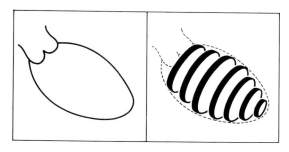

Fig. 3–41. Diagram demonstrating Simpson's rule. The left ventricle is expressed as a series of circular slices. (From Rogers, E.W., Feigenbaum, H., and Weyman, A.E.: Echocardiography for quantitation of cardiac chambers. *In* Progress in Cardiology. Vol. 8. Edited by P.N. Yu and J.F. Goodwin. Philadelphia, Lea & Febiger, 1979.)

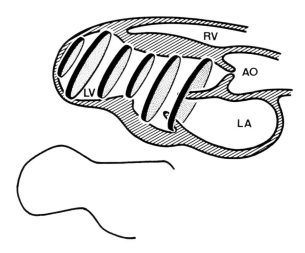

Fig. 3–42. Diagram demonstrating the use of Simpson's rule. Note the series of circular slices in the case of a left ventricular aneurysm. LV = left ventricle; AO = aorta; LA = left atrium; RV = right ventricle. (From Rogers, E.W., Feigenbaum, H., and Weyman, A.E.: Echocardiography for quantitation of cardiac chambers. *In* Progress in Cardiology. Vol. 8. Edited by P.N. Yu and J.F. Goodwin. Philadelphia, Lea & Febiger, 1979.)

of ventricular volume. Merely adding the volume of the individual slices provides a measure of the volume of the entire cavity. Of course, an irregularly shaped ventricle requires more subdivisions or slices than does a regularly shaped chamber.

Because two-dimensional echocardiography has the capability of obtaining multi-ple slices through the left ventricle, Simpson's rule is proving to be a popular method for measuring ventricular volumes. Figure 3–43A shows how one could theoretically use two-dimensional echocardiography to obtain left ventricular volume using Simpson's rule. By moving the transducer linearly across a known width of the heart (H), one can calculate the volume.[102] One can even do a similar examination with a sector scan technique, shown in Figure 3–43B. In this case, to calculate the width and volume of each slice, one needs to know the angle at which the transducer is directed. Slices made by changing the angle of the transducer require more complicated calculations than do linear slices (Fig. 3–43A). Unfortunately, because of the interference of ribs, a simple examination, such as that shown in Figure 3–43A, is not practical except in young infants where the ribs do not obstruct the examination. In adult echocardiography, one must usually examine the left ventricle, as depicted in Figure 3–44. One now must obtain slices using sector scanning from more than one interspace. Such an effort requires many complex calculations to accurately estimate the corresponding volumes.

Because of these limitations some investigators are using modified approaches to Simpson's rule. One approach is to obtain an apical two-chamber examination of the ventricle and to combine it with a short-axis left ventricular examination at the level of the papillary muscles.[103] The endocardial borders of the two views are traced, and then a computer uses a modification of Simpson's rule to calculate the volumes. Each projection is divided into 20 sections along the common axis, since the two views are orthogonal to each other. As expected, the mathematics involved are somewhat complicated.[103]

There is increasing interest in a simplified mathematical model of the left ventricle for calculating volumes using two-dimensional echocardiography.[103a,104,104a] The left ventricle can be described as a "bullet," which is a cylinder and half a prolate ellipse. The basal half of the left ventricle is the cylinder, and the apical half is the partial prolate ellipse. The volume formula is five-sixths the cross-

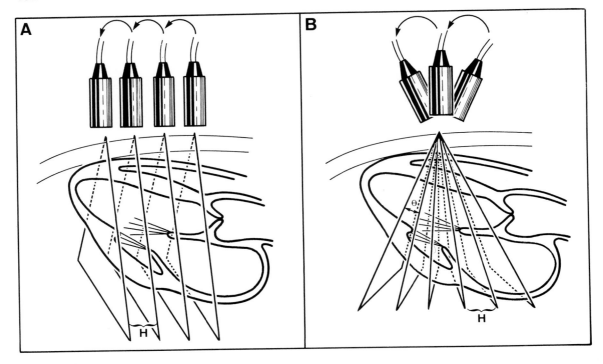

Fig. 3–43.   Diagram of Simpson's rule. *A*, Parallel slices of the left ventricle are obtained by moving the transducer linearly across the heart. *B*, Divergent short-axis scans are obtained by angulating the transducer between scans. H = distance between echocardiographic slices. (From Rogers, E.W., Feigenbaum, H., and Weyman, A.E.: Echocardiography for quantitation of cardiac chambers. *In* Progress in Cardiology. Vol. 8. Edited by P.N. Yu and J.F. Goodwin. Philadelphia, Lea & Febiger, 1979.)

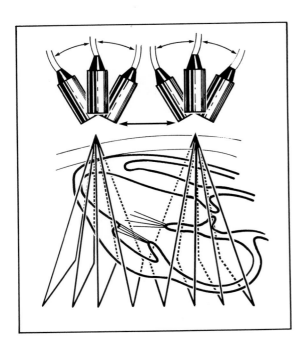

Fig. 3–44.   Multiple short-axis left ventricular scans using displacement and angulation of the transducer between scans. (From Rogers, E.W., Feigenbaum, H., and Weyman, A.E.: Echocardiography for quantitation of cardiac chambers. *In* Progress in Cardiology. Vol. 8. Edited by P.N. Yu and J.F. Goodwin. Philadelphia, Lea & Febiger, 1979.)

sectional area of the cylinder times the length of the total object (V = 5/6 AL). The area would be the cross-sectional area of a short-axis left ventricular examination at the level of the papillary muscles. The long axis of the left ventricle can be measured from the apex to the atrioventricular annulus using either an apical two-chamber or four-chamber two-dimensional study or a parasternal apical examination. The simplicity of this approach makes it an attractive possibility for routine clinical use.

All findings thus far with regard to calculating ventricular volumes using two-dimensional echocardiography must be considered as being in the investigative stages. The preliminary data that use two-dimensional echocardiography to calculate left ventricular volume are encouraging and will stimulate further investigations. However, these techniques require further confirmation before widespread clinical applications can be made. Some of these calculations are complicated and most undoubtedly require a minicomputer or microprocessor as well as a means of introducing the raw data into the computer. A light pen or joystick tracing on a video monitor or a sonic pen or bit pad tracing of a hard-copy recording is commonly used. Unfortunately, the calculations can be no better than the raw data.

Clinical Examples

Despite all proposed echocardiographic measurements, it is usually possible to visually assess the left ventricular status on the M-mode echocardiogram without complicated measurements. For example, Figure 3–45 shows an M-mode scan of a patient with a normal left ventricle. A relatively simple diastolic dimension indicates a measurement of approximately 5 cm. The amplitude of motion of both the posterior ventricular wall and the interventricular septum is quite good. Both walls thicken properly with systole. The mitral E point-septal separation is only a few millimeters. The opening and closing of the mitral valve is brisk and uninterrupted. One could safely say that this ventricle is functioning normally. Figure 3–46 shows a left ventricular echocardiogram of a patient with a clearly dilated ventricle. The diastolic dimension is approximately 7 cm. Neither the septum nor the posterior ventricular wall moves well. The total amplitude of motion and the rates of motion are clearly reduced. One would have no difficulty diag-

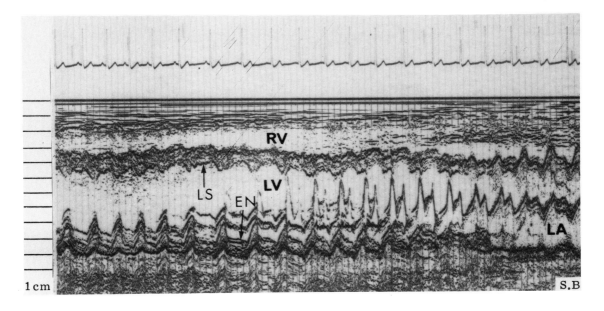

Fig. 3–45. M-mode echocardiographic scan of the left ventricle (LV) in a normal subject. RV = right ventricle; LS = left septum; EN = posterior left ventricular endocardium; LA = left atrium.

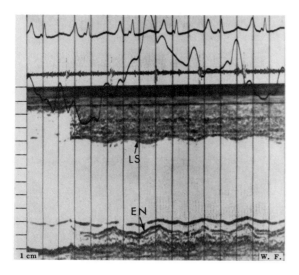

Fig. 3–46. M-mode echocardiogram of a patient with a dilated, poorly contracting left ventricle. LS = left septum; EN = posterior left ventricular endocardium.

nosing diffuse impairment of both the posterior and left ventricular walls in this patient with a dilated congestive cardiomyopathy. The echocardiogram of another patient with a cardiomyopathy is seen in Figure 3–47. Again, there is a dilated left ventricle with poor posterior ventricular wall motion. Some septal motion (LS) remains, but it is appreciably reduced. The separation between the mitral and septal echoes is large. There is abnormal closure of the mitral valve that is clearly visible even on this slow M-mode scan. Thus many echocardiographic findings indicate a poorly functioning left ventricle. Figure 3–48 shows another dilated ventricle that measures almost 7 cm in diastole. In this case, the motion of the walls is not reduced. There is excessive motion of the interventricular septum, and the excursion of the mitral valve is large. The distance between the E point of the mitral valve and the septum is

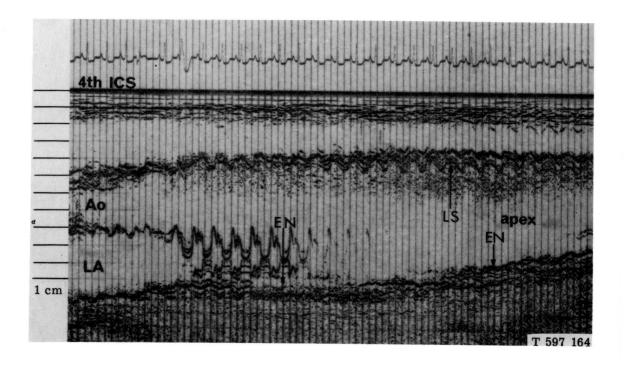

Fig. 3–47. M-mode scan of a patient with a dilated, poorly functioning left ventricle. Little, if any, motion of the posterior left ventricular endocardium (EN) exists. The left septum (LS) continues to move normally. Abnormal closure of the mitral valve can be noted. AO = aorta; LA = left atrium. (From Feigenbaum, H.: Echocardiography. *In* Heart Disease. Edited by E. Braunwald. Philadelphia, W.B. Saunders Co., 1980.)

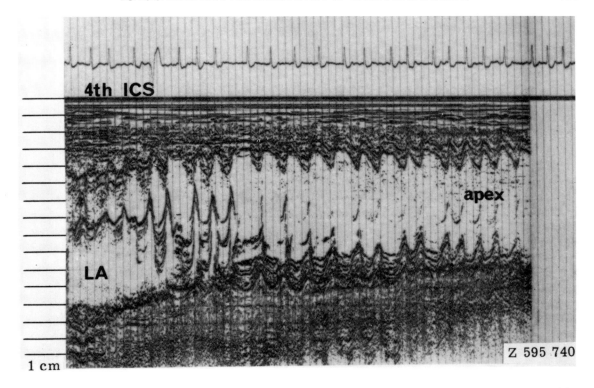

Fig. 3–48.   M-mode scan of the left ventricle in a patient with mitral regurgitation, who has a dilated but vigorously contracting left ventricle. LA = left atrium.

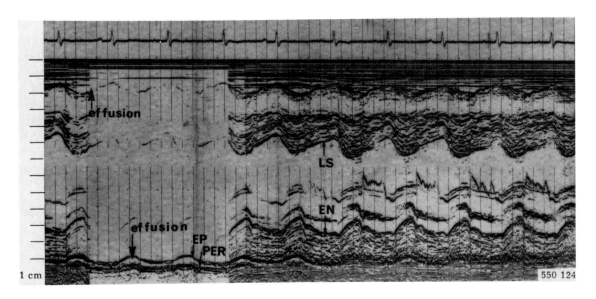

Fig. 3–49.   Left ventricular echocardiogram of a patient with left ventricular hypertrophy and a small pericardial effusion. Note the markedly increased thickness of the septum and the posterior left ventricular wall. LS = left septum; EN = posterior left ventricular endocardium; EP = posterior left ventricular epicardium; PER = pericardium. (From Chang, S.: M-mode Echocardiographic Techniques and Pattern Recognition. Philadelphia, Lea & Febiger, 1976.)

barely more than 5 mm. This dilated ventricle is contracting vigorously as a result of a
left ventricular volume overload. The
echocardiogram in Figure 3–49 shows a
markedly hypertrophied posterior left ventricular wall and interventricular septum.
There is also a minimal amount of pericardial
effusion. The thick walls are striking. The
diastolic thickness is about 1.8 cm, far beyond the upper limits of normal (see Appendix).

These examples illustrate gross abnormalities and demonstrate the potential usefulness of M-mode echocardiography in assessing the status of the left ventricle. More
subtle changes require more sophisticated
measurements, but for routine use most patients can probably be managed with relatively simple measurements, such as diastolic cavity dimension, diastolic wall thickness, mitral E point-septal separation, and
posterior and septal wall motion.

The M-mode echocardiographic examination has proved quite useful in patients with
uniformly functioning ventricles. The principal difficulties with this examination have
been in patients with segmental wall disease. It is neither feasible nor practical to
examine all segments of the left ventricle
with M-mode echocardiography. Thus two-
dimensional echocardiography, because of
its spatial orientation, offers the opportunity
to examine areas, such as the apex and the
medial and lateral walls, that are otherwise
unavailable for the M-mode study. As a result, much of the interest in using two-
dimensional echocardiography to examine
the left ventricle is in reference to patients
with ischemic heart disease. Since most of
the chapter on coronary artery disease deals
with the echocardiographic examination of
the ischemic left ventricle, the use of two-
dimensional echocardiography in coronary
artery disease is discussed in that chapter.

The two-dimensional echocardiographic
examination of the left ventricle can also be
useful in patients without coronary artery
disease. One may debate the advantages of
the two-dimensional examination over those
of the M-mode study. To date, detailed comparison of the two techniques in the nonischemic ventricle has not been made. One

can certainly gain a better appreciation of the
shape of the left ventricle with the two-
dimensional technique. The shape of the
cavity may be altered by segmental disease
and aneurysm formation, and dilatation of
the right ventricle also distorts the shape of
the left ventricle (Fig. 3–23). The left ventricle is no longer a perfect circle in the short-
axis view. Probably the principal benefit of
the two-dimensional examination of the
nonischemic ventricle is to identify the distortion in shape, especially if M-mode left
ventricular measurements are made. For
example, routine M-mode measurements
between the septum and posterior ventricular wall clearly underestimate the true size
and volume of the left ventricular cavity illustrated in Figure 3–23.

Although left ventricular dilatation, hypertrophy, and abnormal contraction patterns
are readily identified in the M-mode examination, these alterations can also be seen in
the two-dimensional examination. Figure
3–50 shows a two-dimensional study of a patient with a dilated ventricle. There is a
marked difference in cavity size between
diastole (A) and systole (B), consistent with a
large stroke volume in this patient with a left
ventricular volume overload. Viewing this
recording in real time affords a dramatic
example of a vigorously contracting, yet dilated, ventricle. A dilated but poorly contracting ventricle is depicted in Figure 3–51.
There is little difference in cavity size between diastole and systole. Again one must
appreciate that in real time the lack of motion
of the ventricle would be striking.

Figure 3–52 shows another left ventricular
abnormality. In this example, the walls of the
ventricle are markedly hypertrophied, and
in systole, there is almost complete cavity
obliteration. It must be emphasized, however, that most of these observations could
be made on the M-mode examination; in fact,
measuring the size of the ventricle and the
thickness of the ventricular walls is considerably easier and more convenient with the
M-mode technique.

There have been attempts to identify the
tissues of the left ventricular walls as well as
to measure thickness and motion by way of
two-dimensional echocardiography. Most of

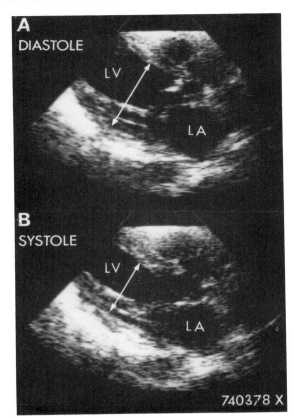

Fig. 3–50. Long-axis parasternal examination of the left ventricle (LV) in a patient with a volume over-load and a well-contracting ventricle. The left ven-tricular cavity *(arrows)* decreases markedly from dias-tole, *A*, to systole, *B*. LA = left atrium.

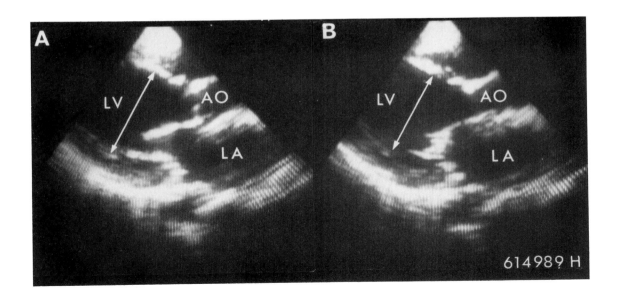

Fig. 3–51.   Long-axis parasternal examination of the left ventricle (LV) in a patient with a dilated and poorly contracting ventricle. Very little difference in cavity size *(arrows)* exists from diastole, *A*, to systole, *B*. AO = aorta; LA = left atrium.

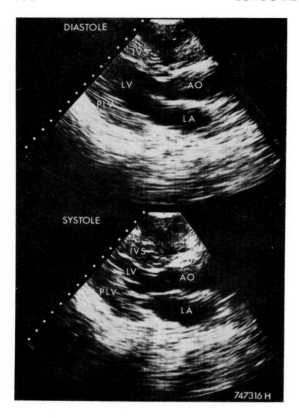

Fig. 3–52.   Long-axis parasternal two-dimensional echocardiogram of a hypertrophied left ventricle. The interventricular septum (IVS) and posterior left ventricular wall (PLV) are thick, and the cavity (LV) is almost obliterated in systole. AO = aorta; LA = left atrium.

these efforts are still in the investigative stages. The only application that has clinical relevance is with regard to identifying myocardial scar. Since this phenomenon occurs most often with coronary artery disease, the topic is discussed in more detail in that chapter.

Effects of Physiologic States and Interventions on the Left Ventricular Echocardiogram

Investigators have used left ventricular echocardiographic measurements to examine normal physiologic states, such as pregnancy,[112,113] aging,[114–116] and the effects of training and deconditioning.[116a] Athletes involved in a variety of activities have been studied echocardiographically.[117,117a,118–123] Those athletes involved in isometric activi-

ties, such as weight lifting or wrestling, have thick cardiac walls,[120] whereas those involved in endurance activities, such as running, have dilated chambers with normal wall thickness.[117a,119] Investigators are also using interventions such as exercise to study the physiology of the ventricle.[44,124–129] There are many technical difficulties in examining the left ventricle during active exercise (see Chapter 2). However, results sufficiently indicate that this type of examination is feasible in selected individuals. The data thus far are not conclusive, but echocardiography is a possible means of gaining information concerning the left ventricle during exercise.[130]

Isometric stress, usually handgrip, has also been used with echocardiography.[124,131,132] Fewer technical problems exist in the echocardiographic recordings, but this form of exercise has limitations regarding its physiologic effects. The Valsalva maneuver has also been suggested as an intervention that can be combined with echocardiography to help define left ventricular function.[133–135] An intriguing stress that has been proposed is to produce a premature ventricular systole by using an external mechanical device over the cardiac apex.[136,137] This device produces a brief blow to the cardiac apex that usually results in a premature ventricular systole, enabling one to look at the post-extrasystolic potentiation of ventricular function. Evidence suggests that the abnormal ventricle shows a significant increase in ventricular performance following the pause of the premature beat. The normally contracting ventricle may not change appreciably. Other investigators have examined the echocardiographic effects of post-stimulation potentiation using a more conventional pacing catheter to produce the premature contraction.[138]

Interventions by way of drugs have been used both in normal patients and in those with various forms of heart disease.[138a,138b] Such studies have been conducted acutely or chronically to see the effect of these drugs, with the echocardiogram as a monitor.[138c–g,138m] In addition, serial echocardiographic studies have been used to judge the effects of potentially toxic cardiac drugs, such as Adriamycin[138h,138l] or general anesthesia.[138i] One report demonstrated serial echocardiographic changes with acute carbon monoxide poisoning.[138j] To be discussed in the chapter on valvular heart disease are several proposed criteria for judging ventricular function and for determining when valvular surgery is required. The reliability of these measurements is still under investigation.[138k]

Technical Difficulties

As with all aspects of echocardiography, significant technical difficulties must be appreciated when examining the left ventricle. As mentioned, dropout of myocardial echoes is particularly troublesome. Unfortunately, the dropout is usually present in those views currently advocated for calculating ventricular volume. The short-axis and apical views have the most frequent incidence of echo dropout because these examinations depend on lateral resolution and the recording of relatively weak, scattered echoes. When relying on lateral resolution or scattered echoes, the signal-to-noise ratio must be extremely good. Thus measurements from these views can be obtained from acoustically satisfactory patients, but with more difficult patients the signal-to-noise ratio is inadequate for recording the desired weaker echoes. It is hoped that with improved instrumentation and possible alterations in transducer design, this problem will be overcome. In addition, it may be possible to develop techniques that depend more on axial rather than lateral resolution in order to yield a higher number of satisfactory recordings.

The problem of overlying lung tissue is well recognized by echocardiographers. Figure 3–8 demonstrates how overlying lung obliterates the lateral border of the left ventricle during a short-axis study. This problem is common and can be partially overcome by making the measurements during expiration or by moving to a slightly lower interspace to avoid the lung.

RIGHT VENTRICLE

The echocardiographic examination of the right ventricle has many limitations. This observation is not surprising when one considers the inherent difficulties in examining this chamber echocardiographically. Much of the right ventricle lies directly beneath the sternum, the chamber has an irregular shape, the walls are trabeculated, and the location of the chamber within the chest may vary significantly, depending on the position of the patient. Despite these formidable problems, echocardiography can reveal useful information concerning the status of the right ventricle, and although right ventricular measurements are admittedly crude, they are helpful in selected patients.

M-mode Examination

With the transducer positioned along the left sternal border and directed toward the left ventricle, the ultrasonic beam traverses a small portion of the right ventricle (Fig. 3–53).[139] Using a standard 2.25-mHz transducer, the anterior right ventricular wall (ARV) is often indistinctly seen. One fre-

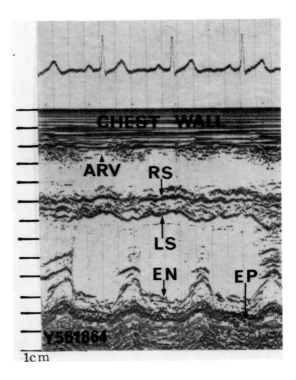

Fig. 3–53. M-mode echocardiogram through the right and left ventricles. ARV = anterior right ventricular wall; RS = right septum; LS = left septum; EN = posterior left ventricular endocardium; EP = posterior left ventricular epicardium.

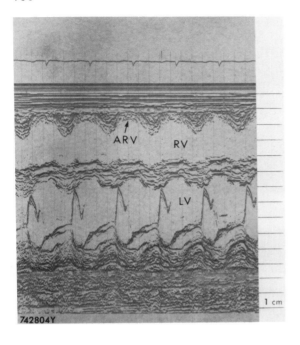

Fig. 3–54. M-mode echocardiogram demonstrating the anterior right ventricular wall (ARV). RV = right ventricle; LV = left ventricle.

quently sees only a band of fuzzy echoes that may exhibit some motion with cardiac action. With more careful angulation of the transducer and especially if one uses a high-frequency transducer, it is often possible to record more distinct echoes from the anterior right ventricular wall (Fig. 3–54). With this M-mode examination, the posterior border of the right ventricular cavity is delineated by the right side of the interventricular septum (RS). One can measure the distance between the anterior right ventricular wall and the right septal echo to estimate the size of the right ventricle. Although every effort should be made to clearly identify an anterior right ventricular wall in those patients in whom the right ventricular wall echoes are not clearly seen, echocardiographers estimate that the anterior right ventricular wall is located about 5 mm from the chest wall. That the right ventricular wall is frequently indistinct is but one reason why the right ventricular measurement is only a gross estimation of its overall size. Another limitation of

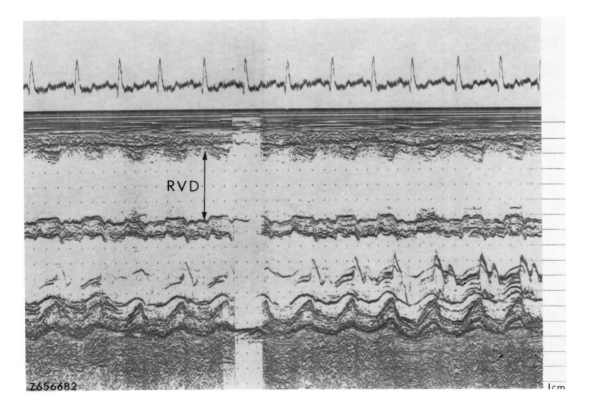

Fig. 3–55. M-mode echocardiogram showing a dilated right ventricle. RVD = right ventricular dimension.

the echocardiographic measurement of the right ventricle is that the dimension is much larger if the patient is in the left lateral position. Thus, in order to standardize the examination, the measurement should be taken with the patient supine. Despite these limitations one can still use this crude measurement to obtain a fairly reliable indication of right ventricular dilatation. Figure 3–55 shows an example of a patient with marked right ventricular dilatation. The distance between the anterior right ventricular wall and the interventricular septum is more than 4 cm, which is clearly beyond the upper limits of normal (see Appendix).

Besides determining right ventricular dilatation, the standard M-mode echocardiogram is also useful in the diagnosis of a hypoplastic right ventricle. Figure 3–56 shows a patient with tricuspid atresia whereby a small space is noted between the right side of the septum (RS) and the chest wall. The anterior right ventricular wall is not clearly identified. Even though the right ventricular dimension is not totally accurate and has many limitations, its overall utility is still significant. One must remember that the ultrasonic measurement measures only that

portion of the right ventricle lying anterior to the interventricular septum. This area corresponds primarily to the right ventricular outflow tract.

Because the anterior right ventricular wall in the adult patient is usually difficult to record using a 2.25-mHz transducer, right ventricular wall thickness has been an infrequent measurement. However, with pediatric echocardiography the frequent occurrence of right ventricular hypertrophy plus the higher-frequency transducer used in such examinations make right ventricular wall thickness a more common echocardiographic measurement.[140] Even in some adults it is possible to note the thickness of the right ventricular wall. Figure 3–57 shows a patient with chronic obstructive lung disease whose right ventricular free wall is obviously hypertrophied, even with a 2.25-mHz transducer. An even more marked degree of right ventricular hypertrophy is seen in Figure 3–58. There has been increasing interest in using echocardiography to measure right ventricular free wall thickness.[141-146] One study showed that with careful adjustment of the gain and depth compensation controls it was possible to re-

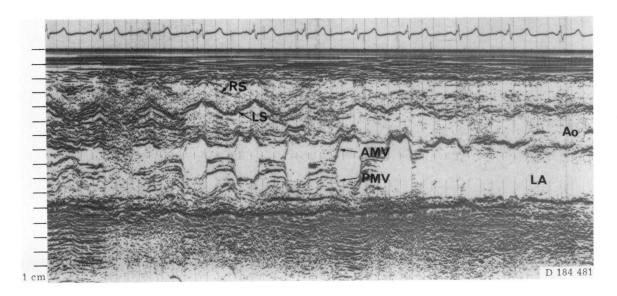

Fig. 3–56. M-mode echocardiographic scan from a patient with tricuspid atresia and a hypoplastic right ventricle. Very little potential space exists between the right septum (RS) and the chest wall echoes. LS = left septum; AMV = anterior mitral valve leaflet; PMV = posterior mitral valve leaflet; AO = aorta; LA = left atrium.

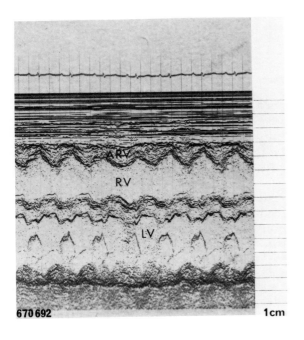

Fig. 3–57. M-mode echocardiogram of a patient with chronic obstructive lung disease and a hypertrophied anterior right ventricular wall (ARV). RV = right ventricle; LV = left ventricle.

cord the right ventricular wall thickness both in systole and diastole and that there was an excellent correlation with necropsy measurements of right ventricular wall thickness.[146] The R value in adults was 0.8. In another study of infants and children with congenital heart disease, it was possible to examine the right ventricular wall in 62 of 82 children. The echocardiographic and anatomic measurements correlated with an R value of 0.93. Yet another author stated that it was possible to record echoes from the anterior right ventricular wall using a 5-mHz transducer in 80 percent of adult patients.[145] Several studies suggested that the sub-xiphoid or subcostal approach might even be more successful in recording echoes from the free wall of the right ventricle.[141–143] A 2.25-mHz transducer may be more successful in the subcostal approach since the right ventricle is farther from the transducer.

Two-dimensional Examination

Two-dimensional echocardiography provides multiple views of the right ventricle.

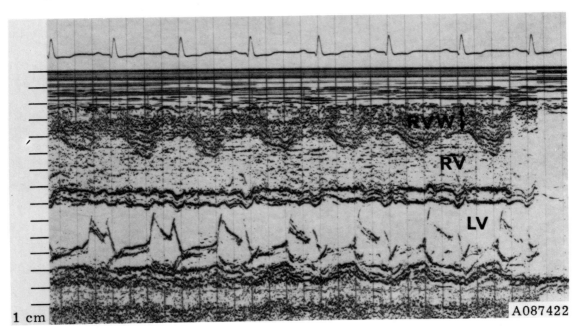

Fig. 3–58. Echocardiographic tracing of a patient with marked right ventricular hypertrophy. The mass of echoes (RVW) below the chest wall is thick and undoubtedly originates from the anterior right ventricular wall. Whether or not all echoes originate from the right ventricle is debatable; however, it is highly probable that the right ventricular wall is indeed thickened and that much of the mass of echoes originates from this hypertrophied wall. The right ventricular cavity (RV) is also dilated. LV = left ventricle.

No single parasternal study provides a complete examination of this chamber. Because of the unusual shape, one must examine the ventricle from several planes of the left sternal border as the right ventricle curves around the left ventricle and aorta. Despite the limitations in examining the right ventricle from the left sternal border, useful information can be obtained. Figure 3–59 shows the effect of a dilated right ventricle on the left ventricle when examined in the short-axis presentation. There is a semiquantitative increase in the size of the right ventricle with an absolute distortion of the shape of the left ventricle. The distortion in shape may be throughout the cardiac cycle, as it was in Figure 3–23, or it may occur only during diastole, as in Figure 3–59. A short-axis parasternal examination of the right ventricle may also be particularly helpful in looking at the right ventricular outflow tract. This determination is especially important in congenital heart disease, such as tetralogy of Fallot (see Chapter 7). Evidence indicates that the two-dimensional examination is better than the M-mode study in evaluating the outflow tract following surgical repair of tetralogy of Fallot.

Better views of the right ventricle can be obtained with either the apical or subcostal approaches. Figure 3–60 is an apical four-chamber view demonstrating the right ventricular cavity. Investigators have suggested techniques that use the apical four-chamber view for measuring the size of the right ventricle.[147] Figure 3–60 can be compared with the echocardiograms in Figure 3–61, in which the right ventricle is dilated. The total echo-free area of the right ventricle is considerably larger than that of the left ventricle, especially when compared to Figure 3–60. In addition, as in Figure 3–58, there is distortion of the interventricular septum, especially in diastole (Fig. 3–61B). The subcostal approach allows another way to examine the right ventricle (Fig. 3–62). This examination,

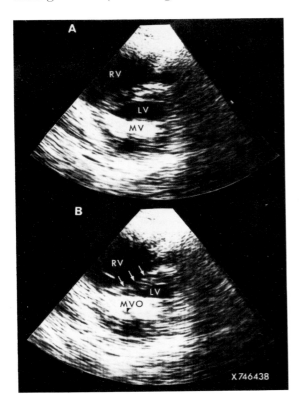

Fig. 3–59. Short-axis, parasternal two-dimensional echocardiograms through the right ventricle (RV) and left ventricle (LV) at the level of the mitral valve (MV) in a patient with several mitral stenosis and a dilated right ventricle. During early diastole, B, the interventricular septum (arrows) indents into the left ventricle, distorting the shape of the left ventricular cavity.

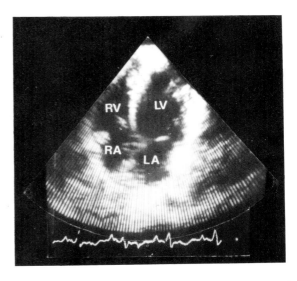

Fig. 3–60. Apical four-chamber view. RV = right ventricle; LV = left ventricle; RA = right atrium; LA = left atrium. (From Feigenbaum, H.: Echocardiography. In Heart Disease. Edited by E. Braunwald. Philadelphia, W.B. Saunders Co., 1980.)

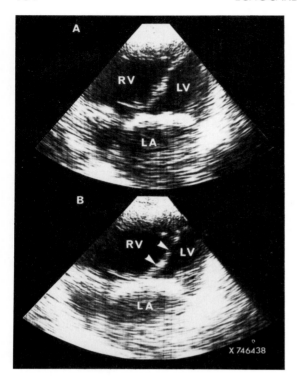

Fig. 3–61.   Apical four-chamber views of a patient with mitral stenosis and marked right ventricular dilatation. During early diastole, *B*, the septum indents toward the left ventricle *(arrows)*.

used with greater frequency in pediatric echocardiography, renders a qualitative estimate of the size of the right ventricle.[148]

Quantitating right ventricular volume is not easy, principally because of the marked complexity of the shape of the ventricle, which has been suggested as that of a pyramid.[147] Another problem is that even with the apical four-chamber view it is not always possible to record the entire right ventricular chamber in one examination. Thus considerably more work is necessary before two-dimensional echocardiography can quantitate the volume of the right ventricle.

Echocardiographic Findings with Overload of the Right Ventricle

A pressure overload of the right ventricle is primarily detected by hypertrophy of the right ventricular free wall. Occasionally, hypertrophy of the interventricular septum is also a consequence of chronic right ventricular pressure overload.[149] A pressure overload may also produce right ventricular dilatation with an increase in the right ventricular echocardiographic dimension. Figure 3–63 shows some early data comparing

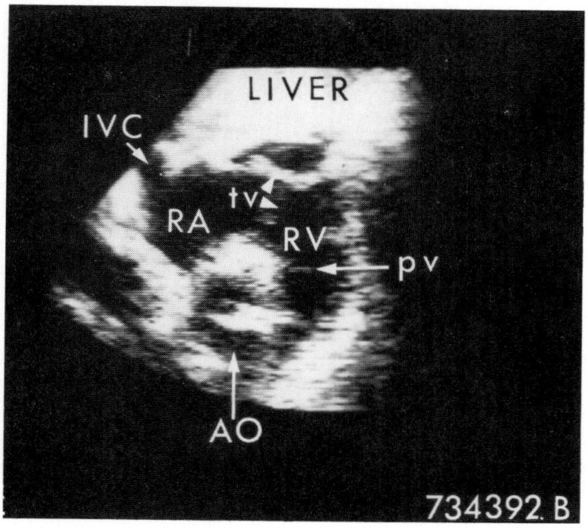

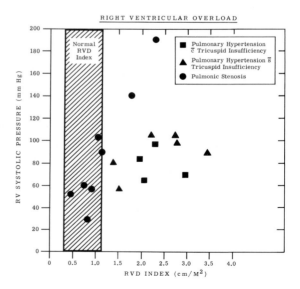

Fig. 3–62.   Subcostal examination. IVC = inferior vena cava; RA = right atrium; tv = tricuspid valve; RV = right ventricle; pv = pulmonary valve; AO = aorta.

Fig. 3–63.   Correlation of right ventricular dimension index (RVD) to right ventricular (RV) systolic pressure in patients with a right ventricular overload.

the echocardiographic estimate of the right ventricle against the right ventricular systolic pressure. In patients with pulmonic stenosis, the right ventricular pressure had to exceed 120 mmHg before an increase in right ventricular dimension was noted. However, in patients with acquired pulmonary hypertension, especially with tricuspid regurgitation, the right ventricle dilated echocardiographically at much lower systolic pressures.

Right ventricular volume overload more consistently produces dilatation of the right ventricle.[139,150,151] Most echocardiographic data with regard to right ventricular volume overload have been obtained from patients with atrial septal defect. These patients almost invariably have dilatation of the right ventricle as evidenced by an increase in the standard right ventricular dimension. The

other finding with a right ventricular volume overload is a peculiar motion of the interventricular septum.[139,150-153] The principal abnormality seen on the M-mode echocardiogram is a rapid anterior motion of the interventricular septum with the onset of ventricular systole (Fig. 3–64, arrow). This observation has fascinated echocardiographers, and a variety of theories have been proposed as to the mechanism of this pattern of motion. Studies using two-dimensional echocardiography indicate that a likely explanation for this abnormal motion is that there is an alteration in the configuration of the interventricular septum during diastole (Fig. 3–65).[154-157] The increased diastolic filling of the right ventricle apparently produces an indentation of the septum toward the left ventricle (Fig. 3–65B). With ventricular systole this indentation is rapidly

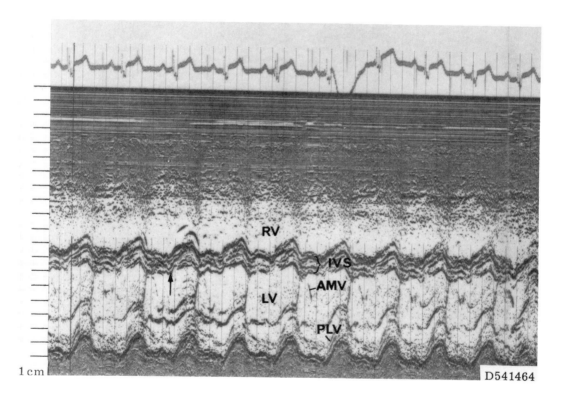

1 cm

D541464

Fig. 3–64.   Echocardiogram of the interventricular septum (IVS) in a patient with an atrial septal defect and a large left-to-right shunt. With ventricular depolarization *(arrow)*, there is a rapid upward motion of the septum. During ventricular ejection the septum gradually moves anteriorly and then posteriorly with ventricular relaxation. RV = right ventricle; LV = left ventricle; AMV = anterior mitral valve leaflet; PLV = posterior left ventricular wall. (From Dillon, J.C., Chang, S., and Feigenbaum, H.: Echocardiographic manifestations of left bundle branch block pattern. Circulation, 49:876, 1974.)

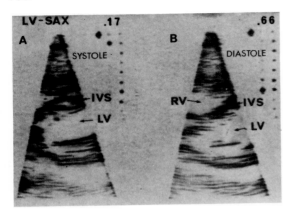

Fig. 3–65. Short-axis two-dimensional echocardiograms of the left ventricle and interventricular septum in a patient with an atrial septal defect and left-to-right shunt. *A,* At end-systole, the interventricular septum (IVS) is curved, and the left ventricle (LV) is essentially circular. *B,* With diastole, the interventricular septum flattens, and the shape of the left ventricle is distorted. RV = right ventricle. (From Weyman, A.E., et al.: Mechanism of abnormal septal motion in patients with right ventricular volume overload. Circulation, *54*:179, 1976.)

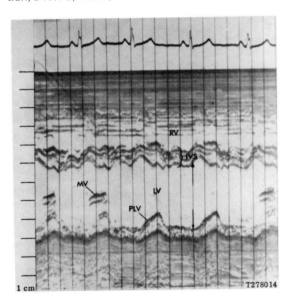

Fig. 3–66. M-mode echocardiogram of a patient with an atrial septal defect that reveals a confusing pattern of the interventricular septal motion. During much of ventricular ejection, as indicated by the motion of the posterior left ventricular wall (PLV), the left side of the septum is actually moving downward or in apposition to the posterior wall. The only abnormality is the anterior septal motion immediately after depolarization *(arrows).* MV = mitral valve; LV = left ventricle; RV = right ventricle; IVS = interventricular septum.

corrected, and the septum moves toward the right ventricle.[154,158,159]

This explanation for the abnormal septal motion in right ventricular volume overload clarifies some of the confusion concerning septal motion during ventricular ejection. In Figure 3–66, the interventricular septum moves normally toward the left ventricle during much of ventricular ejection. Although this patient has a right ventricular volume overload, the septal motion appears superficially normal. However, when examining the onset of ventricular systole (arrow), there is rapid anterior displacement of the septum similar to that seen in Figure 3–64. Thus, irrespective of how the septum moves during ventricular ejection, the motion during isovolumic contraction when the septum resumes its normal curvature (Fig. 3–65A) is the important criterion for the echocardiographic diagnosis.[29] A possible explanation for this mechanism is based on the hypothesis that interventricular septal motion reflects the relative filling of the two ventricles.

This theory can be extended to other conditions besides right ventricular volume overload. There is normally a brief posterior or downward displacement of the interventricular septum with the onset of diastole (Fig. 3–67, arrow). In certain conditions, such as mitral stenosis, this diastolic dip may be exaggerated (Fig. 3–68, arrow). Evidence indicates that this exaggerated diastolic dip in mitral stenosis again is due to unequal filling of the two ventricles and to distortion of the shape of the right ventricle.[160] Figure 3–59 is a short-axis two-dimensional echocardiogram of the left ventricle of a patient with severe mitral stenosis. During ventricular systole (Fig. 3–59A), the ventricle is circular in configuration; however, with the onset of diastole there is a marked indentation of the interventricular septum that distorts the shape of the ventricle (Fig. 3–59B, arrows). The explanation for this distortion is that the mitral stenosis restricts the filling of the left ventricle in early diastole, whereas the unobstructed tricuspid valve permits rapid filling of that ventricle. Thus in early diastole the right ventricle is filling much more rapidly than is the left, and the

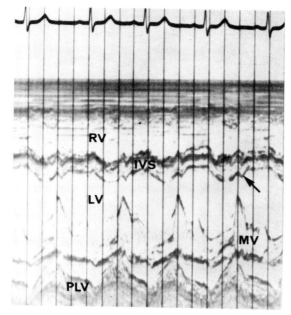

Fig. 3–67. Echocardiogram of a normal interventricular septum (IVS) demonstrating early diastolic dip *(arrow)*. RV = right ventricle; LV = left ventricle; MV = mitral valve; PLV = posterior left ventricular wall. (From Chang, S.: M-mode Echocardiographic Techniques and Pattern Recognition. Philadelphia, Lea & Febiger, 1976.)

septum bulges toward the left ventricle. It is possible that normally the more compliant right ventricle fills more rapidly than the stiffer left ventricle and that this unequal rate of filling produces the normal diastolic dip (Fig. 3–67). An alternate explanation for the diastolic dip is "twisting" of the heart at end-diastole and "untwisting" with the onset of diastole.[161]

This concept of septal motion can possibly be extended to left ventricular volume overload as well. The empirical observation is that patients with left ventricular volume overload have exaggerated septal motion. With increased diastolic filling of the left ventricle, one expects a bulging of the septum toward the right ventricle during diastole. The increased left ventricular stroke volume would then produce exaggerated septal excursion with systole. Although this aspect of the theory seems plausible, there is no proof regarding its validity.

Although there are several alternate explanations for the abnormal septal motion seen with right ventricular volume overload,[152,153,162-166] none of these are uni-

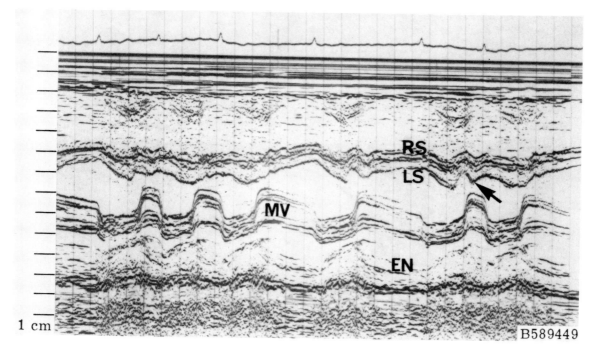

Fig. 3–68. M-mode echocardiogram of a patient with mitral stenosis demonstrating an exaggerated early diastolic dip *(arrow)*. RS = right septum; LS = left septum; MV = mitral valve; EN = posterior left ventricular endocardium.

versally accepted. Irrespective of the exact mechanism, the combination of abnormal septal motion and right ventricular dilatation has been a useful diagnostic sign of right ventricular volume overload. There is some question in the literature as to the reliability and sensitivity of this finding in certain disease states.[167,168] Atrial septal defect has been the condition most often utilized for testing these criteria. Although this topic is discussed in more detail in the chapter on congenital heart disease, it is safe to say that only rarely does a patient with an atrial septal defect and a left-to-right shunt approaching 2:1 have a totally normal M-mode echocardiogram.

The important technical detail to remember when evaluating septal motion is that distortion of the septum occurs in the body and basal portion of the heart. The indentations noted in Figures 3–58 and 3–64 are not seen at the apex. Thus septal motion is best evaluated with an M-mode scan at the level of the tips of the mitral valve or chordae. Assessing septal motion closer to the aorta is difficult because it is influenced by aortic motion. Thus septal motion should be evaluated at approximately the same level on the M-mode echocardiogram as it is when measuring right or left ventricular cavity dimensions.

LEFT ATRIUM

Thus far the discussions have begun with a description of the M-mode examination and then the two-dimensional technique. This approach has been used principally because M-mode echocardiography antedates the two-dimensional examination. In addition, it is easier to describe the function of a stationary ultrasonic beam than it is to describe a beam that moves rapidly and sections the heart. Theoretically, as one understands the principles of two-dimensional or cross-sectional imaging of the heart, it is probably more appropriate to assess the two-dimensional features of the ultrasonic recordings before discussing the M-mode examination. Since the two-dimensional examination of the left atrium has been particularly informative with regard to the M-mode examination, the order in which the left atrium is discussed will be reversed. The two-dimensional examination of this chamber is described first and is followed by discussion of the M-mode technique. It is anticipated that with increased use of instruments that provide equally good M-mode and two-dimensional recordings, the two-dimensional study will probably routinely precede the M-mode examination.

Two-dimensional Examination

Two-dimensional studies of the left atrium can be obtained with the transducer in almost any position on the chest. This chamber is commonly visualized with the transducer placed along the left sternal border (parasternal), at the apex, or in the subcostal position. Although the suprasternal two-dimen-

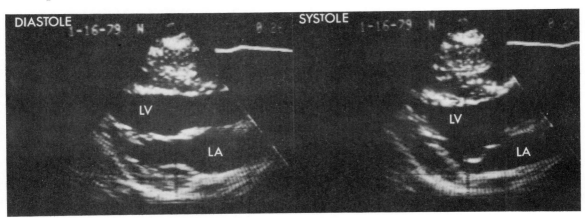

Fig. 3–69.   Long-axis, parasternal two-dimensional echocardiogram of the left ventricle (LV) and left atrium (LA) in diastole and systole.

sional study has principally been used to examine the aorta and pulmonary artery, it is also possible to obtain a two-dimensional view of the left atrium from this approach.

Figure 3–69 shows a long-axis parasternal examination of the left atrium. A short-axis parasternal examination is demonstrated in Figure 3–70. The medial border of the left atrium is comprised of the interatrial septum.[169] The lateral border is not always distinctly recorded as noted in this figure. However, the left atrial border is occasionally clear, and one can identify the left atrial appendage (LAA, Fig. 3–71).

The left atrium may also be recorded in the two apical views. Figure 3–72 demonstrates the left atrial chamber in the apical four-chamber view. Figure 3–73 shows the same atrium in the apical two-chamber view. Occasionally it is possible to see the pulmonary veins entering the left atrium in the apical four-chamber view. The subcostal examination provides another way of visualizing the left atrial chamber (Fig. 3–74).

Thus it is possible to examine the left atrium from multiple directions. Fortunately, since the left atrium is basically spherical, any one of these examinations usually suffices. In the few situations where the left

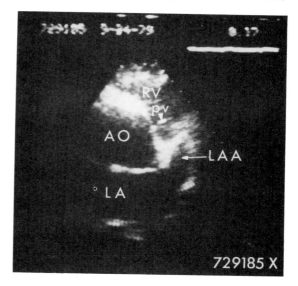

Fig. 3–71. Short-axis, parasternal two-dimensional echocardiogram of the left atrium (LA) demonstrating the left atrial appendage (LAA). AO = aorta; RV = right ventricle; pv = pulmonary valve.

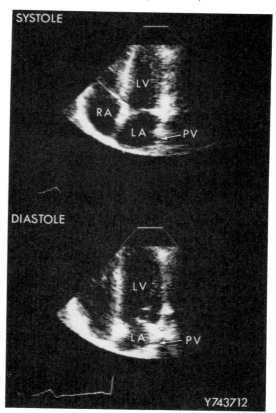

Fig. 3–72. Apical four-chamber echocardiogram demonstrating the change in left atrial size (LA) from systole to diastole. LV = left ventricle; RA = right atrium; PV = pulmonary vein.

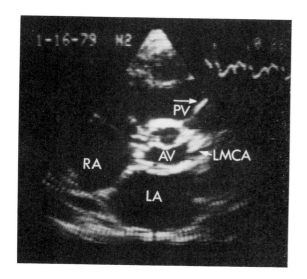

Fig. 3–70. Short-axis, parasternal examination of the left atrium (LA). RA = right atrium; AV = aortic valve; PV = pulmonary valve; LMCA = left main coronary artery.

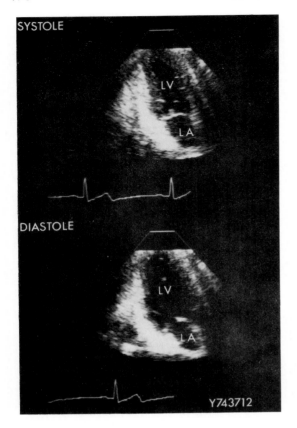

Fig. 3–73. Apical two-chamber echocardiogram demonstrating the change in size of the left atrium (LA) from systole to diastole. LV = left ventricle.

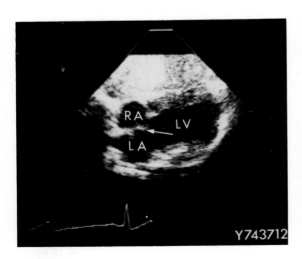

Fig. 3–74. Subcostal two-dimensional echocardiogram demonstrating the left atrium (LA), right atrium (RA), left ventricle (LV), and the interatrial septum *(arrow)*.

atrium does not assume a spherical configuration, more than one view is necessary to totally appreciate the status of this chamber. Figure 3–75 shows the usual manner in which the left atrium dilates. The chamber becomes even more spherical than is normal, and both the long-axis and short-axis views are quite circular. In the long-axis view, the aorta is displaced anteriorly and the posterior left atrial wall is displaced posteriorly. In the short-axis view, the interatrial septum is displaced to the right.

A potential problem that has arisen with regard to judging the left atrium with two-dimensional echocardiography is that of side lobes. A frequent location for side lobe production is the posterior atrioventricular

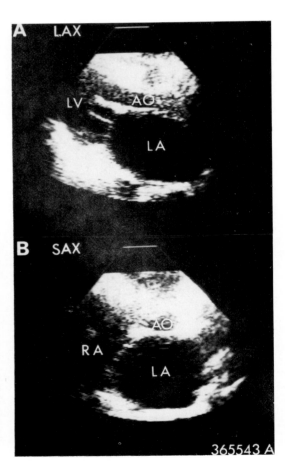

Fig. 3–75. Parasternal long-axis (LAX) and short-axis (SAX) two-dimensional echocardiograms of a patient with a markedly dilated left atrium (LA). AO = aorta; LV = left ventricle; RA = right atrium.

groove. A band of curved, bright echoes may originate from that area of the heart. With a normal-sized left atrium, the band of echoes occurs at the level of the posterior left atrial wall and is usually obscured by echoes posterior to the left atrium. However, if the left atrium is enlarged, as in Figure 3–76, the posterior displacement of the atrial wall permits visualization of the side lobe echoes within the cavity of the left atrium. Fortunately, if one recognizes the side lobes, the angle of the transducer can be changed slightly to eliminate or diminish the side lobes.

Another frequently seen and confusing echocardiogram is demonstrated in Figure 3–77. The left atrium is dilated, and there is a band of faint echoes immediately anterior to the posterior left atrial wall (Fig. 3–77A, arrows). The origin of these echoes is not entirely clear. A similar band of echoes is frequently seen in M-mode tracings as well. One possibility is that some of these echoes may result from relatively stagnant, slow-moving blood in this area of the dilated left

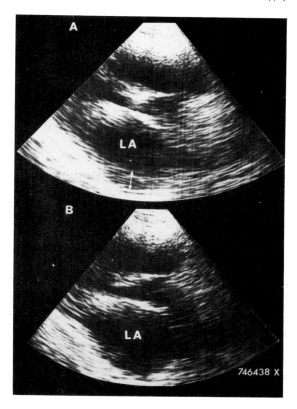

Fig. 3–77. Long-axis parasternal views of the left atrium demonstrating a band of faint echoes (arrows) along the posterior left atrial wall, A. These echoes can be eliminated by changes in angulation and a decrease in gain, B.

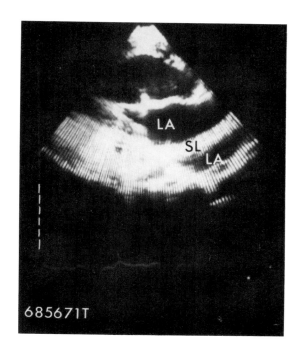

Fig. 3–76. Long-axis parasternal echocardiogram of a patient with a dilated left atrium (LA) showing how a side lobe artifact (SL) can appear within the echo-free cavity of the left atrium.

atrium. An alternate explanation is that this band of echoes could represent side lobe artifacts similar to those seen in Figure 3–76. Figure 3–77B shows how the band of echoes can be minimized or eliminated with slight changes in angulation of the transducer.

In Figures 3–69, 3–72, and 3–73, one can see a definite change in the size of the left atrium from systole to diastole. The left atrium is largest at end-systole immediately before the mitral valve opens and reaches its smallest volume at end-diastole following atrial systole. Attempts at measuring left atrial volume from the two-dimensional echocardiogram have been made.[170] Unfortunately, this technique is still in a preliminary stage and requires confirmation. As noted in the discussion of the M-mode examination, the left atrial M-mode dimension is one of the basic M-mode measurements. Although there are limitations, this measurement has withstood the test of time and is used routinely. As long as the left atrium enlarges in a symmetric fashion, as seen in Figure 3–75, one can see why a single dimension through the center of the chamber gives an accurate assessment of its size and volume. However, the left atrium may not always enlarge symmetrically,[171] or it may be compressed by an enlarged aorta or be distorted by a chest deformity. Thus the simple anterior-posterior dimension may be misleading. In such cases, the two-dimensional technique may indeed more accurately assess left atrial volume than would a single M-mode dimension. One possible approach is to qualitatively assess the shape of the atrium with the two-dimensional study. If the chamber is spherical, then one can merely use the M-mode examination for quantitative measurements. If, however, the two-dimensional study demonstrates a nonspherical left atrium, then either two-dimensional echocardiography or a modified M-mode approach may provide a more accurate assessment of chamber volume.

M-mode Examination

As the ultrasonic beam is directed superiorly and medially from the mitral valve and left ventricle, the transducer points toward the base of the heart, which consists of the aorta and left atrium (AO and LA, Fig. 3–78). The aorta is readily identified by the two parallel-moving echoes that move upward in systole and downward in diastole. Posterior to the aorta lies the left atrium (LA, Fig. 3–78). As the ultrasonic beam moves from the vicinity of the left ventricle into the left atrium, the posterior cardiac wall echoes change their motion. Behind the mitral valve echoes we see the posterior left ventricular wall moving anteriorly with systole and posteriorly with diastole. In the body of the left atrium (LA), the posterior cardiac echo moves minimally and represents the posterior wall of the left atrium. Between these two areas is a transition zone whereby the posterior cardiac echoes change their pattern of motion so that with ventricular systole the wall moves posteriorly rather than anteriorly. This area coincides with the disappearance of the posterior mitral valve echo and represents that portion of the left atrium

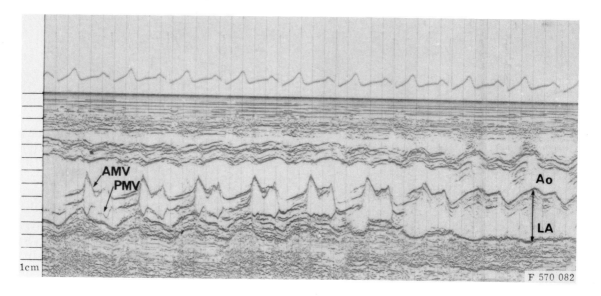

Fig. 3–78.   M-mode echocardiographic scan from the left ventricle and mitral valve leaflets to the aorta (AO) and left atrium (LA). The standard left atrial dimension *(arrow)* represents the distance between the atrial side of the posterior aortic wall and the anterior surface of the posterior left atrial echo at the level of the aortic valve leaflets. AMV = anterior mitral valve leaflet; PMV = posterior mitral valve leaflet. (From Chang, S.: M-mode Echocardiographic Techniques and Pattern Recognition. Philadelphia, Lea & Febiger, 1976.)

that demonstrates marked changes in the cardiac cycle.

The echocardiographic examination just described permits one to obtain an anterior-posterior dimension of the left atrium.[172–174] Figure 3–78 shows how such a left atrial dimension can be obtained (arrow). In this tracing, the measurement is taken from the trailing edge of the echo dividing the aorta from the left atrium to the leading edge of the echo originating from the posterior left atrial wall. The measurement is taken in the vicinity of the aortic valves and is obtained at the maximum upward motion of the aortic wall, which represents end-systole. According to ASE criteria, the left atrial dimension should be taken from the leading edge of the posterior aortic wall to the leading edge of the posterior left atrial wall (LAD–ASE, Fig. 3–79). As noted in Figures 3–78 and 3–79, the echoes can be very thin, and the differences would represent no more than a millimeter or two. However, with some instruments the width of the posterior aortic wall may be quite significant, especially if axial

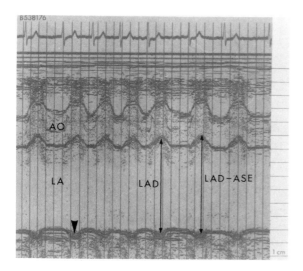

Fig. 3–79. M-mode echocardiogram of the aorta (AO) and left atrium (LA) in a patient with mitral regurgitation exhibiting posterior displacement of the left atrial wall in systole (arrowhead). LAD = left atrial dimension from trailing edge of posterior aortic wall to leading edge of posterior left atrial wall; LAD–ASE = left atrial dimension from leading edge of posterior aortic wall to leading edge of posterior left atrial wall, as recommended by the American Society of Echocardiography.

resolution is poor. Since echocardiographs taken with thin, high-axial resolution instruments are most commonly used and since the ASE criteria are fairly recent, most normal data in the literature are taken from the trailing edge of the posterior aortic wall (LAD, Fig. 3–79) rather than from the leading edge. It is not always easy to clearly identify the posterior left atrial wall to make the proper left atrial dimension. Figure 3–80 demonstrates the confusion that may frequently arise as to where the left atrial dimension should be obtained. Anterior to the posterior left atrial wall are multiple echoes, many of which are relatively indistinct. These echoes seen on the M-mode echocardiogram probably correspond to those demonstrated on the two-dimensional studies in Figure 3–77. The origin of these echoes is still not determined. Occurring most often with dilated left atrium in patients with mitral stenosis, they may originate from relatively stagnant blood layered against the left atrial wall. As indicated in Figure 3–76, an alternate explanation may be artifact partially owing to side lobes. In any case, the correct left atrial dimension is usually more posterior than is the band of indistinct echoes.

The location in the cardiac cycle from which the left atrial dimension is taken has customarily been at end-systole, where the maximum left atrial dimension occurs. This technique was first utilized because this measurement provided the largest left atrial dimension and because the upward motion of the posterior aortic wall was convenient for measurement. Although other areas of the cardiac cycle have been recommended for left atrial dimensions, the end-systolic location continues to be most often used and is recommended by the Society.

Another way of assessing left atrial size is to compare the left atrial dimension with the diameter of the aorta.[175] In the normal patient the diameter of the aorta and that of the left atrium are about equal. As the left atrium dilates, this relationship changes with the left atrial dimension becoming significantly larger than that of the aorta. Figure 3–79 demonstrates a patient with a markedly enlarged left atrium. By any criteria the left

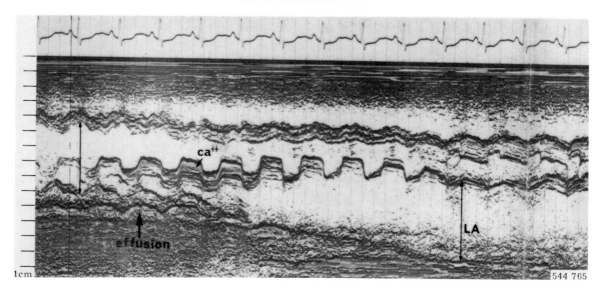

Fig. 3–80.   M-mode scan of a patient with calcific mitral valve and a dilated left atrium (LA). A band of fuzzy echoes are visible along the posterior left atrial wall. (From Chang, S.: M-mode Echocardiographic Techniques and Pattern Recognition. Philadelphia, Lea & Febiger, 1976.)

atrial cavity is well beyond the limits of normal. The diameter is over 6 cm, which is extremely large. Many articles in the literature correlate echocardiography and angiography for judging the size of the left atrium. The correlations have been extremely good with almost all having approximate R values of 0.9. The M-mode left atrial dimension is clearly better than merely looking at the plain chest roentgenogram for judging left atrial enlargement. Although the technique originally recommended correcting the dimension for body surface area, it is debatable whether the body surface area is in fact useful in comparing one individual with another. The aorta-left atrium ratio was recommended as a better technique to correct for size of the patient rather than using the body surface area. As expected, this ratio is used rather extensively in pediatric echocardiography. Other authors believe that merely taking the uncorrected left atrial dimension and comparing it to known normal values (see Appendix) is the best way of judging whether or not the chamber is dilated.[140]

Irrespective of exactly how the left atrium is measured, this echocardiographic dimension has proved useful.[176] The size of the left atrium is important in patients with mitral

valve disease and in patients with chronic left ventricular failure. One study shows the relationship between the echocardiographic measurement of the left atrium and the presence of atrial fibrillation.[177] Another important clinical use of the echocardiographic left atrial measurement is in infants with left-to-right shunts, such as patent ductus arteriosus[178] or ventricular septal defect. These infants may manifest heart failure or respiratory distress,[179,180] and the mere finding of a dilated left atrium may be extremely important diagnostically. In addition, the size of the left atrium gives semiquantitative information as to the size of the shunt.[140,181,182] Figure 3–81 shows serial left atrial echocardiograms from an infant with a patent ductus arteriosus. The preoperative recording shows a dilated left atrium. The dimension is considerably larger than the aorta. Within one hour following closure of the ductus, the size of the left atrium significantly decreases. Twelve hours after surgical closure of the ductus, the left atrium is diminished even further. Closure of a patent ductus may occur spontaneously or with medication. Thus serial echocardiograms can be extremely useful in following patients with this particular problem.

The left atrium may also be examined with

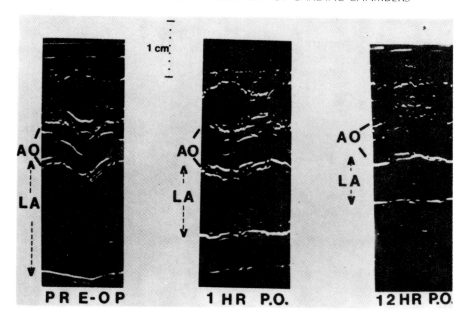

Fig. 3–81.   Serial left atrial echocardiograms of an infant with a patent ductus arteriosus before *(pre-op)* and after *(p.o.)* closure of a patent ductus arteriosus. A dramatic decrease in the size of the left atrium can be noted as soon as one hour after surgery and is further decreased 12 hours after surgery. AO = aorta; LA = left atrium. (From Goldberg, S.J., Allen, H.D., and Sahn, D.J.: Pediatric and Adolescent Echocardiography. Chicago, Year-book Medical Publishers, Inc., 1975.)

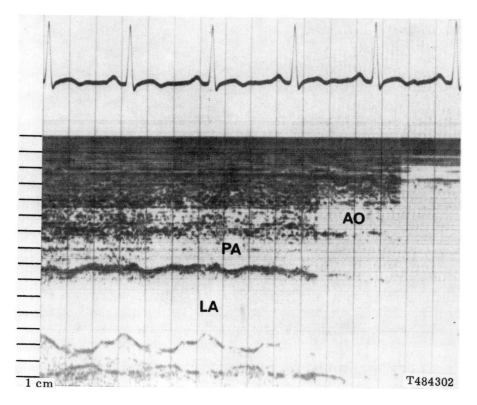

Fig. 3–82.   M-mode echocardiographic appearance of the arch of the aorta (AO), right pulmonary artery (PA), and left atrium (LA) with the transducer pointed inferiorly in the suprasternal notch. This patient had a normal-sized left atrium.

the transducer placed in the suprasternal notch pointed inferiorly and slightly to the left.[183,184] With the transducer in this position, the ultrasonic beam passes through the arch of the aorta, the right pulmonary artery, and the left atrium. Figure 3–82 is an echocardiogram taken with the transducer in the suprasternal notch in a patient with a normal left atrium. A similar examination taken from a patient with a dilated left atrium is shown in Figure 3–83. Although this approach has had relatively little use in examining the left atrium, there may be several patients in whom this left atrial dimension may be a useful supplement to the standard measurement taken from the left sternal border.[140,185] Figure 3–84 shows left atrial measurements taken from the same patient with the transducer placed along the left sternal border and in the suprasternal notch. The left atrial measurement is slightly larger with the suprasternal approach, but the mea-

surements are otherwise comparable. The echocardiograms in Figure 3–85 show a situation in which the two left atrial dimensions are significantly different. In a patient with severe pectus excavatum, there may be considerable difference in the left atrial dimension depending on the orientation of the ultrasonic beam. Because of the chest deformity, there may be a much smaller left atrial dimension with the parasternal approach than with the suprasternal technique. The patient in Figure 3–85, in fact, had a dilated left atrium, and the standard precordial examination would have underestimated the size of this chamber. This patient might have benefitted from an initial two-dimensional examination. The two-dimensional study would have recognized the nonspherical configuration of the left atrium and revealed that a single anterior-posterior M-mode dimension would not provide an accurate assessment of the size of the left atrium.

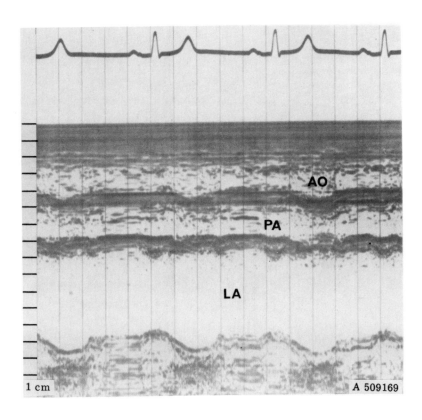

Fig. 3–83.   Echocardiographic examination similar to that in Figure 3–82 except that this patient had a dilated left atrium.

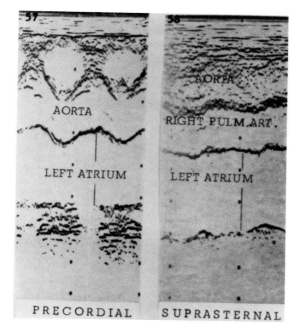

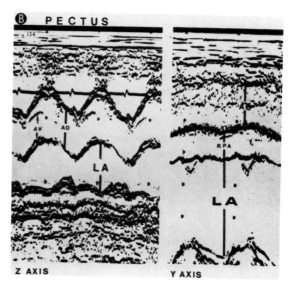

Fig. 3–84. Echocardiographic examination of the left atrium of the same patient using both parasternal (precordial) and suprasternal approaches. (From Goldberg, S.J., Allen, H.D., and Sahn, D.J.: Pediatric and Adolescent Echocardiography. Chicago, Yearbook Medical Publishers, Inc., 1975.)

Fig. 3–85. Parasternal *(z axis)* and suprasternal *(y axis)* left atrial echocardiograms of a patient with pectus excavatum. Because of the chest deformity, the anterior-posterior dimension (z axis) of the left atrium (LA) is significantly smaller than that obtained from the superior-inferior approach (y axis). AO = aorta; AV = aortic valve; RPA = right pulmonary artery. (From Goldberg, S.J., Allen, H.D., and Sahn, D.J.: Pediatric and Adolescent Echocardiography. Chicago, Yearbook Medical Publishers, Inc., 1975.)

Left Atrial Wall Motion

Figure 3–86 is an M-mode scan of a normal left atrium, with the ultrasonic beam passing from the left ventricle into the left atrium. The excursions of the posterior left atrial wall next to the left ventricle (LA) are fairly distinct. As the beam moves superiorly and medially toward the aortic root, the posterior left atrial wall motion is reduced. Since a good recording of the aortic root is necessary for the standard anteroposterior left atrial dimension, this measurement is usually taken at the level at which the posterior left atrial pulsations are dampened and usually absent. Thus left atrial wall motion is usually not appreciated during the typical left atrial examination at the base of the heart. Although little has been written about left atrial wall motion, this motion occasionally provides some useful information.[186,186a] First, the pattern of left atrial wall pulsations must be distinguished from that of left ventricular pulsations.[187] This is easily done

since the two structures move in opposite directions during ventricular systole.

When the ultrasonic beam transects the aorta and aortic valve, the posterior left atrial wall motion is normally negligible. There is virtually no significant posterior left atrial wall motion, even with a dilated chamber. Occasionally, one sees significant pulsations of the posterior left atrial wall in patients with mitral regurgitation (Fig. 3–79, arrowhead).[188] When present at this level, the systolic expansion of the posterior left atrial wall is indicative of mitral regurgitation. Unfortunately, most patients with mitral regurgitation do not demonstrate such systolic expansion.

Patients with mitral regurgitation may have increased motion at the atrioventricular junction. Such motion again may be indicative of increased left atrial stroke volume secondary to mitral regurgitation. However, there must be caution in judging motion of the atrioventricular junction on the M-mode

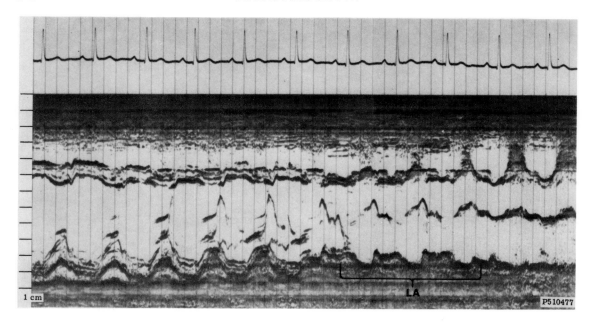

Fig. 3–86.   M-mode scan from the left ventricle to the left atrium. The best excursion of the posterior left atrial wall was seen at the junction between the posterior left ventricular wall and the left atrium (LA).

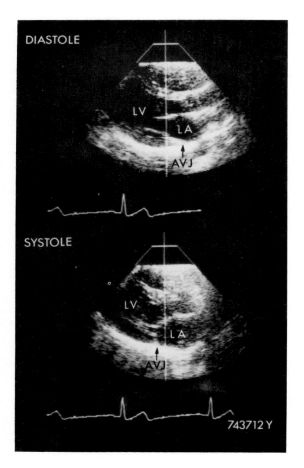

Fig. 3–87.   Long-axis, parasternal two-dimensional echocardiograms demonstrating the mobility of the atrioventricular junction (AVJ) from diastole to systole. The M-mode ultrasonic beam *(white line)* can examine the left ventricular wall in diastole and the left atrial wall in systole without changing the direction of the transducer. LV = left ventricle; LA = left atrium.

echocardiogram. Figure 3–87 demonstrates that there is considerable mobility in the superior-inferior direction of this portion of the heart. The motion seen on the M-mode echocardiogram may be interpreted as anterior-posterior motion of the left atrial wall when in fact one is merely recording different areas of the heart during the cardiac cycle. During systole the atrioventricular junction moves toward the apex of the heart, and the ultrasonic beam may be transecting the left atrium (Fig. 3–87B). With diastole the atrioventricular junction moves toward the base of the heart, and the stationary ultrasonic beam now transects the left ventricle (Fig. 3–87A). Thus at the atrioventricular junction (Fig. 3–86, bracket), one may be recording the left ventricle during diastole and the left atrium during systole.

Numerous reports indicate that if changes in left atrial volume are to be recorded, then the motion of the posterior wall of the aorta, which is the same as that of the anterior wall of the left atrium, should be scrutinized.[189,190] The two-dimensional echocardiograms of the left atrium (Figs. 3–69, 3–72, 3–73) demonstrate that the principal change in left atrial volume is a result of displacement of the aorta and not of motion of the posterior left atrial wall. Thus it is not surprising that the posterior aortic wall has been used to judge both absolute and relative changes in left atrial volume. This topic is discussed in more detail in the following chapter on hemodynamics.

RIGHT ATRIUM

The right atrium has been the neglected chamber in echocardiography, partially because of the difficulty in viewing this chamber. Much of the right atrium lies directly beneath the sternum and is somewhat difficult to examine echocardiographically. Although there have been some efforts to study the right atrium by way of M-mode echocardiography, most of the recent interest in examining this chamber is with two-dimensional echocardiography. The M-mode observations have principally documented the location of the interatrial septum, and thus prove that one can see portions of the right atrial cavity by way of the M-mode technique.[191] Both the left and right parasternal transducer positions have been used to make these M-mode observations. An M-mode technique has even been described for obtaining a right atrial dimension with the transducer along the left sternal border.[192–194]

It is much easier to see the right atrium by way of two-dimensional echocardiography. The left parasternal examination of the right ventricular inflow tract routinely records a large portion of the right atrium (Fig. 3–88). The apical four-chamber view also provides a reasonably good assessment of the right atrial cavity (Figs. 3–60, 3–72).[147–194a] In fact, a technique for measuring the size of the right atrium by using the apical four-chamber view has been described.[147] Figure 3–89 demonstrates an apical four-chamber view of the right atrium and shows a dramatic

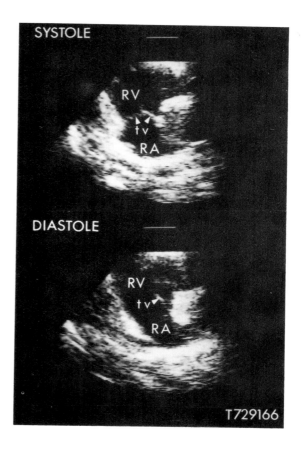

Fig. 3–88. Long-axis parasternal examination of the right ventricle (RV), the tricuspid valve (tv), and the right atrium (RA) in systole and diastole.

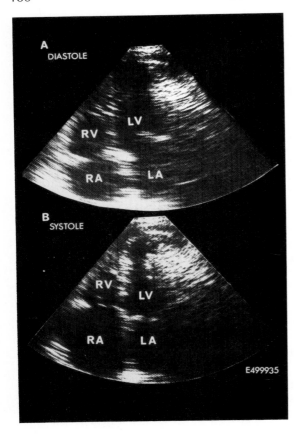

Fig. 3–89. Apical four-chamber views demonstrating a dramatic change in the size of the right atrium (RA) from diastole, *A*, to systole, *B*, in a patient with tricuspid stenosis and regurgitation. RV = right ventricle; LV = left ventricle; LA = left atrium.

change in the right atrial volume from diastole to systole. This patient had tricuspid stenosis and regurgitation with a large right atrial stroke volume. The subcostal approach can also be used to record the right atrial cavity (Fig. 3–74). However, this approach has not been suggested for quantitative assessment of the right atrium.

Thus echocardiographic recording of the right atrium is being done routinely with the two-dimensional approach. A semiquantitative assessment of the size of the right atrium is quite feasible. It is hoped that some reproducible technique for judging the size of the right atrium is forthcoming. The two-dimensional examination is of sufficient clarity to identify the inferior vena cava draining into the right atrium and to identify such structures as the eustachian valve. Because of the unusual location of the right atrium from an echocardiographic point of view, one can anticipate that the two-dimensional technique will become the examination of choice for assessing this chamber.

REFERENCES

1. Corya, B.C., Feigenbaum, H., Rasmussen, S., and Black, M.J.: Anterior left ventricular wall echoes in coronary artery disease. Linear scanning with a single element transducer. Am. J. Cardiol., 34:652, 1974.
2. Chang, S. and Feigenbaum, H.: Subxiphoid echocardiography. J. Clin. Ultrasound, 1:14, 1973.
3. Chang, S., Feigenbaum, H., and Dillon, J.C.: Subxiphoid echocardiography: a review. Chest, 68:233, 1975.
4. Starling, M.R., Crawford, M.H., O'Rourke, R.A., Groves, B.M., and Amon, K.W.: Accuracy of subxiphoid echocardiography for assessing left ventricular size and performance. Circulation, 61:367, 1980.
5. Popp, R.L. and Harrison, D.C.: Ultrasonic cardiac echography for determining stroke volume and valvular regurgitation. Circulation, 41:493, 1970.
6. Pombo, J.F., Troy, B.L., and Russell, R.O., Jr.: Left ventricular volumes and ejection fraction by echocardiography. Circulation, 43:480, 1971.
7. Feigenbaum, H., Wolfe, S.B., Popp, R.L., Haine, C.L., and Dodge, H.T.: Correlation of ultrasound with angiocardiography in measuring left ventricular diastolic volume. Am. J. Cardiol., 23:111, 1969. (Abstract)
8. Feigenbaum, H., et al.: Ultrasound measurements of the left ventricle: a correlative study with angiocardiography. Arch. Intern. Med., 129:461, 1972.
9. Fortuin, N.J., Hood, W.P., Jr., and Craige, E.: Evaluation of left ventricular function by echocardiography. Circulation, 46:26, 1972.
10. Gibson, D.G.: Estimation of left ventricular size by echocardiography. Br. Heart J., 35:128, 1973.
11. Abbasi, A.S., MacAlpin, R.N., Eber, L.M., and Pearce, M.L.: Left ventricular hypertrophy diagnosed by echocardiography. N. Engl. J. Med., 289:118, 1973.
12. Askanas, A., Rajszys, R., and Sandowski, Z.: Measurement of the thickness of the left ventricular wall in man using the ultrasound technique. Pol. Med. J., 9:62, 1970.
13. Feigenbaum, H., Popp, R.L., Chip, J.N., and Haine, C.L.: Left ventricular wall thickness measured by ultrasound. Arch. Intern. Med., 121:391, 1968.
14. Grossman, W., McLaurin, L.P., Moos, S.P., Stefadouros, M.A., and Young, D.T.: Wall thickness and diastolic properties of the left ventricle. Circulation, 49:129, 1974.
15. Sjogren, A.L., Hytonen, I., and Frick, M.H.: Ultrasonic measurements of left ventricular wall thickness. Chest, 57:37, 1970.
16. Troy, B.L., Pombo, J., and Rackley, C.E.: Measurement of left ventricular wall thickness and mass by echocardiography. Circulation, 45:602, 1972.

17. Wirth, J. and Wenzelides, K.: Heart muscle thickening measurement with ultrasound. Cor. Vasa., *12*:112, 1970.

18. Gaasch, W.H.: Left ventricular radius to wall thickness ratio. Am. J. Cardiol., *43*:1189, 1979.

19. Gutgesell, H.P., Paquet, M., Duff, D.F., and McNamara, D.G.: Evaluation of left ventricular size and function by echocardiography. Results in normal children. Circulation, *56*:457, 1977.

20. Chen, W. and Gibson, D.: Relation of isovolumic relaxation to left ventricular wall movement in man. Br. Heart J., *42*:51, 1979.

21. Marsh, J.D., Green, L.H., Wynne, J., Cohn, P.F., and Grossman, W.: Linearity of left ventricular end-systolic pressure-dimension relations in man, and sensitivity to inotropic state. Circulation (Suppl. II), *58*:23, 1978. (Abstract)

22. Dumesnil, J.G., Shoucri, R.M., Laurenceau, J-L., and Turcot, J.: A mathematical model of the dynamic geometry of the intact left ventricle and its applications to clinical data. Circulation, *59*:1024, 1979.

23. Sahn, D.J., DeMaria, A., Kisslo, J., and Weyman, A.: Recommendations regarding quantitation in M-mode echocardiography: results of a survey of echocardiographic measurements. Circulation, *58*:1072, 1978.

24. Crawford, M.H., Grant, D., O'Rourke, R.A., Starling, M.R., and Groves, B.M.: Accuracy and reproducibility of new M-mode echocardiographic recommendations for measuring left ventricular dimensions. Circulation, *61*:137, 1980.

25. Gibson, D.G.: Measurement of left ventricular volumes in man by echocardiography—comparison with biplane angiographs. Br. Heart J., *33*:614, 1971.

26. Chapelle, M. and Mensch, B.: Etude des variations du diametre ventriculaire gauche chez l'homme par echocardiographic transthoracique. Arch. Mal. Coeur, *11*:1505, 1969.

27. Fortuin, N.J., Hood, W.P., Jr., Sherman, E., and Craige, E.: Determinations of left ventricular volumes by ultrasound. Circulation, *44*:575, 1971.

28. Teichholz, L.E., Kreulen, T., Herman, M.V., and Gorlin, R.: Problems in echocardiographic volume determinations: echocardiographic-angiographic correlations in the presence or absence of asynergy. Am. J. Cardiol., *37*:7, 1976.

29. Bhatt, D.R., Isabel-Jones, J.B., Villoria, G.J., Nakazawa, M., Yabek, S.M., Marks, R.A., and Jarmakani, J.M.: Accuracy of echocardiography in assessing left ventricular dimensions and volume. Circulation, *57*:699, 1978.

30. Antani, J.A., Wayne, H.H., and Kuzman, W.J.: Ejection phase indexes by invasive and noninvasive methods: an apexcardiographic, echocardiographic, and ventriculographic correlative study. Am. J. Cardiol., *43*:239, 1979.

31. Martin, M.A.: Assessment of correction formula for echocardiographic estimation of left ventricular volume. Br. Heart J., *40*:294, 1978.

32. Baba, K., Kaneko, H., Echigo, S., Kamiya, T., Ohta, M., Kozuka, T., Nagata, M., and Beppu, S.: Comparative studies between angiocardiographic and echocardiographic methods for evaluating left ventricular function in children with heart disease. J. Cardiogr., *8*:439, 1978.

33. Kronik, G., Slany, J., and Mosslacher, H.: Comparative value of eight M-mode echocardiographic formulas for determining left ventricular stroke volume. A correlative study with thermodilution and left ventricular single-plane cineangiography. Circulation, *60*:1308, 1979.

34. Reference deleted.

35. Tamura, T., Natsume, T., Nishida, K., Machii, K., Yamaguchi, T., Umeda, T., and Matsuda, M.: Echocardiographic left ventricular volume determination by direct measurements of the major and minor axes. J. Cardiogr., *6*:653, 1976.

36. Benzing, G., Stockert, J., Nave, E., and Kaplan, S.: Evaluation of left ventricular performance: circumferential fiber shortening and tension. Circulation, *49*:925, 1974.

37. Cooper, R., Karliner, J.S., O'Rourke, R.A., Peterson, K.L., and Leopold, G.R.: Ultrasound determinations of mean fiber-shortening rate in man. Am. J. Cardiol., *29*:257, 1972.

38. Cooper, R.H., O'Rourke, R.A., Karliner, J.S., Peterson, K.L., and Leopold, G.R.: Comparison of ultrasound and cineangiographic measurements of the mean rate of circumferential shortening in man. Circulation, *46*:914, 1972.

39. Ludbrook, P., Karliner, J.S., Peterson, K., Leopold, G., and O'Rourke, R.A.: Comparison of ultrasound and cineangiographic measurements of left ventricular performance in patients with and without wall motion abnormalities. Br. Heart J., *35*:1026, 1973.

40. Paraskos, J.A., Grossman, W., Saltz, S., Dalen, J.E., and Dexter, L.: A noninvasive technique for the determination of circumferential fiber shortening in man. Circ. Res., *29*:610, 1971.

41. Quinones, M.A., Gaasch, W.H., and Alexander, J.K.: Echocardiographic assessment of left ventricular function: with special reference to normalized velocities. Circulation, *50*:42, 1974.

42. Quinones, M.A., Gaasch, W.H., and Alexander, J.K.: Influence of acute changes in preload, afterload, contractile state, and heart rate on ejection and isovolumic indices of myocardial contractility in man. Circulation, *53*:293, 1976.

43. Mathey, D.G., Decoodt, P.R., Allen, H.N., and Swan, H.J.C.: Abnormal left ventricular contraction pattern in the systolic click-late systolic murmur syndrome. Circulation, *56*:311, 1977.

44. Weiss, J.L., Weisfeldt, M.L., Mason, S.J., Garrison, J.B., Livengood, S.V., and Fortuin, N.J.: Evidence of Frank-Starling effect in man during severe semisupine exercise. Circulation, *59*:655, 1979.

45. Quinones, M.A., Pickering, E., and Alexander, J.K.: Percentage of shortening of the echocardiographic left ventricular dimension. Its use in determining ejection fraction and stroke volume. Chest, *74*:59, 1978.

46. Orlando, E., D'Antuono, G., Cipolla, C., et al.: Analysis of left ventricular wall motion by means of ultrasound. G. Ital. Cardiol., *2*:234, 1972.

47. Pernod, J., Terdjman, M., Kermaree, J., and Haguenauer, G.: Myocardial contraction: study by ultrasonic echography (results in 200 normal patients). Nouv. Presse Med., *2*:2393, 1973.

48. St. John-Sutton, M.G., Tajik, A.J., Gibson, D.G., Brown, D.J., Seward, J.B., and Giuliani, E.R.: Echocardiographic assessment of left ventricular filling and septal and posterior wall dynamics in idiopathic hypertrophic subaortic stenosis. Circulation, *57*:512, 1978.

49. Upton, M.T., Gibson, D.G., and Brown, D.J.:

Echocardiographic assessment of abnormal left ventricular relaxation in man. Br. Heart J., 38:1001, 1976.

50. Traill, T.A., Gibson, D.G., and Brown, D.J.: Study of left ventricular wall thickness and dimension changes using echocardiography. Br. Heart J., 40:162, 1978.

51. Gibson, D.G., Brown, D.J., and Logan-Sinclair, R.B.: Analysis of regional left ventricular wall movement by phased array echocardiography. Br. Heart J., 40:1334, 1978.

51a.Friedman, M.J., Sahn, D.J., Burris, H.A., Allen, H.D., and Goldberg, S.J.: Computerized echocardiographic analysis to detect abnormal systolic and diastolic left ventricular function in children with aortic stenosis. Am. J. Cardiol., 44:478, 1979.

52. Corya, B.C., Rasmussen, S., Feigenbaum, H., Knoebel, S.B., and Black, M.J.: Systolic thickening and thinning of the septum and posterior wall in patients with coronary artery disease, congestive cardiomyopathy, and atrial septal defect. Circulation, 55:109, 1977.

53. Mirro, M.J., Rogers, E.W., Weyman, A.E., and Feigenbaum, H.: Angular displacement of the papillary muscles during the cardiac cycle. Circulation, 60:327, 1979.

54. Sanderson, J.E., Traill, T.A., St. John-Sutton, M.G., Brown, D.J., Gibson, D.G., and Goodwin, J.F.: Left ventricular relaxation and filling in hypertrophic cardiomyopathy: an echocardiographic study. Br. Heart J., 40:596, 1978.

55. St. John-Sutton, M.G., Traill, T.A., Ghafour, A.S., Brown, D.J., and Gibson, D.G.: Echocardiographic assessment of left ventricular filling after mitral valve surgery. Br. Heart J., 39:1283, 1977.

56. Siegert, R., Hanrath, P., Bleifeld, W., Kupper, W., and Mathey, D.: Abnormal relaxation and diastolic filling pattern in different forms of LV hypertrophy. Circulation (Suppl. II), 58:52, 1978. (Abstract)

57. Doran, J.H., Traill, T.A., Brown, D.J., and Gibson, D.G.: Detection of abnormal left ventricular wall movement during isovolumic contraction and early relaxation: comparison of echo- and angiocardiography. Br. Heart J., 40:367, 1978.

58. Lewis, B.S., Moskowitz, S.E., and Gotsman, M.S.: Left ventricular wall thickness during the isovolumic relaxation period. Isr. J. Med. Sci., 14:436, 1978.

59. Anderson, P.A.W., Manring, A., Serwer, G.A., Benson, D.W., Edwards, S.B., Armstrong, B.E., Sterba, R.J., and Floyd, R.D.: The force-interval relationship of the left ventricle. Circulation, 60:334, 1979.

60. Hess, O.M., Grimm, J., and Krayenbuehl, H.P.: Diastolic simple elastic and viscoelastic properties of the left ventricle in man. Circulation, 59:1178, 1979.

61. Spotnitz, H.M., Bregman, D., Bowman, F.O., Edie, R.N., Reemtsma, K., King, D.L., Hoffman, B.F., and Malm, J.R.: Effects of open heart surgery on end-diastolic pressure-diameter relations of the human left ventricle. Circulation, 59:662, 1979.

62. Gibson, D.G. and Brown, D.J.: Assessment of left ventricular systolic function in man from simultaneous echocardiographic and pressure measurements. Br. Heart J., 38:8, 1976.

63. Reference deleted.

64. Devereux, R.B. and Reichek, N.: Echocardiographic determination of left ventricular mass in man. Anatomic validation of the method. Circulation, 55:613, 1977.

65. Sasayama, S., Franklin, D., Ross, J., Kemper, W.S., and McKown, D.: Dynamic changes in left ventricular wall thickness and their use in analyzing cardiac function in the conscious dog: a study based on a modified ultrasonic technique. Am. J. Cardiol., 38:870, 1976.

66. McFarland, T.M., Alam, M., Goldstein, S., Pickard, S.D., and Stein, P.D.: Echocardiographic diagnosis of left ventricular hypertrophy. Circulation, 57:1140, 1978.

67. Bennett, D.H. and Evans, D.W.: Correlation of left ventricular mass determined by echocardiography with vectorcardiographic and electrocardiographic voltage measurements. Br. Heart J., 36:981, 1974.

68. Machida, K., Yasukochi, H., Tada, S., Oshima, M., and Hackimori, K.: Ultrasonic measurements of left ventricular volume, mass, and velocity of posterior wall movement in children. Nippon Acta Radiol., 33:617, 1973.

69. Troy, B.L., Pombo, J., and Rackley, C.E.: Measurement of left ventricular wall thickness and mass by echocardiography. Circulation, 45:602, 1972.

70. Glanz, S., Hellenbrand, W.E., Berman, M.A., and Talner, N.S.: Echocardiographic assessment of the severity of aortic stenosis in children and adolescents. Am. J. Cardiol., 38:620, 1976.

71. Aziz, K.U., vanGrondelle, A., Paul, M.H., and Muster, A.J.: Echocardiographic assessment of the relation between left ventricular wall and cavity dimensions and peak systolic pressure in children with aortic stenosis. Am. J. Cardiol., 40:775, 1977.

72. Gaasch, W.H., Andrias, W., and Levine, H.J.: Chronic aortic regurgitation: the effect of aortic valve replacement on left ventricular volume, mass, and function. Circulation, 58:825, 1978.

73. Blackwood, R.A., Bloom, K.R., and Williams, C.M.: Aortic stenosis in children. Experience with echocardiographic predictions of severity. Circulation, 57:263, 1978.

74. Schwartz, A., Vignola, P.A., Walker, H.J., King, M.E., and Goldblatt, A.: Echocardiographic estimation of aortic-valve gradient in aortic stenosis. Ann. Intern. Med., 89:329, 1978.

75. Brenner, J.I. and Waugh, R.A.: Effect of phasic respiration on left ventricular dimension and performance in a normal population. Circulation, 57:122, 1978.

76. Belenkie, I.: Beat-to-beat variability of echocardiographic measurements of left ventricular end diastolic diameter and performance. J. Clin. Ultrasound, 7:263, 1979.

77. Rogers, E.W., Mirro, M.J., Godley, R.W., Caldwell, R.L., Weyman, A.E., and Feigenbaum, H.: Abnormalities of left ventricular geometry and rotation in endocardial cushion defect. Circulation (Suppl. II) 60:145, 1979. (Abstract)

78. Schieken, R.M. and Kerber, R.E.: Echocardiographic abnormalities in acute rheumatic fever. Am. J. Cardiol., 38:458, 1976.

79. Schuler, G., Peterson, K.L., Johnson, A., Francis, G., Dennish, G., Utley, J., Daily, P.O., Ashburn, W., and Ross, J., Jr.: Temporal response of left

ventricular performance to mitral valve surgery. Circulation, 59:1218, 1979.

80. Stefadouros, M.A. and Canedo, M.I.: Reproducibility of echocardiographic estimates of left ventricular dimensions. Br. Heart J., 39:390, 1977.
81. Vignola, P.A., Bloch, A., Kaplan, A.D., Walker, H.J., Chiotellis, P.N., and Myers, G.S.: Interobserver variability in echocardiography. J. Clin. Ultrasound, 5:238, 1977.
82. Feigenbaum, H., Dillon, J.C., Haine, C.L., and Chang, S.: Effect of elevated atrial component of left ventricular pressure on mitral valve closure. Am. J. Cardiol., 25:95, 1970. (Abstract)
83. Nimura, Y., Matsumoto, M., Shimada, H., Nagata, S., Oyama, S., Takahashi, Y., Able, H., Kitabatake, A., and Matsuo, H.: Unusual configuration of ultrasound cardiogram of mitral valve observed in some cases with myocardial disease of unknown cause. Med. Ultrasonics, 9:108, 1971.
84. Ambrose, J.A., Teichholz, L.E., Meller, J., Weintraub, W., Pichard, A.D., Smith, H., Jr., Martinez, E.E., and Herman, M.V.: The influence of left ventricular late diastolic filling on the A wave of the left ventricular pressure trace. Circulation, 60:510, 1979.
85. Konecke, L.L., Feigenbaum, H., Chang, S., Corya, B.C., and Fischer, J.C.: Abnormal mitral valve motion in patients with elevated left ventricular diastolic pressures. Circulation, 47:989, 1973.
86. Lewis, J.R., Parker, J.O., and Burggraf, G.W.: Mitral valve motion and changes in left ventricular end-diastolic pressure: a correlative study of the PR–AC interval. Am. J. Cardiol., 42:383, 1978.
87. Massie, B.M., Schiller, N.B., Ratshin, R.A., and Parmley, W.W.: Mitral-septal separation: new echocardiographic index of left ventricular function. Am. J. Cardiol., 39:1008, 1977.
88. D'Cruz, I.A., Lalmalani, G.G., Sambasivan, V., Cohen, H.C., and Glick, G.: The superiority of mitral E point-ventricular septum separation to other echocardiographic indicators of left ventricular performance. Clin. Cardiol., 2:140, 1979.
89. Reference deleted.
90. Lew, W., Henning, H., Schelbert, H., and Karliner, J.S.: Assessment of mitral valve E point-septal separation as an index of left ventricular function in acute and chronic ischemic heart disease. Am. J. Cardiol., 41:436, 1978. (Abstract)
91. Upton, M.T., Gibson, D.G., and Brown, D.J.: Instantaneous mitral valve leaflet velocity and its relation to left ventricular wall movement in normal subjects. Br. Heart J., 38:51, 1976.
92. Jugdutt, B.I., Lee, S.J.K., and McFarlane, D.: Noninvasive assessment of left ventricular function from the mitral valve echogram. Relation to final anterior mitral leaflet closing velocity to peak dp/dt and aortic velocity. Circulation, 58:861, 1978.
93. Kurata, E., Fujino, T., Kanaya, S., Ito, M., Fujino, M., Yamada, K., Hamanaka, Y., Kinoshita, R., and Ueno, T.: Isometric contraction and relaxation times of the left ventricle in patients with myocardial infarction measured by bi-directional echocardiography. J. Cardiogr., 9:65, 1979.
94. Hirschfeld, S., Meyer, R., Korfhagen, J., Kaplan, S., and Liebman, J.: The isovolumic contraction time of the left ventricle: an echocardiographic study. Circulation, 54:751, 1976.

95. Johnson, G.L., Meyer, R.A., Schwartz, D.C., Korfhagen, J., and Kaplan, S.: Left ventricular function by echocardiography in children with fixed aortic stenosis. Am. J. Cardiol., 38:611, 1976.
95a. Hanrath, P., Mathey, D.G., Siegert, R., and Bleifeld, W.: Left ventricular relaxation and filling pattern in different forms of left ventricular hypertrophy: an echocardiographic study. Am. J. Cardiol., 45:15, 1980.
96. Ito, M., Fujino, T., Kurata, E., Kanaya, S., Imanishi, S., Yasuda, H., Fujino, M., and Ueno, T.: Isometric contraction and relaxation times of the right and left ventricles in patients with right ventricular overload measured by bidirectional echocardiography. J. Cardiogr., 7:357, 1977.
97. Ito, M., Fujino, T., Kurata, E., Kanaya, S., Fujino, M., Imanishi, S., Yasuda, H., and Ueno, T.: Isometric contraction and relaxation times of right and left ventricles in normal subjects and in patients with right ventricular overloading measured with bidirectional echocardiography. Jpn. Heart J., 19:203, 1978.
98. Hickman, H.O., Weyman, A.E., Wann, L.S., Phillips, J.F., Dillon, J.C., Feigenbaum, H., and Marshall, J.: Cross-sectional echocardiography of the cardiac apex. Circulation (Suppl. III), 56:153, 1977. (Abstract)
99. Weyman, A.E., Peskoe, S.M., Williams, E.S., Dillon, J.C., and Feigenbaum, H.: Detection of left ventricular aneurysms by cross-sectional echocardiography. Circulation, 54:936, 1976.
100. Fukaya, T., Tomita, Y., Baba, K., Owaki, T., and Yoshikawa, J.: Computer-aided system analyzing left ventricular volume by real time cross-sectional echocardiograms. J. Cardiogr., 8:431, 1978.
101. Carr, K.W., Engler, R.L., Forsythe, J.R., Johnson, A.D., and Gosink, B.: Measurement of left ventricular ejection fraction by mechanical cross-sectional echocardiography. Circulation, 59:1196, 1979.
102. Eaton, L.W., Maughan, W.L., Shoukas, A.D., and Weiss, J.L.: Accurate volume determination in the isolated ejecting canine left ventricle by two-dimensional echocardiography. Circulation, 60:320, 1979.
103. Schiller, N.B., Acquatella, H., Ports, T.A., Drew, D., Goerke, J., Ringertz, H., Silverman, N.H., Brundage, B., Botvinick, E.H., Boswell, R., Carlsson, E., and Parmley, W.W.: Left ventricular volume from paired biplane two-dimensional echocardiography. Circulation, 60:547, 1979.
103a. Wyatt, H.L., et al.: Cross-sectional echocardiography. II. Analysis of mathematical models for quantifying volume of the formalin-fixed left ventricle. Circulation, 61:1119, 1980.
104. Gueret, P., Wyatt, H.L., Meerbaum, S., and Corday, E.: A practical two-dimensional echocardiographic model to assess volume in the ischemic left ventricle. Am. J. Cardiol., 45:471, 1980. (Abstract)
104a. Helak, J., Reichek, N., Pearlman, E., Weber, K., Pietra, G., and Kastor, J.A.: Quantitation of human left ventricular (LV) mass and volume by cross-sectional echocardiography: in vitro anatomic validation. Am. J. Cardiol., 45:470, 1980. (Abstract)
105. Wyatt, H.L., Heng, M.K., Meerbaum, S., Hestenes, J., Davidson, R., and Corday, E.: Quantification of volumes in asymmetric left ventricles by

2–D echocardiography. Circulation (Suppl. II), 58:188, 1978. (Abstract)

106. Wyatt, H.L., Heng, M., Meerbaum, S., Davidson, R., Lee, S–S., and Corday, E.: Quantitative left ventricular analysis in dogs with the phased array sector scan. Circulation (Suppl. III), 56:152, 1977. (Abstract)

107. Reference deleted.

108. Bommer, W., Chun, T., Kwan, O.L., Neumann, A., Mason, D.T., and DeMaria, A.N.: Biplane apex echocardiography versus biplane cineangiography in the assessment of left ventricular volume and function: validation by direct measurements. Am. J. Cardiol., 45:471, 1980. (Abstract)

109. Helak, J., Reichek, N., Pearlman, E., Weber, K., Guiseppe, P., and Kastor, J.A.: Quantitation of human left ventricular (LV) mass and volume by cross-sectional echocardiography: in vitro anatomic validation. Am. J. Cardiol., 45:470, 1980. (Abstract)

110. Wyatt, H.L., Heng, M.K., Meerbaum, S., Hestenes, J.D., Cobo, J.M., Davidson, R.M., and Corday, E.: Cross-sectional echocardiography. I. Analysis of mathematic models for quantifying mass of the left ventricle in dogs. Circulation, 60:1104, 1979.

111. Ueda, K., Kuwaki, K., and Inoue, K.: Three-dimensional display and volume determination of the left ventricle by two-dimensional echocardiography. Am. J. Cardiol., 45:471, 1980. (Abstract)

112. Joffe, C.D.: Cardiovascular physiology of normal pregnancy as assessed by echocardiography. Circulation (Suppl. III), 56:25, 1977. (Abstract)

113. Rubler, S., Damani, P.M., and Pinto, E.R.: Cardiac size and performance during pregnancy estimated with echocardiography. Am. J. Cardiol., 40:534, 1977.

114. Yin, F.C.P., Raizes, G.S., Guarnieri, T., Spurgeon, H.A., Lakatta, E.G., Fortuin, N.J., and Weisfeldt, M.L.: Age-associated decrease in ventricular response to hemodynamic stress during beta-adrenergic blockade. Br. Heart J., 40:1349, 1978.

115. Gerstenblith, G., Frederiksen, J., Yin, F.C.P., Fortuin, N.J., Lakatta, E.G., and Weisfeldt, M.L.: Echocardiographic assessment of a normal adult aging population. Circulation, 56:273, 1977.

116. Gardin, J.M., Henry, W.L., Savage, D.D., and Epstein, S.E.: Echocardiographic evaluation of an older population without clinically apparent heart disease. Am. J. Cardiol., 39:277, 1977. (Abstract)

116a. Ehsani, A.A., Hagberg, J.M., and Hickson, R.C.: Rapid changes in left ventricular dimensions and mass in response to physical conditioning and deconditioning. Am. J. Cardiol., 42:52, 1978.

117. Roeske, W.R., O'Rourke, R.A., Klein, A., Leopold, G., and Karliner, J.S.: Noninvasive evaluation of ventricular hypertrophy in professional athletes. Circulation, 53:286, 1976.

117a. Raskoff, W.J., Goldman, S., and Cohn, K.: The "Athletic Heart." Prevalence and physiological significance of left ventricular enlargement in distance runners. J.A.M.A., 236:158, 1976.

118. DeMaria, A.N., Neumann, A., Lee, G., Fowler, W., and Mason, D.T.: Alterations in ventricular mass and performance induced by exercise training in man evaluated by echocardiography. Circulation, 57:237, 1978.

119. Gilbert, C.A., Nutter, D.O., Felner, J.M., Perkins, J.V., Heymsfield, S.B., and Schlant, R.C.:

Echocardiographic study of cardiac dimensions and function in the endurance-trained athlete. Am. J. Cardiol., 40:528, 1977.

120. Menapace, F.J., Hammer, W.J., Kessler, K.K., Ritzer, T., Bove, A.A., Warner, H.H., and Spann, J.F.: Echocardiographic measurements of left ventricular wall thickness in weight lifters: a problem with the definition of ASH. Am. J. Cardiol., 39:276, 1977. (Abstract)

121. Laurenceau, J-L., Turcot, J., and Dumesnil, J.: Echocardiographic findings in Olympic athletes. Circulation (Suppl. III), 56:25, 1977. (Abstract)

122. Allen, H.D., Goldberg, S.J., Sahn, D.J., Schy, N., and Wojcik, R.: A quantitative echocardiographic study of champion childhood swimmers. Circulation, 55:142, 1977.

123. Ikaheimo, M.J., Palatsi, I.J., and Takkunen, J.T.: Noninvasive evaluation of the athletic heart: sprinters versus endurance runners. Am. J. Cardiol., 44:24, 1979.

124. Crawford, M.H., White, D.H., and Amon, K.W.: Echocardiographic evaluation of left ventricular size and performance during handgrip and supine and upright bicycle exercise. Circulation, 59:1188, 1979.

125. Imataka, K., Kato, Y., Tomono, S., Ueda, S., Natsume, T., and Yazaki, Y.: Changes in left ventricular dimension during supine exercise assessed by continuous recording of echocardiograms: an effect of beta-adrenergic blockade. J. Cardiogr., 8:729, 1978.

126. Weiss, J.L., Weisfeldt, M.L., Mason, S.J., Garrison, J.B., Livengood, S.V., and Fortuin, N.J.: Evidence of Frank-Starling effect in man during severe semisupine exercise. Circulation, 59:655, 1979.

127. Noda, H., Ogita, K., Amono, N., Koro, T., Ito, Y., Akaike, A., and Kogure, T.: Echocardiographic estimation of left ventricular responses to supine bicycle exercise: a study of normal subjects. J. Cardiogr., 8:237, 1978.

128. Ajisaka, R., Itoh, H., Niwa, A., Iizumi, T., Fujiwara, H., Taniguchi, K., and Takeuchi, J.: Echocardiographic study of left and right ventricular functions during dynamic exercise by subxiphoid approach. J. Cardiogr., 8:737, 1978.

129. Stein, R.A., Michielli, D., Fox, E.L., and Krasnow, N.: Continuous ventricular dimensions in man during supine exercise and recovery. Am. J. Cardiol., 41:655, 1978.

130. Mason, S.J., Weiss, J.L., Weisfeldt, M.L., Garrison, J.B., and Fortuin, N.J.: Exercise echocardiography: detection of wall motion abnormalities during ischemia. Circulation, 59:50, 1979.

131. Laird, W.P., Fixler, D.E., and Huffines, F.D.: Cardiovascular response to isometric exercise in normal adolescents. Circulation, 59:651, 1979.

132. Laird, W.P., Fixler, D.E., and Huffines, F.D.: Cardiovascular response to isometric exercise in normal adolescents. Circulation, 59:651, 1979.

133. Parisi, A.F., Harrington, B.S., Askenazi, J., Pratt, R.C., and McIntyre, K.M.: Echocardiographic evaluation of the Valsalva maneuver in healthy subjects and patients with and without heart failure. Circulation, 54:921, 1976.

134. Robertson, D., Stevens, R.M., Friesinger, G.C., and Oates, J.A.: The effect of the Valsalva maneuver on echocardiographic dimensions in man. Circulation, 55:596, 1977.

135. Yokoyama, H., Ishizawa, K., Okada, M., Mat-

sumori, A., and Kawashita, K.: Alterations in left ventricular systolic time intervals induced by Valsalva maneuver: an echocardiographic-mechanocardiographic correlative study. J. Cardiogr., 7:49, 1977.

136. Angoff, G.H., Wistran, D., Sloss, L.J., Markis, J.E., Come, P.C., Zoll, P.M., and Cohn, P.F.: Value of a noninvasively induced ventricular extrasystole during echocardiographic and phonocardiographic assessment of patients with idiopathic hypertrophic subaortic stenosis. Am. J. Cardiol., 42:919, 1978.

137. Cohn, P.F., Angoff, G.H., Zoll, P.M., Sloss, L.J., Markis, J.E., Graboys, T.B., Green, L.H., and Braunwald, E.: A new, noninvasive technique for inducing post-extrasystolic potentiation during echocardiography. Circulation, 56:598, 1977.

138. Gomes, J.A.C., Carambas, C.R., Matthews, L.M., Moran, H.E., and Damato, A.N.: Inotropic effect of post-stimulation potentiation in man: an echocardiographic study. Am. J. Cardiol., 43:745, 1979.

138a.Gomes, J.A.C., Carambas, C.R., Moran, H.E., Dhatt, M.S., Calon, A.H., Caracta, A.R., and Damato, A.N.: The effect of isosorbide dinitrate on left ventricular size, wall stress, and left ventricular function in chronic refractory heart failure. Am. J. Med., 65:794, 1978.

138b.Hardarson, T. and Wright, K.E.: Effect of sublingual nitroglycerin on cardiac performance in patients with coronary artery disease and non-dyskinetic left ventricular contraction. Br. Heart J., 38:1272, 1976.

138c.Gomes, J.A.C., Moran, H.E., Dhatt, M.S., Caracta, A.R., Reddy, C.P., and Damato, A.N.: Echocardiographic evaluation of ventricular performance in refractory heart failure after long acting vasodilator therapy. Circulation (Suppl. II), 54:99, 1976. (Abstract)

138d.Crawford, M.H., Karliner, J.S., O'Rourke, R.A., and Amon, K.W.: Favorable effects of oral maintenance digoxin therapy on left ventricular performance in normal subjects: echocardiographic study. Am. J. Cardiol., 38:843, 1976.

138e.Martin, M.A. and Fieller, N.R.J.: Echocardiography in cardiovascular drug assessment. Br. Heart J., 41:536, 1979.

138f.Ryan, W.F. and Karliner, J.S.: Effects of tocainide on left ventricular performance at rest and during acute alterations in heart rate and systemic arterial pressure: an echocardiographic study. Br. Heart J., 41:175, 1979.

138g.LeJemtel, T.H., Keung, E., Sonnenblick, E.H., Ribner, H.S., Matsumoto, M., Davis, R., Schwartz, W., Alousi, A.A., and Davolos, D.: Amrinone: a new non-glycosidic, non-adrenergic cardiotonic agent effective in the treatment of intractable myocardial failure in man. Circulation, 59:1098, 1979.

138h.Fortuin, N.J. and Pawsey, C.G.K.: The evaluation of left ventricular function by echocardiography. Am. J. Med., 63:1, 1977.

138i.Lendrum, B.L., Adelman, D.E., Wong, A., Carr, I., and Thornton, J.: Echocardiographic determination of the effects of general anesthesia on left ventricular performance. Am. J. Cardiol., 39:311, 1977. (Abstract)

138j.Corya, B.C., Black, M.J., and McHenry, P.L.: Echocardiographic findings after acute carbon monoxide poisoning. Br. Heart J., 38:712, 1976.

138k.Johnson, A.D., Alpert, J.S., Francis, G.S., Vieweg, V.R., Ockene, I., and Hagan, A.D.: Assessment of left ventricular function in severe aortic regurgitation. Circulation, 54:975, 1976.

138l.Bjorkhem, G. and Garwicz, S.: Echocardiographic assessment of left ventricular function during the injection of Adriamycin. Acta Paediatr. Scand., 66:595, 1977.

138m.Stefan, G.: Echocardiographic evaluation of left ventricular function during therapy with cardiovascularly effective drugs. Z. Kardiol., 65:669, 1976.

139. Popp, R.L., Wolfe, S.B., Hirata, T., and Feigenbaum, H.: Estimation of right and left ventricular size by ultrasound. A study of the echoes from the interventricular septum. Am. J. Cardiol., 24:523, 1969.

140. Goldberg, S.J., Allen, H.D., and Sahn, D.J.: In Pediatric and Adolescent Echocardiography. Chicago, Year Book Medical Publishers, Inc., 1975.

141. Matsukubo, H., Matsuura, T., Endo, N., Asayama, J., Watanabe, T., Furukawa, K., Kunishige, H., Katsume, H., and Ijichi, H.: Echocardiographic measurement of right ventricular wall thickness: a new application of subxiphoid echocardiography. Circulation, 56:278, 1977.

142. Ueda, K., Saito, A., and Nakano, H.: Electrocardiography and echocardiography in the determination of right ventricular dimension and anterior wall thickness in infants and children with congenital heart disease. J. Cardiogr., 8:47, 1978.

143. Matsukubo, H., Furukawa, K., Watanabe, T., Asayama, J., Katsume, H., Kunishige, H., Endo, N., Matsuura, T., and Ijichi, H.: Echocardiographic measurement of right ventricular wall motion by subxiphoid echocardiography. J. Cardiogr., 6:15, 1976.

144. Prakash, R. and Lindsay, P.: Determination of right ventricular wall thickness by echocardiography. J.A.M.A., 239:638, 1978.

145. Tsuda, T., Sawayama, Kawai, N., Nezuo, S., and Kikawa, K.: Echocardiographic measurement of right ventricular wall thickness in adults by anterior approach. J. Cardiogr., 8:417, 1978.

146. Prakash, R.: Determination of right ventricular wall thickness in systole and diastole. Echocardiographic and necropsy correlation in 32 patients. Br. Heart J., 40:1257, 1978.

147. Bommer, W., Weinert, L., Neumann, A., Neef, J., Mason, D.T., and DeMaria, A.: Determination of right atrial and right ventricular size by two-dimensional echocardiography. Circulation, 60:91, 1979.

148. Sahn, D.J., Sobol, R.G., and Allen, H.D.: Subxiphoid real-time cross-sectional echocardiography for imaging the right ventricle and right ventricular outflow tract. Am. J. Cardiol., 41:354, 1978. (Abstract)

149. Maron, B.J., Edwards, J.E., Moller, J.H., and Epstein, S.E.: Prevalence and characteristics of disproportionate ventricular septal thickening in infants with congenital heart disease. Circulation, 59:126, 1979.

150. Diamond, M.A., Dillon, J.C., Haine, C.L., Chang, S., and Feigenbaum, H.: Echocardiographic features of atrial septal defect. Circulation, 43:129, 1971.

151. Tajik, A.J., Gau, G.T., Ritter, D.G., et al.: Echocar-

diographic pattern of right ventricular diastolic volume overload in children. Circulation, 46:36, 1972.

152. Kerber, R.E., Dippel, W.F., and Abboud, F.M.: Abnormal motion of the interventricular septum in right ventricular volume overload. Experimental and clinical echocardiographic studies. Circulation, 48:86, 1973.

153. Meyer, R.A., Schwartz, D.C., Benzing, G., and Kaplan, S.: Ventricular septum in right ventricular volume overload: an echocardiographic study. Am. J. Cardiol., 30:349, 1972.

154. Weyman, A.E., Wann, L.S., Feigenbaum, H., and Dillon, J.C.: Mechanism of abnormal septal motion in patients with right ventricular volume overload: a cross-sectional echocardiographic study. Circulation, 54:179, 1976.

155. Fukui, Y., Kato, T., Hibi, N., Arakawa, T., Nishimura, K., Tatematsu, H., Miwa, A., Tada, H., and Kambe, T.: Clinical study on atrial septal defect by means of ultrasono-cardiotomography: with special reference to the backward deviation of interventricular septum. J. Cardiogr., 6:519, 1976.

156. Tomoda, H.: Real-time, two-dimensional echocardiographic assessment of interventricular septal performance. J. Cardiogr., 6:527, 1976.

157. Kabasawa, T., Ohno, M., Kamei, K., Yazawa, Y., Satoh, H., Kasahara, T., Shu, T., Higuma, N., Ozawa, T., Tamura, K., and Murooka, H.: Study of volume and/or pressure overload by real time, two-dimensional echocardiography: motion of the interventricular septum and motion and shape of the left ventricular cavity. J. Cardiogr., 8:55, 1978.

158. Hayashida, N., Umeda, T., Furuta, S., and Machii, K.: Echocardiographic study on interventricular septal movement in atrial septal defect. J. Cardiogr., 6:349, 1976.

159. Kabasawa, T., Ohno, M., Kamei, K., Yazawa, Y., Satoh, H., Kasahara, T., Shu, T., Higuma, N., Ozawa, T., Tamura, K., and Murooka, H.: Study of volume and/or pressure overload by real time, two-dimensional echocardiography: motion of the interventricular septum and motion and shape of the left ventricular cavity. J. Cardiogr., 8:55, 1978.

160. Weyman, A.E., Heger, J.J., Kronik, G., Wann, L.S., Dillon, J.C., and Feigenbaum, H.: Mechanism of paradoxical early diastolic septal motion in patients with mitral stenosis: cross-sectional echocardiographic study. Am. J. Cardiol., 40:691, 1977.

161. McDonald, I.G., Feigenbaum, H., and Chang, S.: Analysis of left ventricular wall motion by reflected ultrasound: application to assessment of myocardial function. Circulation, 46:14, 1972.

162. Hagan, A.D., Francis, G.S., Sahn, D.J., Karliner, J., Friedman, W.F., and O'Rourke, R.: Ultrasound evaluation of systolic anterior septal motion in patients with and without right ventricular volume overload. Circulation, 50:248, 1974.

163. Pearlman, A.S., Clark, C.E., Henry, W.L., Morganroth, J., Itscoitz, S.B., and Epstein, S.E.: Determinants of ventricular septal motion: influence of relative right and left ventricular size. Circulation, 54:83, 1976.

164. Laurenceau, J.L. and Dumesnil, J.G.: Right and left ventricular dimensions as determinants of ventricular septal motion. Chest, 69:388, 1976.

165. Mueller, T.N., Kerber, R.E., and Marcus, M.L.:

Comparison of interventricular septal motion studied by ventriculography and echocardiography in patients with atrial septal defect. Br. Heart J., 40:984, 1978.

166. Matsuzaki, M., Maeda, S., Yorozu, T., Fukagawa, K., Ozaki, M., Ikee, Y., Sasada, T., Mise, J., Tanikado, O., Shimizu, M., and Nomoto, R.: A study of abnormal interventricular septal motion: influence of position of interventricular septum in end-diastole. J. Cardiogr., 7:153, 1977.

167. Bahler, A.S., Meller, J., Brik, H., Herman, M.V., and Teichholz, L.E.: Paradoxical motion of the interventricular septum with right ventricular dilatation in the absence of shunting. Am. J. Cardiol., 38:654, 1976.

168. Eslami, B., Roitman, D., Karp, R.B., and Sheffield, L.T.: Paradoxical septal motion in a patient with pulmonic stenosis. Chest, 67:244, 1975.

169. Dillon, J.C., Weyman, A.E., Feigenbaum, H., Eggleton, R.C., and Johnston, K.: Cross-sectional echocardiographic examination of the interatrial septum. Circulation, 55:115, 1977.

170. Schabelman, S., Schiller, N., Ports, T., Silverman, N., and Parmley, W.: Left atrial volume by two-dimensional echocardiography. Circulation (Supp. II), 58:188, 1978. (Abstract)

171. Lemire, F., Tajik, A.J., and Hagler, D.J.: Asymmetric left atrial enlargement: an echocardiographic observation. Chest, 69:779, 1976.

172. Hirata, T., Wolfe, S.B., Popp, R.L., Helmen, C.H., and Feigenbaum, H.: Estimation of left atrial size using ultrasound. Am. Heart J., 78:43, 1969.

173. Lundstrom, N.R. and Mortensson, W.: Clinical applications of echocardiography in infants and children. II. Estimation of aortic root diameter and left atrial size: a comparison between echocardiography and angiocardiography. Acta Paediatr. Scand., 63:33, 1974.

174. TenCate, F.J., Kloster, F.E., VanDorp, W.G., Meester, G.T., and Roelandt, J.: Dimensions and volumes of left atrium and ventricle determined by single beam echocardiography. Br. Heart J., 36:737, 1974.

175. Lester, L.A., Vitullo, D., Sodt, P., Hutcheon, N., and Arcilla, R.: An evaluation of the left atrial/aortic root ratio in children with ventricular septal defect. Circulation, 60:364, 1979.

176. Kronzon, I. and Mehta, S.S.: Giant left atrium. Chest, 65:677, 1974.

177. Henry, W.L., Morganroth, J., Pearlman, A.S., Clark, C.E., Redwood, D.R., Itscoitz, S.B., and Epstein, S.E.: Relation between echocardiographically determined left atrial size and atrial fibrillation. Circulation, 53:273, 1976.

178. Silverman, N.H., Lewis, A.B., Heymann, M.A., and Rudolph, A.M.: Echocardiographic assessment of ductus arteriosus in premature infants. Circulation, 50:821, 1974.

179. Baylen, B., Meyer, R.A., and Kaplan, S.: Echocardiographic assessment of patent ductus arteriosus in prematures with respiratory distress. Circulation (Suppl. III), 50:16, 1974. (Abstract)

180. Goldberg, S.J., Allen, H.D., Sahn, D.J., Friedman, W.F., and Harris, T.: A prospective 2½ year experience with echocardiographic evaluation of prematures with patent ductus arteriosus (PDA) and respiratory distress syndrome (RDS). Am. J. Cardiol., 35:139, 1975. (Abstract)

181. Carter, W.H. and Bowman, C.R.: Estimation of

shunt flow in isolated ventricular septal defect by echocardiogram. Circulation (Suppl IV), 48:64, 1973. (Abstract)

182. Laird, W.P. and Fixler, D.E.: Echocardiographic estimation of pulmonary, systemic flow in children with patent ductus arteriosus. Circulation (Suppl. III), 50:184, 1974. (Abstract)

183. Goldberg, B.B.: Suprasternal ultrasonography. J.A.M.A., 215:245, 1971.

184. Ueda, K., Saito, A., and Nakano, H.: Measurement of the dimensions of the great vessels and the left atrium by suprasternal notch echocardiography. J. Cardiogr., 8:409, 1978.

185. Allen, H.D. and Goldberg, S.J.: Usefulness of biaxial left atrial dimension measurements by echocardiography. J. Clin. Ultrasound, 2:222, 1974. (Abstract)

186. Sasse, L.: Echocardiography of left atrial wall. J.A.M.A., 228:1667, 1974.

186a.Yoshikawa, J., Kato, H., Owaki, T., and Tanaka, K.: Study of posterior left atrial wall motion by echocardiography and its clinical application. Jpn. Heart J., 16:683, 1975.

187. Winsberg, F. and Goldman, H.S.: Echo patterns of cardiac posterior wall. Invest. Radiol., 4:173, 1969.

188. Patton, R., Dragatakis, L., Marpole, D., and Sniderman, A.: The posterior left atrial echocardiogram of mitral regurgitation. Circulation, 57:1134, 1978.

189. Strunk, B.L., Fitzgerald, J.W., Lipton, M., Popp, R.L., and Barry, W.H.: The posterior aortic wall echocardiogram: its relationship to left atrial volume change. Circulation, 54:744, 1976.

190. Akgun, G. and Layton, C.: Aortic root and left atrial wall motion: an echocardiographic study. Br. Heart J., 39:1082, 1977.

191. Gramiak, R. and Nanda, N.C.: Structure identification in echocardiography. In Cardiac Ultrasound. Edited by R. Gramiak and R. Waag. St. Louis, C.V. Mosby Co., 1975.

192. Saito, A., Ueda, K., and Nakano, H.: Echocardiographic determination of right atrial dimension. J. Cardiogr., 8:37, 1978.

193. Saito, A., Ueda, K., and Nakano, H.: Echocardiographic determination of right atrial dimension. J. Cardiogr., 8:425, 1978.

194. Asayama, J., Matsuura, T., Endo, N., Matsukubo, H., and Furukawa, K.: Idiopathic enlargement of the right atrium. Am. J. Cardiol., 40:620, 1977.

194a.Kushner, F.G., Lam, W., and Morganroth, J.: Apex sector echocardiography in evaluation of the right atrium in patients with mitral stenosis and atrial septal defect. Am. J. Cardiol., 42:733, 1978.

Hemodynamic Information Derived from Echocardiography

One of the many unique features of echocardiography is that it can provide an excellent recording of functional anatomy. With M-mode echocardiography, the data acquisition rate is so rapid, usually 1,000 samples per second, that the motion of various cardiac structures can be recorded in a way not possible with any other technique. The echocardiographic recording of functional anatomy has improved our understanding of cardiac physiology and has provided clinical clues to altered hemodynamics. This chapter discusses some reported echocardiographic findings that may alert the echocardiographer to changes in blood flow or intravascular pressure. It must be emphasized, however, that echocardiography does not directly measure flow or pressure. All ultrasonic information is indirect and, as with any indirect measurement, is relatively insensitive. Thus, although the echocardiographic findings are indeed helpful, the various limitations must also be considered.

ECHOCARDIOGRAPHIC REFLECTORS OF BLOOD FLOW

Echocardiography does not directly measure blood flow. Techniques such as Doppler or contrast echocardiography, however, come close to obtaining truly physiologic data. Most clinical echocardiographic reflectors of blood flow depend on observing the pattern of motion of various cardiac structures on the M-mode echocardiogram. Although these techniques are indirect, they have advantages over some of the other clinical methods for measuring blood flow, especially stroke volume. Attempts to calculate stroke volume by measuring absolute volumes may require geometric assumptions that are frequently incorrect. The echocardiographic measurements of stroke volume or blood flow that utilize the pattern of motion of cardiac valves or walls do not have this problem of assuming certain geometric shapes.

Mitral Valve

Echocardiography began with the description of mitral valve motion on the M-mode echocardiogram. Thus it is not surprising that the first attempts to obtain physiologic information should be from altered motion of the anterior leaflet of the mitral valve. Before discussing the possible ways in which the mitral valve M-mode echocardiogram can reflect changes in mitral valve blood flow, I will review normal mitral valve motion.

Figure 4–1 demonstrates the diastolic pattern of motion of a normal mitral valve. The valve opens rapidly in early diastole from points D to E; then there is fairly rapid closure from point E to a nadir at F. Following the F point the valve often partially reopens during the mid-diastolic phase of ventricular filling. Following atrial systole the valve reopens, reaching a peak at the A point just before ventricular systole.[1] With atrial relaxation the valve begins to close, and with the onset of ventricular systole, point B, the valve completes its closure at point C.[2] The closure from A to C is rapid and smooth, and

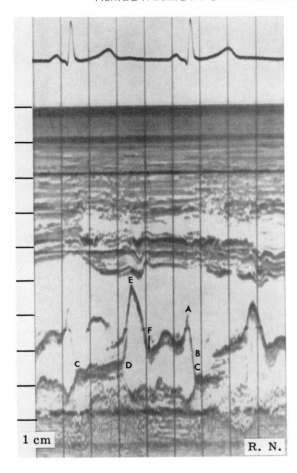

Fig. 4–1. M-mode echocardiogram of a normal mitral valve. Note pattern of motion.

which the leaflets are attached.[11–14] During ventricular diastole, the leaflets move apart as blood flows from the left atrium into the left ventricle. One feature of mitral valve motion that was first clearly demonstrated by echocardiography is the closure of the valve during early diastole. This diastolic, or E to F, slope has been an important measurement in M-mode echocardiography ever since its beginnings. A reduced E to F slope was originally the principal diagnostic feature of mitral stenosis (see Chapter 6). Unfortunately, the E to F slope has proved to be a relatively unreliable sign for judging the severity of mitral stenosis. However, the mechanism for closure of the mitral valve in early diastole has intrigued investigators since it was first described.

Figure 4–2 diagrammatically shows one theory behind the early diastolic closure of the mitral valve.[15] These investigators believed that with the opening of the mitral valve (Fig. 4–2II), vortices occurred behind the leaflets and forced the valve to close. The manner in which the leaflets closed was a function of the amount and velocity of blood flowing through the mitral orifice and also of the location of the leaflets with respect to the adjacent walls.[15,16] The normal anterior mitral valve leaflet had a greater closing motion than did the posterior leaflet because the distance between the anterior leaflet and the interventricular septal wall was greater than it was between the posterior leaflet and the posterior left ventricular wall.

The diastolic closure velocity of the mitral valve was probably the first echocardiographic reflector of altered hemodynamics. In patients with mitral stenosis and a decreased rate of filling of the ventricle, there was a predictable decrease in the E to F slope (Fig. 4–3). It later became apparent that the E to F slope might be decreased in other conditions (Fig. 4–4). The rate of filling of the left ventricle may be decreased in patients without mitral stenosis and may also produce a reduced closing velocity of the mitral valve. The most popular theory is that decreased left ventricular compliance or increased left ventricular stiffness is responsible for the decreased E to F slope in these patients.[12,17–20] However, diastolic mitral

the point at which ventricular systole occurs, point B, is frequently inapparent. The posterior mitral leaflet moves as a virtual mirror image of the anterior leaflet. The amplitude of motion is significantly less. During systole, from C to D, the mitral valve gradually moves upward or in an anterior motion.

Ever since the mid-1950s, when Edler first described the motion of an anterior mitral leaflet,[3–5] investigators have attempted to explain the pattern of motion exhibited by the valve.[6,7] There is evidence that the leaflet motion follows the pattern of blood flow through the mitral orifice.[8–10] During ventricular systole, when the valve is closed and the leaflets are together, the gradual anterior motion of the two leaflets is probably secondary to the motion of the mitral annulus to

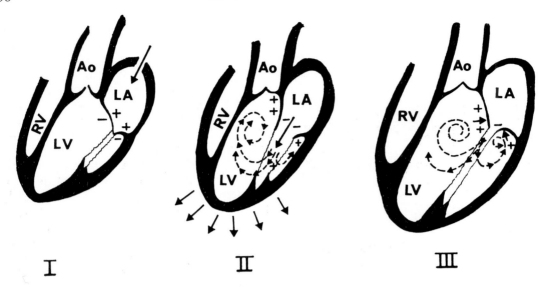

I   II   III

Fig. 4–2.   Diagram demonstrating one theory for the mid-diastolic closure of the mitral valve. With the inflow of blood during early diastole, *II*, vortices of blood occur behind the leaflets and force them to close, *III*. The rate of closure of the leaflets is a function of the blood flowing through the mitral orifice and of the location of the leaflets with respect to the adjacent walls. AO = aorta; RV = right ventricle; LV = left ventricle; LA = left atrium. (From Madeira, H.C., et al.: Echocardiographic assessment of left ventricular volume overload. Br. Heart J., 36:1175, 1974.)

valve motion may also be reduced in patients with pulmonary hypertension and no apparent left ventricular compliance difficulty.[21–23] Thus, although the E to F slope is a common measurement frequently used as an indicator of altered hemodynamics,[12,20,24] the sign is nonspecific and has many limitations. One technical limitation is that the slope is frequently not a straight line (Fig. 4–5B). With a decrease in the duration of diastole, the more rapid portion of the E to F slope (F'–F, Fig. 4–5B) might not be recorded (Fig. 4–5A), and one would obtain a totally different E to F measurement. Even with mitral stenosis, the diastolic slope may vary.

The D to E slope has also been mentioned as a possible indicator of the velocity of blood flow between the left atrium and left ventricle.[25] This observation, largely ignored for many years, was resurrected when examples of rather striking alterations in the D to E slope were noted in patients with low flow states. Figure 4–6 shows a patient with a decreased D to E slope. This decreased rate of opening of the mitral valve was initially thought to be due to an elevated left ventricular diastolic pressure. It became appar-

ent later that the D to E slope was probably more flow related than pressure related. Several examples were found in patients who had normal left ventricular diastolic pressures but extremely low cardiac output. Frequently, patients with a decreased D to E slope have accentuated A waves. This accentuation is usually just relative to a diminutive E point but may also be absolutely increased. One receives the impression that in this type of patient atrial systole is responsible for a higher percentage of left ventricular filling.

An extreme example of a decreased D to E slope is noted in Figure 4–7. In this patient there is no recognizable E point. There is slight downward motion of the posterior mitral leaflet during early diastole. However, the maximum separation of the leaflets occurs with atrial systole. This patient had severe aortic regurgitation with high left ventricular diastolic pressures and low cardiac output. Thus multiple factors were responsible for the virtually absent D to E slope, e.g., regurgitant jet hitting the valve, high initial diastolic pressures, and decreased left atrial filling. Figure 4–8 shows another

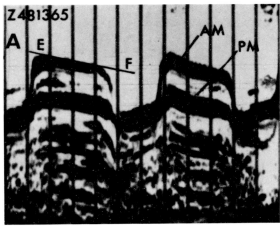

A

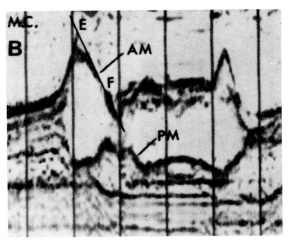

Fig. 4–3. Echocardiograms of the anterior (AM) and posterior (PM) mitral valve leaflets in a patient with mitral stenosis, A, and in a patient with a normal mitral valve, B. (From Duchak, J.M., Jr., Chang, S., and Feigenbaum, H.: The posterior mitral valve echo and the echocardiographic diagnosis of mitral stenosis. Am. J. Cardiol., 29:628, 1972.)

B

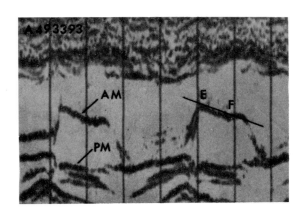

Fig. 4–4. Mitral valve echocardiogram of a patient with a diminished E to F slope of the anterior mitral leaflet (AM) but no evidence of mitral stenosis. Despite the diminished E to F slope, the leaflets were thin, and the posterior mitral leaflet (PM) moved normally. (From Duchak, J.M., Jr., Chang, S., and Feigenbaum, H.: The posterior mitral valve echo and the echocardiographic diagnosis of mitral stenosis. Am. J. Cardiol., 29:628, 1972.)

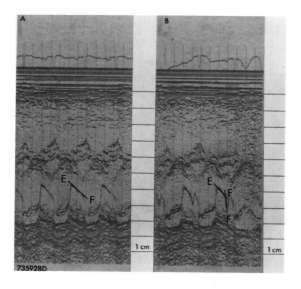

Fig. 4–5. Mitral valve echocardiogram demonstrating how the E to F slope is frequently not a single slope. Often a more rapid closure rate (F′ − F, *B*) is present. When the heart rate is rapid and the diastolic filling period is short, this more rapid diastolic slope may not be recorded, *A.*

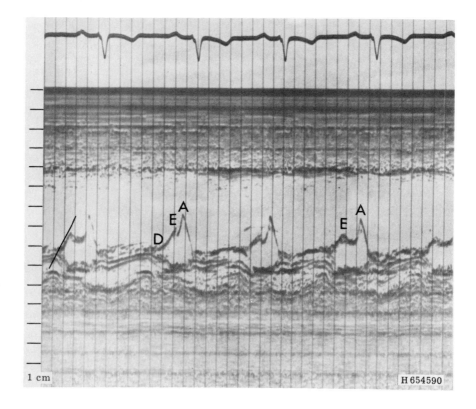

Fig. 4–6. Mitral valve echocardiogram of a patient with left ventricular failure, low cardiac output, and elevated left ventricular diastolic pressure. The velocity of opening of the mitral valve (D to E slope) is reduced, and the atrial component to mitral valve motion is accentuated.

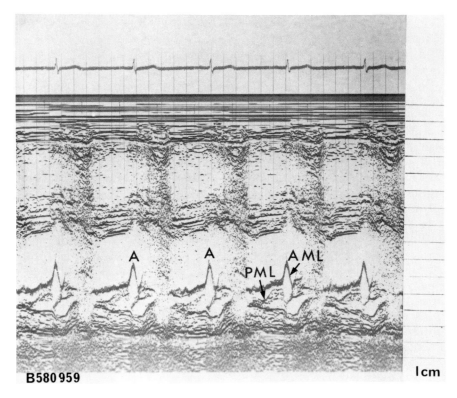

Fig. 4–7.   M-mode recording of a patient with such a markedly reduced initial mitral valve opening that no appreciable E point is present. Slight posterior displacement of the posterior mitral leaflet (PML) is visible in early diastole. The maximum opening of the mitral valve occurs with atrial systole (A). AML = anterior mitral leaflet.

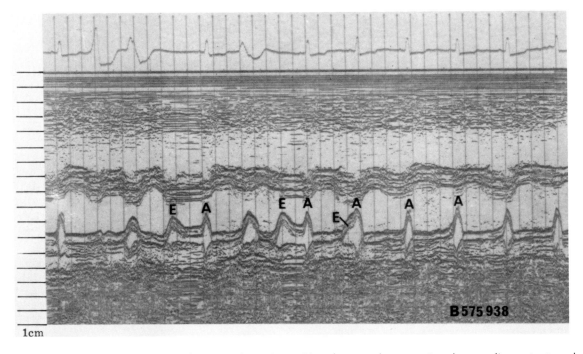

Fig. 4–8.   Mitral valve echocardiogram of a patient with pulmonary hypertension, low cardiac output, and frequent ventricular premature beats. During sinus rhythm the mitral valve opens only with atrial contraction.

example of a markedly decreased E point in a patient with no aortic regurgitation.[26] The patient had pulmonary hypertension and low cardiac output with normal left ventricular diastolic pressures. The E point is seen only with a long pause following a premature ventricular systole.

Another empirical observation with reference to the mitral valve and blood flow is that the total amplitude of mitral motion is decreased in patients with low stroke volumes. Figure 4–9 shows two patients with differing amplitudes of mitral valve motion. The patient in Figure 4–9A had a relatively high flow through the mitral orifice, whereas the patient in Figure 4–9B had a low cardiac output and a small stroke volume. Although mitral valve motion is best recorded on the M-mode echocardiogram, mitral leaflet motion can also be readily appreciated in real-time two-dimensional echocardiography. Extremes in mitral valve excursion and motion are apparent on the two-dimensional studies, and it is usually a reliable and simple observation to note a low cardiac output in a patient whose mitral valve barely opens in real time.

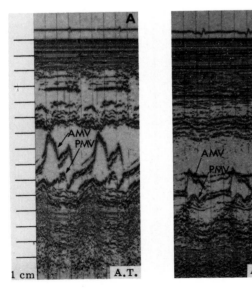

Fig. 4–9.   Mitral valve echocardiogram of a patient with high mitral valve flow, A, and of a patient with low mitral valve flow, B. Calibrations are the same for both recordings. AMV = anterior mitral valve leaflet; PMV = posterior mitral valve leaflet.

These observations have led several investigators to attempt using the mitral valve opening or separation as an indicator of blood flow.[27-30] Initially, the area inscribed between the mitral leaflets was planimetered.[28] Although the early results were promising, there were many difficulties and the actual measurements were cumbersome. A more practical technique for using the mitral valve separation was recently described and is illustrated in Figure 4–10.[29,30] The echocardiographic measurements utilized the separation of the anterior and posterior mitral leaflets at the E points. For convenience the authors measured from "outside to outside," that is, from the leading edge of the anterior leaflet to the trailing edge of the posterior leaflet. In addition, an M-mode scan of the mitral valve was obtained and the maximum mitral leaflet separation was used for this determination. They also used the echocardiographic D to E slope in their formula. The other two measurements used for calculating mitral valve flow were the heart rate in beats per minute and the electrocardiographic P–R interval in seconds. The resultant formula for calculating mitral valve stroke volume was $SV = \left(\dfrac{E-E}{HR} + P-R \right) \times 100 + 2\, \dfrac{D-E}{HR}$ (Fig. 4–10B).

There are many advantages to this technique for measuring mitral valve flow. The raw data are fairly simple to obtain. Even in a relatively poor echocardiogram it is usually possible to identify the E to E separation and the D to E slope. One does not have to planimeter the echocardiogram. There is a theoretical basis for this formula. Initial mitral valve separation, E to E' distance, and the D to E slope both indicate blood flow into the ventricle in early diastole. This portion of diastole normally represents most of the mitral blood flow. There must be some recognition of mid-diastolic flow. Normally this flow is relatively low, and is primarily a function of the diastolic filling period. The duration of diastole correlates fairly well with heart rate, and thus mid-diastolic flow is accounted for by heart rate in the formula. The third contribution to ventricular filling is atrial systole. There are experimental data in the literature demonstrating that the con-

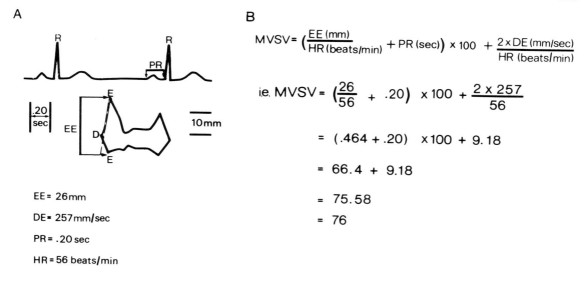

Fig. 4–10.   A, Diagram illustrating variables used in one technique to calculate stroke volume from the mitral valve echogram and the electrocardiogram. EE is measured from the outermost echoes. DE represents the most rapid slope from the D to E points. Heart rate (HR) is calculated by dividing 60 by the R–R interval in second increments. B, Formula for calculating mitral valve stroke volume (MVSV). (From Rasmussen, S., et al.: Stroke volume calculated from the mitral valve echogram in patients with and without ventricular dyssynergy. Circulation, 58:125, 1978. By permission of the American Heart Association, Inc.)

tribution of atrial filling is largely a function of the atrioventricular conduction time or the electrocardiographic P–R interval. With a short P–R interval less time is available for filling of the ventricle with atrial systole. Thus the formula takes into account the three main phases of ventricular filling. Another feature that makes this formula attractive is that although the units are dissimilar the resulting echocardiographic number for stroke volume or mitral valve flow comes close to the actual stroke volume measurement. This fact, though fortuitous, does add a degree of convenience as no regression equation is necessary.

Figure 4–11 shows the statistical relationship between the mitral valve stroke volume, determined by this echocardiographic formula, and the corresponding stroke volume determined by the Fick and thermodilution techniques. The correlation is excellent, and the margin of error in the estimate is acceptable when considered against the margin of error in the Fick and thermodilution techniques. The ultrasonic technique appears more accurate in the low flow states than under high flow conditions. There is more

scatter when the stroke volume exceeds 90 ml. This application for measuring mitral valve flow has been confirmed by a group of investigators[30] and, it is hoped, will be substantiated by others.

There are limitations to using the mitral valve to record mitral flow. Any anatomic restriction of mitral valve motion alters its value in reflecting flow. Mitral stenosis is one situation in which leaflet motion does not reflect the flow of blood though the valve. Even with a flail or disrupted valve there is some question whether the flow is accurately estimated by the pattern of valve motion. With aortic regurgitation there is distortion of the shape of the valve as the regurgitant jet restricts full opening of the anterior leaflet (see Chapter 6). Thus there would again be some question over whether valve motion accurately reflects flow. Another restriction to this approach would be in a patient with an unusually small ventricle whereby the mitral leaflets abut against the walls of the chamber and cannot separate fully.

One should remember that the mitral valve reflects flow through the orifice and

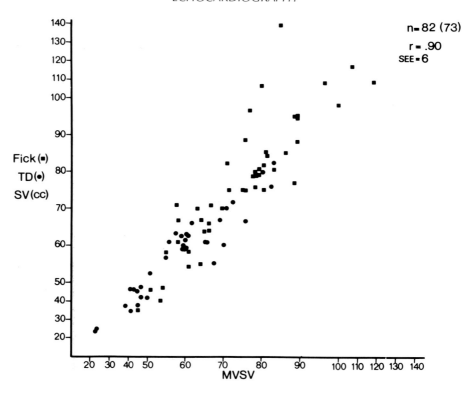

Fig. 4–11.   Graph plotting mitral valve stroke volume (MVSV), calculated from the mitral valve echocardiogram versus stroke volume (SV), determined by the Fick or thermodilution (TD) techniques.

not necessarily left ventricular stroke volume. For example, in aortic regurgitation the total left ventricular stroke volume would include the regurgitant volume, whereas the mitral valve stroke volume would not. With aortic regurgitation, the mitral valve flow theoretically reflects the effective stroke volume, which is the total left ventricular stroke volume minus the regurgitant fraction. Unfortunately, because of possible distortion of the mitral valve by the regurgitant jet, the usefulness of estimating mitral valve flow is limited in these patients. With mitral regurgitation the mitral valve flow theoretically includes the regurgitant fraction plus the effective cardiac output and equals total left ventricular stroke volume. Again, this use is limited because of possible anatomic distortion of the valve that produced the mitral regurgitation. Probably the best application of using the mitral valve to calculate mitral valve flow or stroke volume is in patients without intrinsic valvular disease,

such as those with coronary artery disease or congestive cardiomyopathy.

Tricuspid Valve

The mitral and tricuspid valves are similar in their patterns of motion. Figure 4–12 demonstrates an M-mode echocardiogram of a normal tricuspid valve. Usually only the anterior leaflet is recorded, and the valve echo may drop out frequently throughout the cardiac cycle. It is much easier to record a complete mitral valve than it is a complete tricuspid valve. This is one reason why more has been written on the mitral valve than on the tricuspid valve. There is a tendency to apply information on the mitral valve to the tricuspid valve. Many changes in motion observed with the mitral valve have also been noted with the tricuspid valve. For example, Figure 4–13 shows a recording of a tricuspid valve that has a slow, almost absent, D to E slope. One would like to assume that this

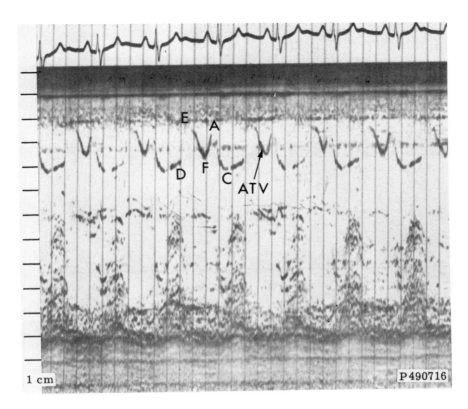

Fig. 4–12.   Normal tricuspid valve echocardiogram. The pattern of motion of the anterior tricuspid leaflet (ATV) is essentially the same as that of the anterior mitral leaflet.

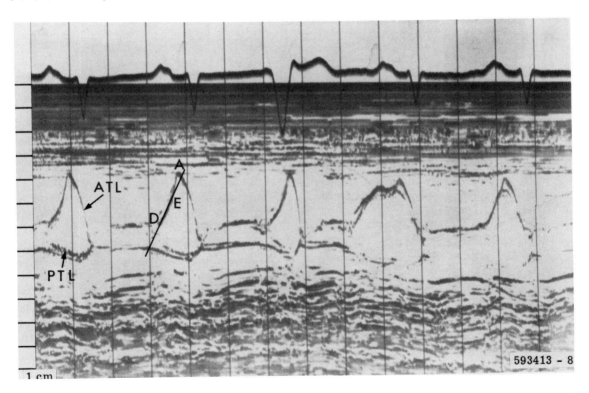

Fig. 4–13.   Tricuspid valve echocardiogram of a patient with right ventricular dysfunction and a decreased D to E slope. ATL = anterior tricuspid valve leaflet; PTL = posterior tricuspid valve leaflet.

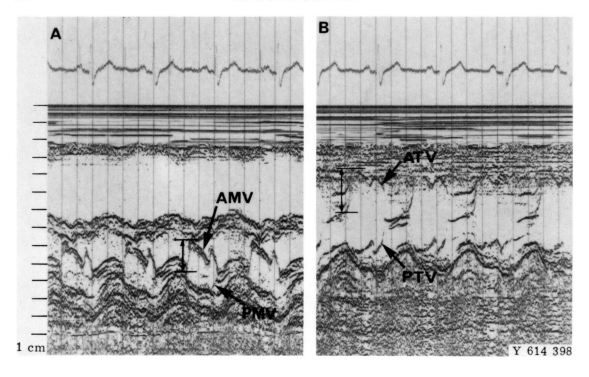

Fig. 4–14.   M-mode scans comparing mitral, *A*, and tricuspid, *B*, valve echograms of a patient with an atrial septal defect and a large left-to-right shunt. The amplitude of opening of the anterior tricuspid valve leaflet (ATV) is greater than that of the anterior mitral valve leaflet (AMV). In addition, the separation between the anterior and posterior leaflets is greater for the tricuspid valve than for the mitral valve. PMV = posterior mitral valve leaflet; PTV = posterior tricuspid valve leaflet. (From Chang, S.: M-mode Echocardiographic Techniques and Pattern Recognition. Philadelphia, Lea & Febiger, 1976.)

finding has a significance similar to that noted with the mitral valve. Unfortunately, data supporting this possibility are not available. However, it is reasonable to assume that a distorted pattern of motion, as seen in Figure 4–13, suggests altered right ventricular hemodynamics and possibly a decreased rate of initial filling of the right ventricle.

Echocardiographers have also suggested that increased separation of the tricuspid leaflets represents increased flow through the tricuspid valve. Figure 4–14 shows a patient with an atrial septal defect. The separation of the tricuspid valve leaflets is significantly greater than that of the mitral leaflets. In addition, the total amplitude of motion of the anterior tricuspid leaflet is greater than that of the anterior mitral leaflet. Although a few studies suggest that an increased amplitude of motion of the anterior tricuspid valve is indicative of increased

flow through that valve, this observation has not been confirmed. In addition, trying to judge relative flow through the tricuspid and mitral orifices from the amplitude of motion of the respective valve has not proved too reliable. It must be remembered that the tricuspid valve is frequently recorded at an acute angle. The valve lies in a more superficial position and is almost directly under the sternum. Thus the amplitude of motion may be influenced by the angle of the ultrasonic beam.

The tricuspid valve is recorded more easily and hence more frequently with two-dimensional echocardiography. The full excursion of the tricuspid valve may at times be better appreciated with the real-time examination. As with the mitral valve, one can obtain a semiquantitative estimate of the flow across the valve by noting the motion of the leaflets in real time.

Aortic Valve

Figure 4–15 demonstrates an M-mode echocardiogram of a normal aortic valve. Two of the leaflets are seen in systole. With the onset of ejection of blood through the aortic valve, they separate briskly, remain roughly parallel to each other throughout systole, and close abruptly at the end of ejection. As indicated in this figure, the separation of the leaflets is approximately 1.5 to 2 cm. Aortic valve motion may also reflect the amount of blood flowing through that orifice. Figure 4–16 demonstrates an aortic valve echocardiogram of a patient with atrial fibrillation. There is marked variation in the aortic valve motion depending on the preceding

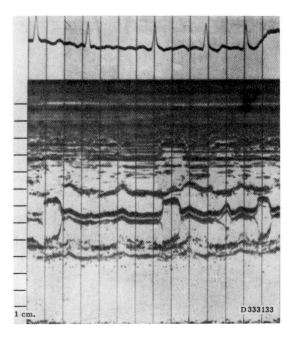

Fig. 4–16.   Aortic valve echocardiogram of a patient with atrial fibrillation. With a short R–R interval, the separation of the leaflets in systole is either diminished or absent.

R–R interval. Following the second echocardiographic QRS complex, there is no opening of the aortic valve. This finding would certainly be compatible with the pulse deficit that commonly occurs with atrial fibrillation. The lack of aortic valve opening has even been reported in a patient with a pulmonary embolus and severe paradoxical pulse.[31] Figure 4–17 shows another pattern of aortic valve motion seen in patients with abnormal flow. The initial separation of the leaflets is much greater than the separation just prior to closure of the valve. In Figure 4–15 the leaflets remain maximally opened throughout systole as blood flows through the leaflets. In Figure 4–17 there is gradual closure of the valve during systole. This finding would suggest that the amount of blood is gradually decreasing throughout systole. It appears that the blood flow cannot be sustained at an equal rate throughout systole. This finding is usually indicative of reduced ventricular function or reduced stroke volume. An alternate situation exists in patients with mitral regurgitation whereby the

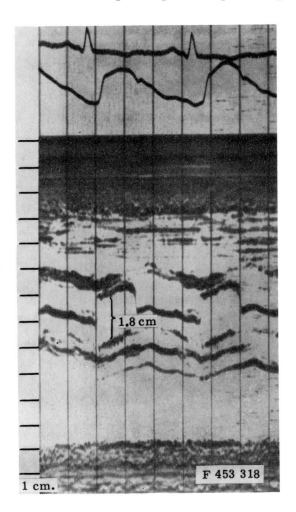

Fig. 4–15.   Echocardiogram of a normal aortic valve. The leaflets are 1.8 cm apart during ventricular systole.

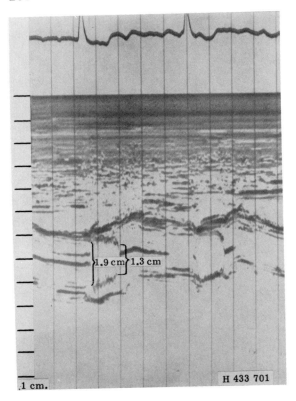

Fig. 4–17. Echocardiogram of the aortic valve in a patient with mitral regurgitation and decreased cardiac output. The leaflets separate normally with the onset of ventricular ejection; however, they gradually close throughout systole.

blood may be flowing back into the left atrium during the latter part of systole.

Yet another example whereby aortic valve motion reflects altered flow into the aorta is seen in Figure 4–18. In this patient the flow initially is brisk with fairly wide separation of the leaflets; however, shortly after maximum opening there is immediate partial closure of the valve (arrow). This aortic valve motion indicates a sudden decrease in flow in early systole. This patient had hypertrophic subaortic stenosis. A somewhat similar pattern of motion can be seen in Figure 4–19 in a patient with discrete subaortic stenosis. In both figures there appears to be an abrupt decrease in blood flow shortly after the initial wide separation of the leaflets in early systole. With hypertrophic subaortic stenosis the valve frequently reopens in late systole (Fig. 4–18). The proposed mecha-

nism of aortic valve motion seen in both hypertrophic and discrete subaortic stenosis is that the subvalvular obstruction exerts its effect in blood flow shortly after the explosive initial ejection of blood. It is possible that the subvalvular obstruction becomes greater as the ventricular volume decreases during ejection.

Unfortunately, the pattern of motion seen with subaortic obstruction is nonspecific since conditions other than subaortic stenosis produce somewhat similar aortic

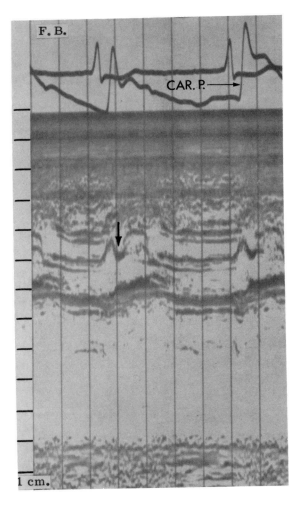

Fig. 4–18. Aortic valve echocardiogram of a patient with hypertrophic subaortic stenosis. During mid-systole the aortic valve closes *(arrow)* secondary to the subvalvular obstruction. The valve reopens before diastole begins. (From Feigenbaum, H.: Clinical applications of echocardiography. Prog. Cardiovasc. Dis., *14*:531, 1972.)

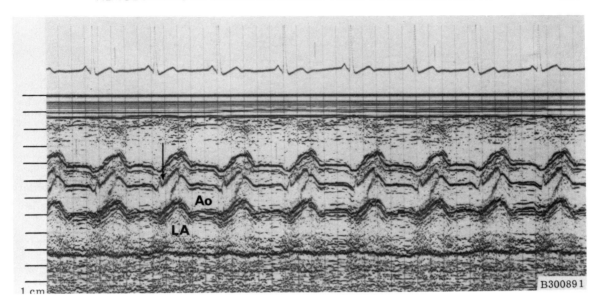

Fig. 4–19.   M-mode echocardiogram of the aortic valve in a patient with discrete subaortic stenosis. Closure of the anterior aortic leaflet *(arrow)* can be noted immediately following the initial opening. Gradual closure is seen throughout systole. Note also the fine systolic fluttering of the aortic valve leaflets. AO = aorta; LA = left atrium.

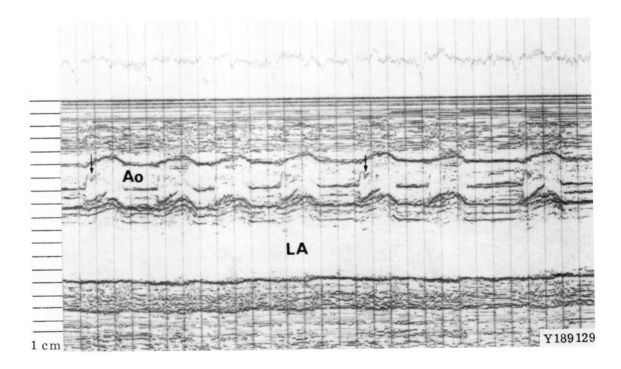

Fig. 4–20.   Early systolic closure of the aortic valve *(arrow)* noted in a patient with mitral regurgitation. AO = aorta; LA = left atrium.

valve echocardiograms.[32] Figure 4–20 shows early systolic closure of the aortic valve (arrows) in a patient with mitral regurgitation and no subaortic obstruction. A possible explanation is that the early systolic closure reflects the reduced aortic flow resulting from regurgitant blood flowing into the left atrium. A similar situation can occur with a ventricular septal defect. One might also see early systolic closure in patients with a dilated aorta. These patients may have relative subaortic obstruction and may also have vortices produced in the dilated aorta that partially close the aortic valve, much as the normal mitral valve closes in early diastole.

With evidence that the aortic valve motion reflects flow through that orifice, it is not surprising that attempts to quantitate aortic valve flow from the aortic valve echocardiogram have been made. Several studies have shown a correlation between the amplitude and duration of aortic valve separation and left ventricular stroke volume by measuring the area inscribed by the aortic valve leaflets.[33–35] More recent studies again measured the separation of the aortic valve leaflets, also including the amplitude of motion of the posterior aortic wall (Fig. 4–21).[36] The actual measurements were the separation of the aortic leaflets at the onset of opening (1), the separation just prior to closure (2), the ejection time as measured by the total duration that the aortic valve leaflets were open (ET), and the amplitude of motion of the posterior aortic wall (AA). The aortic valve stroke volume was equal to the average aortic valve separation (initial aortic leaflet separation and final separation divided by two) times the ejection time, plus the aortic wall amplitude. The actual formula was AVSV = (average AVO × ET) × 100 + AA, where the AVSV = aortic valve stroke volume, AVO = aortic valve opening, ET = ejection time, and AA = aortic amplitude. Initial experience provides a correlation with Fick and thermodilution techniques for stroke volume with an R value in excess of 0.9.

These aortic valve techniques are attractive and would provide complementary measurements to the mitral valve flow measured from the mitral valve echocardiogram. However, more experience is necessary to

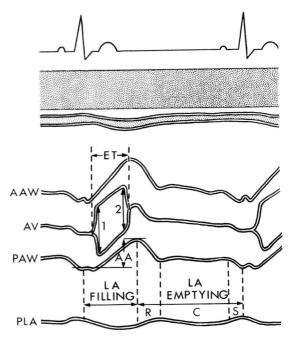

Fig. 4–21. Diagram of an M-mode echocardiogram of the aortic valve (AV) and left atrium (LA) demonstrating several measurements that can be made from this type of recording. Ejection time (ET) can be measured between the opening and closing point of the aortic valve. Separation of the aortic valve leaflets can be measured at the onset, 1 and at the end, 2, of ejection. The amplitude of motion (AA) of the posterior aortic wall (PAW) can be obtained. The posterior aortic wall motion reflects left atrial volume changes. Left atrial emptying can be divided into a rapid filling phase (R), a conduit phase (C), and a filling owing to atrial systole phase (S). AAW = anterior aortic wall; PLA = posterior left atrial wall.

determine the reliability of these aortic valve flow measurements, especially in high flow states where the velocity of aortic blood flow increases.

Aortic Wall Motion

One of the attempts to measure aortic valve flow by way of the aortic valve included aortic wall amplitude.[36] The aortic wall amplitude improved the statistical correlation with the flow through the aortic valve. This finding is not surprising since a relationship between aortic wall amplitude and cardiac output is well recognized.[37,38] Figure 4–22 shows an M-mode aortic valve

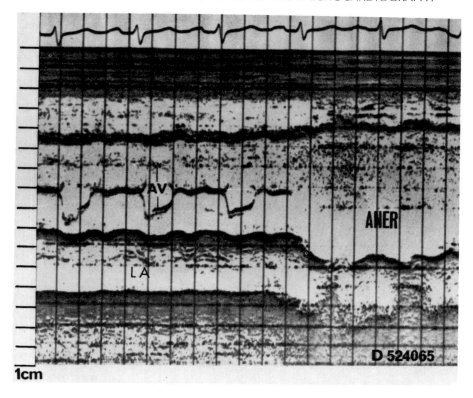

1cm

Fig. 4–22.   M-mode echocardiogram of a patient with an aortic aneurysm (ANER). Note how the posterior aortic wall motion reflects changes within the aorta rather than volume changes of the left atrium. AV = aortic valve; LA = left atrium.

echocardiogram of a patient with a low cardiac output, in which the reduced amplitude of aortic wall motion is apparent. Another study used aortic wall motion, ejection time, and the mitral valve B to C slope to calculate stroke volume.[39] More recent investigators have emphasized the relationship of aortic motion to changes in left atrial volume.[40–45]

Ever since the left atrium was first recorded echocardiographically, it was obvious that the posterior wall of the aorta also represented the anterior wall of the left atrium.[47] Since the posterior left atrial wall rarely shows any significant motion, the change in left atrial volume is best reflected by the motion of its anterior wall, which is the same as the posterior aortic wall. Although few efforts have been made to measure absolute left atrial volumes by way of aortic wall motion, the pattern of left atrial filling and emptying has been assessed by looking at the aortic root.

As noted in Figure 4–21, the posterior aortic wall (PAW) moves downward fairly rapidly with the onset of diastole. During mid-diastole there is relatively little motion of the aortic wall. Following atrial systole there is again a downward displacement of the wall toward the left atrium. This pattern of wall motion can be interpreted as a sudden decrease in left atrial volume in early diastole as the mitral valve opens and blood flows from the left atrium into the left ventricle. This phase of left atrial emptying has been labeled the "rapid emptying phase" (R, Fig. 4–21).[40] During mid-diastole the blood flowing from the left atrium to the left ventricle is about equal to that coming into the left atrium through the pulmonary veins. This phase has been called the "conduit phase" (C, Fig. 4–21). With atrial systole the left atrium actively contracts and produces the "systolic phase of atrial emptying" (S, Fig. 4–21). During ventricular systole the mitral valve is closed and the left atrium fills with blood coming from the pulmonary veins (LA filling). If left atrial emptying is restricted, as might occur with mitral stenosis, the rapid filling phase is decreased.[41,42] This decrease may also occur if left ventricular filling is restricted because of decreased compliance of the left ventricle.[45] There is evidence that the rate at which the aortic wall moves posteriorly in early diastole (first derivative of aortic root motion) is related to transmitral flow.[48] One study suggests dividing the diastolic pattern of aortic wall motion into thirds to determine the ratio of emptying of the left atrium.[41] Normally the amplitude of the first third of diastole should exceed 40 percent of total amplitude of left atrial emptying. A reduced left atrial emptying index could be due to obstruction at the mitral orifice, either from mitral stenosis or a malfunctioning prosthetic valve,[41] or to abnormal filling of the ventricle as a result of intrinsic myocardial disease of that chamber.[45] Other studies have examined the percentage and slope of left atrial emptying with atrial systole. The investigators found that patients with a decreased left ventricular compliance had an increased percentage of left atrial emptying following atrial systole.[44,49]

It should be remembered that these measurements are obtained from the posterior wall of the aorta and that intrinsic disease in the aorta and the ejection of blood into the aorta may also affect posterior aortic wall motion. Figure 4–22 is an echocardiogram of a patient with an aortic aneurysm. During ventricular ejection the aorta expands and the posterior aortic wall moves downward toward the left atrium. Thus wall motion in this patient is influenced more by blood flowing into the aorta than by blood flowing into the left atrium. The left atrial filling probably produces displacement of atrial walls not recorded on this M-mode examination.

Doppler Echocardiography

Doppler ultrasound comes close to measuring blood flow directly. The returning Doppler signal from a column of moving blood is related to the velocity at which the blood is flowing. If one knows the angle of the ultrasonic beam to the column of blood,

one can calculate fairly accurately the velocity of flow. Theoretically, if one knew the velocity of flow in addition to the cross-sectional area of the vascular container through which the blood was flowing, then the absolute blood flow could be calculated. This reasoning is still theoretical because many technical problems have made actual measurement of blood flow by way of Doppler echocardiography difficult. First, even with two-dimensional echocardiography it is not easy to accurately determine the angle of the ultrasonic beam to the moving column of blood. Minor changes in the angle of the ultrasonic beam may produce major changes in the Doppler signal. It is best to record the Doppler signal when the ultrasonic beam is parallel to the blood flow, a technique exactly opposite to that employed when using ultrasound for imaging. The best echoes for imaging occur when the ultrasonic beam is perpendicular to those structures being recorded. Thus combining imaging echocardiography, either M-mode or two-dimensional, has some geometric difficulties. Despite these limitations and the fact that absolute blood flow has yet to be measured by way of Doppler techniques, the literature is filled with clinical applications of Doppler ultrasound for determining central intravascular blood flow. The most frequently used technique is to place the Doppler transducer in the suprasternal notch and to record the pattern of flow in the aorta.[50–55] Figure 4–23 demonstrates how one can record a Doppler signal from either the ascending or descending portion of the aorta. The rapid flow of blood in the aorta during systole produces an appropriate Doppler signal. In an examination of the ascending aorta, the flow moves toward the transducer while in the descending aorta the flow moves away from the transducer. With a directional Doppler system the signal frequently rises above the baseline when the flow is toward the transducer and is inscribed below the baseline when flow is away from the transducer. Many suprasternal techniques for estimating blood flow velocity use continuous-wave ultrasound. More recently, pulsed Doppler echocardiography has been used for these same purposes.

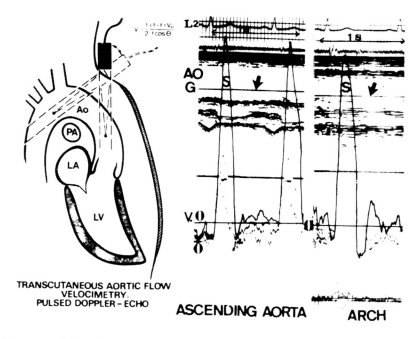

$$V = \frac{1(f-f)V_0}{2 \ f\cos\theta}$$

TRANSCUTANEOUS AORTIC FLOW
VELOCIMETRY.
PULSED DOPPLER – ECHO

ASCENDING AORTA   ARCH

Fig. 4–23.   Diagram and Doppler echocardiogram demonstrating how a Doppler signal can be obtained from the ascending aorta (AO) and arch of the aorta with the transducer in the suprasternal notch. PA = pulmonary artery; LA = left atrium; LV = left ventricle; G = location of Doppler sampling gate; S = systole. (From Veyrat, C., et al.: Validity of echo-pulsed Doppler velocimetry for assessing the diagnosis and severity of aortic valve disease and prosthetic valve function. *In* Echocardiology. Edited by C.T. Lancee. The Hague, Martinus Nijhoff, 1979.)

The pattern of blood flow can be readily apparent when using the suprasternal technique. For example, this examination can detect changes in blood flow velocity in patients with hypertrophic subaortic stenosis.[56] In addition, one could conceivably monitor an individual patient to look for changes in velocity following interventions or while following the course of an acutely ill patient.[53] Theoretically, if one could combine the Doppler technique with two-dimensional echocardiography, which would give a cross-sectional area of the aorta, one could calculate absolute blood flow in the aorta. Instrumentation is beginning to become commercially available for this purpose, and only time will tell whether this theoretical technique becomes a reality.

Besides attempts to measure absolute blood flow, Doppler echocardiography can demonstrate differences in types of blood flow. Probably the most promising application thus far is in the use of Doppler echocardiography to distinguish between laminar and turbulent, or disturbed, blood flow.[56a] Laminar flow is characterized by blood flowing in one direction. Turbulent flow produces eddy currents in multiple directions. This application of Doppler echocardiography has demonstrated value in detecting certain valvular abnormalities and intracardiac shunts. More recent work with multigated, color-encoded Doppler (see Chapter 1) is exciting and promises to provide even more ultrasonic techniques for recording intravascular blood flow.

Contrast Echocardiography

Contrast echocardiography was initially used in echocardiography to help identify the cardiac structures. This technique was next applied to the detection of intracardiac shunts. An intriguing, relatively new application for contrast echocardiography is to use it as an indicator dilution technique for evaluating blood flow.[57] A peripheral venous injection can be made and the contrast-producing bubbles can be studied as they traverse the right side of the heart. As expected, in a patient having good cardiac output the microbubbles pass through the right side of the heart quickly with a rapid clearance time. In patients with decreased cardiac output and/or poor right-sided hemodynamics, the washout of the echoes is much slower. A video densitometer is used to measure the change in contrast intensity from the passing microbubbles, and a washout, or clearance, curve of the contrast echoes is inscribed. The preliminary findings indicate that the clearance contrast of echoes is related fairly well to the rate of blood flow through the right side. This research remains unconfirmed and awaits further investigation before its clinical utility is established. Thus far this application of contrast echocardiography has been limited to the right side of the heart because the contrast-producing bubbles are too large to pass through capillaries. Researchers are trying to develop an echo-producing contrast substance that can pass through the pulmonary capillaries and produce echoes on the left side of the heart with a peripheral or right-sided injection.

EFFECT OF ALTERED INTRAVASCULAR PRESSURE ON THE ECHOCARDIOGRAM

The use of echocardiography to predict changes in cardiac pressure do not have the same degree of sensitivity and accuracy as do the echocardiographic reflectors of blood flow. The echocardiographic findings that reflect alterations in intravascular pressure are more indirect and hence are relatively insensitive. Despite these limitations, however, the observations are still of clinical value and can frequently be helpful in the diagnosis and management of a specific patient.

Elevated Left Ventricular Systolic Pressure

An increase in the afterload of the left ventricle produces an increase in the systolic left ventricular pressure. Such an increase in afterload may be a result of obstruction to left ventricular outflow or of an increase in systemic peripheral resistance. Irrespective of the cause, the common consequence of a chronically increased afterload is hypertrophy of the left ventricular walls and an increase in total left ventricular mass. Several groups have shown a good relationship between echocardiographic left ventricular hypertrophy and the systolic left ventricular pressure.[58-66] This research has been conducted primarily in children with valvular aortic stenosis. Some groups have used either the diastolic or systolic wall thickness, whereas others have used a ratio between the wall thickness and the left ventricular diameter.[58,60,62,64,65] Yet other groups have attempted to calculate total left ventricular mass. In children without left ventricular dilatation, the correlation between the echocardiographic findings of left ventricular hypertrophy, either in diastole or systole, and the left ventricular systolic pressure has been reasonably good. These studies suggest that one can merely subtract the systemic systolic blood pressure, as determined by sphygmomanometry, to determine the pressure gradient across the aortic valve. Whether this technique is accurate for estimating left ventricular systolic pressure is still unsettled. Apparently in children the technique is considered reasonably valid and is used by many pediatric echocardiographers. However, it is well known that when the ventricle begins to dilate, the technique is no longer dependable. In addition, little data indicate this technique is valid in adults. The echocardiographic findings can probably help to categorize even adult patients. Patients with elevated left ventricular systolic pressures undoubtedly have thicker walls than do patients with normal left ventricular systolic pressure. However, it is unlikely that a statistical relationship exists between the absolute wall thickness and the systolic pressure. Thus few echocardiographers attempt to estimate left ventricular systolic pressure in adult patients.

Elevated Left Ventricular Diastolic Pressure

A change in mitral valve motion in patients with elevated left ventricular diastolic pressure was one of the earliest echocardiographic observations to predict altered hemodynamics. One such observation was that in patients with elevated left ventricular diastolic pressure secondary to aortic regur-

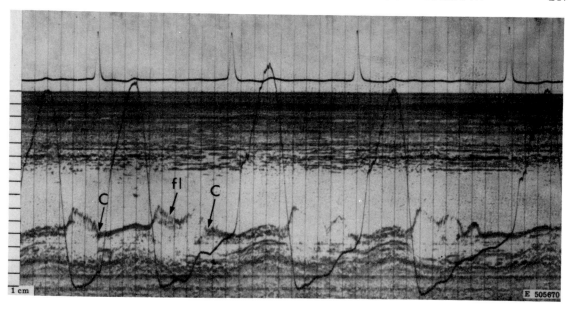

Fig. 4–24. Simultaneous left ventricular pressure and mitral valve echocardiogram in a patient with severe aortic regurgitation and atrial fibrillation. With a prolonged diastolic interval and a high left ventricular diastolic pressure, closure (C) of the mitral valve occurs before the onset of electrical depolarization. Fluttering (fl) of the mitral leaflet can be noted.

gitation there was premature closure of the mitral valve.[67–70,70a] Figure 4–24 shows a simultaneous mitral valve echocardiogram that reveals left ventricular pressure in a patient with severe aortic regurgitation and atrial fibrillation. The anterior mitral leaflet shows fluttering of the valve during diastole This phenomenon, a sign of aortic regurgitation, is discussed further in Chapter 6. Figure 4–24 shows that closure of the mitral valve (C) varies from cycle to cycle. The first cardiac cycle is relatively short, and mitral valve closure occurs immediately after the onset of electrical depolarization. Left ventricular diastolic pressure is low. The interval between the first and second cardiac complexes is much longer. In this case, closure of the valve (C) clearly precedes the onset of ventricular systole, and left ventricular diastolic pressure is considerably higher than in the preceding cardiac cycle. The next two cardiac intervals are again relatively long, and premature closure of the mitral valve again precedes the onset of electrical depolarization. This finding is most striking before the last cardiac complex at which time closure of the mitral valve is markedly pre-

mature. This premature closure most likely occurs because the regurgitant aortic blood elevates the left ventricular diastolic pressure beyond that of the left atrial pressure, and thus the mitral valve closes.[67,68]

Figure 4–25 shows another example of a patient with severe aortic regurgitation. This time the patient is in sinus rhythm, which is more usual. Again the two leaflets abruptly approach each other prior to the onset of electrical depolarization (C'). There is actually a small amount of separation between the leaflets from C' until after ventricular systole at point C. However, the mitral valve is functionally closed at C', and this echocardiogram shows effective premature closure similar to that seen in Figure 4–24. Again this phenomenon is probably the result of massive aortic regurgitation and a high left ventricular diastolic pressure. Note the mitral valve fluttering secondary to the regurgitation (f1). Premature mitral valve closure is a clinically useful sign because it has been shown to be a bad prognostic finding in patients with acute aortic regurgitation secondary to bacterial endocarditis.[71] This echocardiographic observation may be one

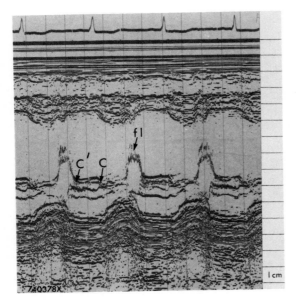

Fig. 4–25.   Mitral valve echocardiogram of a patient with severe aortic regurgitation. The valve is almost completely closed (C′) long before the onset of ventricular systole. Atrial contraction has little effect in reopening the valve. Complete closure occurs with ventricular systole (C). Note fluttering of the mitral valve (fl).

of the first signs that indicate a possible need for surgical replacement of the aortic valve.[67,68] One might argue over whether this premature closure is totally a function of rising left ventricular diastolic pressure or whether it is due to the back flow of blood from the aortic regurgitation. This question is difficult to answer since all factors are interrelated. Mid-diastolic closure of the mitral valve secondary to aortic regurgitation may also be noted (see Chapter 6), but following atrial systole premature closure does not occur unless the left ventricular diastolic pressure is significantly elevated.

Other examples of altered mitral valve motion in patients with abnormal cardiac pressures have been noted.[72] Figure 4–26 diagrammatically shows the relationship between mitral valve motion and left ventricular pressure in a normal subject and in a patient with an elevated left ventricular diastolic pressure. In a normal individual (Fig. 4–26A), the left ventricular diastolic pressure is initially low and gradually rises dur-

ing diastole, and there is a slight variation in left atrial pressure during this period. The corresponding mitral valve shows rapid opening from D to E. Closure of the mitral valve, from A to C, is smooth and of brief duration. Figure 4–26B shows a situation that may occur in patients with an elevated left ventricular diastolic pressure as a result of a marked rise in pressure following atrial systole.[73] These patients often have poor left ventricular compliance owing to hypertrophy, fibrosis, or ischemia.[72] Following atrial systole, there is a rapid rise in left atrial pressure followed by an almost immediate similar rise in left ventricular pressure. As a result, the two pressures cross earlier than usual, and the onset of mitral valve closure is premature, that is, the A point occurs earlier than usual. Immediately before ventricular systole, the two pressures are nearly equal and mitral valve closure is interrupted, as noted by a plateau, or notch, between A and C.[73–75] Complete closure of the mitral valve occurs at a higher left ventricular pressure and is delayed. The end result is a prolongation of the A to C interval and a "plateau," "notch," or "B bump" between the A and C points. Since the duration of the A to C inter-

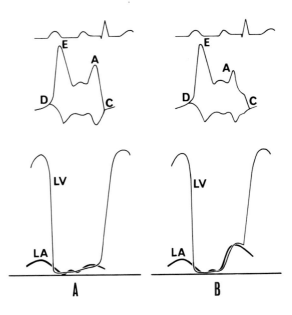

Fig. 4–26.   Diagrams illustrating how the mitral valve echocardiogram may reflect changes in left ventricular diastolic pressure (see text for details).

val depends on atrioventricular conduction, a measure of the electrocardiographic P–R interval minus the echocardiographic A–C interval was used to correct for the effect of atrioventricular conduction. In an early study, this P–R minus A–C interval was noted as useful in identifying those patients with elevated left ventricular diastolic pressures. Subsequent experience revealed many limitations to this measurement. First, patients who had a short P–R interval, less than 150 msec, would frequently have abnormal P–R minus A–C intervals, despite the fact that the left ventricular diastolic pressures were normal. Thus the PR–AC interval proved unreliable in patients with short P–R intervals. In addition, it became apparent that the A–C interval was probably not totally dependent on abnormal pressure. Prolongation of the C point was probably a function of ventricular contraction as well as pressure. Finally, it should be emphasized that no one has yet demonstrated a correlation between echocardiographic mitral valve motion and left ventricular diastolic pressure.[73,76] The abnormal closure may help identify groups of individuals who probably have elevated left ventricular diastolic pressures, but one cannot predict absolute pressure from this echocardiographic finding. Probably the most reliable echocardiographic sign is the plateau, or B bump, between the A–C intervals. This finding most likely indicates some equalization of left ventricular and left atrial pressures and a temporary cessation of flow prior to ventricular systole usually as a result of an elevated atrial component of the diastolic pressure. As with almost all echocardiographic measurements that reflect pressure changes, abnormal mitral valve closure is a relatively insensitive indicator of an elevated left ventricular diastolic pressure. Most echocardiographers have found that a left ventricular end-diastolic pressure of about 20 mmHg is usually necessary before abnormal closure is seen.

Another difficulty with using the mitral valve closure for detecting abnormal ventricular pressure is that this echocardiographic sign is not always apparent. Figure 4–27 demonstrates the typical pattern of ab-

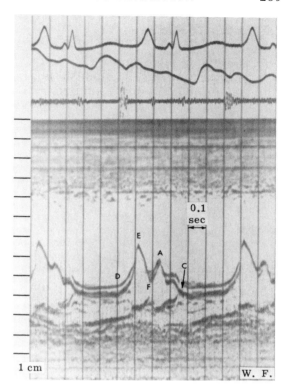

Fig. 4–27. Mitral valve echocardiogram of a patient with an elevated left ventricular end-diastolic pressure secondary to poor left ventricular compliance and an elevated atrial component of the left ventricular pressure. Closure of the mitral valve (A–C) is prolonged and interrupted.

normal mitral valve closure in a patient with left ventricular dysfunction and an elevated diastolic pressure. The abnormal closure pattern in Figure 4–28 is more subtle. The A wave is actually partially obscured by the E point, and the abnormal closure pattern is not as obvious. Although the pattern in Figure 4–29 should not be as confusing, it can be missed unless the echocardiographer closely examines the electrocardiogram. The true A wave may be misinterpreted as mid-diastolic reopening, and the B bump may be erroneously interpreted as the A wave.

The mitral valve D to E slope was also thought to be a reflector of elevated initial diastolic pressure. As already indicated, the D to E slope is probably influenced more by flow than by pressure. Thus, although the D to E slope may be reduced in patients who have initially elevated diastolic pressure, the

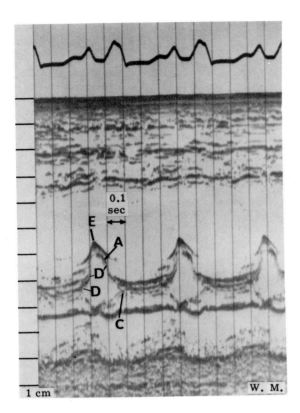

Fig. 4–28. Mitral valve echocardiogram of a patient with elevated left ventricular diastolic pressure in whom the E and A points occur almsot simultaneously. The C point is delayed, and the A–C interval is prolonged. The initial opening slope (D–D′) is reduced.

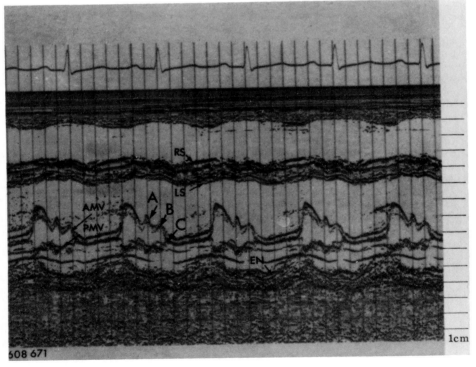

Fig. 4–29. Mitral valve echocardiogram of a patient with elevated left ventricular diastolic pressure in whom the B notch is prominent and superficially resembles an A wave. The patient has a prolonged P–R interval, and the A wave occurs earlier than usual. AMV = anterior mitral valve leaflet; PMV = posterior mitral valve leaflet; RS = right side of interventricular septum; LS = left side of interventricular septum; EN = posterior left ventricular endocardium.

210

abnormal echocardiographic finding is probably a consequence of the altered flow rather than of the elevated pressure.

A recent case study described a patient with severely elevated left ventricular diastolic pressure secondary to aortic regurgitation in whom premature opening of the aortic valve had occurred.[77] Figure 4–30 is from that report and shows opening of the aortic valve prior to the onset of ventricular systole. The presumptive mechanism is that the left ventricular diastolic pressure was so high that it exceeded the aortic pressure at end-diastole and the aortic valve opened.

There are specific situations in which the left ventricular diastolic pressure is elevated and echocardiography may be of some value. One such situation is constrictive pericarditis. This entity is described in more detail in the chapter on pericardial disease. There have been alterations in left ventricular wall motion, mitral valve motion, and interventricular septal motion reported in the literature in patients with constrictive pericarditis. Unfortunately, none of these measurements are highly reliable as an isolated finding. These abnormalities are more reliable when they appear in a constellation of abnormalities. The pattern of left ventricular posterior wall motion during diastole may prove to be the most reliable sign. With constriction, filling of the ventricle following the initial rapid filling is restricted because of the thickened, nonstretching pericardium. As a result, the diastolic slope of the posterior wall motion during diastole is flat. This motion probably corresponds with the rapid rise and plateau in left ventricular diastolic pressure, i.e., square root sign. There are patients without constrictive pericarditis who may also exhibit this flat motion during mid-diastole. In patients with acute left ventricular dilatation or even in a normal subject with a high stroke volume, the pericardium is relatively constricting and the echocardiogram may show flat, mid-diastolic left ventricular wall motion. Thus this finding is again nonspecific.

Elevated Right Ventricular Systolic Pressure

The two causes of an elevated right ventricular systolic pressure are obstruction to the right ventricular outflow tract or elevated pulmonary artery pressure. One consequence of a chronically elevated right ventricular systolic pressure is right ventricular hypertrophy. Some investigators have attempted to use the thickness of the right ventricular wall as a predictor of right ventricular systolic pressure.[78,79] This technique is somewhat similar to that used for estimating systolic left ventricular pressure by measuring left ventricular wall thickness. As with the left-sided measurement, using right ventricular wall thickness to estimate the systolic pressure is limited primarily to pediatric patients. The right ventricular wall thickness does not record well in adults. The 2.25-mHz transducer usually used for adult echocardiography does not have sufficient resolution in the near field to permit accurate measurement of the right ventricular wall (see Chapter 3). In unusual situations the right ventricular wall thickness may be clearly hypertrophied and can reliably predict an elevated right ventricular systolic pressure even in adults. The situation may occur with either right ventricular outflow obstruction or pulmonary hypertension.

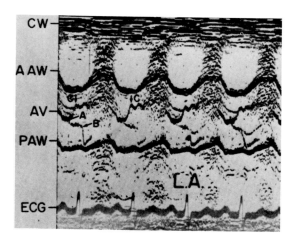

Fig. 4–30. Premature opening of the aortic valve (AV) in a patient with severe aortic regurgitation. The valve opens *(arrow)* before the onset of electrical depolarization (C). Additional opening of the valve occurs with ventricular ejection (B). CW = chest wall; AAW = anterior aortic wall; PAW = posterior aortic wall; LA = left atrium; ECG = electrocardiogram. (From Pietro, D.A., et al.: Premature opening of the aortic valve: an index of highly advanced aortic regurgitation. J. Clin. Ultrasound, 6:170, 1978.)

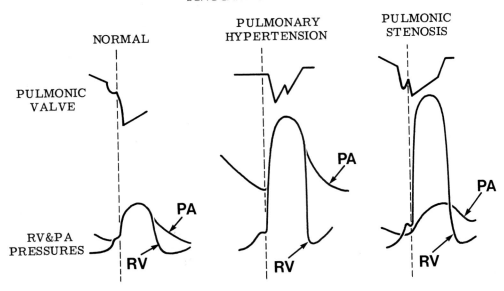

Fig. 4–31. Diagrams demonstrating the relationship between pulmonic valve motion and pressures within the right ventricle and pulmonary artery. RV = right ventricle; PA = pulmonary artery.

The pulmonary valve can provide information that may be helpful in judging right ventricular systolic pressure. Figure 4–31 diagrammatically shows the relationship between pulmonic valve motion and elevated right ventricular systolic pressure. With pulmonary hypertension, both right ventricular and pulmonary artery systolic pressures are elevated. In addition, the pulmonary artery diastolic pressure is elevated disproportionate to any rise in right ventricular diastolic pressure. With pulmonic stenosis, the right ventricular systolic and frequently diastolic pressures are elevated, whereas the systolic and diastolic pulmonary artery pressures are normal or reduced. Thus the relationship between the two pressures is different. The atrial component of the right ventricular diastolic pressure may be elevated and may actually exceed the pulmonary artery pressure. As a result, the atrial component of the pulmonary valve motion is accentuated (Fig. 4–31).[79a]

Figure 4–31 is primarily shown to provide an understanding of how pulmonary valve motion can reflect alterations in right-sided pressures. The pulmonary valve motion depicted in this diagram is not absolute. There are significant limitations to the patterns of motion seen both in patients with pulmonary hypertension and pulmonic stenosis. The exaggerated A wave with pulmonic stenosis is quite insensitive and only occurs in patients with at least moderate pulmonic stenosis. In addition, exaggerated A waves may occur in patients without pulmonic stenosis.[79b] If there is a large right ventricular stroke volume owing to a variety of causes, exaggerated A waves may again be detected.[79c] Figure 4–32 demonstrates a patient with exaggerated A waves secondary to pulmonic stenosis. The termination of the A wave, which is the B point, varies considerably with respiration. As a result, the measurement of the A wave must consider respiration. Thus A wave measurements are frequently given as maximum A waves with quiet respiration. This illustration also notes the technical difficulties in recording the pulmonary valve.

Several abnormalities of the pulmonary valve have been suggested as indicators of pulmonary hypertension.[79d-g] One since discredited sign is a flat diastolic slope, or E to F slope, of the pulmonary valve. This diastolic slope has proved nonspecific, and its reliability in predicting pulmonary hypertension is so poor that it should probably be no

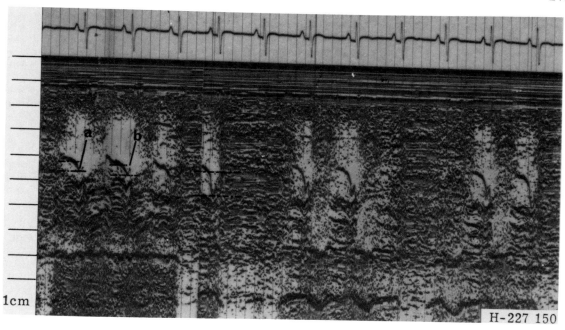

Fig. 4–32. Pulmonary valve echocardiogram of a patient with pulmonic stenosis. Note marked variation in the depths of the A wave and in the position of the B point. As depicted by the respiratory interference, with inspiration the A wave is exaggerated, with the total depth approximating 9 mm (fourth complex).

longer used.[80,81,81a] It has been noted that a negative or upward sloping diastolic slope may be more reliable in predicting pulmonary hypertension, but this observation has not been confirmed. An absent or diminished A wave is a fairly frequent finding in pulmonary hypertension and presumably is due to an elevated pulmonary artery diastolic pressure (Figs. 4–31 and 4–33). However, if there is right ventricular failure, the A wave may reappear as the atrial component of the right ventricular diastolic pressure increases (Fig. 4–34).[79d,81b] Thus the presence of a normal-sized A wave does not exclude pulmonary hypertension, especially when right ventricular failure is suspected. Another observation that has not received wide acceptance is the lack of variation in the A-wave depth in patients with pulmonary hypertension.[79c] The A wave normally varies significantly in amplitude with respiration. With pulmonary hypertension the degree of variation tends to decrease. Unfortunately, the pulmonary valve A wave is also influenced by motion of the aorta, which in turn is a function of left atrial emptying.[81] Thus it is

not surprising that the pulmonary A wave is not completely reliable in predicting pulmonary hypertension.[82]

The pre-ejection period and the opening velocity of the pulmonary valve are also measurements used for determining pulmonary hypertension. The right ventricular pressure requires more time to exceed the pulmonary artery pressure so that the pulmonary valve can open. Often, the valve then opens more rapidly. These measurements are more difficult to make and require strip-chart recordings of 100 mm/sec. Recent experimental data question the reliability of pulmonary valve opening velocity and pre-ejection period to predict pulmonary hypertension.[83] Midsystolic closure, or "notching," is a valuable sign for pulmonary hypertension.[79e,79g] Figure 4–33 demonstrates a pulmonary valve in a patient with pulmonary hypertension. The midsystolic notch (n) is clearly visible. One can also see the lack of an A wave. A variation of the midsystolic notch is shown in Figure 4–34. The notch is not quite as apparent because the reopening of the valve in the latter half of systole is not

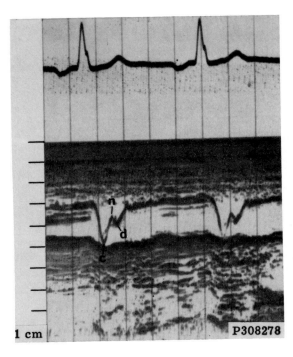

Fig. 4–33. Characteristic motion of the posterior pulmonary valve leaflet in a patient with pulmonary hypertension. This tracing demonstrates the absence of an *A* wave (a), negative *E–F* slope, and midsystolic notching (n) of the leaflet. (From Weyman, A.E., et al.: Echocardiographic patterns of pulmonic valve motion with pulmonary hypertension. Circulation, 50:905, 1974.)

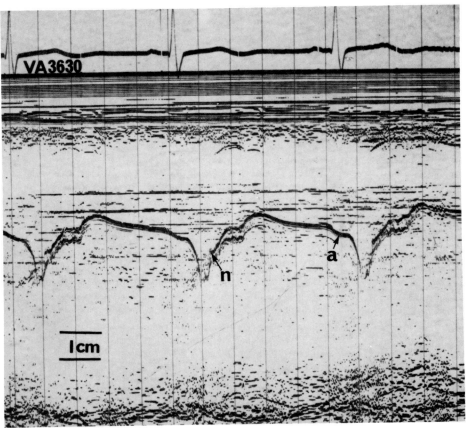

Fig. 4–34. Pulmonary valve echocardiogram of a patient with pulmonary hypertension and right ventricular failure. Despite the pulmonary hypertension, a small A wave (a) is still present. Midsystolic notching (n), though present, is less obvious because the valve does not reopen in late systole as much as it did in Figure 4–33.

as striking as in Figure 4–22. Figure 4–35 shows another patient with pulmonary hypertension. This pulmonary valve echocardiogram demonstrates both anterior (APV) and posterior (PPV) pulmonary leaflets and illustrates how the midsystolic notch (arrow) can vary from beat to beat.

The explanation for the midsystolic notch of the pulmonary valve with pulmonary hypertension is not known;[84] however, when present, the notch is one of the more reliable signs of pulmonary hypertension.[82] The biggest problem with this sign is that it is not always present. There is also a rare false positive (Fig. 4–36). The pulmonary valve in Figure 4–36 has an obvious midsystolic notch. However, this patient did not have pulmonary hypertension.[85] He had a dilated pulmonary artery and normal right-sided

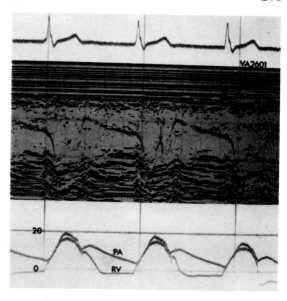

Fig. 4–36. Pulmonary valve echocardiogram and pulmonary artery (PA) and right ventricular (RV) pressures in a patient with a midsystolic pulmonary valve notch (N) and no pulmonary hypertension. The patient had idiopathic dilatation of the pulmonary artery and normal pulmonary artery pressure. (From Bauman, W., et al.: Mid-systolic notching of the pulmonary valve in the absence of pulmonary hypertension. Am. J. Cardiol., 43:1049, 1979.)

pressures. The pulmonary artery dilatation was idiopathic. The midsystolic closure presumably was due to eddy currents formed within the dilated pulmonary artery in systole. These eddy currents partially closed the valve in midsystole. A similar finding may be seen occasionally with the aortic valve in patients with aortic dilatation. Thus the pulmonary valve echocardiogram is definitely useful in detecting pulmonary hypertension, although with many significant limitations. The measurements are insensitive. A pulmonary mean pressure of 20 mmHg or more is necessary before one can expect any change in pulmonary valve motion. In addition, there are potential false positives and false negatives for all signs.

The right ventricular systolic pressure, or the pulmonary artery pressure has been estimated using systolic time intervals derived from the M-mode echocardiogram.[86–91] The right ventricular ejection time and pre-ejection period can be measured by record-

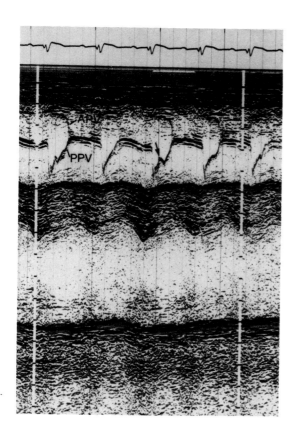

Fig. 4–35. M-mode recording of the anterior (APV) and posterior (PPV) pulmonary valve leaflets in a patient with pulmonary hypertension. Midsystolic notching (arrow) is seen intermittently in the posterior leaflet.

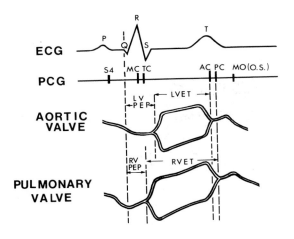

Fig. 4–37. Diagram of the aortic and pulmonary valve M-mode echocardiograms showing how left-sided and right-sided systolic time intervals can be measured. MC = mitral closure; TC = tricuspid closure; AC = aortic closure; PC = pulmonic closure; MO = mitral opening; PEP = pre-ejection period; LV = left ventricle; RV = right ventricle; ET = ejection time; PCG = phonocardiogram.

ing the pulmonary valve together with an electrocardiogram (Fig. 4–37). As mentioned, the right ventricle pre-ejection period lengthens with pulmonary hypertension. In addition, the right ventricular ejection time shortens with earlier closure of the pulmonary valve. Thus the PEP/RVET ratio increases with pulmonary hypertension. This ratio supposedly even reflects the pressure in a banded pulmonary artery and can be used to judge the adequacy of the surgical procedure.[91a] As expected, this technique has been popular in pediatric echocardiography. The application requires a complete recording of the pulmonary valve. When the pulmonary valve can be recorded, the PEP/RVET measurements supposedly correlate well with the pulmonary artery pressure; however, reports have refuted the usefulness of systolic time intervals in predicting pulmonary artery pressures, especially in patients with ventricular septal defects.[83,92]

Elevated Right Ventricular Diastolic Pressure

The similarity between the tricuspid and mitral valves prompts echocardiographers to transfer their knowledge about the mitral valve to the tricuspid valve.[93,94] In patients with elevated right ventricular diastolic pressure, it is not uncommon to see abnormal closure of the tricuspid valve, as noted in Figure 4–38. This abnormal tricuspid valve superficially resembles the mitral valve in Figure 4–27. Data in the literature indicate that the abnormal tricuspid valve closure identifies patients whose left ventricular diastolic pressures are elevated.

Occasionally, the right ventricular diastolic pressure may be elevated to the point that it influences pulmonary valve motion. An elevated left ventricular diastolic pressure rarely produces diastolic opening of the aortic valve (Fig. 4–30) because of the usually high aortic diastolic pressure.[95,96] However, since the pulmonary artery diastolic pressure is relatively low, an elevated right ventricular diastolic pressure occasionally produces premature opening of the pulmonary valve prior to atrial systole. Figure 4–39 shows a patient whose pulmonary valve opens with a significant downward motion (arrow) prior to the usual location of the A dip (dotted line). This particular patient had a ruptured sinus of Valsalva aneurysm with blood flowing from the aorta directly into the right atrium. The sudden increase in blood and transmission of pressure from the aorta into the right atrium caused markedly elevated right atrial and right ventricular pressures which, as they exceeded the pulmonary artery pressure, opened the valve. Following surgical correction of the aneurysm, the pulmonary valve motion returned to normal (Fig. 4–39B). A variety of other conditions that produce a marked increase in right ventricular or right atrial pressures in diastole may produce the same phenomenon. This sign has been noted in patients with constrictive pericarditis, tricuspid regurgitation, or severe right heart failure.[95,96]

There are other situations in which right ventricular diastolic pressure is elevated. Such conditions include constrictive pericarditis or cardiac tamponade. These problems are discussed in more detail in the chapter on pericardial disease. As mentioned, premature pulmonary valve opening is one sign that may occur with constrictive pericarditis.[95–97] Other echocardiographic signs indicating elevated right ventricular

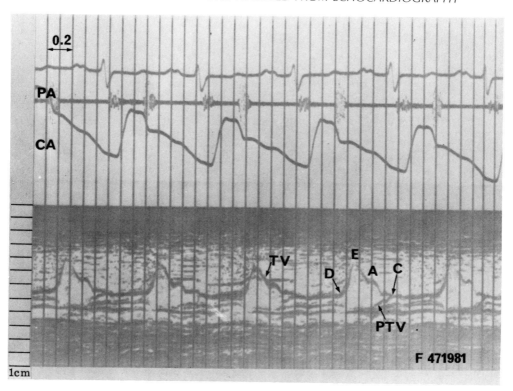

Fig. 4–38. Echocardiogram of the tricuspid valve in a patient with pulmonary hypertension and an elevated right ventricular diastolic pressure. Closure of the tricuspid valve (C) is delayed with a prolonged A-C interval. PA = phonocardiogram in the pulmonic area; CA = carotid pulse; TV = anterior tricuspid valve leaflet; PTV = posterior tricuspid valve leaflet. (From Chang, S.: M-mode Echocardiographic Techniques and Pattern Recognition. Philadelphia, Lea & Febiger, 1976.)

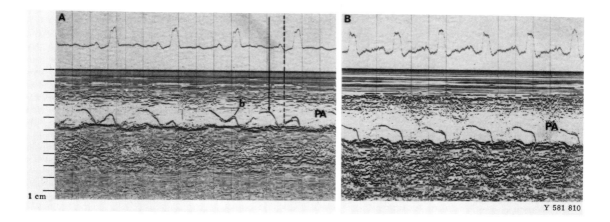

Fig. 4–39. A, Pre-operative pulmonary valve echocardiogram in a patient with a sinus of Valsalva aneurysm that ruptured into the right atrium. The valve can be seen opening in early diastole (solid arrow) well before the onset of atrial systole. The leaflet is almost fully opened at the onset of atrial systole (dotted line). B, Following surgical closure of the fistula, the diastolic pulmonary valve opening is no longer present. (From Weyman, A.E., et al.: Premature pulmonic valve opening following sinus of Valsalva aneurysm rupture into the right atrium. Circulation, 51:556, 1975. By permission of the American Heart Association, Inc.)

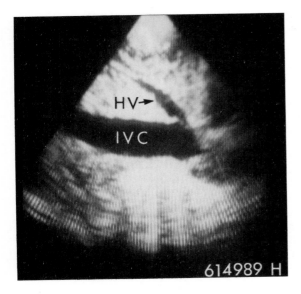

Fig. 4–40. Subcostal two-dimensional echocardiogram of a dilated inferior vena cava (IVC) and hepatic vein (HV) in a patient with right heart failure and elevated right atrial pressure.

diastolic pressures owing to constriction or tamponade have not been very reliable and have produced considerable confusion in the literature.

Right ventricular diastolic and right atrial pressures can be reflected by the systemic veins. The clinical assessment of venous pressure is a time-honored bedside examination. Echocardiography offers the opportunity to examine the inferior vena cava to note the effects of elevated right atrial pressure on this vessel. Figure 4–40 shows a two-dimensional echocardiogram of the inferior vena cava in a patient with right heart failure and elevated systemic venous pressure. Dilatation of the systemic vein is striking.

REFERENCES

1. DeMaria, A.N., Lies, J.E., King, J.F., Miller, R.R., Amsterdam, E.A., and Mason, D.T.: Echographic assessment of atrial transport, mitral movement, and ventricular performance following electroversion of supra-ventricular arrhythmias. Circulation, 51:273, 1975.
2. Zaky, A., Steinmetz, E.F., and Feigenbaum, H.: Role of atrium in closure of mitral valve in man. Am. J. Physiol., 217:1952, 1969.
3. Edler, I.: Ultrasound cardiogram in mitral valve disease. Acta Chir. Scand., 111:230, 1956.
4. Edler, I. and Gustafson, A.: Ultrasonic cardiogram in mitral stenosis. Acta Med. Scand., 159:85, 1957.
5. Edler, I., Hertz, C.H., Gustafson, A., Karlefors, T., and Christensson, B.: The movements of the heart valves recorded by ultrasound. Nord. Med., 64:1178, 1960.
6. Salerni, R., Reddy, P.S., Sherman, M.E., O'Toole, J.D., Leon, D.F., and Shaver, J.A.: Pressure and sound correlates of the mitral valve echocardiogram in mitral stenosis. Circulation, 58:119, 1978.
7. Shiina, A., Matsumoto, Y., Kawasaki, K., Tsuchiya, M., Itoh, K., Hokamaki, H., Miyata, K., Tomita, T., Matsumoto, Y., Yaginuma, T., and Hosoda, S.: Analysis of opening and closing motion of the mitral valve by simultaneous echocardiogram and pressure tracing across the valve. J. Cardiogr., 6:661, 1976.
8. Pohost, G.M., Dinsmore, R.E., Rubenstein, J.J., O'Keefe, D.D., Grantham, N., Scully, H.E., Beierholm, E.A., Frederiksen, J.W., Weisfeldt, M.L., and Daggest, W.M.: The echocardiogram of the anterior leaflet of the mitral valve: correlation with hemodynamic and cineroentgenographic studies in dogs. Circulation, 51:88, 1975.
9. Rubenstein, J.J., Pohost, G.M., Dinsmore, R.E., and Harthorne, J.W.: The echocardiographic determination of mitral valve opening and closure: correlation with hemodynamic studies in man. Circulation, 51:98, 1975.
10. Laiken, S.L., Johnson, A.D., Bhargava, V., and Rigo, P.: Instantaneous transmitral blood flow and anterior mitral leaflet motion in man. Circulation, 59:476, 1979.
11. Chakorn, S.A., Siggers, D.C., Wharton, C.F.P., and Deuchar, D.C.: Study of normal and abnormal movements of mitral valve ring using reflected ultrasound. Br. Heart J., 34:480, 1972.
12. Layton, C., Gent, G., Pridie, R., McDonald, A., and Brigden, W.: Diastolic closure rate of normal mitral valve. Br. Heart J., 35:1066, 1973.
13. Zaky, A., Grabhorn, L., and Feigenbaum, H.: Movement of the mitral ring: a study of ultrasoundcardiography. Cardiovasc. Res., 1:121, 1967.
14. Zaky, A., Nasser, W.K., and Feigenbaum, H.: Study of mitral valve action recorded by reflected ultrasound and its application in the diagnosis of mitral stenosis. Circulation, 37:789, 1968.
15. Madeira, H.C., Ziady, G., Oakley, C.M., and Pridie, R.B.: Echocardiographic assessment of left ventricular volume overload. Br. Heart J., 36:1175, 1974.
16. Vignola, P.A., Walker, H.J., Pohost, G.M., and Zir, L.M.: Relation between phasic mitral flow and the echocardiogram of the mitral valve in man. Br. Heart J., 39:1292, 1977.
17. DeMaria, A., Miller, R.R., Amsterdam, E.A., Markson, W., and Mason, D.T.: Mitral valve early diastolic closing velocity on echogram: relation to sequential diastolic flow and ventricular compliance. Am. J. Cardiol., 37:693, 1976.
18. Quinones, M.A., Gaasch, W.H., Waisser, E., and Alexander, J.K.: Reduction in the rate of diastolic descent of the mitral valve echogram in patients with altered left ventricular diastolic pressure-volume relations. Circulation, 49:246, 1974.
19. DeMaria, A.N., Miller, R.R., Amsterdam, E.A., Markson, W., and Mason, D.T.: Mitral valve early diastolic closing velocity in the echocardiogram: relation to sequential diastolic flow and ventricular compliance. Am. J. Cardiol., 37:693, 1976.

20. Vignola, P.A., Walker, H.J., Gold, H.K., and Leinbach, R.C.: Alteration of the left ventricular pressure-volume relationship in man and its effect on the mitral echocardiographic early diastolic closure slope. Circulation, 58:586, 1977.

21. Duchak, J.M., Jr., Chang, S., and Feigenbaum, H.: The posterior mitral valve echo and the echocardiographic diagnosis of mitral stenosis. Am. J. Cardiol., 29:628, 1972.

22. Goodman, D.J., Harrison, D.C., and Popp, R.L.: Echocardiographic features of primary pulmonary hypertension. Am. Heart J., 86:847, 1973.

23. McLaurin, L.P., Gibson, T.C., Waider, W., Grossman, W., and Craige, E.: An appraisal of mitral valve echocardiograms mimicking mitral stenosis in conditions with right ventricular pressure overload. Circulation, 48:801, 1973.

24. Laniado, S., Yellin, E., Kotler, M., Levy, L., Stadler, J., and Terdiman, R.: A study of the dynamic relations between the mitral valve echogram and phasic mitral flow. Circulation, 51:104, 1975.

25. Pennock, R., Kingsley, B., Kawai, N., Kimbiris, D., and Segal, B.L.: Stroke volume and cardiac output measured by echocardiography. Am. J. Cardiol., 25:121, 1970. (Abstract)

26. Glasser, S.P.: Illustrative echocardiogram: late mitral valve opening in aortic regurgitation. Chest, 70:70, 1976.

27. Lee, F.C.S., Talbot, L., and Abbott, J.A.: Echocardiographic determination of cardiac output from mitral or aortic valve motion. Circulation (Suppl. II), 54:84, 1976. (Abstract)

28. Fischer, J.C., Chang, S., Konecke, L.L., and Feigenbaum, H.: Echocardiographic determination of mitral valve flow. Am. J. Cardiol., 29:262, 1972. (Abstract)

29. Rasmussen, S., Corya, B.C., Feigenbaum, H., Black, M.J., Lovelace, D.E., Phillips, J.F., Noble, R.J., and Knoebel, S.B.: Stroke volume calculated from the mitral valve echogram in patients with and without ventricular dyssynergy. Circulation, 58:125, 1978.

30. Scheele, W., Kraus, R., Allen, H.N., Halpern, S.W.: Use of M-mode echocardiography to determine stroke volume. Am. J. Cardiol., 43:411, 1979. (Abstract)

31. Winer, H., Kronzon, I., and Glassman, E.: Echocardiographic findings in severe paradoxical pulse due to pulmonary embolization. Am. J. Cardiol., 40:808, 1977.

32. Okumachi, F., Komine, Y., Yamaoka, S., Takagi, Y., Yanagihara, K., Kato, H., Owaki, T., and Yoshikawa, J.: Diagnostic significance of aortic valve motion. J. Cardiogr., 8:367, 1978.

33. Yeh, H.C., Winsberg, F., and Mercer, E.M.: Echocardiographic aortic valve orifice dimensions: its use in evaluating aortic stenosis and cardiac output. J. Clin. Ultrasound, 1:182, 1973.

34. Jacobs, W.R., Croke, R.P., Loeb, H.S., and Gunnar, R.M.: Echocardiographic aortic ejection area as a reflection of left ventricular stroke volume. J. Clin. Ultrasound, 7:369, 1979.

35. Laniado, S., Yellin, E., Terdiman, R., Meytes, I., and Stadler, J.: Hemodynamic correlates of the normal aortic valve echogram. A study of sound, flow, and motion. Circulation, 54:729, 1976.

36. Rasmussen, S., Corya, B.C., Lovelace, E., Black, M.J., and Phillips, J.F.: Forward stroke volume derived from aortic valve echograms. Clin. Res., 27:672A, 1979. (Abstract)

37. Morioka, S., Tomonaga, G., Hoshino, T., Motomura, M., Shimono, Y., and Kusukawa, R.: Systolic aortic root motion and left ventricular stroke volume. J. Cardiogr., 8:223, 1978.

38. Pratt, R.C., Parisi, A.F., Harrington, J.J., and Sasahara, A.A.: The influence of left ventricular stroke volume on aortic root motion: an echocardiographic study. Circulation, 53:947, 1976.

39. Lalani, A.V. and Lee, S.J.K.: Echocardiographic measurement of cardiac output using the mitral valve and aortic root echo. Circulation, 54:738, 1976.

40. Strunk, B.L., Fitzgerald, J.W., Lipton, M., Popp, R.L., and Barry, W.H.: The posterior aortic wall echocardiogram: its relationship to left atrial volume change. Circulation, 54:744, 1976.

41. Strunk, B.L., London, E.J., Fitzgerald, J., Popp, R.L., and Barry, W.H.: The assessment of mitral stenosis and prosthetic mitral valve obstruction, using the posterior aortic wall echocardiogram. Circulation, 55:885, 1977.

42. Akgun, G. and Layton, C.: Aortic root and left atrial wall motion: an echocardiographic study. Br. Heart J., 39:1082, 1977.

43. Yorozu, T., Matsuzaki, M., Sasada, T., Ehara, K., Ishida, K., Fukagawa, K., Tanikado, O., Shimizu, M., Nomoto, R., and Kusukawa, R.: Echocardiographic estimation of stroke volume and mitral regurgitant volume using new parameter from aortic posterior wall motion. J. Cardiogr., 8:473, 1978.

44. Tye, K-H., Desser, K.B., and Benchimol, A.: Relation between apexcardiographic a wave and posterior aortic wall motion. Am. J. Cardiol., 43:24, 1979.

45. Hall, R.J.C., Clark, S.E., and Brown, D.: Evaluation of posterior aortic wall echogram in diagnosis of mitral valve disease. Br. Heart J., 41:522, 1979.

46. Reference deleted.

47. Hirata, T., Wolfe, S.B., Popp, R.L., Helmen, C.H., and Feigenbaum, H.: Estimation of left atrial size using ultrasound. Am. Heart J., 78:43, 1969.

48. Teichholz, L., Caputo, G., Ambrose, J., Knopsler, B., Martinez, E., and Herman, M.: First derivative of diastolic aortic root motion as a measure of transmitral flow. Am. J. Cardiol., 45:436, 1980. (Abstract)

49. Ambrose, J., Martinez, E., Teichholz, L., Meller, J., Pichard, A., and Herman, M.: The slope of the posterior aortic root during atrial systole—an index of left ventricular chamber stiffness. Circulation (Suppl. II), 60:121, 1979. (Abstract)

50. Colocousis, J.S., Huntsman, L.L., and Curreri, P.W.: Estimation of stroke volume changes by ultrasonic Doppler. Circulation, 56:914, 1977.

51. Huntsman, L.L. and Colocousis, J.S.: Stroke volume monitoring by ultrasonic Doppler. Circulation (Suppl. II), 58:234, 1978. (Abstract)

52. Sequeira, R.F., Light, L.H., Gross, G., and Raftery, E.B.: Transcutaneous aortovelography: a quantitative evaluation. Br. Heart J., 38:443, 1976.

53. Buchtal, A., Hanson, G.C., and Peisach, A.R.: Transcutaneous aortovelography: potentially useful technique in management of critically ill patients. Br. Heart J., 38:451, 1976.

54. Veyrat, C., Cholot, G., Abitbol, G., and Kalmanson, D.: Validity of echo-pulsed Doppler velocimetry for assessing the diagnosis and severity of aortic valve disease and prosthetic valve function. In Echocardiology. Edited by C.T. Lancee. The Hague, Martinus Nijhoff, 1979.

55. Colocousis, J.S. and Huntsman, L.L.: Stroke vol-

ume estimation by non-invasive Doppler. Circulation (Suppl. III), 56:219, 1977. (Abstract)

56. Joyner, C.R., Jr., Harrison, F.S., Jr., and Gruber, J.W.: Diagnosis of hypertrophic subaortic stenosis with a Doppler velocity flow detector. Ann. Intern. Med., 74:692, 1971.

56a.Baker, D.W.V. and Johnson, S.L.: Doppler echocardiography. In Cardiac Ultrasound. Edited by R. Gramiak, et al. St. Louis, C.V. Mosby Co., 1975.

57. Bommer, W., Neef, J., Neumann, A., Weinert, L., Lee, G., Mason, D.T., and DeMaria, A.N.: Indicator-dilution curves obtained by photometric analysis of two-dimensional echo-contrast studies. Am. J. Cardiol., 41:370, 1978. (Abstract)

58. Glanz, S., Hellenbrand, W.E., Berman, M.A., and Talner, N.S.: Echocardiographic assessment of the severity of aortic stenosis in children and adolescents. Am. J. Cardiol., 38:620, 1976.

59. Schwartz, A., Vignola, P.A., Walker, H.J., King, M.E., and Goldblatt, A.: Echocardiographic estimation of aortic valve gradient in aortic stenosis. Ann. Intern. Med., 89:329, 1978.

60. Blackwood, R.A., Bloom, K.R., and Williams, C.M.: Aortic stenosis in children. Experience with echocardiographic predictions of severity. Circulation, 57:263, 1978.

61. Johnson, G.L., Meyer, R.A., Schwartz, D.C., Korfhagen, J., and Kaplan, S.: Echocardiographic evaluation of fixed left ventricular outlet obstruction in children. Circulation, 56:299, 1977.

62. Bass, J.L., Einzig, S., Hong, C.Y., and Moller, J.H.: Echocardiographic screening to assess the severity of congenital aortic valve stenosis in children. Am. J. Cardiol., 44:82, 1979.

63. Johnson, G.L., Meyer, R.A., Schwartz, D.C., Korfhagen, J., and Kaplan, S.: Left ventricular function by echocardiography in children with fixed aortic stenosis. Am. J. Cardiol., 38:611, 1976.

64. Mokotoff, D.M., Quinones, M.A., Winters, W.L., and Miller, R.R.: Non-invasive quantification of severity of aortic stenosis by echocardiographic wall thickness-radius ratio. Am. J. Cardiol., 43:406, 1979. (Abstract)

65. Gewitz, M.H., Werner, J.C., Kleinman, C.S., Hellenbrand, W.E., and Talner, N.S.: Role of echocardiography in aortic stenosis: pre- and postoperative studies. Am. J. Cardiol., 43:67, 1979.

66. Aziz, K.U., van Grondelle, A., Paul, M.H., and Muster, A.J.: Echocardiographic assessment of the relation between left ventricular wall and cavity dimensions and peak systolic pressure in children with aortic stenosis. Am. J. Cardiol., 40:775, 1977.

67 Botvinick, E.H., Schiller, N.B., Wickramasekaran, R., Klausner, S.C., and Gertz, E.: Echocardiographic demonstration of early mitral valve closure in severe aortic insufficiency: its clinical implications. Circulation, 51:836, 1975.

68. Pridie, R.B., Beham, R., and Oakley, C.M.: Echocardiography of the mitral valve in aortic valve disease. Br. Heart J., 33:296, 1971.

69. Oki, T., Matsuhisa, M., Tsuyuguchi, N., Kondo, C., Matsumura, K., Niki, T., Mori, H., and Sawada, S.: Echo patterns of the anterior leaflet of the mitral valve in patients with aortic insufficiency. J. Cardiogr., 6:307, 1976.

70. Ambrose, J.A., Meller, J., Teichholz, L.E., and Herman, M.V.: Premature closure of the mitral valve. Echocardiographic clue for the diagnosis of aortic dissection. Chest, 73:121, 1978.

70a.Fox, S., Kotler, M.N., Segal, B.L., and Parry, W.: Echocardiographic diagnosis of acute aortic valve endocarditis and its complications. Arch. Intern. Med., 137:85, 1977.

71. Mann, T., McLaurin, L., Grossman, W., and Craige, E.: Assessing the hemodynamic severity of acute aortic regurgitation due to infective endocarditis. N. Engl. J. Med., 293:108, 1975.

72. Konecke, L.L., Feigenbaum, H., Chang, S., Corya, B.C., and Fischer, J.C.: Abnormal mitral valve motion in patients with elevated left ventricular diastolic pressures. Circulation, 47:989, 1973.

73. Ambrose, J.A., Teichholz, L.E., Meller, J., Weintraub, W., Pichard, A.D., Smith, H., Jr., Martinez, E.E., and Herman, M.V.: The influence of left ventricular late diastolic filling on the A wave of the left ventricular pressure trace. Circulation, 60:510, 1979.

74. Feigenbaum, H., Dillon, J.C., Haine, C.L., and Chang, S.: Effect of elevated atrial component of left ventricular pressure on mitral valve closure. Am. J. Cardiol., 25:95, 1970. (Abstract)

75. Nimura, Y., Matsumoto, M., Shimada, H., Nagata, S., Oyama, S., Takahashi, Y., Abe, H., Kitabatake, A., and Matsuo, H.: Unusual configuration of ultrasound cardiogram of mitral valve observed in some cases with myocardial disease of unknown cause. Med. Ultrasonics, 9:108, 1971.

76. Lewis, J.R., Parker, J.O., and Burggraf, G.W.: Mitral valve motion and changes in left ventricular end-diastolic pressure: a correlative study of the PR–AC interval. Am. J. Cardiol., 42:383, 1978.

77. Pietro, D.A., Parisi, A.F., Harrington, J.J., and Askenazi, J.: Premature opening of the aortic valve: an index of highly advanced aortic regurgitation. J. Clin. Ultrasound, 6:170, 1978.

78. Nakano, H., Saito, A., and Ueda, K.: Echocardiographic estimation of right ventricular peak systolic pressure in children with heart disease. J. Cardiogr., 9:83, 1979.

79a.Weyman, A.E., Dillon, J.C., Feigenbaum, H., and Chang, S.: Echocardiographic patterns of pulmonic valve motion in pulmonic stenosis. Am. J. Cardiol., 34:644, 1974.

79b.Goldberg, S.J., Allen, H.D., and Sahn, D.J.: Pediatric and Adolescent Echocardiography. Chicago, Year Book Medical Publishers, Inc., 1975.

79c.Weyman, A.E.: Pulmonary valve echo motion in clinical practice. Am. J. Med., 62:843, 1977.

79d.Nanda, N.C., Gramiak, R., Robinson, T.I., and Shah, P.M.: Echocardiographic evaluation of pulmonary hypertension. Circulation, 50:575, 1974.

79e.Weyman, A.E., Dillon, J.C., Feigenbaum, H., and Chang, S.: Echocardiographic patterns of pulmonary valve motion with pulmonary hypertension. Circulation, 50:905, 1974.

79f.Belenkov, Iu. N. and Atkov, O. Iu.: Echocardiographic signs of pulmonary hypertension. Kardiologiia, 16:34, 1976.

79g.Shiina, A., Yaginuma, T., Matsumoto, Y., Kawasaki, K., Tsuchiya, M., Miyata, K., Tomita, T., Matsumoto, Y., Kawai, N., and Hosoda, S.: Echocardiographic analysis of pulmonic and aortic valve motion by simultaneous recordings of flow velocity and intravascular pressure: genesis of mid-systolic semi-closure of the pulmonic valve in patients with pulmonary hypertension. J. Cardiogr., 7:599, 1977.

80. Lew, W. and Karliner, J.S.: Assessment of pulmonary valve echogram in normal subjects and in pa-

tients with pulmonary arterial hypertension. Br. Heart J., *42*:147, 1979.

81. Pocoski, D.J. and Shah, P.M.: Physiologic correlates of echocardiographic pulmonary valve motion in diastole. Circulation, 58:1064, 1978.

81a. Hada, Y., Sakamoto, T., Hayashi, T., Ichiyasu, H., and Amano, K.: Echocardiogram of the pulmonary valve: variability of the pattern and the related technical problems. Jpn. Heart J., *18*:298, 1977.

81b. Sulbaran, T. A., Garcia, E., Dear, W.E., Guttin, J., Pechacek, L.W., and Hall, R.J.: Severe pulmonary hypertension with significant "A" dip on pulmonic valve echocardiogram. Cardiovasc. Dis., *4*:172, 1977.

82. Acquatella, H., Schiller, N.B., Sharpe, D.N., and Chatterjee, K.: Lack of correlation between echocardiographic pulmonary valve morphology and simultaneous pulmonary arterial pressure. Am. J. Cardiol., 43:946, 1979.

83. Kerber, R.E., Martins, J.B., Barnes, R., Manuel, W.J., and Maximov, M.: Effects of acute hemodynamic alterations on pulmonic valve motion: experimental and clinical echocardiographic studies. Circulation, 60:1074, 1979.

84. Tahara, M. and Tanaka, H.: Hemodynamic determinants of systolic pulmonary valve echogram in experimental pulmonary hypertension. Circulation (Suppl. II), 60:790, 1979. (Abstract)

85. Bauman, W., Wann, L.S., Childress, R., Weyman, A.E., Feigenbaum, H., and Dillon, J.C.: Midsystolic notching of the pulmonary valve in the absence of pulmonary hypertension. Am. J. Cardiol., 43:1049, 1979.

86. Hirschfeld, S., Meyer, R., Schwartz, D.C., Korfhagen, J., and Kaplan, S.: Measurement of right and left ventricular systolic time intervals by echocardiography. Circulation, 51:304, 1975.

87. Riggs, T., Hirschfeld, S., Borkat, G., Knoke, J., and Liebman, J.: Assessment of the pulmonary vascular bed by echocardiographic right ventricular systolic time intervals. Circulation, 57:939, 1978.

88. Mills, P., Amara, I., McLaurin, L., Koch, G., and Craige, E.: Dual echocardiographic right ventricular isovolumic contraction in estimation of pulmonary artery pressure. Circulation (Suppl. III), 56:67, 1977. (Abstract)

89. Spooner, E.W., Perry, B.L., Stern, A.M., and Sigmann, J.M.: Estimation of pulmonary/systemic resistance ratios from echocardiographic systolic time intervals in young patients with congenital or acquired heart disease. Am. J. Cardiol., 42:810, 1978.

90. Johnson, G.L., Meyer, R.A., Korfhagen, J., Schwartz, D.C., and Kaplan, S.: Echocardiographic assessment of pulmonary arterial pressure in children with complete right bundle branch block. Am. J. Cardiol., 41:1264, 1978.

91. Gutgesell, H.P., Pinsky, W.W., Duff, D.F., Adams, J., and McNamara, D.G.: Left and right ventricular systolic time intervals in the newborn. Usefulness and limitation in distinguishing respiratory disease from transposition of the great arteries. Br. Heart J., 42:27, 1979.

91a. Garcia, E.J., Riggs, T., Hirschfeld, S., and Liebman, J.: Echocardiographic assessment of the adequacy of pulmonary arterial banding. Am. J. Cardiol., 44:487, 1979.

92. Silverman, N.H., Snider, A.R., and Rudolph A.M.: Evaluation of pulmonary hypertension by M-mode echocardiography in children with ventricular septal defects. Circulation, 61:1125, 1980.

93. Starling, M.R., Crawford, M.H., Walsh, R.A., and O'Rourke, R.A.: Value of the tricuspid valve echogram for estimating right ventricular end-diastolic pressure during vasodilator therapy. Am. J. Cardiol., 45:966, 1980.

94. Fujii, J., Morita, K., Watanabe, H., and Kato, K.: Tricuspid valve echograms in various right heart diseases. Cardiovasc. Sound Bull., 5:241, 1975.

95. Wann, L.S., Weyman, A.E., Dillon, J.C., and Feigenbaum, H.: Premature pulmonary valve opening. Circulation, 55:128, 1977.

96. Nishimoto, M., Tanaka, C., Oku, H., Ikuno, Y., Kawai, S., Furukawa, K., Takeuchi, K., and Shiota, K.: Presystolic pulmonary valve opening in constrictive pericarditis. J. Cardiogr., 7:55, 1977.

97. Hada, Y., Sakamoto, T., Hayashi, T., Ichiyasu, H., and Amano, K.: Echocardiogram of normal pulmonary valve. Physiological data and effect of atrial contraction on the valve motion. Jpn. Heart J., *18*:421, 1977.

Echocardiographic Findings with Altered Electrical Activation

Because of its rapid sampling rate, M-mode echocardiography provides an excellent opportunity to study cardiac motion. This motion is influenced not only by anatomic and hemodynamic abnormalities, but also by changes in electrical activation. Many of the changes in motion are too subtle to be detected by angiographic or radionuclide techniques. Even real-time two-dimensional echocardiography has a relatively slow sampling rate compared with that of M-mode echocardiography. The rapid sampling rate and the use of time as one of the dimensions make M-mode echocardiography an ideal diagnostic and investigative tool for noting functional changes that occur with altered electrical activation.[1] The following discussion is not intended to be an exhaustive review of all possible relationships between the echocardiogram and electrocardiogram. It should, however, provide some principles and examples of how changes in cardiac electrical activity can influence the echocardiogram.

ABNORMAL VENTRICULAR DEPOLARIZATION

Bundle Branch Block

Patients with left bundle branch block serve as an excellent example of how altered electrical depolarization can influence cardiac motion. The echocardiographic findings in patients with left bundle branch block involve changes in the motion of the interventricular septum.[1a,2–4,4a,5,5a] Figure 5–1 briefly

reviews normal interventricular septal motion. Following electrical depolarization there may be a brief anterior motion of the interventricular septum. This motion is then followed immediately by downward displacement of the septum toward the left ventricular cavity during ventricular ejection.

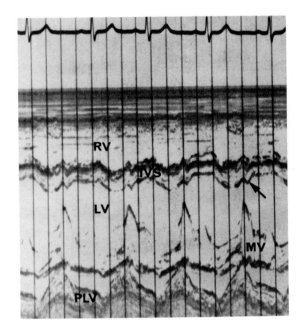

Fig. 5–1. M-mode echocardiogram of a normal interventricular septum (IVS). In early diastole there is a brief diastolic downward dip *(arrow)* shortly after the opening of the mitral valve (MV). RV = right ventricle; LV = left ventricle; PLV = posterior left ventricular wall. (From Chang, S.: M-mode Echocardiographic Techniques and Pattern Recognition. Philadelphia, Lea & Febiger, 1976.)

With ventricular relaxation the septum moves anteriorly toward the right ventricle. Shortly after the initial mitral valve opening, or E point, there is a brief downward dip of the septum toward the left ventricle (arrow). This dip is immediately followed by resumption of the anterior motion of the interventricular septum as diastole continues. Figure 5–2 demonstrates the echocardiographic findings with left bundle branch block. Shortly after the onset of electrical depolarization (heavy vertical line at right), there is a rapid downward dip of the left septum (LS)

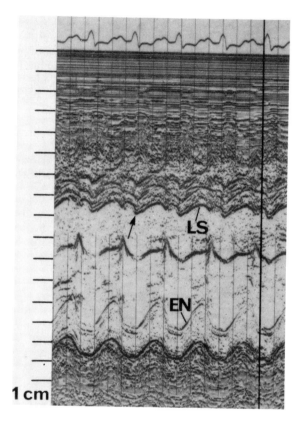

Fig. 5–2. M-mode echocardiogram of the left ventricle in a patient with left bundle branch block. Following the onset of electrical depolarization (heavy vertical line at right) there is a rapid downward displacement of the left septum (LS) followed by an upward motion during ventricular ejection. This motion produces a downward beaking (arrow) shortly after electrical depolarization and paradoxical septal motion during ventricular ejection. EN = posterior left ventricular endocardium. (From Dillon, J.C., et al.: Echocardiographic manifestations of left bundle branch block pattern. Circulation, 49:876, 1974.)

followed by a gradual anterior displacement of the interventricular septum throughout ventricular ejection. There may be a slight downward dip of the septum corresponding to the E point of the mitral valve. The principal echocardiographic feature of left bundle branch block is the downward motion of the interventricular septum with the onset of electrical depolarization (Fig. 5–2, arrow).

The abnormal anterior motion of the interventricular septum during ventricular ejection may be an important hemodynamic consequence of this electrical abnormality. As expected, the abnormal septal motion during ejection alters overall ventricular function. The extent to which this abnormal systolic motion occurs has been examined with two-dimensional echocardiography.[6] Since this portion of the interventricular septum is not often recorded with the routine right anterior oblique left ventricular angiogram, the abnormal function produced by left bundle branch block pattern is not commonly recognized as an important hemodynamic factor.

The abnormal septal motion during ventricular ejection is not always as striking as in Figure 5–2. Figure 5–3 demonstrates another echocardiogram of a patient with left bundle branch block. The abnormal posterior displacement of the septum with the onset of electrical depolarization is again noted (arrows). This downward dip, or beaking, is followed by another downward, more gradual motion of the septum toward the left ventricle. Thus, during ventricular ejection the septum is moving toward the left ventricle rather than paradoxically as in Figure 5–2. A somewhat larger early diastolic dip is also noted in Figure 5–3. The mechanical or hemodynamic effects of the left bundle branch block would not be as adverse to overall ventricular function in the patient in Figure 5–3 as it would in the patient in Figure 5–2. Thus, although septal motion is usually paradoxical during ventricular ejection in left bundle branch block, this situation is not always present. However, the early systolic downward dip, or beaking, immediately following electrical depolarization is a consistent and diagnostic finding in this abnormality.

Few studies have attempted to delineate

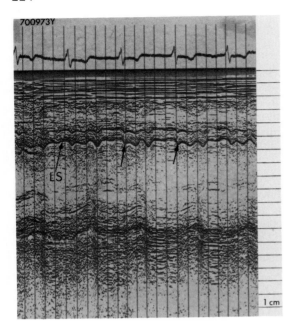

Fig. 5–3. M-mode echocardiogram of the inter-ventricular septum in a patient with left bundle branch block. Note again the posterior beaking *(arrows)* following the onset of electrical depolarization. The septal motion during ventricular ejection is more normal or downward rather than anterior or paradoxical as in Figure 5–2. LS = left septum.

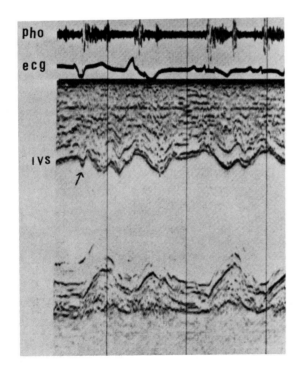

Fig. 5–4. Left ventricular echocardiogram demonstrating the septal motion in a patient with a pacemaker in the right ventricle. The first electrocardiographic complex is a paced beat. The aberrant depolarization produces an early beaking *(arrow)* of the interventricular septum (IVS) similar to that seen with left bundle branch block. Pho = phonocardiogram. (From Zoneraich, S.O. and Rhee, J.J.: Echocardiographic evaluation of septal motion in patients with artificial pacemakers: echocardiographic correlations. Am. Heart J., 93:596, 1977.)

the mechanism of the abnormal septal motion in left bundle branch block. Most investigators assume that the abnormal contraction pattern is secondary to the altered path of depolarization.[7] Pacing the right ventricle produces both electrocardiographic and echocardiographic patterns similar to left bundle branch block.[7a] Figure 5–4 shows a paced beat with a pacemaker in the right ventricle. Following the paced electrical depolarization there is an early systolic dip in the septum (arrow) identical to that seen in left bundle branch block. During ventricular ejection the septal motion is normal and moves downward toward the left ventricle. A subsequent premature ventricular systole produces no abnormal septal motion. The last two electrical complexes are normally conducted beats and septal motion is normal.[8-10] In one study that investigated right ventricular pacing by way of electrocardiography and echocardiography, the authors reported that the septal motion varied depending on where the right ventricle was stimulated. If the right ventricular apex was paced, then one saw the septal beaking but not the paradoxical motion during ejection (Fig. 5–4). However, if the right ventricular outflow tract was paced, then the septal motion was similar to a left bundle branch block with paradoxical motion during ejection.[10]

Interventricular septal motion is grossly normal in right bundle branch block. In one study, however, complete right bundle branch block produced delayed opening of a pulmonary valve, and in three out of twenty patients delayed tricuspid valve closure was detected.[11] Another study of patients with postoperative right bundle branch block reported an early systolic anterior motion of the septum following electrical depolarization.[12] These authors believed that this was an exaggerated amount of anterior motion. Both these observations on right bundle branch block have not been confirmed.

Wolff-Parkinson-White (WPW) Syndrome

Many articles in the literature describe the echocardiographic findings associated with Wolff-Parkinson-White syndrome.[13-22,22a] With so-called type B Wolff-Parkinson-

White syndrome one may find an echocardiogram similar to that found in left bundle branch block. Following electrical depolarization, a sharp, brief, downward or posterior dip of the interventricular septum may appear (Fig. 5–5, arrow).[13-17,19-22,22a] The frequency with which this echocardiographic pattern is observed in type B WPW varies in the literature. In one study only four out of

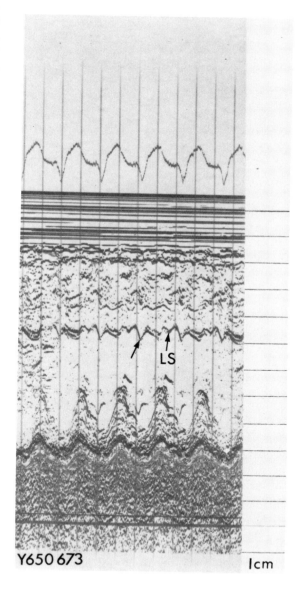

Fig. 5–5. Echocardiogram of the interventricular septum demonstrating an early systolic downward beaking (arrow) in a patient with type B Wolff-Parkinson-White syndrome. LS = left side of interventricular septum.

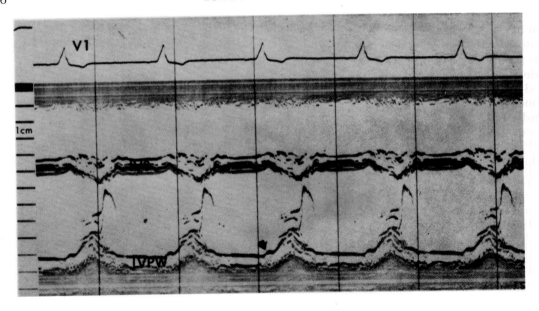

Fig. 5–6.   Left ventricular echocardiogram in a patient with type A Wolff-Parkinson-White syndrome. Note premature contraction or anterior motion *(arrow)* in left ventricular posterior wall (LVPW) echoes. IVS = interventricular septum. (From DeMaria, A.N., et al.: Alterations in ventricular contraction pattern in the Wolff-Parkinson-White syndrome. Circulation, *53*:249, 1976.)

twenty-two patients demonstrated the abnormal septal motion.[17] However, other series had frequencies as high as eight out of eleven.[22] Some authors have noted an exaggerated diastolic dip in patients with type B WPW syndrome.[20]

In patients with type A WPW syndrome, abnormal motion of the posterior ventricular wall may be detected (Fig. 5–6).[19,22–24] The consistent finding is a brief anterior displacement of the posterior left ventricular wall following the onset of electrical depolarization (Fig. 5–6, arrow). The frequency with which this echocardiographic pattern occurs in patients with type A WPW again varies in the literature. One group of investigators could not find this abnormality in any of their patients,[20] whereas in another study abnormal left ventricular posterior wall motion could be detected in all 20 patients with type A WPW.[19] It should be emphasized that the abnormal motion seen with type A WPW may be extremely subtle and thus warrants careful examination.[24] Figure 5–7 shows an unusual patient with WPW who has an abnormal early systolic motion of

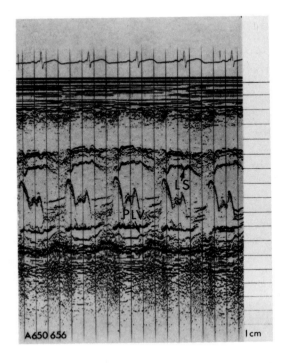

Fig. 5–7.   Echocardiogram of the left ventricle in a patient with Wolff-Parkinson-White syndrome who shows abnormal early systolic motion of the left septum (LS) and the posterior left ventricular wall (PLV).

both the posterior left ventricular wall (PLV) and the interventricular septum (LS). Variations of type A and type B are to be expected. As knowledge of this electrophysiologic abnormality increases, multiple types are being discovered, with the location of the bypass varying from patient to patient.

ECTOPIC RHYTHM

Ventricular Ectopy

Premature ventricular beats primarily influence the echocardiogram by the hemodynamic consequence of the premature systole. One might also expect an alteration in motion of either the interventricular septum or the posterior ventricular wall with spontaneous ventricular ectopy because of the abnormal path of depolarization, as with left bundle branch block, WPW, or electrical pacing. Such echocardiographic changes have not been described to date but, as will

be noted, these changes may occur. Thus far, only the hemodynamic consequences of premature ventricular beats have been noted by echocardiographers.

Figure 5–8 represents a common finding with a premature ventricular systole. The premature beat (heavy arrow) occurs before atrial depolarization, thus the A wave of the mitral valve is aborted in that cardiac cycle. Systolic motion of the interventricular septum (LS) and the posterior left ventricular wall (PLV) is diminished. Diastolic filling, as noted by the mitral valve, is reduced following the premature beat. However, the ventricular dimension between the septum and the posterior left ventricular wall increases since the ventricle was inadequately emptied with the premature beat. With the next ventricular depolarization there is a vigorous ejection with increased motion of the septum and the posterior left ventricular endocardium. The diastolic filling following

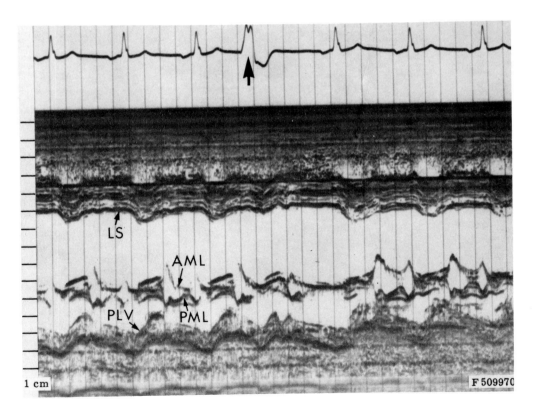

Fig. 5–8. M-mode echocardiogram of the left ventricle and mitral valve showing the effect of a premature ventricular systole *(heavy arrow)*. LS = left septum; PLV = posterior left ventricular wall; PML = posterior mitral leaflet; AML = anterior mitral leaflet.

that systole shows an increased separation of the anterior and posterior mitral leaflets that is indicative of an increasing flow of blood into the ventricle.

Figure 5–9 demonstrates the hemodynamic events as reflected by the mitral valve in a patient with two consecutive premature ventricular systoles (heavy arrows). The mitral valve pattern shows abnormal hemodynamics despite the normally conducted beats. Following the first electrical depolarization, the D to E slope is markedly reduced, and there is barely any E point with the second diastolic interval. The first premature ventricular systole occurs when the mitral valve would ordinarily open during diastole. The premature beats prevents the opening. The second premature ectopic beat again prevents the opening of the valve until a

sufficiently long interval occurs following the second premature ventricular beat. Partially because the mitral valve has been closed for such a long time (undoubtedly with increased blood volume in the left atrium), mitral valve motion following the premature beats is more normal with a brisker D to E slope and an obvious E point.

Figure 5–10 demonstrates the hemodynamic consequences of premature ventricular beats on the aortic valve. This recording also graphically demonstrates the influence of the interval between the premature beat and the preceding normally conducted complex. Following the first premature beat (1), the aortic valve opening is clearly reduced in both amplitude and duration. Premature beat 2 occurs following two normally conducted beats and is slightly farther away

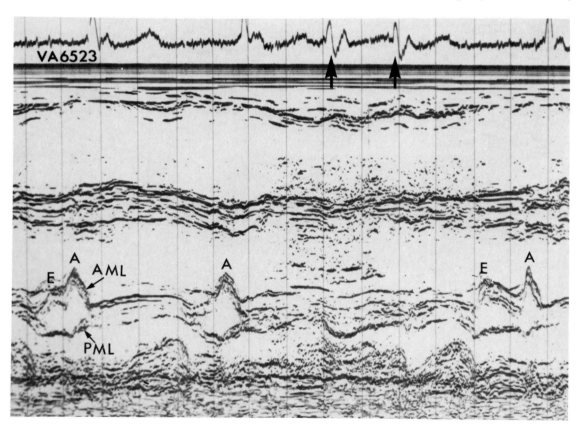

Fig. 5–9. Mitral valve echocardiogram showing the effect of two consecutive premature ventricular systoles (heavy arrows). The basic mitral valve motion is abnormal with a markedly decreased D to E slope and a diminished E point. No mitral opening is detected with the ventricular premature beats. Following the long pause of the second premature beat a more normal mitral valve is recorded. AML = anterior mitral leaflet; PML = posterior mitral leaflet.

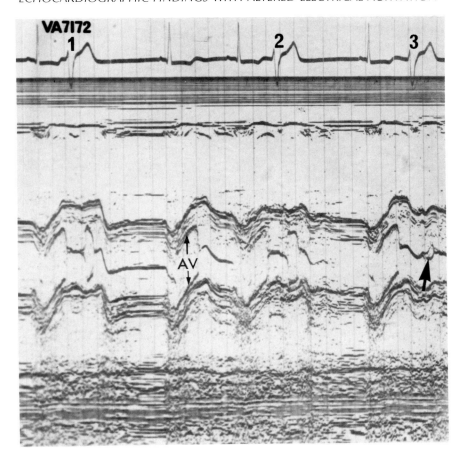

Fig. 5–10. Aortic valve echocardiogram showing the effect of premature ventricular systoles on aortic valve (AV) motion. Following the third premature ventricular systole, 3, the aortic valve barely opens (heavy arrow).

from the preceding normal beat than is premature beat 1. The aortic valve motion following the second premature beat is clearly reduced but is more normal than that following the first premature beat. There is even a brief interval at which time both aortic leaflets are parallel to each other while open. The most interesting finding is that following premature beat 3, the aortic valve barely opens (heavy arrow). One could speculate over why the third premature beat produced such miminal blood flow into the aorta. The sequence of normal and premature beats preceding the third premature beat was undoubtedly a factor. However, irrespective of the exact mechanism, this figure clearly demonstrates how hemodynamic consequences of ventricular premature systoles can be detected echocardiographically.

The pulmonary valve echocardiogram may also reflect the hemodynamic consequences of premature ventricular beats. Figure 5–11 is an artist's rendition of an actual electrocardiogram and echocardiogram with the proposed hemodynamic explanation for the observation as indicated by the pulmonary artery and right ventricular pressures. The interesting empirical finding is that following a single premature ventricular systole, no A wave is noted in the pulmonary valve, (Fig. 5–11A). However, when two premature systoles occur consecutively (Fig. 5–11B), a prominent A wave appears on the pulmonary valve echocardiogram. As suspected from the pulmonary valve echocardiogram in Figure 5–11A, the patient had pulmonary hypertension since no A wave was detectable on the pulmonary valve trac-

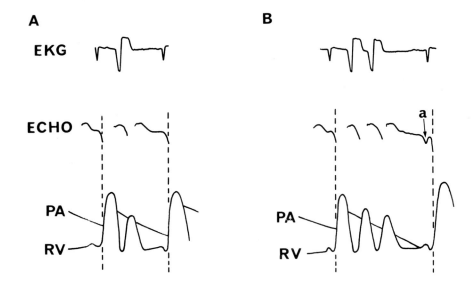

Fig. 5–11. Tracings demonstrating the effect of premature ventricular systoles on the pulmonary valve echocardiogram. *A*, The patient has pulmonary hypertension and no A wave is present with a single premature ventricular systole and a long diastolic pause. *B*, With two consecutive ventricular beats, however, the pulmonary artery pressure drops sufficiently so that with atrial contraction the right ventricular pressure can exceed the pulmonary artery pressure, and an A wave (a) can be recorded. PA = pulmonary artery; RV = right ventricle.

ing. However, an A wave did appear following the two consecutive premature systoles. The explanation for the A wave in Figure 5–11B is that the premature beats and the long diastolic interval permitted the diastolic pulmonary artery pressure to drop sufficiently so that atrial contraction could elevate the right ventricular pressure sufficiently to open the pulmonary valve. The echocardiogram in Figure 5–11 not only represents an interesting example of the influence of premature ventricular systoles on the echocardiogram, but it also offers clinical evidence that the A wave on the pulmonary valve echocardiogram is a function of the interrelationship of the pulmonary artery and right ventricular pressures.

Premature ventricular systoles may also produce peculiar configurations of the interventricular septum.[24a] Figure 5–12 shows an example of how septal motion can be distorted by premature ventricular systoles. Following normal electrical depolarization the septal motion in this area of the heart is flat. There is an early diastolic dip immediately prior to the full opening of the mitral valve. There is a second diastolic dip

in midsystole; thus this patient's septal motion is abnormal despite normal depolarization. However, following a ventricular premature beat there is a striking downward or posterior displacement of the interventricular septum (arrow). This dip is followed by a marked anterior motion of the septum during ventricular systole. The exact explanation for this peculiar septal motion is not certain, but the motion resembles that observed in left bundle branch block (Fig. 5–2) and may be due to the abnormal depolarization.

A somewhat more common finding with premature ventricular systoles is noted in Figure 5–13. In this patient the septal motion following a normal beat is normal. The unusual finding is that following the premature ventricular systoles there is an exaggerated diastolic septal dip (arrows). The diastolic dip is partially the result of the flat to absent systolic motion of the septum following ventricular ejection. Thus the diastolic dip, which is actually not much deeper than the normal diastolic dip, is more obvious because of the flat septum during ejection. A potential misinterpretation is mistaking the diastolic dip for systolic septal motion.

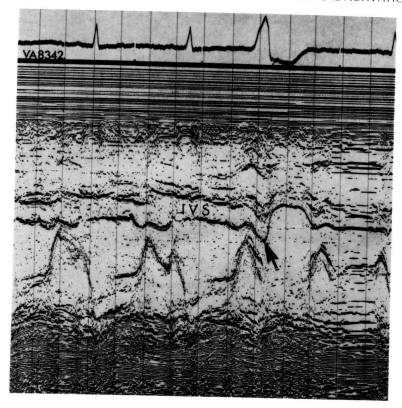

Fig. 5–12. M-mode echocardiogram of the interventricular septum (IVS) demonstrating a systolic downward beaking *(arrow)* of the septum and paradoxical motion during ejection with a premature ventricular systole.

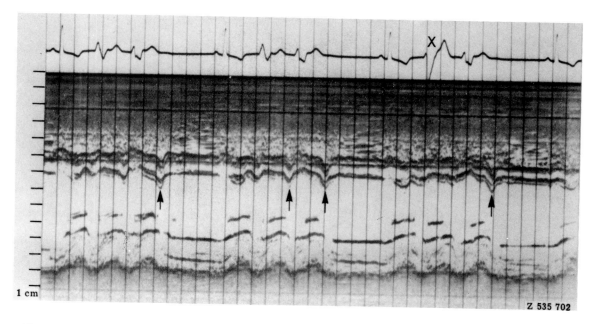

Fig. 5–13. M-mode examination demonstrating exaggerated diastolic septal dips *(arrows)* in a patient with premature ventricular systoles (see text for details).

These brief downward displacements of the septum are clearly diastolic events. A somewhat interesting but unexplained feature is that a prominent diastolic dip does not occur following the premature systole that has a different pattern of depolarization (X).

Supraventricular Ectopy

Before discussing supraventricular ectopic rhythms it should be apparent that sinus arrhythmia, which is a normal variant, distorts the echocardiogram. Figure 5–14 demonstrates the changes in mitral valve motion that occur with varying R–R intervals. The principal difference is the length of the mid-diastolic filling period. It is interesting that mitral valve motion in early diastole and late diastole is unchanged by the varying diastolic intervals. The height of the E and A points are essentially equal in all cardiac complexes. This observation helps to justify some of the formulas used for calculating mitral valve flow from the mitral valve echocardiogram (see Chapter 4).

Premature atrial systoles have similar effects on the echocardiogram as do premature ventricular systoles. Figure 5–15 demonstrates the effect of premature atrial systoles on the mitral valve echocardiogram. Despite the marked variation in the mitral valve motion, only three premature atrial systoles were recorded in this tracing. Three normally conducted beats occur between each atrial premature beat. The resultant A wave of the second premature atrial systole (2) is superimposed on the E point. Following ventricular systole, the mitral valve closes. The subsequent diastolic filling period shows a decreased separation of the leaflets and an indistinct E point. The next normal depolarization produces a vigorous ventricular systole, and the following mitral valve opening is brisk with an increased E point separation. Because of the heart rate and possibly some left ventricular dysfunction, the subsequent A wave is superimposed on the down slope of the closing mitral valve. The following diastolic interval produces an alternating effect of the mitral valve with decreased diastolic separation, possibly as a consequence of the vigorous ventricular contraction and filling of the preceding cycle. More normal mechanical contraction and relaxation occur with the third normally conducted beat. The subsequent diastole is prematurely ended by the third premature

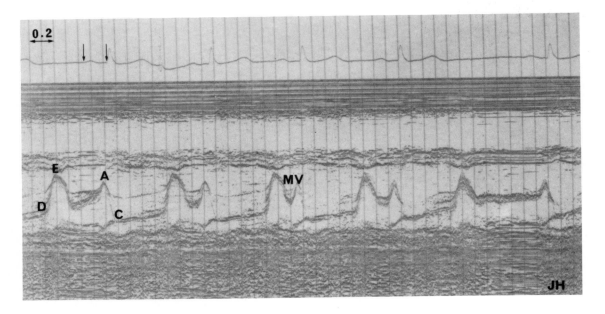

Fig. 5–14. Mitral valve echocardiogram demonstrating the effect of sinus arrhythmia on mitral valve (MV) motion. The principal effect of an increased R–R interval is the duration of diastasis. The heights of the E and A points are not influenced.

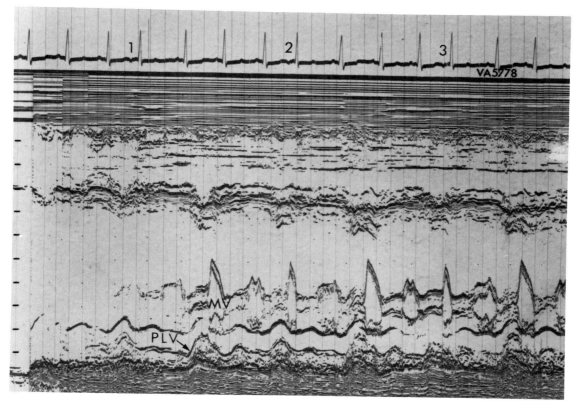

Fig. 5–15.   The effect of atrial premature beats on an M-mode echocardiogram of the left ventricle and mitral valve (MV). PLV = posterior left ventricular wall (see text for details).

atrial systole (3), and then the cycle is repeated. Figure 5–15 is yet another example of how echocardiography can help decipher the hemodynamic consequences of arrhythmias.

Figure 5–16 demonstrates the effect of a burst of supraventricular tachycardia on the left ventricle. The patient has atrial fibrillation with occasional premature ventricular systole (Fig. 5–16A). During a burst of supraventricular tachycardia, which probably is only accelerated atrioventricular conduction and rapid ventricular response (Fig. 5–16B), there is a striking decrease in septal and posterior wall motion (arrows) and a decrease in the left ventricular diastolic dimension. The interesting clinical counterpart is that the patient became extremely short of breath during these bursts of supraventricular tachycardia and died suddenly at home two weeks after this echocardiogram was taken.

Most echocardiographic literature on supraventricular tachycardia relates to patients with atrial fibrillation and atrial flutter. Figure 5–17 demonstrates that patients with atrial fibrillation or atrial flutter frequently show striking oscillations of the mitral valve (arrows).[7] It should be noted that the posterior mitral leaflet (PML) also oscillates at the same frequency as the anterior mitral leaflet (AML) and moves in an opposite direction to that of the anterior leaflet. Thus, although organized atrial activity is not evident on this electrocardiogram, there apparently are well-organized atrial contractions that produce sufficient blood flow to open the mitral valve with each atrial systole. Thus, although the electrocardiogram shows classic atrial fibrillation, one might argue that the left atrium is actually in a flutter rhythm. There is evidence that with electrocardiographic atrial fibrillation, one atrium may be fibrillating while the other is in flutter. Echocardiog-

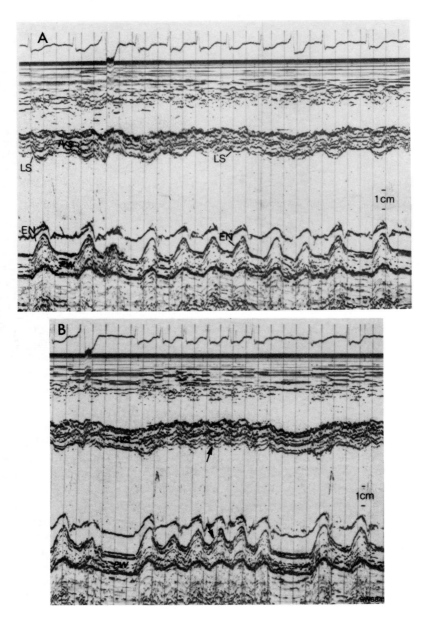

Fig. 5–16.   The effect of a supraventricular tachycardia on the M-mode echocardiogram. The patient has atrial fibrillation with an occasional premature ventricular systole, A. With a burst of supraventricular tachycardia, the septal and posterior left ventricular wall motion (arrows) is reduced, B. The left ventricular diastolic dimension also decreases. LS = left septum; EN = posterior left ventricular endocardium; IVS = interventricular septum; PW = posterior wall.

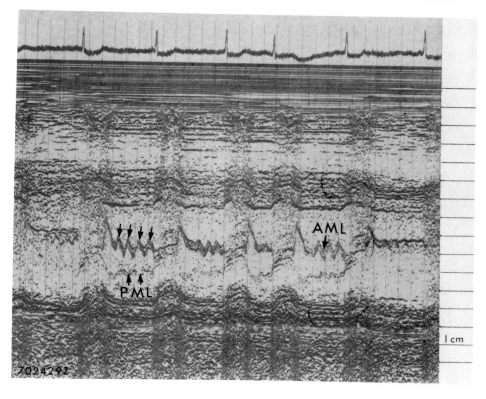

Fig. 5–17.   The effect of atrial flutter on the mitral valve echocardiogram. With atrial systole the anterior (AML) and posterior (PML) mitral leaflets separate, indicating flow through the orifice *(arrows)*.

raphy has been used to try to determine whether the atria are in the same electrical state.[7] For example, in Figure 5–17 it is quite possible that the right atrium may be in atrial fibrillation and the left atrium in flutter. One may be able to establish that fact by recording the tricuspid valve and by finding no organized atrial activity sufficient to produce opening of the tricuspid valve with atrial contractions.[25-27] Dual echocardiography with recording of simultaneous mitral and tricuspid valves is one technique that has been recommended for evaluating the atria with various atrial arrhythmias.[25]

Occasionally, the oscillations seen on the echocardiogram may not represent atrial contractions and opening of the atrioventricular valves owing to atrial systole. Figure 5–18 shows undulating motion on the echocardiogram corresponding to the fibrillatory waves on the electrocardiogram. What distinguishes the echocardiogram in this figure from that in Figure 5–17 is that the entire heart is oscillating. Oscillations of the left septum (LS), and the posterior left ventricular wall (PLV) can also be seen, as can the obvious undulating motion of the mitral valve. In addition, the motion of the anterior mitral leaflet (AML) and the posterior mitral leaflet (PML) is in the same direction, and the leaflets do not separate following the F waves. Thus the motion observed on the echocardiogram probably represents rocking or moving of the entire heart with the fibrillation and not necessarily propulsion of blood through the mitral valve with each atrial systole. Other echocardiographic observations noted with atrial arrhythmias are oscillations of the left atrial wall[28,29] premature closure of the mitral valve.[30]

ABNORMAL ATRIOVENTRICULAR CONDUCTION

Prolonged atrioventricular conduction, or heart block, can alter the echocardiogram in a fairly predictable manner. Echocardio-

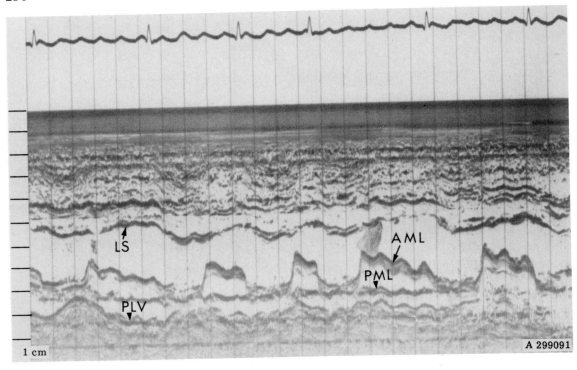

Fig. 5–18.   M-mode echocardiogram of the left ventricle and mitral valve in a patient with atrial flutter-fibrillation. Note undulating movements of the mitral leaflets and the ventricular walls. LS = left septum; AML = anterior mitral leaflet; PML = posterior mitral leaflet; PLV = posterior left ventricular wall.

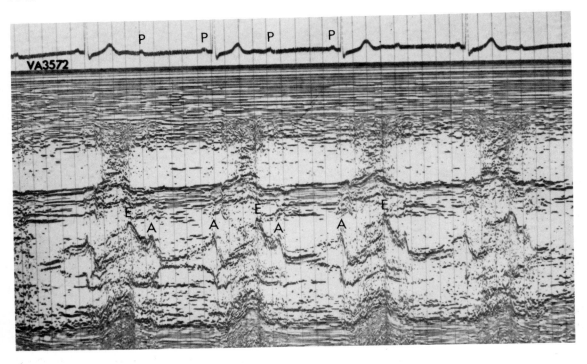

Fig. 5–19.   Mitral valve echocardiogram in a patient with heart block and 2:1 conduction. The mitral valve A waves follow each electrocardiographic P wave.

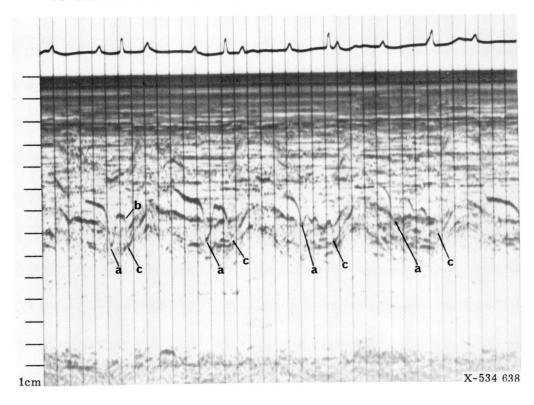

Fig. 5–20.   The effect of complete heart block on the pulmonary valve echocardiogram. Large A waves (a) are seen corresponding with each electrocardiographic P wave. The opening of the mitral valve with ventricular systole (c) follows each ventricular depolarization. b = onset of pulmonary valve opening with ventricular systole. (From Weyman, A.E., et al.: Echocardiographic patterns of pulmonary valve motion in valvular pulmonary stenosis. Am. J. Cardiol., 34:644, 1974.)

graphic events that are dependent on atrial systole follow the contractions of the atria and are not synchronous with ventricular contraction if heart block is present.[31] Figure 5–19 substantiates the fact that the mitral valve closes with atrial relaxation as well as with ventricular systole. Thus it is not surprising to find a virtually closed mitral valve before ventricular systole in a patient with first-degree heart block and a prolonged P–R interval. In fact, heart block is one of the causes of premature mitral valve closure.

Figure 5–20 shows a pulmonary valve echocardiogram of a patient with complete heart block. Again the consequences of atrial contraction, namely the A dips of the pulmonary valve, follow each P wave on the electrocardiogram. The C point, which represents opening of the valve following ventricular systole, remains related to ventricu-

lar depolarization. In occasional cases where the atrial depolarization is not apparent on the electrocardiogram, it is sometimes possible to identify the P wave by way of echocardiographic valve motion. Thus the echocardiogram may help in the diagnosis of arrhythmias in rare situations.

REFERENCES

1. DeMaria, A.N. and Mason, D.T.: Echocardiographic evaluation of disturbances of cardiac rhythm and conduction. Chest, 71:439, 1977.
1a. Dillon, J.C., Chang, S., and Feigenbaum, H.: Echocardiographic manifestations of left bundle branch block. Circulation, 49:876, 1974.
2. Abbasi, A.S., Eber, L.M., MacAlpin, R.N., and Kattus, A.A.: Paradoxical motion of the interventricular septum in left bundle branch block. Circulation, 49:423, 1974.
3. McDonald, I.G., Feigenbaum, H., and Chang, S.: Analysis of left ventricular wall motion by reflected ultrasound: application to assessment of myocardial function. Circulation, 46:14, 1972.

238 ECHOCARDIOGRAPHY

4. McDonald, I.G.: Echocardiographic demonstration of abnormal motion of the interventricular septum in left bundle branch block. Circulation, 48:272, 1973.

4a. Burch, G.E., Giles, T.D., and Martinez, E.C.: Echocardiographic abnormalities of interventricular septum associated with absent Q syndrome. J.A.M.A., 228:1665, 1974.

5. Fujii, J., Watanabe, H., Watanabe, T., Takahashi, N., Ohta, A., and Kato, K.: M-mode and cross-sectional echocardiographic study of the left ventricular wall motions in complete left bundle branch block. Br. Heart J., 42:255, 1979.

5a. DeMaria, A.N., Vismara, L.A., Vera, Z., Miller, R.R., Amsterdam, E.A., and Mason, D.T.: Hemodynamic effects of cardiac arrhythmias. Angiology, 28:427, 1977.

6. Bommer, W., Weinert, L., Neef, J., Neumann, A., Vera, Z., Mason, D.T., Klein, R., and DeMaria, A.N.: The magnitude and temporal sequence of abnormal septal contraction in left bundle branch block: evaluation by two-dimensional echocardiography. Clin. Res., 26:221a, 1978. (Abstract)

7. Endo, N., Shimada, E., Asano, H., and Yamane, Y.: Paradoxical septal motion in left bundle branch block. J. Cardiogr., 7:313, 1977.

7a. Tsuji, Y., Matsukubo, H., Inoue, D., Furukawa, K., Watanabe, T., Tohara, M., Katsume, H., Endo, N., Matsuura, T., and Kunishige, H.: Study of ventricular wall movements in patients with left bundle branch block by echocardiography. J. Cardiogr., 8:745, 1978.

8. Fujino, T., Ito, M., Kanaya, S., Ito, S., Fukumoto, T., Kawamura, T., Yasuda, H., Fukushima, I., Tetsuo, M., Hirata, T., and Mashiba, H.: Abnormal septal motion in the cases with various intraventricular conduction disturbances. Cardiovasc. Sound Bull., 5:77, 1975.

9. Zoneraich, S., Zoneraich, O., and Rhee, J.J.: Echocardiographic evaluation of septal motion in patients with artificial pacemakers: vectorcardiographic correlations. Am. Heart J., 93:596, 1977.

10. Gomes, J.A.C., Damato, A.N., Akhtar, M., Dhatt, M.S., Calon, A.H., Reddy, C.P., and Moran, H.E.: Ventricular septal motion and left ventricular dimensions during abnormal ventricular activation. Am. J. Cardiol., 39:641, 1977.

11. Brooks, N., Leech, G., and Leatham, A.: Complete right bundle-branch block. Echophonocardiographic study of first heart sound and right ventricular contraction times. Br. Heart J., 41:637, 1979.

12. Shapiro, J., Boxer, R., and Krongrad, E.: Echocardiographic observations in patients with postoperative right bundle branch block pattern. Circulation (Suppl. II), 54:46, 1976. (Abstract)

13. Chandra, M.S., Kerber, R.E., Brown, D.D., and Funk, D.C.: Echocardiography in Wolff-Parkinson-White syndrome. Circulation, 53:943, 1976.

14. DeMaria, A.N., Vera, Z., Neumann, A., and Mason, D.T.: Alterations in ventricular contraction pattern in the Wolff-Parkinson-White syndrome. Circulation, 53:249, 1976.

15. Dohmen, H., Roelandt, J., Durrer, D., Wellens, H.: Wall motion abnormalities in WPW syndrome studied with echo. Circulation (Suppl. II), 52:34, 1975. (Abstract)

16. Theroux, P., Francis, G., Hagan, A., Johnson, A., and O'Rourke, R.: Echocardiographic study of in-terventricular septal motion in the Wolff-Parkinson-White syndrome. Circulation (Suppl. II), 52:70, 1975. (Abstract)

17. Lebovitz, J.A., Mandel, W.J., Laks, M.M., Kraus, R., and Weinstein, S.: Relationship between the electrical (electrocardiographic) and mechanical (echocardiographic) events in Wolff-Parkinson-White syndrome. Chest, 71:463, 1977.

18. Gimbel, K.S.: Left ventricular wall motion in patients with the Wolff-Parkinson-White syndrome. Am. Heart J., 93:160, 1977.

19. Hishida, H., Sotobata, I., Koike, Y., Okumura, M., and Mizuno, Y.: Echocardiographic patterns of ventricular contraction in the Wolff-Parkinson-White syndrome. Circulation, 54:567, 1976.

20. Francis, G.S., Theroux, P., O'Rourke, R.A., Hagan, A.D., and Johnson, A.D.: An echocardiographic study of interventricular septal motion in the Wolff-Parkinson-White syndrome. Circulation, 54:174, 1976.

21. Chandra, M.S., Kerber, R.E., Brown, D.D., and Funk, D.C.: Echocardiography in Wolff-Parkinson-White syndrome. Circulation, 53:943, 1976.

22. Ticzon, A.R., Damato, A.N., Caracta, A.R., Russo, G., Foster, J.R., and Lau, S.H.: Interventricular septal motion during preexcitation and normal conduction in Wolff-Parkinson-White syndrome. Am. J. Cardiol., 37:840, 1976.

22a. Sasse, L. and Del Puerto, H.A.: Echocardiography of ventricular septal movement in Wolff-Parkinson-White syndrome. Arch. Inst. Cardiol. Mex., 46:445, 1976.

23. Berman, N.D., Gilbert, B.W., McLaughlin, P.R., and Morch, J.E.: Mitral stenosis with posterior diastolic movement of posterior leaflet. Can. Med. Assoc. J., 112:976, 1975.

24. Stevenson, J.G.: Type A WPW Echo. Circulation, 54:161, 1976. (Letter)

24a. Weiss, N., Chaval, S., and Ludbrook, P.A.: Echocardiographic recognition of paradoxical interventricular septal motion associated with right ventricular premature beats. Circulation (Suppl. III), 50:250, 1974. (Abstract)

25. Fujii, J., Foster, J.R., Mills, P.G., Moos, S., and Craige, E.: Dual echocardiographic determination of atrial contraction sequence in atrial flutter and other related atrial arrhythmias. Circulation, 58:314, 1978.

26. Fujii, J., Watanabe, H., Kuboki, M., and Kato, K.: Echocardiographic study of atrial flutter. Jpn. Circ. J., 41:1393, 1977.

27. Procacci, P.M., Levites, R., Kotler, M.N., and Anderson, G.J.: Dissimilar atrial rhythm diagnosed by echocardiography. Chest, 73:429, 1978.

28. Fujii, J., Watanabe, H., Kuboki, M., Morita, K., and Kato, K.: Echocardiograms of the left atrial wall, mitral valve, and tricuspid valve in atrial flutter. Cardiovasc. Sound Bull., 5:751, 1975.

29. Sasse, L. and Frolich, C.R.: Suprasternal notch echocardiography and atrial arrhythmias. Cardiovasc. Dis., 6:61, 1979.

30. Greenberg, M., Herman, L.S., and Cohen, M.V.: Mitral valve closure in atrial flutter. Circulation, 59:902, 1979.

31. D'Cruz, I.A., Prabhu, R., Cohen, H.C., and Glick, G.: Echocardiographic features of second degree atrioventricular block. Chest, 72:459, 1977.

CHAPTER 6

Acquired Valvular Heart Disease

Echocardiography is the examination of choice when recording the functional anatomy of the cardiac valves. One of the principal advantages of echocardiography is its ability to visualize intracardiac structures such as valves. The rapid sampling rate of M-mode echocardiography permits an excellent recording of the motion of the individual valves. The spatial orientation inherent in two-dimensional echocardiography provides an opportunity to study the shape of the valves during the cardiac cycle and in various disease states. Thus it is not surprising that one of the principal uses of echocardiography is for patients with valvular heart disease. Although much of clinical cardiology assesses valvular heart disease by detecting the consequences of the valvular abnormality on hemodynamics or cardiac chambers, echocardiography directly records the abnormal valvular anatomy. Thus in some respects echocardiography permits a more direct diagnosis of valvular heart disease than any other cardiologic procedure.

MITRAL VALVE DISEASE

Mitral Stenosis

Echocardiography was first clinically used for the detection of mitral stenosis. The initial observation was that normally the anterior mitral leaflet partially closed shortly after initial opening with a peak at the E point. The diastolic, or E to F, slope was steep (Fig. 6–1B). In patients with mitral stenosis, this early diastolic closure either did not occur or occurred at a much slower rate.[1,2] Thus the mid-diastolic closing velocity of the valve or the E to F slope was mark-

edly diminished (Fig. 6–1A). The explanation for this observation was that the E to F slope was a function of the rate of left ventricular filling.[3] Normally, the left atrium rapidly emptied blood into the left ventricle so that in mid-diastole there was relatively little mitral flow and the valve tended to

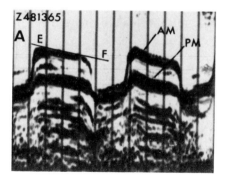

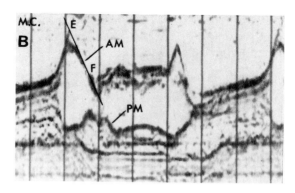

Fig. 6–1. Mitral valve echocardiogram of the anterior (AM) and posterior (PM) mitral valve leaflets in A, a patient with mitral stenosis and B, in a normal subject. Note E to F slopes. (From Duchak, J.M., Chang, S., and Feigenbaum, H.: The posterior mitral valve echo and the echocardiographic diagnosis of mitral stenosis. Am. J. Cardiol., 29:628, 1972.)

close. With mitral stenosis, filling of the ventricle was slow and the valve was held open by the persistent pressure gradient between the left atrium and the left ventricle. The abnormal E to F slope in mitral stenosis has been confirmed by numerous investigators since Edler's original observation.[4-8] Several investigators found a quantitative relationship between the degree of mitral stenosis and the closing velocity or E to F slope.

There is relatively little question that the E to F slope is altered in mitral stenosis and that it is at least partially a function of the degree of stenosis. For example, Figure 6–2 shows a patient before and after a successful mitral commissurotomy. In the preoperative echocardiogram (Fig. 6–2A), there is a flat E to F slope of the anterior mitral leaflet that is much more rapid following the commissurotomy (Fig. 6–2B). In addition, several investigators have detected mitral restenosis by serial reductions in the E to F slope.[9] Thus, when following a given individual, the

diastolic closing velocity can be a useful quantitative measurement in patients with mitral stenosis.[6,9-11]

Unfortunately, the diastolic closing velocity is not a specific finding limited only to mitral stenosis. As indicated in Chapter 4, mitral valve motion is influenced by many hemodynamic factors. Figure 6–3 shows a patient with a flat E to F slope with no evidence of mitral stenosis. This patient had aortic stenosis and insufficiency. Such a flat E to F slope is a fairly common finding in patients with aortic valve disease. The change in valve motion is believed to be due to a decreased rate of left ventricular filling as a result of reduced left ventricular compliance.[12,13] Because of this frequent alteration of the E to F slope in patients without mitral stenosis, the validity of using this echocardiographic measurement for quantitating mitral stenosis was reevaluated. Many of the original studies used patients with wide ranges of mitral valve areas, including normal patients.[7] When the range of

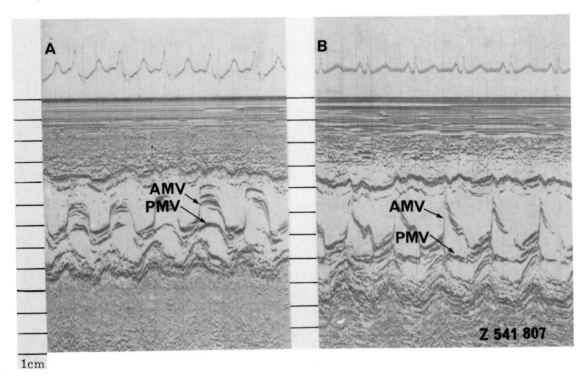

Fig. 6–2. Mitral valve echocardiogram of a patient with mitral stenosis before, A, and after, B, successful mitral commissurotomy. AMV = anterior mitral valve leaflet; PMV = posterior mitral valve leaflet. (From Chang, S.: M-mode Echocardiographic Techniques and Pattern Recognition. Philadelphia, Lea & Febiger, 1976.)

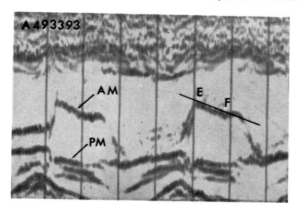

Fig. 6–3. Mitral valve echocardiogram of a patient with a diminished diastolic slope of the anterior mitral leaflet (AM) with no evidence of mitral stenosis. Despite the diminished E to F slope, the leaflets are thin and the posterior mitral leaflet (PM) moves normally. (From Duchak, J.M., Chang, S., and Feigenbaum, H.: The posterior mitral valve echo and the echocardiographic diagnosis of mitral stenosis. Am. J. Cardiol., 29:628, 1972.)

valve orifices was reduced by studying only patients with mitral stenosis, then the correlation was much worse. The correlation between the diastolic E to F slope and the degree of mitral stenosis was not as good as noted in the earlier studies.[14,15] What was surprising was how poor the correlation actually was. In some studies the correlation was so bad that it was not even statistically significant.[14] The poor correlation between the diastolic slope and the degree of mitral stenosis when comparing one patient with another was so consistent that most echocardiographers no longer use this measurement for quantitating the degree of obstruction. It should be emphasized, however, that this measurement still has value when following a given individual, such as in Figure 6–2.

Another finding on the M-mode echocardiogram that is helpful in the diagnosis of mitral stenosis is the pattern of motion of the posterior mitral leaflet.[12] As shown in Figure 6–1B, the normal posterior mitral leaflet is a virtual mirror image of the anterior leaflet. When the valve opens in diastole, the posterior leaflet moves downward while the anterior leaflet moves upward. Figure 6–1A illustrates the situation in the case of mitral stenosis. The most striking qualitative

change is that, with early diastole, the posterior leaflet now moves upward in the same direction as the anterior leaflet. From a strictly empirical point of view, this echocardiographic finding is useful and usually helps in the qualitative diagnosis of mitral stenosis, especially in such a confusing situation as shown in Figure 6–3. In this figure, the anterior leaflet is compatible with mitral stenosis because of the reduced E to F slope; however, the posterior leaflet moves downward in normal fashion. Although most echocardiographers know that the posterior leaflet is supposed to move upward with mitral stenosis and downward normally, the more important point is that the separation of the leaflets is diminished. The fact that the posterior leaflet actually moves upward with diastole is interesting and probably indicates fusion of the commissures in which the two leaflets partially function as a single unit. The larger, more mobile anterior leaflet probably pulls the posterior leaflet anteriorly during diastole. In Figure 6–2A, the preoperative echocardiogram shows a diminished separation between the two leaflets during diastole with the posterior mitral leaflet moving slightly anteriorly during diastole. Following an unusually good mitral commissurotomy, the posterior leaflet returns to normal, and the separation between the leaflets is significantly improved.

It should be emphasized that all patients with mitral stenosis do not necessarily have anterior motion of the posterior leaflet during diastole.[16–20,20a] Figure 6–4 shows a patient with some degree of mitral stenosis. The patient underwent a mitral commissurotomy, but still had hemodynamically significant residual mitral stenosis. The posterior mitral leaflet clearly moves downward in diastole. The anterior motion of the anterior leaflet is certainly less than normal, and the separation between the two leaflets is also less than normal. In addition, the E to F slope is reduced. Thus, although the pattern of motion of the posterior leaflet is helpful and quite reliable in most patients, some patients may show downward motion of the posterior leaflet, even in the presence of mitral stenosis. In one study, 10 percent of all patients with mitral stenosis showed down-

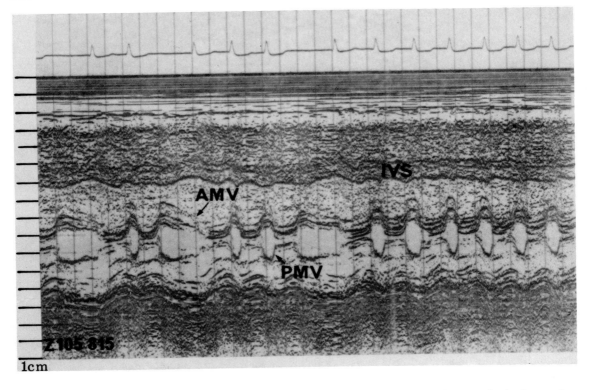

1cm

Fig. 6–4.   Mitral valve echocardiogram of a patient with rheumatic mitral valve disease who had a previous mitral commissurotomy and some residual mitral stenosis. Despite the thickened and relatively immobile anterior mitral leaflet (AMV), the posterior mitral valve (PMV) is thinner and moves downward with diastole. IVS = interventricular septum. (From Chang, S.: M-mode Echocardiographic Techniques and Pattern Recognition. Philadelphia, Lea & Febiger, 1976.)

ward motion of the posterior leaflet during diastole,[17] and in another series 17 percent of such patients demonstrated this type of posterior mitral leaflet motion.[18] In the second study the authors found an increased incidence of posterior motion of the posterior mitral leaflet when the mitral stenosis was also associated with aortic stenosis.[18]

In addition to decreased diastolic closing slope and abnormal posterior mitral leaflet motion, the third M-mode sign for the diagnosis of mitral stenosis is thickening of the leaflets. In all examples of mitral stenosis illustrated thus far (Figs. 6–1A, 6–2, 6–4), the mitral valve leaflets are thickened. The diagnosis of a thickened valve is partially subjective and can be best appreciated by comparing the diseased valves with their normal counterparts (Figs. 6–1B and 6–3). When judging the thicknesses of the mitral valve, it is best to evaluate the echoes when

the valve is maximally open. During this phase of the cardiac cycle the leaflets are reasonably perpendicular to the ultrasonic beam and there is a minimum of extra echoes because the beam is transecting the valve tangentially. For example, multiple mitral valve echoes are commonly seen in systole with or without mitral stenosis merely because the closed valve is almost parallel to the ultrasonic beam.

Using the three M-mode criteria of reduced diastolic filling, abnormal posterior mitral leaflet motion, and thickening of the leaflets, there should be few patients in whom the qualitative diagnosis of mitral stenosis cannot be made with M-mode echocardiography. In those few cases in which the M-mode technique is not definitive, two-dimensional echocardiography can help with the qualitative diagnosis of mitral stenosis by showing doming of the mitral

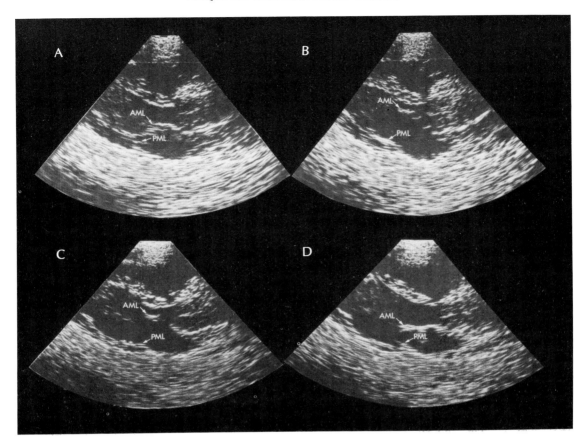

Fig. 6–5. Long-axis, parasternal two-dimensional echocardiograms of a normal mitral valve showing the position of the anterior (AML) and posterior (PML) leaflets during the cardiac cycle. A = systole, B,C,D = phases of diastole.

valve during diastole. Figure 6–5 illustrates sequential two-dimensional long-axis views of the mitral valve in systole (A), initial diastole (B), and later phases of diastole (C and D). During diastole the two leaflets are frequently parallel to each other and are relatively straight. Figure 6–6 shows long-axis two-dimensional views of the mitral valve in a patient with mitral stenosis. The principal diagnostic feature of mitral stenosis in this view is doming of the anterior mitral leaflet in diastole. Doming indicates that the valve cannot accommodate all of the blood available for delivery into the left ventricle. Thus the body of the leaflets separates more widely than do the edges. Doming is one of the main two-dimensional features of any stenotic valve.

The mitral valve may also open poorly in patients who have a low cardiac output (Fig. 6–7). If the mitral valve is intrinsically normal, however, the anterior leaflet does not dome (Fig. 6–7B). Thus two-dimensional echocardiography can assist in the qualitative diagnosis of mitral stenosis, although M-mode echocardiography should be sufficient in most cases.

Since the E to F slope has been discredited as a means of quantitating mitral stenosis, many efforts have been made to find alternate echocardiographic methods for quantitating the degree of mitral stenosis. Theoretically, one might use the separation between the anterior and mitral leaflets to measure the degree of stenosis. However, the separation between the two leaflets varies depending on the angle of the beam. For example, in Figure 6–8 the separation be-

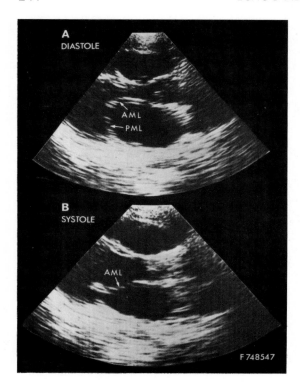

Fig. 6–6.   Long-axis two-dimensional echocardiograms of a stenotic mitral valve in diastole, A, and systole, B. Diastolic doming of the mitral valve is diagnostic for mitral stenosis. AML = anterior mitral leaflet; PML = posterior mitral leaflet.

tween the mitral leaflets is about 3 cm when the mitral valve is examined near its base. However, as the beam moves toward the apex, the separation is much less. One might argue that the separation closest to the apex may represent a true diameter of the mitral orifice. This might have been the case, but with the advent of two-dimensional echocardiography, the M-mode technique for measuring the separation between the anterior mitral leaflets never became popular.

One of the first applications for two-dimensional echocardiography was the demonstration that this technique provided a means of quantitating mitral stenosis.[14,15,21–23] In some respects, this examination is similar to looking at the separation between the leaflets, except the two-dimensional approach attempts to examine the area of the mitral valve orifice. Figure 6–9 demonstrates short-axis, two-dimensional views of a stenotic mitral valve in diastole and systole. The small orifice inscribed by the thickened mitral valve can be appreciated (MVO, Fig. 6–9). Figure 6–10 demonstrates how the orifice can be measured using the two-dimensional technique. Several independent studies have now demonstrated that the mitral valve area measured in this way correlates well

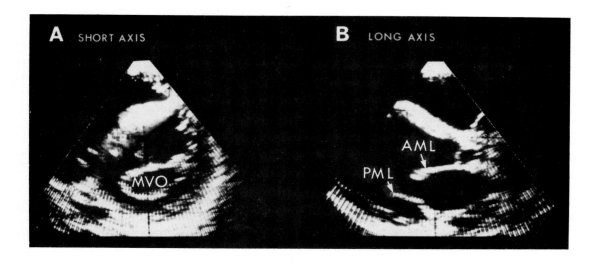

Fig. 6–7.   Short-axis, A, and long-axis, B, two-dimensional echocardiograms of a mitral valve in a patient with cardiomyopathy and low cardiac output. The short-axis mitral valve orifice (MVO) is decreased, and there is no doming of the mitral leaflets in the long-axis view. AML = anterior mitral leaflet; PML = posterior mitral leaflet.

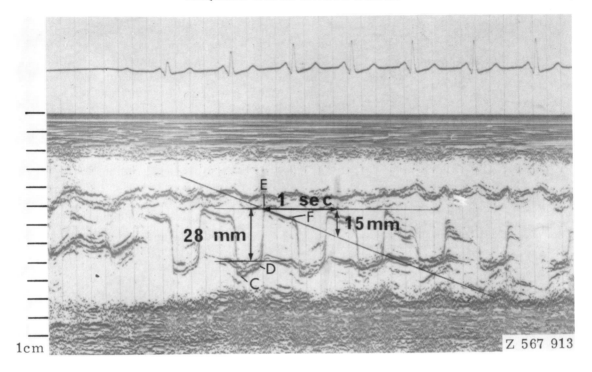

Fig. 6–8. Echocardiogram of a mitral valve in a patient with moderate mitral stenosis and a pliable mitral valve. Note how the diastolic closing velocity, or E to F slope, is measured and how one may measure the amplitude of opening of the mitral leaflet, or D to E amplitude. (From Chang, S.: M-mode Echocardiographic Techniques and Pattern Recognition. Philadelphia, Lea & Febiger, 1976.)

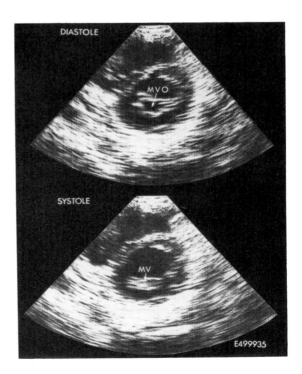

Fig. 6–9. Short-axis two-dimensional echocardiograms of a patient with mitral stenosis. Note the diastolic mitral valve orifice (MVO). In systole the leaflets come together, and the orifice is obliterated.

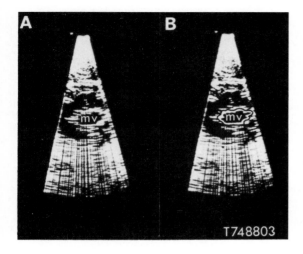

Fig. 6–10. Short-axis two-dimensional echocardiograms of a stenotic mitral valve. Note how the mitral orifice (MV) can be measured in *B*.

with the degree of mitral stenosis. Figure 6–11 shows the relationship between the two-dimensional echocardiographic measurement of mitral valve area and a similar calculation by way of hemodynamic information obtained by cardiac catheterization.[24] There is a wide range of valve areas in 75 patients, some of whom had predominant mitral regurgitation. If one restricts the patients to only those with pure mitral stenosis, the range of valve area is reduced and the correlation is not as good (Fig. 6–12). This correlation is still better than when using the mitral E to F slope and is statistically significant. However, there are patients who clearly have a poor predictive value. The lack of correlation in some patients could partially be a result of the gold standard used. Although the mitral valve area calcu-

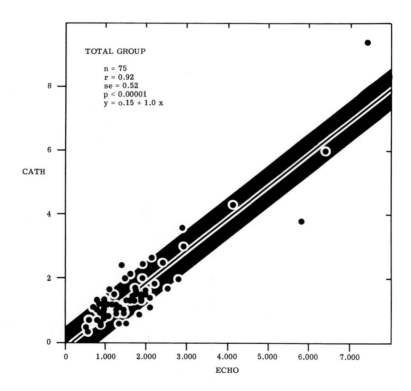

Fig. 6–11. Graph demonstrating the relationship between the mitral valve orifice, measured by two-dimensional echocardiography (ECHO), and the orifice measure at cardiac catheterization (CATH).

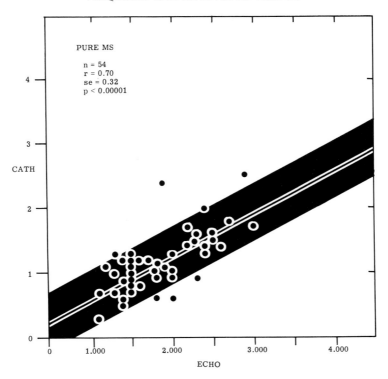

Fig. 6–12.   Graph showing the correlation between the two-dimensional echocardiographic measurement of the mitral valve orifice (ECHO) compared with a similar measurement made at catheterization (CATH) in patients with pure mitral stenosis.

lated by way of cardiac catheterization is the standard by which we manage patients clinically, there are known potential errors in this measurement. In a relatively small number of patients, the two-dimensional measurements were compared with direct anatomic assessment of valve area. The ultrasonic technique correlated extremely well and possibly even better than did the hemodynamically derived measurements.

There are obvious limitations to the two-dimensional measurement of the mitral valve area. Patients with low cardiac output will have a reduced mitral orifice (Fig. 6–7A). However, the qualitative diagnosis should be clearly evident, and the size of the orifice owing to low cardiac output is still larger than with even mild mitral stenosis. One potential technical error is that the measurement is influenced by any dropout of echoes. The mitral orifice in Figure 6–9 is not totally complete. The examiner must fill in some gaps where echoes are missing.

Another problem is that the lateral resolution of all echocardiographic systems is less than ideal, and the echoes from the lateral and medial walls of the mitral orifice appear wider than they really are.[22] For example, in Figure 6–13 the patient has a densely calcified mitral valve and one can barely see any remnant of a valve orifice in diastole (MVO, Fig. 6–13B). Although the patient had severe mitral stenosis, one could not actually measure a valve orifice, which is undoubtedly larger than it appears in this figure. Some two-dimensional echocardiographic systems are more gain-sensitive than others.[22] Thus the valve orifice can be significantly influenced by the gain settings (Fig. 6–14). Fortunately, not all echocardiographic systems are as gain-sensitive as the one with which Figure 6–14 was made. In addition, this recording was artificially produced by purposely turning the gain to its maximum setting. One would not ordinarily distort the picture in such a fashion.

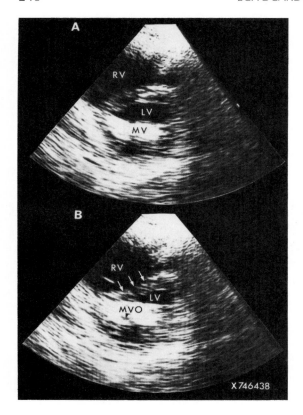

Fig. 6–13. Short-axis two-dimensional echocardiogram of a patient with calcific mitral stenosis. In diastole, *B*, the mitral valve orifice (MVO) is barely visible. There is also an indentation of the interventricular septum *(arrows)* toward the left ventricle in early diastole. RV = right ventricle; LV = left ventricle.

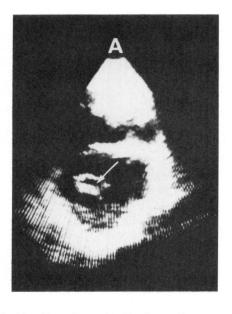
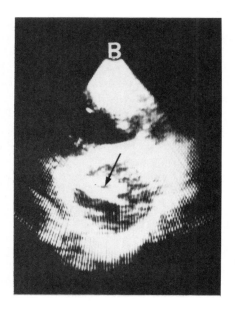

Fig. 6–14.   Two-dimensional echocardiograms of a stenotic mitral valve with two different gain settings. Note how the apparent mitral valve orifice is much smaller with a high-gain setting, *B*.

There are other technical details that must be considered when using two-dimensional echocardiography to measure the mitral valve orifice. For example, the stenotic mitral valve assumes the shape of a funnel. If one slices the valve too closely to the aorta, one obtains a falsely large mitral valve orifice. Figure 6–15 demonstrates how one could possibly record two different mitral orifices. The left study shows the true mitral orifice and the right study a falsely large orifice obtained with improper technique.

Despite these many limitations, estimating the severity of mitral stenosis by way of the two-dimensional examination has many advantages, and this technique remains quite popular. This examination comes closest to directly measuring the actual anatomic abnormality. The measurement is uninfluenced by accompanying mitral regurgitation. It is not surprising, therefore, that the ultrasonic measurement correlates quite well with the pathologist's or surgeon's findings during their examination of the valve. Most limitations can be overcome by careful technique and gain control. It is hoped that improvements in transducer design and instrumentation will improve lateral resolution and the accuracy of the measurements.

Alternate echocardiographic techniques are described in the literature for quantitating the degree of mitral stenosis. One author suggests calculating a mitral valve closure index.[25,26] Such an index is obtained by taking the difference in the separation between the anterior mitral leaflets from the M-mode echocardiogram in early diastole and immediately prior to atrial systole when the patient is in sinus rhythm. The difference is then divided by the initial separation and multiplied by the diastolic filling period. The resultant index estimates the rapidity with which the mitral valve closes. This author found this index to be reliable in predicting the degree of mitral stenosis.[25] In a follow-up study, this author found the mitral valve closing index helpful in judging the results of mitral valvulotomy.[26]

Another M-mode technique based on the physiologic consequences of mitral stenosis is a left atrial emptying index by way of the posterior aortic wall echo.[27] Figure 6–16 demonstrates the principle behind the left atrial emptying index. The motion of the posterior aortic wall reflects the filling and emp-

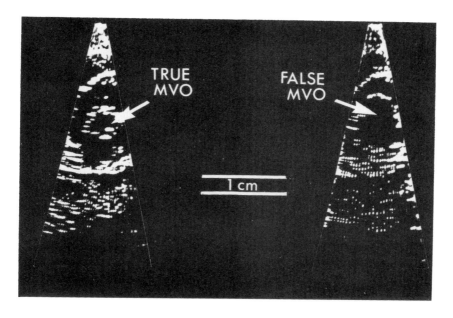

Fig. 6–15. Short-axis two-dimensional studies of the same patient with mitral stenosis. The true mitral valve orifice (MVO) is located at the edges of the leaflets. Note in the righthand study how a two-dimensional slice closer to the base of the heart will produce a falsely large mitral valve orifice.

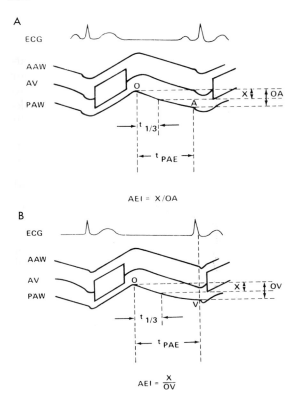

Fig. 6–16. Diagram demonstrating how a left atrial emptying index (AEI) can be calculated from the posterior aortic wall echocardiogram. A represents the calculation with sinus rhythm and B the method for measuring the index in patients with atrial fibrillation. The time of passive atrial emptying (t_{PAE}) occurs between points O and A with sinus rhythm and between points O and V with atrial fibrillation. (From Strunk, B.L., et al.: The assessment of mitral stenosis and prosthetic mitral valve obstruction, using the posterior aortic wall echocardiogram. Circulation, 55:885, 1977. By permission of the American Heart Association, Inc.)

tying patterns of the left atrium (see Chapter 4). Normally, the left atrium empties rapidly, and there is an early diastolic downward motion of the posterior aortic wall. With impaired left atrial emptying, the aortic wall motion is reduced during the rapid emptying phase, or the first third of diastole. The left atrial emptying index is calculated by dividing the diastolic period prior to atrial systole into thirds (Fig. 6–16A). If the first third of diastole does not represent at least 40 percent of the total amplitude of the aortic wall motion during diastole, then restricted ven-

tricular filling is present. A reasonable correlation between the left atrial index and the severity of mitral stenosis has been demonstrated.[27] As with any physiologic measurement, the left atrial emptying index is not specific. Patients who have abnormal left ventricular filling patterns owing to intrinsic myocardial disease may also have reduced left atrial emptying indices. If the patient is in atrial fibrillation (Fig. 6–16B), then the measurement is taken until the onset of ventricular systole.

In addition to making qualitative and quantitative diagnoses of mitral stenosis, echocardiography has been used to judge the suitability of the valve for commissurotomy. A factor that must be considered is the valve's pliability. Pliability can be estimated echocardiographically by judging the total amplitude of motion of the anterior mitral leaflet. Figure 6–8 shows how the amplitude of valve motion can be measured. In this particular tracing, the measurement is taken from the onset of diastole to the peak opening of diastole, the D to E amplitude.[28] Some echocardiographers measure from the onset of systole to the onset of diastole, the C to E amplitude.[10,29] The American Society of Echocardiography has recommended using the D to E amplitude rather than the C to E amplitude since the mitral motion from C to D is actually a function of mitral annulus motion.[3] The maximum amplitude in Figure 6–8 is 28 mm. This echocardiogram also shows how the amplitude varies with the direction of the ultrasonic beam. Deeper within the left ventricle, the amplitude of motion is considerably less. As a rule, a mitral valve with a maximum amplitude of 20 mm or more is usually considered pliable. Figure 6–17 shows another patient with mitral stenosis. The entire mitral valve is scanned as the ultrasonic beam moves from the left ventricle to the aorta and left atrium. The maximum amplitude from the anterior mitral leaflet is clearly less than 2 cm, and this valve would be classified as nonpliable.

The suitability for commissurotomy is also judged by the thickening, fibrosis, or calcification of the valve. As indicated, the qualitative diagnosis of mitral stenosis requires some thickening of the valve, at least in the

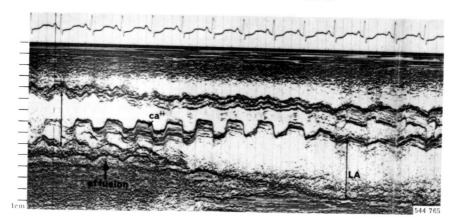

Fig. 6–17. M-mode scan of a patient with a calcified (Ca++) and immobile mitral valve. LA = left atrium. (From Chang, S.: M-mode Echocardiographic Techniques and Pattern Recognition. Philadelphia, Lea & Febiger, 1976.)

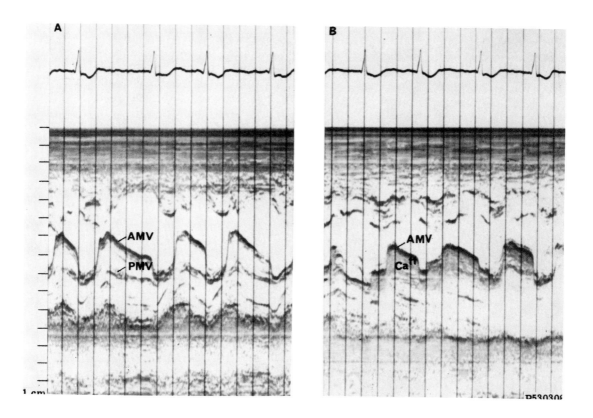

Fig. 6–18. Mitral valve echocardiograms of a patient with mitral stenosis. When a different area of the mitral valve is recorded, *A*, the calcium visible in *B* is not noted. AMV = anterior mitral valve leaflet; PMV = posterior mitral valve leaflet; Ca++ = calcium. (From Chang, S.: M-mode Echocardiographic Techniques and Pattern Recognition. Philadelphia, Lea & Febiger, 1976.)

adult patient. As expected, the degree of thickening or fibrosis varies in patients with mitral stenosis. Figure 6–8 is an example of a patient with minimal fibrosis of the valve, whereas Figure 6–17 shows an extreme echo-producing mitral valve that most likely contains calcium.[28,30] Two-dimensional echocardiography can also help assess the degree of fibrosis and calcification. Figures 6–6 and 6–9 show fibrotic but noncalcified mitral valves, whereas Figure 6–13 illustrates a highly calcified mitral valve. Figure 6–18 demonstrates that the degree of fibrosis and calcification of a stenotic valve need not be uniform. It should not be surprising that one area of the valve may be densely fibrotic or calcified, and another area may be much less fibrotic. In Figure 6–18A, although there is obvious fibrosis, no dense calcification is noted. Pliability is at the lowest limits possible for a mitral commissurotomy. When a different portion of the valve is recorded (Fig. 6–18B), one sees a highly echo-producing mitral valve with much less pliability that is most likely calcified. Thus it is imperative that when evaluating patients for mitral commissurotomy, one should examine as much of the mitral valve as possible.

Scanning the entire mitral valve apparatus is important for several reasons. There are increasing reports of subvalvular mitral stenosis primarily involving the chordae and papillary muscles.[31,32] Such obstruction involving the infravalvular apparatus can be extremely important from a management point of view. Although the leaflets may be quite pliable, the chordae and papillary muscles may be fused into a mass of dense fibrous tissue that may be difficult to resect and divide surgically. A few reports demonstrate that two–dimensional echocardiography may be able to detect this subvalvular obstruction.[32] The authors emphasize the necessity for multiple views of the mitral valve when attempting to assess subvalvular obstruction.

There are many secondary changes on the echocardiogram in patients with mitral stenosis. Left atrial dilatation and evidence of pulmonary hypertension are clear-cut findings. Changes in the motion of the interventricular septum are not as frequently recognized. Normally the interventricular system dips toward the left ventricle in early diastole. With mitral stenosis this diastolic dip is exaggerated (Fig. 6–19).[33] There is

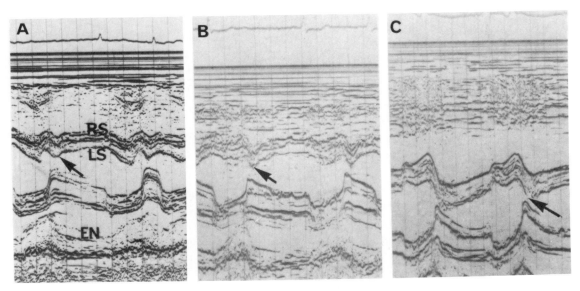

Fig. 6–19. M-mode echocardiograms of three patients with mitral stenosis. The early diastolic dip *(arrows)* of the interventricular septum is varied though prominent in all three patients. RS = right septum, LS = left septum; EN = posterior left ventricular endocardium. (From Weyman, A.E., et al.: Mechanism of paradoxical early diastolic septal motion in patients with mitral stenosis: a cross-sectional echocardiographic study. Am. J. Cardiol., 40:691, 1977.)

even a rough correlation between the severity of this dip and the severity of the mitral obstruction. The patient in Figure 6–19B had more stenosis than did the patient in Figure 6–19A, but less than the patient in Figure 6–19C. A possible explanation for this diastolic dip is offered in Figure 6–13. In this short-axis two-dimensional view of the mitral valve and left ventricle one notes a marked distortion of the interventricular septum during early diastole (Fig. 6–13B, arrows). This distortion of the septum is believed to be due to unequal filling of the two ventricles in early diastole. Because flow into the right ventricle is unobstructed, it fills more rapidly and the septum is pushed toward the more slowly filling left ventricle. When the left ventricular filling catches up, the usual circular shape of the left ventricle is resumed (Fig. 6–13A). This finding represents another example of how interventricular septal motion reflects the filling patterns of both ventricles.

Investigators using Doppler echocardiography have demonstrated that this technique can be helpful in both the qualitative and quantitative evaluation of mitral stenosis.[34–38, 38a] The blood flowing through the stenotic mitral valve represents a turbulent or disturbed flow that produces a fairly distinctive Doppler signal. The pattern of flow through the stenotic valve has quantitative information with regard to the degree of stenosis. The phasic flow pattern that one would expect in the normal individual is lost with significant mitral stenosis. Instead one sees a slow, gradually decreasing flow through a stenotic orifice. One study indicates that the Doppler recording can estimate the pressure gradient across the stenotic valve.[35]

Mitral Regurgitation

Aside from specific causes of mitral regurgitation, such as mitral valve prolapse or flail mitral valve (both discussed later), the echocardiographic signs for mitral regurgitation have been disappointing. Excessive mitral valve motion and a steep E to F slope have been noted in these patients,[4,9,39–41] but for the most part these criteria have not been useful. If the amplitude of motion is unusually great, then this finding would definitely

be compatible with mitral regurgitation, or probably more specifically, with a large mitral valve flow.[42] Unfortunately, large mitral flow could be due to other conditions. When mitral regurgitation is secondary to rheumatic valvular disease, there is always some degree of fibrosis, and valve motion is reduced. As a result, the valve amplitude and E to F slope are rarely greater than normal, even with massive mitral regurgitation.[42,43,43a] Occasionally, with mixed mitral stenosis and mitral regurgitation, but predominant mitral regurgitation, one may see a so-called "ski sloping" with an initial brisk downward E to F slope and then a more gradual, flatter diastolic slope during the latter portion of diastole. Again, this echocardiographic sign is occasionally useful but not totally reliable.

A few investigators have attempted to make the echocardiographic diagnosis of mitral regurgitation by looking at the mitral echoes during systole.[44,45] Occasionally, in patients with mitral regurgitation one may find a separation between the leaflets in systole. This separation was believed to represent failure of the leaflets to coapt, which in turn produced valvular regurgitation.[44] Although this theory is quite plausible, in reality such a technique has many false positives and false negatives. The irregularly shaped mitral valve apparatus is almost parallel to the ultrasonic beam in systole, and the problem of beam width makes this echocardiographic sign unreliable. In most M-mode mitral valve echocardiograms illustrated thus far, one sees multiple echoes in systole. It is extremely difficult to clearly identify those echoes originating from the edges of the leaflets. Often it is impossible to determine whether the echoes originate from the valve leaflets or from the chordae. As a result, most experienced echocardiographers do not rely on separation of the mitral leaflets in systole as a sign of mitral regurgitation even though this sign may occur occasionally.

Despite the inaccuracy of the M-mode examination in judging systolic leaflet separation, one group of investigators has indicated that two-dimensional echocardiography may be able to record the regurgitant mitral orifice in patients with rheumatic mitral regurgitation.[46] They found that with careful analysis of the early systolic frames one could see the regurgitant orifice (RO, Fig. 6–20) in patients with significant regurgitation. The examination utilized short-axis views of the mitral valve that overcame some of the variability in leaflet separation by way of M-mode echocardiography. Unfortunately, this observation has not been confirmed by independent investigators. Since frame-by-frame analysis is required, the technique is admittedly difficult. It must be remembered that the mitral valve apparatus constantly moves from base to apex. The area of the mitral valve that shows the lack of coaptation does not persist within the examining plane throughout systole. Thus one must look at isolated early frames before the valve moves out of the examining plane. In addition, the axial resolution of the instrument must be good. Fortunately, the lateral resolution is not as important for this particular examination. With any instrument that has relatively poor axial resolution one could not hope to make this type of observation. It is hoped that with improved techniques for analyzing individual two-dimensional frames, this technique may become more practical, provided that it is truly valid. For now, this observation remains investigational and is not ready for routine clinical use.

Although echocardiography may have difficulties making a positive diagnosis of rheumatic mitral regurgitation, it is extremely useful in a patient with apparent mitral regurgitation in whom one wishes to determine whether the valvular insufficiency is rheumatic in origin. Patients with rheumatic mitral insufficiency invariably exhibit some degree of stenosis with thickening of the valve and abnormal motion during diastole.[47]

Most echocardiographers depend on the secondary signs of mitral regurgitation for the echocardiographic diagnosis. These signs include the size of the left atrium, pulsations of the left atrial wall, the size of the left ventricle, aortic valve motion, and the pattern of motion of the interventricular septum.[48–51] Figure 6–21 shows an M-mode scan of a patient with mitral regurgitation. The dilated left atrium and left ventricle are clearly visible. In addition, the septal motion is exaggerated. The amplitude of septal motion is approximately 1 cm. Exaggerated septal motion is often seen with a volume overload of the left ventricle.[48,52] An explanation for this excessive motion has not been determined. However, if one wants to develop a unifying theory on septal motion, one can consider the septal motion in patients with left ventricular volume overload to be opposite that noted previously with right ventricular volume overload (see Chapter 3). Assuming that the septum reflects the relative filling patterns of the two ventricles, then it is not surprising that with the excessive inflow of blood into the left ventricle one expects increased anterior motion of the septum in early diastole. With ventricular systole the increased left ventricular stroke volume, which exceeds that of the right ventricle, produces an increased posterior motion of the septum.

Increased septal motion is not specific for mitral regurgitation. As noted later, aortic regurgitation also produces exaggerated septal motion. The exact pattern of septal motion

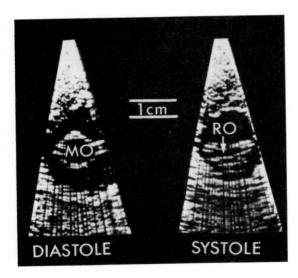

Fig. 6–20. Short-axis mitral valve echocardiogram of a patient with rheumatic mitral regurgitation. The stenotic mitral valve orifice (MO) is recorded in diastole and the regurgitant orifice (RO) in systole as the leaflets fail to coapt properly. (From Wann, L.S., et al.: Cross-sectional echocardiographic detection of rheumatic mitral regurgitation. Am. J. Cardiol., *41*:1258, 1978.)

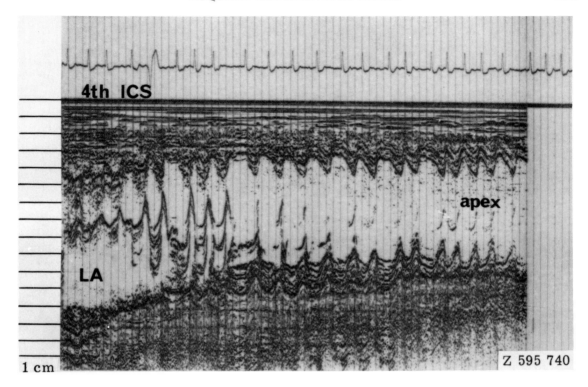

Fig. 6–21. M-mode scan of a patient with mitral regurgitation. The left atrium (LA) and left ventricle are dilated, and the septal motion is exaggerated.

is slightly different with mitral regurgitation and aortic insufficiency, principally in the early diastolic septal dip, which is frequently exaggerated with aortic regurgitation,[53] and may be absent with mitral regurgitation.[51]

Figure 6–22 shows an M-mode left atrial echocardiogram in a patient with mitral regurgitation. In addition to the obviously dilated left atrium, there is also systolic expansion of the posterior left atrial wall.[54,55] When present this sign is helpful in establishing the diagnosis of mitral regurgitation. Unfortunately, these pulsations are not usually seen with mitral regurgitation. One may note exaggerated motion at the junction between the left atrium and left ventricle. Although these pulsations may represent atrial contractions, they more likely show the motion of the atrioventricular ring and are unreliable for the diagnosis of mitral regurgitation.

The posterior aortic wall has also been noted as different in patients with mitral regurgitation.[55] The early, rapid left atrial filling phase with mitral regurgitation may be steep with mitral regurgitation.[56] Thus the left atrial emptying index in the patient illustrated in Figure 6–22 would be high. The onset of the downward motion of the aortic wall in diastole may also be early in patients with mitral regurgitation.[57]

Other M-mode techniques have been described that help in the detection and possible quantitation of mitral regurgitation.[51,58] One such sign is examining the shortening of the left ventricular diameter during the pre-ejection phase.[58] With a competent mitral valve there should be no change in left ventricular volume during isovolumic contraction. With mitral regurgitation, isovolumic contraction does not exist because of the regurgitation of blood into the left atrium. One study noted a significant decrease in the left ventricular diameter during the pre-ejection period in patients with mitral regurgitation.[58] In a recent study, investigators examined the interatrial septum from a right parasternal position and found abnormal mo-

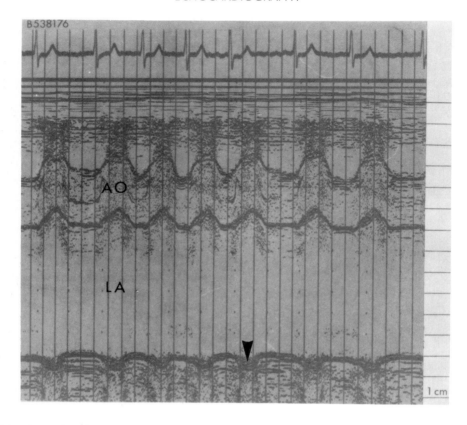

Fig. 6–22.   M-mode echocardiogram of a patient with mitral regurgitation demonstrating a dilated left atrium (LA) and systolic expansion *(arrow)* of the posterior left atrial wall. AO = aorta.

tion and shape of this structure with mitral regurgitation.[59]

The aortic valve motion in patients with mitral regurgitation is frequently abnormal. The aortic valve gradually closes during systole in patients with mitral regurgitation as the flow of blood into the aorta is not sustained (see Chapter 4). Another pattern of the aortic valve is early systolic closure similar to that seen with subaortic obstruction. One could measure regurgitant fraction by way of flow measurements calculated from the aortic valve echocardiogram and possibly total left ventricular stroke volume as judged by either left ventricular dimensions, left atrial chamber sizes, or mitral valve flow (see Chapter 4). Unfortunately, all measurements for calculating total left ventricular stroke volume in the presence of mitral regurgitation have some limitations. However, if the posterior aortic wall, left atrium, left ventricle, and mitral valve all suggest high flow

states and the aortic valve suggests a low flow state, one can expect a sizable mitral regurgitant fraction.

As one might expect, Doppler echocardiography has been proposed as a technique for detecting mitral regurgitation.[34,36,60–62,62a,62b] Figure 6–23 demonstrates a Doppler echocardiographic study of a patient with rheumatic mitral stenosis and regurgitation. The M-mode tracing shows a clearly thickened stenotic mitral valve. The Doppler sampling probe is placed along the atrial side of the mitral valve. The Doppler signal records a band of turbulent flow in systole (arrow). The abnormal flow is indicated by the scatter of dots during systole in contrast to the laminar flow in diastole. Since the Doppler signals are below the baseline, the turbulent flow is away from the transducer or toward the left atrium. The Doppler tracing in this figure would be highly indicative if not diagnostic of mitral regurgitation. Unfortu-

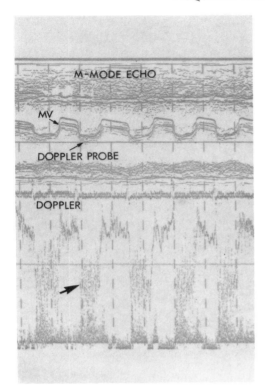

Fig. 6–23. Doppler echocardiogram of a patient with rheumatic mitral regurgitation. The Doppler probe is placed on the atrial side of the mitral valve (MV). Turbulent blood flow moving away from the transducer is visible in systole *(arrow)*. (From Feigenbaum, H.: Echocardiography. *In* Heart Disease. Edited by E. Braunwald. Philadelphia, W.B. Saunders Co., 1980.)

nately, the Doppler study for mitral regurgitation has many limitations yet to be overcome. The examination must be relatively far away from the transducer, and this distance frequently exceeds the capability of the Doppler instrument. The angle necessary for detecting the regurgitant jet may not be optimal for the Doppler examination. With the parasternal examination the regurgitant jet may be perpendicular to the sampling volume and may be missed. One can place the transducer at the apex but, unfortunately, the sampling site is even farther from the transducer. Another problem is that the location and direction of the turbulent jet may vary significantly; it may not be easy to find the jet with the Doppler sample. Finally, Doppler echocardiography has not

been too successful in quantitating the degree of mitral regurgitation. Despite these limitations, there continues to be active investigation into the use of Doppler echocardiography for the detection and possible quantitation of mitral regurgitation. For example, there is a study that demonstrates a correlation between the extent to which the regurgitant Doppler signal is found within the left atrium and the degree of regurgitation.[62a] In view of the difficulties with both M-mode and two-dimensional echocardiography, any contribution that Doppler echocardiography can make is certainly valuable.

Mitral Valve Prolapse

The diagnosis of mitral valve prolapse is probably one of the most important and most confusing applications of echocardiography. The first echocardiographic finding reported with mitral valve prolapse is demonstrated in Figure 6–24. In late ventricular systole, there is posterior displacement of the mitral

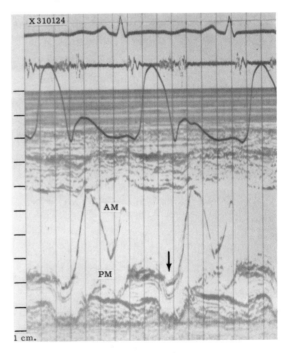

Fig. 6–24. Echocardiogram of a patient with a prolapsed mitral valve. Note the late systolic posterior motion of the anterior (AM) and posterior (PM) mitral valve leaflets *(arrow)*. This abnormal motion corresponds with a late systolic murmur as seen on the phonocardiogram.

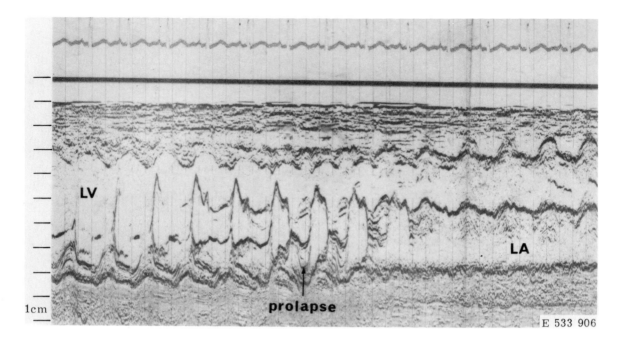

Fig. 6–25.   M-mode scan of the mitral valve in a patient with a prolapsed mitral valve. The characteristic abnormality *(arrow)* is best seen at the junction between the left ventricle (LV) and the left atrium (LA). (From Chang, S.: M-mode Echocardiographic Techniques and Pattern Recognition. Philadelphia, Lea & Febiger, 1976.)

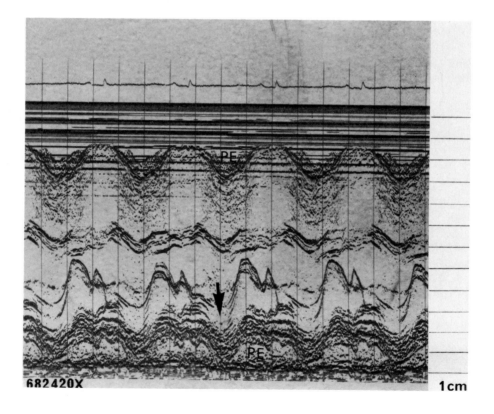

Fig. 6–26.   M-mode echocardiogram of a patient with a large pericardial effusion (PE) with excessive cardiac motion during systole. The entire heart, including the mitral valve apparatus, moves posteriorly with systole, producing artifactual mitral valve prolapse *(arrow)*.

valve, especially the posterior leaflet toward the left atrium (arrow). This posterior or downward displacement of the mitral valve in late systole corresponds with the systolic click and late systolic murmur that are clinical hallmarks of this abnormality. Figure 6–25 demonstrates an M-mode scan showing how the typical M-mode findings for mitral valve prolapse are best seen at the junction between the left ventricle and the left atrium.

The finding of late systolic prolapse, or midsystolic buckling, of the mitral valve has withstood the test of time. With rare exception it has proved quite reliable with relatively few false positives. Figure 6–26 shows a mitral valve with posterior displacement during the latter two-thirds of systole. The mitral valve motion superficially resembles that of mitral valve prolapse. However, this patient has obvious pericardial effusion with

swinging of the entire heart posteriorly during systole. Thus the apparent mitral valve prolapse is merely a function of total cardiac motion. Although this type of echocardiogram could be misinterpreted as mitral valve prolapse, it is not a true false positive.

Much of the confusion with M-mode echocardiography with regard to mitral valve prolapse is in patients with holosystolic prolapse. It was recognized from the beginning that under certain circumstances the late systolic prolapse could become holosystolic. Figure 6–27A demonstrates a patient with late systolic prolapse (arrow). The midsystolic click and late systolic murmur can be seen on the phonocardiogram. With amyl nitrite the patient developed a tachycardia, and the prolapse became holosystolic (Fig. 6–27B). Many patients with mitral valve prolapse only demonstrate the holosystolic variety (Fig. 6–28). With holosystolic pro-

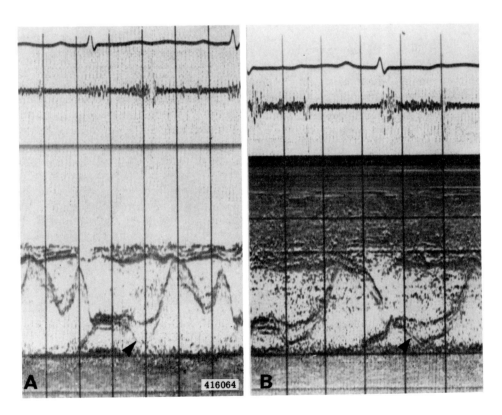

Fig. 6–27. Simultaneous mitral valve echocardiograms and phonocardiograms of a patient with a prolapsed mitral valve before, *A*, and after, *B*, the inhalation of amyl nitrite. With this drug the late systolic prolapse *(arrow, A)* begins earlier, and one sees a holosystolic prolapse and a holosystolic murmur *(arrow, B)*. (From Dillon, J.C., et al.: Use of echocardiography in patients with prolapsed mitral valve. Circulation, *43*:503, 1971.)

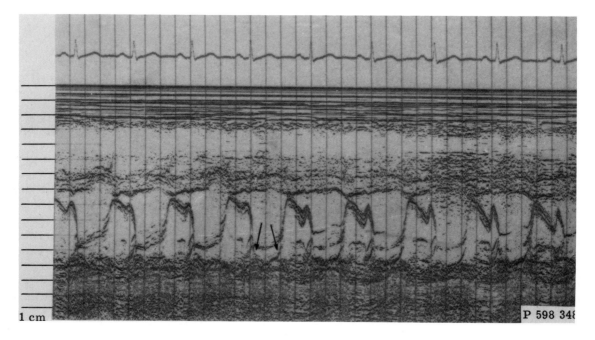

Fig. 6–28. Mitral valve echocardiogram demonstrating holosystolic prolapse *(arrows)*.

lapse, new criteria must be developed to differentiate mitral valve prolapse from a normal variant. A small degree of posterior buckling or bowing of the mitral valve in systole can occur in patients with no apparent evidence of mitral valve prolapse. One proposed criterion is that if the mitral valve leaflet extends below 3 mm of a line drawn between the C and D points, then that patient has mitral valve prolapse. This criterion, however, greatly increases the incidence of mitral valve prolapse within the general population.[63–65] One study using the more liberal criteria for mitral valve prolapse showed up to 18% of healthy young females with evidence of mitral valve prolapse.[64] Thus some echocardiographers have been reluctant to use the 3-mm systolic bowing or hammocking of the mitral valve as the sole criterion for mitral valve prolapse.[66,67]

Another M-mode finding with mitral valve prolapse is anterior motion of the leaflets during systole.[68,69] Figure 6–29 shows a patient with a classic late systolic murmur. The echocardiogram exhibits prominent early anterior systolic motion of the mitral valve. There is also posterior displacement of the mitral leaflets in the latter half of systole.

Because the M-mode echocardiogram is not spatially oriented, it became apparent that the position of the transducer and the direction of the ultrasonic beam could influence the motion of the mitral valve.[70] This problem was most pressing when looking for the hammocking type of mitral valve prolapse. The transducer position probably had less influence on late systolic prolapse or on the systolic anterior motion in Figure 6–29. One group of investigators recommended that mitral valve prolapse only be diagnosed when the ultrasonic beam is perpendicular to the mitral valve with the transducer placed along the left sternal border.[71] This technical detail is helpful in eliminating false positives, but it does not totally solve the problem of what constitutes prolapse, since all hearts are not located in the same spot within the chest and since one cannot always examine the heart from whatever interspace one desires.

Because of the confusion introduced by the M-mode echocardiogram it is not surprising that many investigators attempted to use two-dimensional echocardiography to diagnose mitral valve prolapse.[72–76] Since this valvular abnormality is principally a dis-

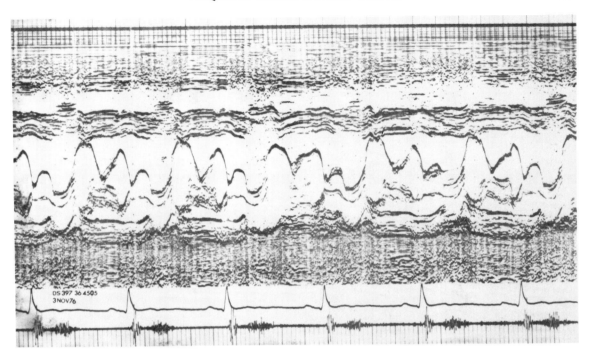

Fig. 6–29.   M-mode echocardiogram of a patient with mitral valve prolapse. In systole there is initial anterior motion of the mitral leaflet and then posterior motion in the latter half of systole corresponding to the late systolic murmur on the phonocardiogram. (Courtesy of William Jacobs, M.D., Chicago, Illinois.)

placement or bulging of the mitral leaflet into the left atrium, it would be expected that the spatial orientation inherent in two-dimensional echocardiography might be helpful in establishing this diagnosis. Figure 6–30 diagrammatically demonstrates the long-axis plane of the normal mitral valve in systole. The dotted line extends from the base of the aortic valve to the atrioventricular junction. This line is roughly parallel to the plane of the atrioventricular ring. The closed normal mitral valve does not reach this plane. Figure 6–31 diagrammatically shows how prolapsing anterior and posterior mitral leaflets may bulge through this plane into the left atrium in systole. Figure 6–32 demonstrates a mitral valve echocardiogram that shows the buckling and bowing of the mitral valve (arrows) in a patient with mitral valve prolapse.[77] The posterior leaflet actually exhibits a sharp hairpin turn as it bends toward the left atrium. The anterior leaflet curves more gradually, producing an almost right-angle bend at the attachment of the anterior

NORMAL

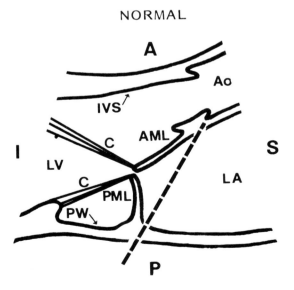

Fig. 6–30.   Diagram demonstrating the relationship of the closed normal mitral valve to the plane of the mitral annulus (dotted line). A = anterior; P = posterior; I = inferior; S = superior; AO = aorta; IVS = interventricular septum; AML = anterior mitral leaflet; C = chordae; PML = posterior mitral leaflet; PW = posterior wall; LA = left atrium; LV = left ventricle.

leaflet and the aorta. The posterior leaflet clearly passes through the arbitrary plane between the root of the aorta and the atrioventricular junction. The anterior leaflet is approximately parallel to this plane, well be-

ANTERIOR AND POSTERIOR LEAFLET PROLAPSE

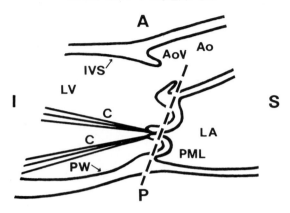

Fig. 6–31. Diagram showing the relationship of a prolapsed mitral valve to the plane of the mitral annulus (dotted line). In systole (S) the leaflets protrude into the left atrium and cross the plane of the annulus. A = anterior; P = posterior; I = inferior; S = superior; Ao = aorta; AoV = aorta valve; IVS = interventricular septum; LV = left ventricle; C = chordae; PW = posterior wall; PML = posterior mitral leaflet; LA = left atrium.

yond the normal location for the closed mitral valve.

One may not find both leaflets to be prolapsed. Figure 6–33 shows a patient whose prolapse is limited to the posterior leaflet. The bulging of the posterior leaflet into the left atrium is fairly obvious, whereas the anterior leaflet position is reasonably normal.

Mitral valve prolapse can also be detected in the four-chamber view.[78] Figure 6–34 demonstrates an apical four-chamber examination of a normal mitral valve. During systole (Fig. 6–34B), there is initial closure of the valve. The bodies of the leaflets are approximately within the plane of the annulus. Shortly after the onset of ventricular ejection, there may be slight bowing of the leaflets immediately below the plane of the annulus (Fig. 6–34C). Figure 6–35 demonstrates a four-chamber view of a patient with mitral valve prolapse. The bulging of the anterior leaflet is distinctly beyond the plane of the annulus (dotted line). No firm criterion has been developed as to when slight bulging beyond the plane of the annulus becomes pathologic.

There are some potential advantages to using the four-chamber rather than the long-axis view for this diagnosis. The four-chamber view permits more frequent visu-

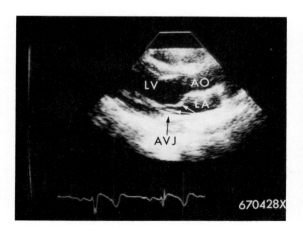

Fig. 6–32. Two-dimensional long-axis echocardiogram of a patient with mitral valve prolapse. Both the anterior and posterior mitral leaflets (arrows) curve into the left atrium (LA). The posterior leaflet makes almost a hairpin turn as it moves to the atrial side of the atrioventricular junction (AVJ). LV = left ventricle; AO = aorta.

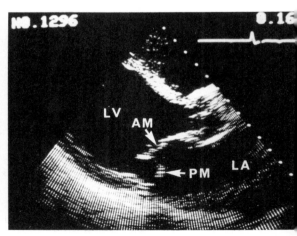

Fig. 6–33. Long-axis parasternal two-dimensional echocardiogram of a patient with prolapse of the posterior mitral leaflet (PM). AM = anterior mitral leaflet; LV = left ventricle; LA = left atrium. (From Machii, K.: Atlas of Cross-sectional Echocardiography. Tokyo, Toshiba Corporation, 1978.)

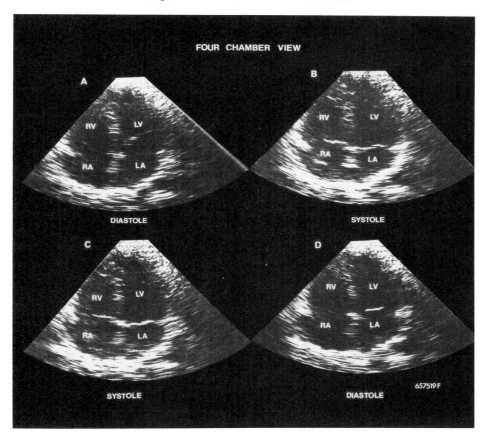

Fig. 6–34. Serial apical four-chamber two-dimensional echocardiograms of a normal mitral valve. At end-systole, C, the closed mitral valve is parallel to the plane of the mitral annulus. RV = right ventricle; RA = right atrium; LV = left ventricle; LA = left atrium.

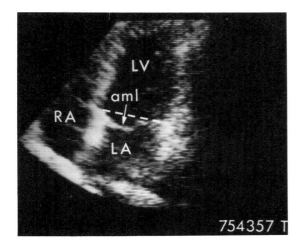

Fig. 6–35. Apical four-chamber echocardiogram of a patient with mitral valve prolapse demonstrating a curved anterior mitral leaflet (aml) that extends beyond the plane of the mitral annulus (dotted line). LV = left ventricle; LA = left atrium, RA = right atrium.

alization of the body of both leaflets since the ultrasonic beam is more perpendicular to the valve in systole. In addition, the direction of the annulus is horizontal and can be readily appreciated in this view. The plane of the annulus in the parasternal long-axis view is angled and is constantly moving because the posterior atrioventricular junction moves vigorously throughout the cardiac cycle.

Both two-dimensional views provide an opportunity to demonstrate the spatial orientation of the mitral valve and can add significant information concerning the presence of mitral valve prolapse. Unfortunately, in some situations, a gray zone still remains between a normal and a prolapsing valve. It should be realized that the two-dimensional criteria are distinctly different from those used in M-mode echocardiography. The M-mode findings depend principally on the pattern of motion, whereas the two-dimensional data depend on spatial orientation of the valve. Thus in many respects the two examinations are complementary; in a confusing patient one may assist the other.

Besides bowing and displacement of the valve, other two-dimensional echocardiographic criteria have been proposed to assist with the diagnosis of mitral valve prolapse. One study noted posterior displacement of the coaptation point of the two leaflets.[76,77] Unfortunately, this technique has not been confirmed, and there is some question as to its reliability. A recent study has reported an abnormal contraction pattern of the interventricular septum in patients with mitral valve prolapse.[79] In the apical four-chamber view, vigorous contraction of the septum produced bending of the septum toward the left ventricle.

Although most clinicians are aware of the distortion of the mitral valve in systole, the pathologist also sees histologic changes in the valve. These changes have been referred to as "myxomatous degeneration." This term may or may not be correct since the principal histologic finding apparently is collagen de-

generation within the leaflets.[80,81] The echocardiogram occasionally reflects the histologic changes. Figure 6–36 shows a patient with mitral valve prolapse who has thickening of the anterior leaflet and a mass of echoes in the vicinity of the posterior mitral leaflet in diastole (arrow). The mass of echoes seen in the vicinity of the posterior mitral leaflet may not only represent a thickened posterior leaflet, but may also be partially a result of the redundant mitral valve folding on itself as it assumes a vertical orientation to the ultrasonic beam.[82] The mass of echoes in this figure can often be confused with a large vegetation or even a tumor.[83] The valve thickening can also be appreciated on the two-dimensional study. Figure 6–37 demonstrates two views of a floppy, prolapsing mitral valve. The anterior

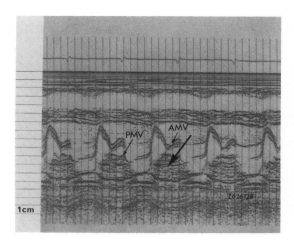

Fig. 6–36. M-mode echocardiogram of a patient with an angiographically and surgically proven mitral valve prolapse. During diastole, multiple echoes (large arrow) occur behind the posterior mitral valve leaflet (PMV). These multiple echoes most likely originate from a vertically oriented, thickened, and/or folded posterior leaflet. During systole the posterior leaflet moves posteriorly toward the left atrial wall. AMV = anterior mitral valve leaflet.

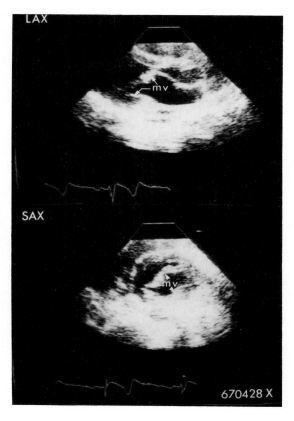

Fig. 6–37. Long-axis (LAX) and short-axis (SAX) two-dimensional echocardiograms of a patient with mitral valve prolapse. The leaflets are thickened and appear redundant in the short-axis view. mv = mitral valve.

leaflet is thickened and appears redundant. The short-axis view also demonstrates the thickening as well as an unusual configuration of the valve.

Papillary Muscle Dysfunction

Attempts have been made to diagnose papillary muscle dysfunction on the basis of M-mode echocardiography. One study associated the clinical syndrome with a decreased mitral valve E to F slope.[84] This finding has not been confirmed by other investigators. Papillary muscle dysfunction can be diagnosed indirectly by clinically identifying a patient with mitral regurgitation, by detecting wall motion abnormalities echocardiographically, and by using echocardiography to exclude other causes for the valvular insufficiency.[85]

A recent observation using two-dimensional echocardiography holds promise in making the direct diagnosis of papillary muscle dysfunction.[86,87] As noted in Figure 6–34, in an examination of the normal mitral valve from the apical four-chamber view, the leaflets line up in a plane approximately parallel to the mitral annulus. With papillary muscle dysfunction the papillary muscle or the adjacent ventricular muscle may be scarred, dyskinetic, or merely dilated so that the leaflet to which the papillary muscle is attached may not be able to close fully. The result may be incomplete closure of the valve. Figure 6–38 demonstrates the echocardiographic finding of incomplete closure in a patient with papillary muscle dysfunction. In systole the closed mitral valve does not reach the plane of the mitral annulus (dotted line). This finding has been noted both in patients with ischemic heart disease[86] and in patients with diffuse cardiomyopathy.[87] Although this observation agrees with our understanding of papillary muscle dysfunction, it must be confirmed by independent investigators before we can establish its reliability in clinical echocardiography.

Flail Mitral Valve

A large number of echocardiographic findings have been described in patients with flail mitral valve. One pattern is indis-

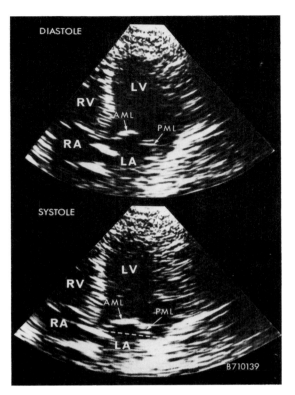

Fig. 6–38. Apical four-chamber echocardiograms of a patient with coronary artery disease and papillary muscle dysfunction. During systole the closed mitral leaflets (AML and PML) fail to reach the plane of the mitral annulus (dotted line). LV = left ventricle; RV = right ventricle; RA = right atrium; LA = left atrium.

tinguishable from marked mitral valve prolapse and usually primarily involves the posterior leaflet.[88] A more common finding is coarse diastolic fluttering of the flail mitral leaflets.[89–93] Figure 6–39 shows a patient who has bacterial endocarditis with torn chordae and a flail anterior leaflet. The fluttering of the anterior leaflet during diastole is chaotic and coarse.

One of the more reliable echocardiographic signs of flail mitral valve appears when recording part of the leaflet in the left atrium.[88,90–92] Figure 6–40 shows an M-mode echocardiogram of a flail valve whereby part of the valve appears within the left atrium during ventricular systole (FML). This echocardiogram exhibits another sign of a flail valve—fine systolic fluttering of the valve. Unfortunately, the fluttering does not repro-

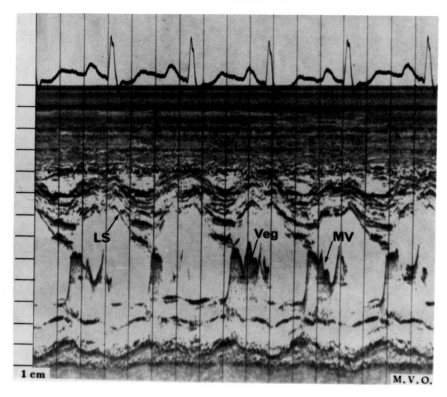

Fig. 6–39. Mitral valve echocardiogram of a patient with torn chordae of the anterior mitral leaflet and vegetations (Veg) secondary to bacterial endocarditis. During diastole the anterior leaflet (MV) exhibits chaotic, coarse fluttering.

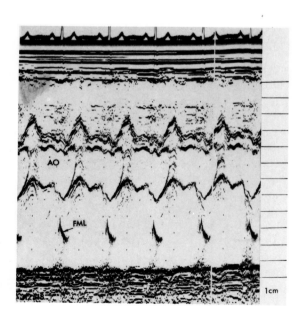

Fig. 6–40. M-mode echocardiogram of the aorta (AO) and left atrium of a patient with a flail mitral leaflet (FML). During systole, part of the flail mitral valve can be seen extending into the left atrial cavity.

duce well in this illustration. Systolic fluttering is repeatedly noted by investigators as a valuable sign of a flail or disrupted mitral valve.[94-97] One study demonstrated that the systolic fluttering most often occurred with torn chordae,[97] or with fenestration of the valve.[94] In this series, a ruptured papillary muscle, which also produces a flail valve, rarely produced systolic fluttering.

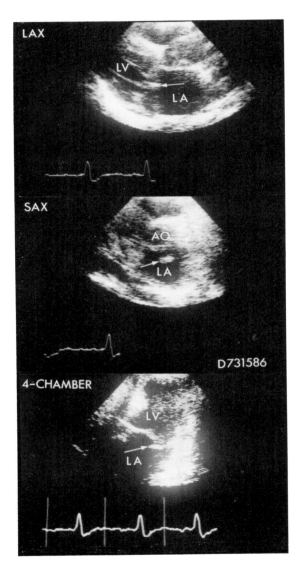

Fig. 6–41. Two-dimensional echocardiograms of a patient with a flail mitral valve. The flail portion of the mitral valve (arrows) can be seen extending into the left atrium in the long-axis (LAX), short-axis (SAX), and four-chamber views. LV = left ventricle; LA = left atrium; AO = aorta.

A flail mitral valve can also be detected with two-dimensional echocardiography.[93,95,95a,98] Extension of part of the valve into the left atrium in systole can be readily noted with this spatially oriented examination.[93,95,98] Figure 6–41 shows three views of a patient with a flail valve. The abnormal portion of the mitral valve (arrow) can be seen within the left atrium during systole in the long-axis, short-axis, and four-chamber views. A feature on the two-dimensional echocardiogram that distinguishes between mitral valve prolapse and flail mitral valve is that with a flail valve the tip of the leaflet points toward the left atrium (Fig. 6–41), whereas with mitral prolapse the tip of the leaflet points toward the left ventricle (Figs. 6–32, 6–35).[95] Thus, if one can identify the direction in which the leaflet curves in systole, one might use this criterion to distinguish between a severely prolapsing valve and a truly flail leaflet. One study found two-dimensional echocardiography to be more sensitive and reliable in the echocardiograms of a flail mitral valve.[98a]

AORTIC VALVE DISEASE

Although isolated aortic valve disease is possibly always congenital and may be a consequence of a bicuspid aortic valve, aortic stenosis and insufficiency are progressive problems that usually affect adults. In addition, these two valvular problems are frequently secondary to rheumatic heart disease. Since rheumatic and congenital aortic valve disease may be indistinguishable echocardiographically, both aortic stenosis and aortic regurgitation are discussed in this chapter. Congenital aortic stenosis, especially in the child, is also discussed in the chapter on congenital heart disease.

Aortic Stenosis

Figure 6–42 demonstrates an M-mode tracing of a normal aortic valve. The leaflets are thin and open widely in systole. Figure 6–43 shows an M-mode aortic valve echocardiogram of a patient with valvular aortic stenosis. The echocardiographic findings include thickening of the valve leaflets as demonstrated by multiple echoes coming from the leaflets, especially during diastole.

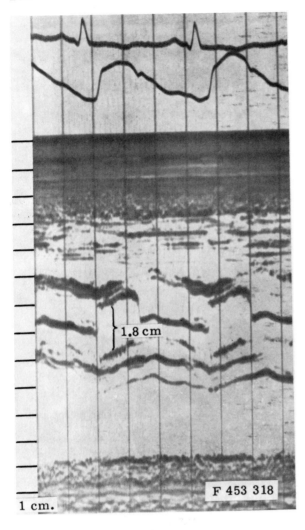

1.8 cm

F 453 318

1 cm.

Fig. 6–42. M-mode tracing of a normal aortic valve. The leaflets are 1.8 cm apart during ventricular systole.

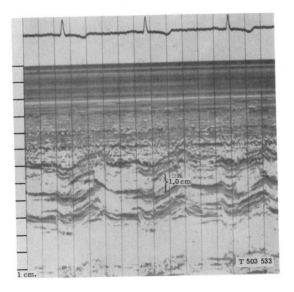

1.0 cm

T 503 533

1 cm.

Fig. 6–43. Aortic valve echocardiogram of a patient with noncalcific aortic stenosis. Note multiple echoes from the valve leaflets, which separate to only 1.0 cm during systole.

There is also restricted motion of the leaflets; if one measured the distance between the leaflets, it would be below normal, that is, approximately 1.5 to 2.5 cm in adults (see Appendix). In Figure 6–43, the dominant echoes during systole are approximately 1.0 cm apart. Even in this exceptionally good aortic valve echocardiogram, one might select other systolic echoes for measurement. Thus the point of measurement of the separation of the aortic valve leaflets can be difficult.[99] Figure 6–44 represents a more typical aortic valve echocardiogram of a patient with aortic stenosis. Multiple echoes are visible within the aortic root, and there is some vague suggestion of leaflet motion during systole. It is almost impossible to clearly identify valve leaflets, let alone to measure the separation between them in systole. Thus, although echocardiographers have attempted to quantitate the degree of aortic stenosis by measuring the systolic separation

of the leaflets, there are many limitations to this type of examination.[99]

Even the qualitative diagnosis of aortic stenosis can be difficult at times. Figure 6–45 shows an aortic valve echocardiogram of a patient with predominant mitral stenosis. There is no hemodynamically significant aortic stenosis, although one cannot rule out mild thickening of the valve. As the relationship of the ultrasonic beam to the aortic valve changes with respiration, the echoes within the aortic root change drastically. One can identify at least two aortic orifices (labeled 1 and 2). Aortic valve echo 1 is suggestive of aortic stenosis. The aortic leaflet appears thickened, and the separation is approximately 1 cm. However, aortic valve echo 2 shows a much wider separation of the leaflets, as do those in the subsequent systoles. There still may be some thickening of the leaflets and possibly mild aortic stenosis; there was definitely no hemodynamically

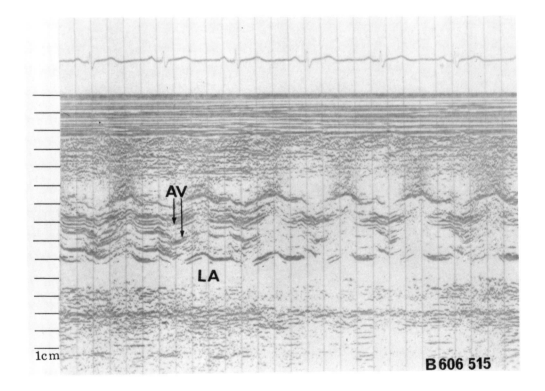

Fig. 6–44.   Fairly typical aortic valve echocardiogram of a patient with aortic stenosis. Thickened aortic leaflets are readily apparent, although the distance between the cusps is difficult to evaluate. AV = aortic valve leaflets; LA = left atrium. (From Chang, S.: M-mode Echocardiographic Techniques and Pattern Recognition. Philadelphia, Lea & Febiger, 1976.)

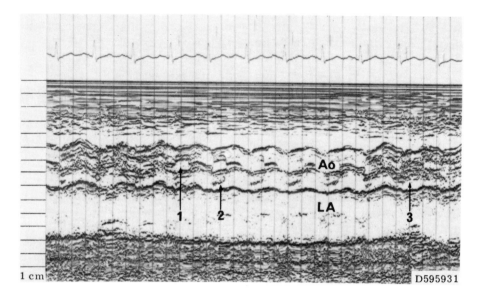

Fig. 6–45.   Aortic valve echocardiogram showing variations in the aortic valve echoes in a patient who had no hemodynamically significant aortic stenosis. AO = aorta; LA = left atrium. (From Chang, S.: M-mode Echocardiographic Techniques and Pattern Recognition. Philadelphia, Lea & Febiger, 1976.)

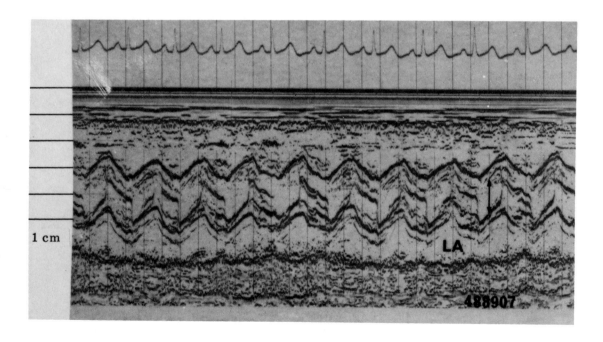

Fig. 6–46.   Echocardiogram of the aortic valve in a four-and-a-half-year-old child with severe congenital aortic stenosis. The apparent separation of the aortic valve leaflets *(arrow)* is within normal limits. LA = left atrium. (From Chang, S.: M-mode Echocardiographic Techniques and Pattern Recognition. Philadelphia, Lea & Febiger, 1976.)

significant aortic stenosis, as might be indicated by the aortic valve echoes labeled 1. To complicate matters further, when the ultrasonic beam did not cross through the center of the aorta, as in the area labeled 3, one merely recorded a mass of echoes within the aorta that closely resembled those echoes seen in Figures 6–43 and 6–44. This mass of echoes most likely is the result of directing the ultrasonic beam tangentially through the aorta.

Another potential problem with the echocardiographic diagnosis of aortic stenosis is in patients with congenital aortic stenosis with minimal fibrosis and no calcification. Because of the domed nature of these valves, echoes from the wide part of the valve, near its attachment to the aorta, are recorded more readily than those originating from the true flow-restricting orifice at the top of the dome. The echoes near the attachment to the aorta separate widely in systole and give the appearance of a normal aortic valve. Figure 6–46 shows an aortic valve echocardiogram of a four-and-a-half year-old child with severe congenital aortic stenosis. One might have difficulty distinguishing this tracing from a normal aortic valve. The dominant valve echoes apparently separate widely (arrow).

Thus, although M-mode echocardiography can be helpful in identifying patients with valvular aortic stenosis, the many limitations must be recognized. When one finds multiple echoes from the aortic leaflets, one can be reasonably assured that he is dealing with a thickened valve. Restricted leaflet motion provides further evidence that some degree of aortic stenosis is present. Attempts to quantitate the degree of stenosis by the appearance of the aortic valve echoes can be frustrating and misleading. A mass of echoes within the aorta should not be labeled aortic stenosis unless some leaflet motion is detected, ensuring that the ultrasonic beam is not merely transecting the aorta tangentially. In children or young adults with congenital aortic stenosis, the aortic valve echocardiogram may be grossly normal despite the presence of severe valvular disease.

Two-dimensional echocardiography can contribute significant information about pa-tients with valvular aortic stenosis.[100,101] This technique can overcome some deficiencies in the M-mode examination. Figure 6–47 demonstrates systolic and diastolic frames from a long-axis two-dimensional study of a normal aortic valve (av). In systole, the aortic valve appears as two thin, parallel lines that lie close to the walls of the aorta (Fig. 6–47A). The echoes coming from the leaflets are straight and parallel to the aortic wall. During diastole the leaflets come together. Most of the valve is parallel to the ultrasonic beam and hence is seen only faintly if at all. The point of coaptation (av, Fig. 6–47B) is recorded as a small linear echo in the middle of the aorta.

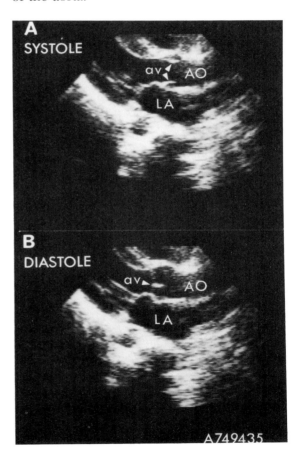

Fig. 6–47. Long-axis two-dimensional examination of a normal aortic valve (av). A, In systole, the opened aortic leaflets are parallel to each other and lie near the wall of the aorta (AO). B, In diastole, the point at which the leaflets coapt is seen as a bright echo within the aorta. Faint echoes from the body of the leaflets may occasionally be seen. LA = left atrium.

With valvular aortic stenosis the valve becomes thickened and is frequently seen in diastole (Fig. 6–48A). A more important sign of valvular aortic stenosis is systolic doming (Fig. 6–48B). The echoes from the leaflets are no longer parallel to the aorta. The edges of the leaflets are curved inward toward the center of the aorta. Doming is probably the most important two-dimensional echocardiographic finding for any form of valvular stenosis. The same type of doming is seen with mitral, pulmonic, and sometimes tricuspid stenoses.

Figure 6–49 shows another long-axis two-dimensional study of a stenotic aortic valve in systole. Doming of the valve is apparent. In addition, the edges of the flow-restricting orifice can be identified. A beam-width artifact shows the edges to be

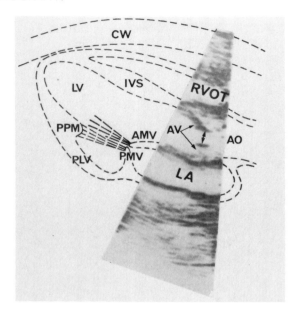

Fig. 6–49. Long-axis two-dimensional echocardiogram of a patient with congenital aortic stenosis. This systolic frame demonstrates the domed valve. The separation between the edges of the leaflets can be measured *(arrows)*. CW = chest wall; IVS = interventricular septum; LV = left ventricle; PPM = posterior papillary muscle; PLV = posterior left ventricular wall; AMV = anterior mitral valve leaflet; PMV = posterior mitral valve leaflet; RVOT = right ventricular outflow tract; LA = left atrium; AV = aortic valve; AO = aorta. (From Weyman, A.E., et al.: Localization of left ventricular outflow obstruction by cross-sectional echocardiography. Am. J. Med., *60*:33, 1976.)

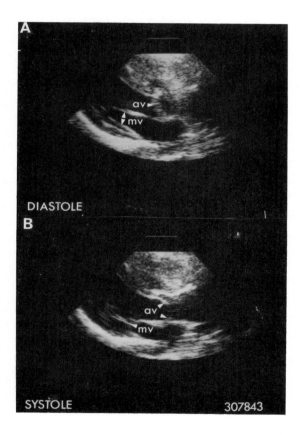

Fig. 6–48. Long-axis two-dimensional echocardiograms of a thickened, stenotic aortic valve (av). *A*, In diastole, the body of the thickened leaflets can be seen. *B*, In systole, doming of the aortic valve is apparent. mv = mitral valve.

slightly wider than the body of the leaflets. This artifact can be helpful in identifying the edge of the structure and can help distinguish a true orifice from echo dropout. Figure 6–49 also shows how the separation of the leaflet edges can be measured for possible quantitation.

Figure 6–50 demonstrates long-axis views of the aortic valve in systole in a patient with calcific aortic stenosis. The two frames demonstrate the variability in aortic leaflet separation that can occur in these often eccentrically oriented orifices. In Figure 6–50A the separation is a barely visible slit (av). By changing the scanning plane one can find a somewhat wider separation (av, Fig. 6–50B).

The aortic valve can also be examined in its short-axis presentation. Because the valve

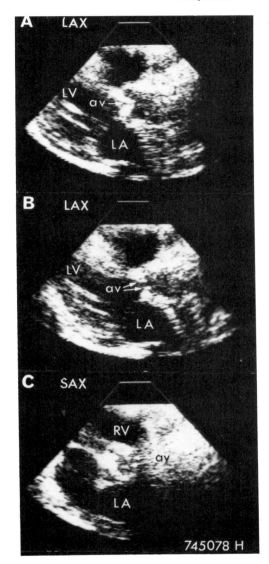

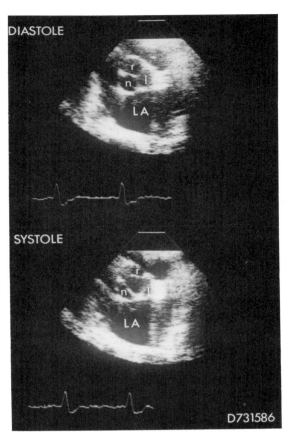

Fig. 6–50. Two-dimensional echocardiograms of a patient with calcific aortic stenosis. A and B are long-axis (LAX) examinations demonstrating the differences in aortic valve separation (av) that can be obtained. C is a short-axis (SAX) examination of the valve. LV = left ventricle; LA = left atrium; RV = right ventricle.

Fig. 6–51. Short-axis two-dimensional echocardiogram of a normal aortic valve. Because the patient has a reduced cardiac output, the orifice is triangular rather than circular in systole. r = right coronary cusp; n = noncoronary cusp; l = left coronary cusp; LA = left atrium.

is relatively small and constantly moves in and out of the examining plane, the short-axis study of the aortic valve is far more difficult than is the short-axis study of the mitral valve. Figure 6–51 demonstrates diastolic and systolic short-axis echocardiograms of a normal aortic valve. During diastole the commissures of the three leaflets are easily seen in the closed position. The separation of the leaflets are apparent in systole. This patient had a low cardiac output; the leaflets, therefore, do not oppose the walls of the aorta, and the orifice is more triangular than circular, which is the normal shape. This short-axis examination is distinctly different from that seen in Figure 6–52. In diastole the commissures of the valve are thickened, and whether there are two or three leaflets is not clearly seen (Fig. 6–52A). The systolic orifice is visible in Figure 6–52B. With calcified valves the orifice is frequently slit-like, and it is difficult to record a complete orifice (Fig. 6–50C).

These examples demonstrate that two-dimensional echocardiography can help de-

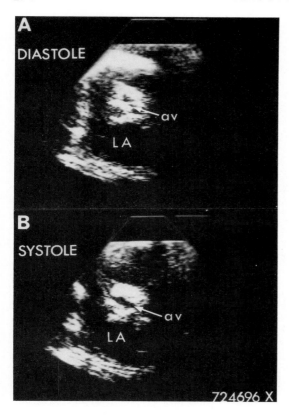

Fig. 6–52. Short-axis two-dimensional echocardiogram of a patient with calcific aortic stenosis. A slit-like orifice is visible in systole, *B*. LA = left atrium; av = aortic valve.

lineate the presence of valvular aortic stenosis. The most significant contribution is with the noncalcified, domed aortic valve. The potential false negative demonstrated in Figure 6–46 should be eliminated with the two-dimensional study. Two-dimensional echocardiography is also useful in examining calcified valves because it excludes the possibility of the ultrasonic beam transecting the aorta tangentially as seen in Figure 6–45. Thus the two-dimensional examination should help in the qualitative evaluation of calcific and noncalcific valvular aortic stenosis.

The usefulness of two-dimensional echocardiography in quantitative aortic stenosis is still uncertain. Data indicate that the separation of the leaflets as seen in the long-axis presentation of the aortic valve (Fig. 6–49) is related to the degree of stenosis.[101] For

example, one would not be surprised to find the aortic stenosis in Fig. 6–48 to be less than that in Figures 6–49 or 6–50. The data thus far suggest that the maximum aortic cusp separation in the long axis can help distinguish mild from moderate or severe aortic stenosis. The principal difficulty is differentiating between patients who have moderate and severe aortic stenosis. Unfortunately, this separation is critical since the advisability of surgery frequently depends on this determination. Thus far there is considerable overlap between patients who have moderate and severe aortic stenosis by merely measuring the separation of aortic leaflets in the long axis.[102]

One might logically study the short-axis examination of the aortic valve and then measure an area as one does with mitral stenosis. If all short-axis studies were as good as Figure 6–52, one might consider such a possibility as practical. Although one group of investigators is proposing such an approach,[103] it is extremely difficult to record a short-axis systolic orifice. More commonly the orifice is irregular (Fig. 6–50C), making it technically impossible to determine its size. Another possible use of the short-axis aortic valve examination is to judge the mobility of the individual leaflets to semiquantitate the degree of stenosis. If the leaflets are completely rigid, the likelihood of significant obstruction is much higher. If one or more of the leaflets is mobile, it is highly unlikely that the degree of obstruction is significant. Of course, gradations exist between these two observations. Thus, to what degree the short-axis aortic valve examination helps in the quantitation of aortic stenosis remains to be determined.

When judging valvular stenosis, especially aortic stenosis, it must be remembered that the clinical and hemodynamic gold standard is frequently a pressure gradient. Figure 6–53 shows a graph correlating aortic valve area against aortic valve gradient, assuming certain fixed parameters. The curve that is plotted is merely theoretical and uses the Gorlin formula for calculating aortic valve area. The reason for showing this graph is to demonstrate the relationship between valve area and pressure gradient. There can

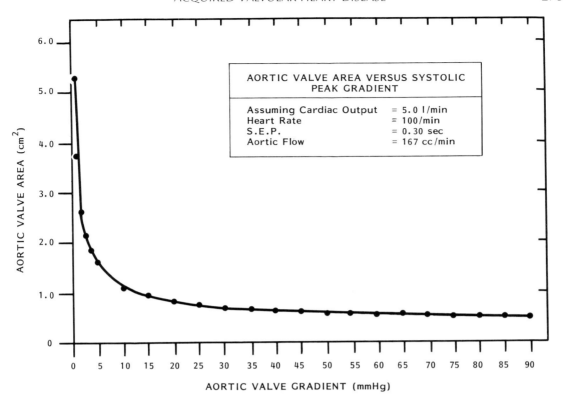

Fig. 6–53. Graph demonstrating the theoretical relationship of aortic valve area and aortic valve gradient with aortic stenosis.

be a significant decrease in aortic valve area before any appreciable aortic valve gradient occurs. There can be a 50% decrease in aortic valve area with a gradient of only 5 mmHg. Even a gradient of 10 mmHg can represent an aortic valve area of 1.0 cm². However, as the aortic valve area decreases from 1.0 cm² to 0.5 cm², the aortic gradient can increase from 10 mmHg to 90 mmHg. This part of the curve is almost flat so that the difference between a 25-mm gradient and a 75-mm gradient corresponds to a minimal change in aortic valve area. From a clinical point of view a 25-mm gradient is often considered mild and not worthy of consideration for valve replacement, whereas a 75-mm gradient would almost always indicate the need for surgery. Two-dimensional echocardiography holds great promise of being able to determine aortic valve area. However, whether it ever attains the sensitivity necessary to detect the small change in aortic valve

area previously mentioned is doubtful. It is even doubtful that the surgeon or pathologist can detect the significant difference between a valve that produces a 25-mm gradient and one that produces a 75-mm gradient. One can probably expect a good correlation between echocardiographic and pathologic studies and a relatively poor relationship between echocardiographic and pressure measurements, especially in aortic stenosis. Unfortunately, we do not know whether valve area or pressure gradient is more important in the management of an individual patient. If valve area is the critical factor it is possible that two-dimensional echocardiography may provide a more accurate measurement since it is uninfluenced by aortic regurgitation and other inaccuracies inherent in the Gorlin formula. However, if the pressure gradient is the critical factor that influences the natural history of patients with aortic stenosis, then it is quite possible that the echocardiographic determination of valve area will not accurately predict this hemodynamic measurement.

There has been considerable interest in using indirect echocardiographic findings for assessing the severity of aortic stenosis. The most popular technique is to judge the thickness or hypertrophy of the left ventricular walls. A fairly popular technique is to compare the thickness of the left ventricular wall with the diameter of the left ventricular chamber.[104-112] Although these measurements have been taken both in diastole and in systole, most echocardiographers use the end-systolic measurement. A formula has been derived for estimating the left ventricular systolic pressure by using the ratio of the left ventricular posterior wall systolic thickness (LVT_s) and the left ventricular systolic dimension (LVD_s). A constant of either $225^{104,110}$ or 245^{112} can be multiplied by the ratio (LVT_s/LVD_s), thus determining an estimation of the peak systolic pressure. Subtracting the systemic pressure, as determined by sphygmomanometry gives the pressure gradient.

The reliability of this technique varies in the literature.[106,112] Most information has been obtained from children with valvular aortic stenosis. Both excellent[110,112] and poor[104,106] correlations with hemodynamics have been reported. Most investigators agree that if the ventricle is dilated, this formula does not reliably predict the pressure.[104] In addition, it does not function as accurately in the postoperative state. There has been relatively little use of this technique in adults with valvular aortic stenosis. These patients more often have dilated ventricles and thus would probably not be reliable subjects for this technique. In any case, left ventricular hypertrophy is certainly an important hemodynamic consequence of significant valvular aortic stenosis. Most echocardiographers look for this finding in their overall evaluation of a patient with aortic stenosis. Whether one can predict the peak systolic pressure or the systolic pressure gradient is debatable and probably limited only to certain patients.

A variety of other echocardiographic signs for judging the severity of aortic stenosis has

been introduced to the literature. One study indicated that the pattern of left ventricular wall motion would be helpful in estimating the severity of aortic stenosis.[113] A slow-rising posterior left ventricular wall during systole was supposedly indicative of hemodynamically significant aortic stenosis. Other techniques that examine left ventricular wall motion both in systole and diastole have been introduced into the literature. However, none of these measurements are popular, having not been independently confirmed thus far.

There is evidence that Doppler echocardiography can be helpful in at least the qualitative assessment of aortic stenosis.[114] The turbulent flow produced by the stenotic jet of blood into the aorta can be readily detected by way of the Doppler technique. There have been efforts to judge the size of the turbulent jet in order to quantitate the stenosis, but this technique has not been confirmed.

Aortic Regurgitation

The echocardiographic recording of the aortic valve occasionally provides clues to the existence of aortic regurgitation. Figure 6–54 shows one of the more reliable but infrequent M-mode findings with valvular aortic regurgitation.[115] Fine diastolic fluttering (arrow) of the aortic valve is seen in this patient with a fenestrated aortic valve. With a ruptured aortic cusp, the diastolic fluttering echoes can also be seen in the left ventricular outflow tract.[116-121] Figure 6–55 demonstrates an M-mode echocardiogram of a patient with bacterial endocarditis and a ruptured aortic valve leaflet. The fine to coarse diastolic fluttering motion can be seen anterior to the mitral valve in the left ventricular outflow tract as well as within the aorta itself. Whether the actual vegetation or part of the aortic valve is fluttering cannot be distinguished from the echocardiogram. In addition, identical appearing echoes have been seen in patients with rupture of the aortic valve secondary to myxomatous degeneration rather than to bacterial endocarditis.[120,122]

Two-dimensional echocardiographic examination of the aortic valve occasionally

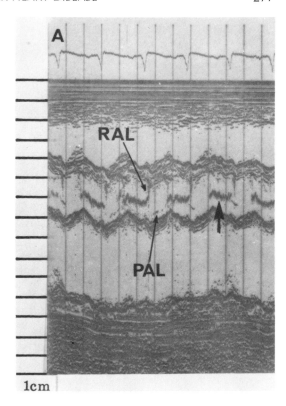

Fig. 6–54. Aortic valve echocardiogram demonstrating fluttering of the aortic valve during diastole *(arrow)* in a patient with a myxomatous degeneration of the aortic valve and marked aortic regurgitation. RAL = right aortic leaflet; PAL = posterior aortic leaflet. (From Estevez, C.N., et al.: Echocardiographic manifestations of aortic cusp rupture in a case of myxomatous degeneration of the aortic valve. Chest, 69:544, 1976.)

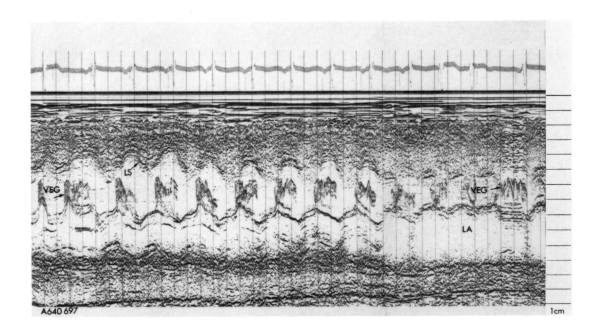

Fig. 6–55. M-mode scan of a patient with bacterial endocarditis and a vegetation on the aortic valve. The oscillating vegetation (VEG) is visible in the left ventricular outflow tract as well as in the vicinity of the aortic valve. LS = left side of interventricular septum; LA = left atrium.

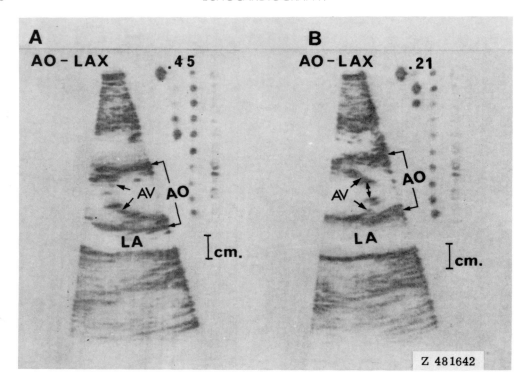

Fig. 6–56.   Long-axis (LAX) two-dimensional echocardiogram of an aortic valve in a patient with congenital aortic stenosis and regurgitation. A, During diastole, there is eversion of the aortic leaflets (AV) away from the aorta (AO). B, A domed, stenotic valve bulging toward the aorta in systole can be noted. LA = left atrium. (From Weyman, A.E., et al.: Cross-sectional echocardiography in assessing the severity of valvular aortic stenosis. Circulation, 52:828, 1975.)

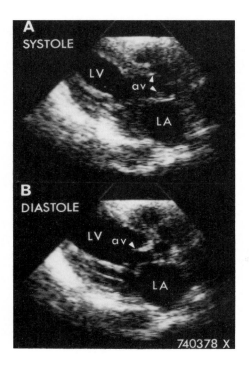

Fig. 6–57.   Long-axis two-dimensional echocardiogram of a patient with bacterial endocarditis and a vegetation on the aortic valve. During diastole, B, a mass of echoes attached to the aortic valve (av) can be seen protruding into the left ventricular outflow tract. LV = left ventricle; LA = left atrium.

provides a clue to the presence of aortic regurgitation. Figure 6–56 shows a patient with congenital aortic stenosis and regurgitation. Note the systolic doming of the valve (Fig. 6–56B). In diastole (Fig. 6–56A), there is reverse motion of the leaflets with herniation into the outflow tract. There are recent reports of similar findings with aortic valve prolapse diagnosed with two-dimensional echocardiography.[123–125] A flail aortic valve with or without vegetation can also be detected with two-dimensional echocardiography. The echocardiograph in Figure 6–57 shows a flail aortic valve and a vegetation. In diastole (Fig. 6–57B), a mass of echoes protrudes into the left ventricular outflow tract and may represent a vegetation and parts of the flail valve alike.

It is tempting at times to diagnose aortic regurgitation by noting failure of the aortic leaflets to coapt properly in diastole.[126] This finding is occasionally noted with both M-mode and two-dimensional techniques.

However, diagnosing aortic regurgitation on this basis encounters the same difficulties as diagnosing mitral regurgitation by examining mitral closure. That the aortic valve is smaller and moves in and out of the examining plane renders such a diagnosis of aortic regurgitation even less reliable than the diagnosis for mitral regurgitation.

The most common echocardiographic finding in patients with aortic regurgitation is the presence of diastolic fluttering of the mitral valve.[127,128] The oscillations are quite rapid and difficult to detect at times. Figure 6–58 is an echocardiograph of a patient with aortic regurgitation and diastolic fluttering of the mitral valve. If the resolution of the recording system is relatively poor, the fluttering may appear as a smudge or mass of echoes rather than as fine oscillations. One may even misinterpret oscillations as a thickened valve. Figure 6–58 also demonstrates that fluttering of the interventricular septum may occur with aortic regurgi-

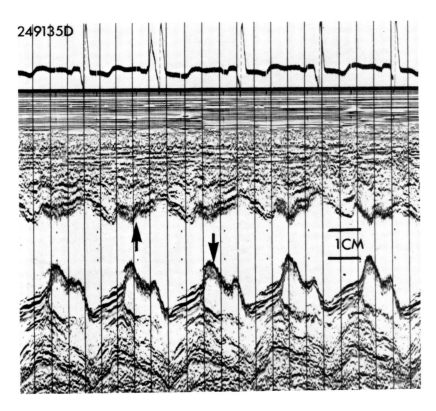

Fig. 6–58. M-mode echocardiogram of a patient with aortic regurgitation. Note fluttering *(arrows)* of the interventricular septum and mitral valve.

tation.[127,129,130] Looking for fluttering of the septal echoes is particularly helpful if there is intrinsic disease of the mitral valve that prevents the usual occurrence of fluttering. There is evidence that when fluttering of the septum occurs, the regurgitant jet passes through the vicinity of the posterior, or noncoronary, cusp.[131]

In patients with mitral stenosis, mitral valve fluttering is more difficult to detect because of the fibrosis. A prosthetic mitral valve does not exhibit fluttering. Although the posterior mitral leaflet does not flutter as often as the anterior leaflet, posterior leaflet fluttering has been reported with aortic regurgitation.

The effect of aortic regurgitation on mitral valve motion can be profound. Besides fluttering, the E point of the mitral valve motion can be altered. Figure 6–59 demonstrates obvious fluttering of the mitral valve in diastole. In addition, there are several echoes during diastole. The one that exhibits the most fluttering also has incomplete opening of the valve in early diastole. Figure 6–60

shows a two-dimensional echocardiogram of the mitral valve in the short-axis presentation in a patient with severe aortic regurgitation. Distortion of the shape of the mitral valve in early diastole is evident. This partial closure of the valve in early diastole probably results from the regurgitant jet hitting the anterior leaflet and suggests that the jet passes through the aortic valve in the vicinity of the anterior right coronary cusp.[131] The two-dimensional study also explains why multiple diastolic echoes might be seen on the M-mode echocardiogram. One mitral leaflet echo opens more fully than the other (Fig. 6–59). Figure 6–61 demonstrates a more extreme form of abnormal mitral valve opening with aortic regurgitation. There is practically no E point, and the valve opens almost entirely with atrial systole (A wave). Such an extreme example is probably not only a function of the regurgitant aortic jet, but also reflects the abnormal filling pattern through the mitral valve in this patient with severe aortic regurgitation.

In patients with elevated left ventricular

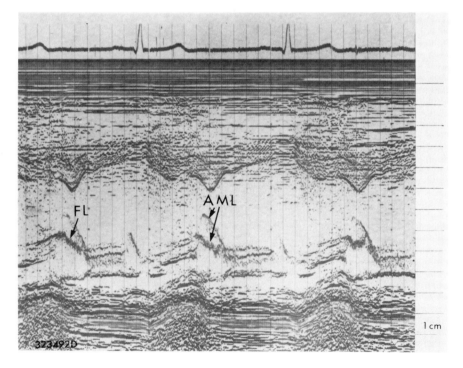

Fig. 6–59.   M-mode echocardiogram of a mtiral valve in a patient with aortic regurgitation. Two different echoes from the anterior mitral leaflet (AML) can be seen. The leaflet with the greater fluttering (FL) also shows incomplete opening during early diastole.

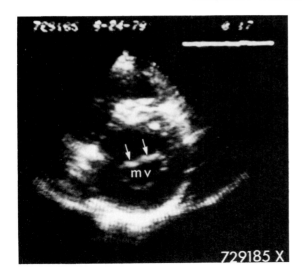

Fig. 6–60. Short-axis two-dimensional mitral valve echocardiogram in a patient with severe aortic regurgitation. The anterior leaflet is pushed posteriorly *(arrows)* by the regurgitant jet of blood. MV = mitral valve.

diastolic pressures, early closure of the mitral valve may occur.[128,131a-e] Figure 6–62 is a mitral valve echocardiogram of a patient with acute aortic regurgitation and severely elevated left ventricular diastolic pressures. The mitral valve is almost completely closed (C') long before ventricular systole (C). Atrial systole causes little if any reopening of the mitral valve.[128] This premature closure is an important clinical sign for elevated diastolic pressures in the setting of acute aortic regurgitation. The diastolic pressure may occasionally be so high with acute aortic regurgitation that the aortic valve may prematurely open (see Chapter 4).[118,132]

The left ventricle has also been extensively studied in patients with aortic regurgitation.[49,50,133-136] Figure 6–63 shows the left ventricular echocardiogram of a patient with aortic regurgitation. Note the obvious left ventricular dilatation on this tracing as well as the markedly increased amplitude of sep-

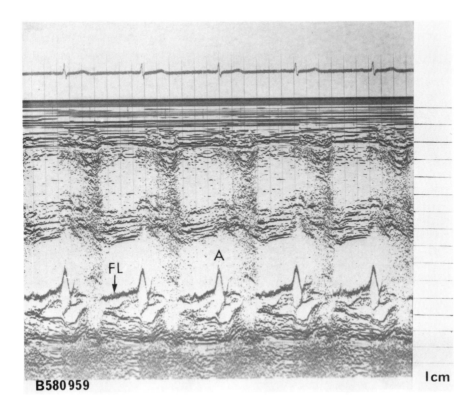

Fig. 6–61. M-mode recording of a mitral valve in a patient with severe aortic regurgitation. Fluttering (FL) of the leaflet can be noted, and there is virtually no opening of the anterior leaflet until atrial systole (A).

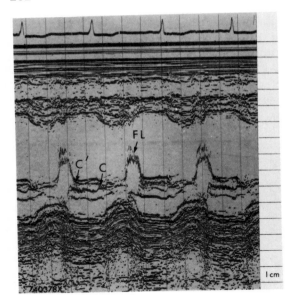

Fig. 6–62. Mitral valve echocardiogram of a patient with acute severe aortic regurgitation. The valve is almost completely closed (C') before ventricular systole. The valve does not reopen with atrial systole and closes completely with ventricular systole (C).

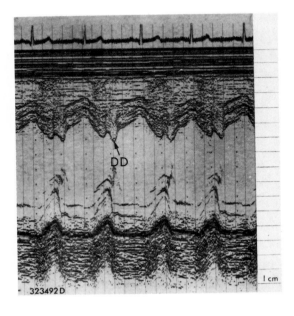

Fig. 6–63. Left ventricular echocardiogram of a patient with aortic regurgitation. The left ventricle is dilated, the septal and posterior walls move excessively, and there is an exaggerated diastolic dip (DD) of the interventricular septum.

tal excursion. Thus the echocardiographic signs of left ventricular volume overload, dilatation of the ventricle, and increased septal motion are common findings in aortic regurgitation. These echocardiographic signs are nonspecific for left ventricular volume overload and are similar to what is observed with mitral regurgitation. However, the septal motion can be different with aortic regurgitation. An exaggerated early diastolic dip (DD, Fig. 6–63) is occasionally seen in these patients. The mechanism for this septal motion is not known. Since there is no isovolumic relaxation period with aortic regurgitation, one would expect the septum to move anteriorly sooner with the onset of diastole.[53] The exaggerated diastolic downward dip could be a function of rebound and/or a relative increase in right ventricular filling as a result of a reduced inflow of blood through the mitral valve. Thus the exaggerated diastolic dip with aortic regurgitation may be similar to that which occurs with mitral stenosis. Irrespective of the explanation, the exaggerated diastolic dip can help distinguish the left ventricular volume overload pattern of aortic regurgitation from that of mitral regurgitation.

Considerable research has attempted to use echocardiography to assess the left ventricle in patients with aortic regurgitation to determine the proper timing for aortic valve replacement.[134,134a,136–138] Fractional shortening, diastolic and systolic dimensions, wall thickness, and wall thickness-cavity dimension ratios have all been proposed as possible echocardiographic signs for judging when intervention should occur.[138] One group of investigators suggests that a left ventricular systolic dimension greater than 55 mm or a percent fractional shortening less than 25% is indicative of a decompensated left ventricle, and aortic valve replacement should be seriously considered.[134,134a] Figure 6–63 is an echocardiogram of a patient with a well-compensated ventricle and severe aortic regurgitation. Figure 6–64 shows an M-mode echocardiogram of a patient with severe aortic regurgitation whose left ventricle is functioning poorly. The ventricle is markedly dilated, and the fractional shortening is much less than in Figure 6–63. Note also the lack of mitral valve opening at the E point in Figure 6–64. The extreme difference between Figures 6–63 and 6–64 can be easily detected by echocardiography. There is debate over whether more subtle differences in ventricular function can be detected echocardiographically by way of any of the proposed measurements.[137] There is evidence that M-mode left ventricular dimensions do not correlate well with ventricular volumes and ejection fraction in patients with aortic regurgitation.[138a] If one chooses to follow a patient with echocardiography to determine left ventricular deterioration, then meticulous care must be taken as to how the left ventricular examination and dimensions are obtained.

There are several Doppler echocardiographic techniques for the detection of aortic regurgitation. Continuous-wave Doppler has been used to record the aortic flow pattern in patients with aortic regurgitation. Normally there is a relatively small amount of flow within the aorta in diastole. The flow is probably a function of the recoil of the elastic aorta. As expected, with aortic regurgitation a much larger flow pattern is seen in diastole with aortic regurgitation. In addition, the direction of the flow is reversed from that seen in systole. One suggested technique takes a ratio of the systolic and diastolic Doppler signal to quantitate the degree of aortic regurgitation.

Pulsed Doppler echocardiography can also be used to detect aortic regurgitation. This examination requires placing the Doppler sample in the left ventricular outflow tract.[139,140] Diastolic flow can be detected in patients with an insufficient aortic valve. Unfortunately, this technique is partially hindered by diastolic flow coming through the mitral valve, making it occasionally difficult to distinguish between the two flow patterns. Quantitation of the aortic regurgitation has been suggested by noting how far into the ventricle the regurgitant

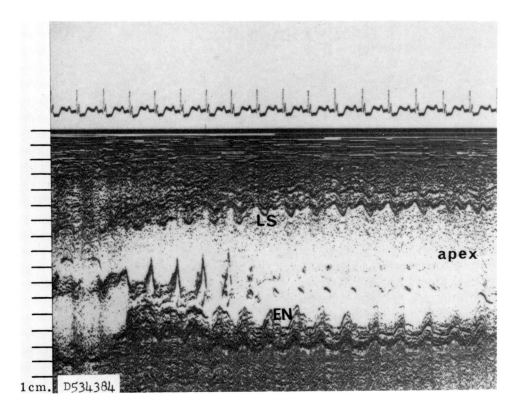

Fig. 6–64. M-mode scan of a patient with severe aortic regurgitation and poor left ventricular function. The left ventricle is dilated, and the septal (LS) and posterior endocardial (EN) echoes do not exhibit excessive motion.

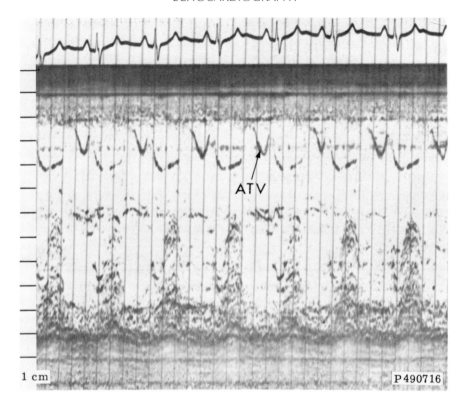

Fig. 6–65.   Normal tricuspid valve M-mode echocardiogram. The pattern of motion of the anterior tricuspid leaflet (ATV) is essentially the same as that of the anterior mitral leaflet.

jet can be detected.[140] The reliability of this observation is unknown.

TRICUSPID VALVE DISEASE

Tricuspid Stenosis

Figure 6–65 shows a normal tricuspid valve M-mode echocardiogram. As usual, the echoes are recorded exclusively from the anterior leaflet of the tricuspid valve (ATV). The valve echo resembles that of the anterior leaflet of the mitral valve.[9] The typical M-shaped appearance during diastole is apparent. The first clinical application of the tricuspid valve echocardiogram was the detection of tricuspid stenosis.[4,9,141] Figure 6–66 shows an echocardiogram of a patient with tricuspid stenosis. The echocardiographic criteria used in the diagnosis of tricuspid stenosis are similar to those used in diagnosing mitral stenosis. The hallmark of this diagnosis is a decreased diastolic slope

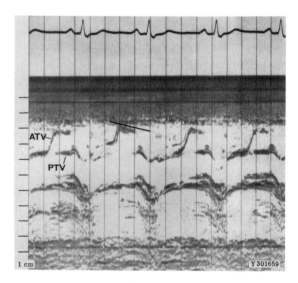

Fig. 6–66.   Tricuspid valve echocardiogram of a patient with tricuspid stenosis. Both anterior (ATV) and posterior (PTV) tricuspid leaflets are recorded. The slope of diastolic closure is diminished, and the overall pattern is similar to that of a stenotic mitral valve.

of the tricuspid valve (Fig. 6–66). In one case report, the echocardiographic diagnosis of tricuspid stenosis secondary to carcinoid syndrome was based on a thickened tricuspid valve and a decreased E to F slope.[142] One can occasionally record the posterior tricuspid valve leaflet and, when present, its motion fits the usual criteria for mitral stenosis in that the posterior leaflet is no longer an exact mirror image of the anterior leaflet. Unfortunately, the posterior tricuspid valve leaflet is infrequently recorded so that this criterion is not useful.

As indicated in the discussion on mitral stenosis, the diastolic slope of the tricuspid valve, as with the mitral valve, is influenced by many factors. Thus a reduced diastolic slope is not pathognomonic for tricuspid stenosis just as it is not pathognomonic for mitral stenosis.[144] Figure 6–67 shows a tricuspid valve echocardiogram with a clearly diminished diastolic slope. This patient underwent cardiac catheterization, and with simultaneous right ventricular and right at-

rial pressures, no gradient could be demonstrated across the tricuspid valve. The patient had mitral stenosis and pulmonary hypertension. Whether the altered diastolic slope was due to reduced right ventricular filling because of pulmonary hypertension and low cardiac output is not known. Thus, as with mitral stenosis, a decreased diastolic slope of the tricuspid valve is compatible with, but unfortunately not diagnostic of, tricuspid stenosis. Even a more rapid diastolic slope may not be entirely reliable in excluding the diagnosis of tricuspid stenosis. Figure 6–68A demonstrates a tricuspid valve echocardiogram that looks reasonably normal. The diastolic slope, though not excessively steep, would not be judged as unusually flat. Figure 6–68B shows simultaneous right atrial and right ventricular pressures that reveal a pressure gradient across the tricuspid valve in this patient with tricuspid stenosis. An adequate explanation for the unusually normal filling pattern of the tricuspid valve is unknown. Thus the

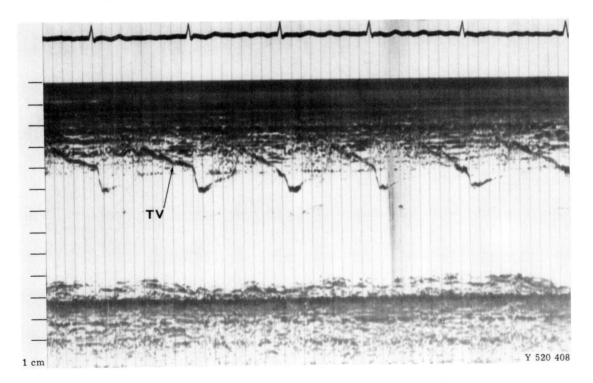

1 cm   Y 520 408

Fig. 6–67.   Tricuspid valve (TV) echocardiogram exhibiting a decreased diastolic slope in a patient with no evidence of tricuspid stenosis. (From Chang, S.: M-mode Echocardiographic Techniques and Pattern Recognition. Philadelphia, Lea & Febiger, 1976.)

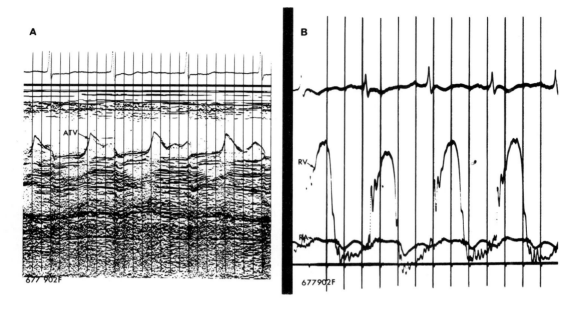

Fig. 6–68. A, Tricuspid valve echocardiogram and B, simultaneous right ventricular (RV) and right atrial (RA) pressures in a patient with tricuspid stenosis. Despite the apparent pressure gradient across the tricuspid valve, the diastolic slope of the anterior tricuspid valve leaflet (ATV) is only mildly reduced.

M-mode examination for tricuspid stenosis is fraught with many difficulties. The appearance of the tricuspid valve can only be suggestive but not diagnostic of excluding or detecting this valvular problem.

There have been no reports to date that use two-dimensional echocardiography for the detection of tricuspid stenosis. However, one might expect this technique to have some advantages over the M-mode examination. Figure 6–69 shows a systolic and diastolic two-dimensional echocardiogram of a patient with tricuspid stenosis. This short-axis study is taken at the level of the base of the heart. The tricuspid valve is visible between the right atrium and the right ventricle. In systole the closed tricuspid valve is possibly slightly thickened, otherwise no abnormality can be detected. However, in diastole there is doming of the septal leaflet because it does not open fully. Although the doming was visible in other views of the tricuspid valve, the recordings were not sufficiently good for illustration. Thus, just as with mitral, aortic, and pulmonic stenoses, diastolic doming may prove a useful sign in the diagnosis of tricuspid stenosis.

Tricuspid Regurgitation

Tricuspid regurgitation is a cause for right ventricular volume overload.[145] The M-mode echocardiogram may reflect this hemodynamic abnormality by a dilated right ventricle and abnormal septal motion. Figure 6–70 is an echocardiograph of a patient with tricuspid regurgitation that shows early systolic paradoxical or anterior motion of the interventricular septum.[146] Although not clearly visible here, the right ventricle is also dilated.

Several reports have demonstrated the usefulness of contrast echocardiography in the diagnosis of tricuspid regurgitation.[148,149] Both two-dimensional and M-mode techniques have been used for this application. Several abnormal patterns of the contrast-producing echoes have been described. Occasionally, one can recognize echoes moving back and forth through the regurgitant tricuspid orifice.[149] Possibly a more reliable sign for tricuspid regurgitation is the appearance of regurgitation contrast echoes in the inferior vena cava during systole.[148,150] The contrast injection must be made in an upper-extremity vein. There are other

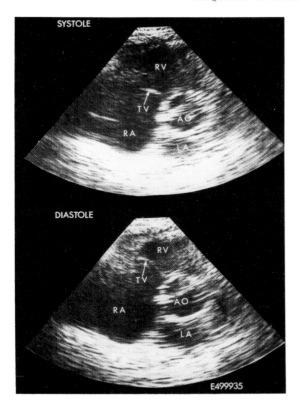

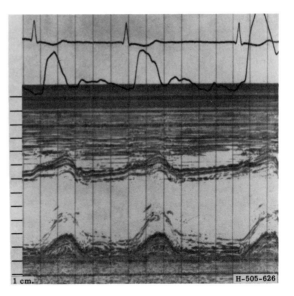

Fig. 6–70.   Left ventricular echocardiogram showing abnormal septal motion in a patient with tricuspid regurgitation. With ventricular depolarization anterior motion exists briefly. During early ventricular ejection the septal motion is flat, and anterior motion occurs in late systole.

Fig. 6–69.   Short-axis two-dimensional echocardiograms of the base of the heart and the tricuspid valve in a patient with tricuspid stenosis. Doming of the tricuspid valve (TV) is visible in diastole. RV = right ventricle; RA = right atrium; AO = aorta; LA = left atrium.

causes of contrast echoes appearing in the inferior vena cava. Cardiac tamponade or right heart failure may produce this finding, but the echoes usually appear in the inferior vena cava before ventricular systole. Since timing is critical, the M-mode recording is more reliable. Arrhythmias are a source of false positives.

Another echocardiographic sign of tricuspid regurgitation is excessive systolic pulsations of the hepatic vein detected by way of either the M-mode or two-dimensional examinations. Distortion of shape and motion of the interatrial septum has also been reported with tricuspid regurgitation.[59]

Doppler echocardiography has been used for the detection of tricuspid regurgitation.[151,152] The finding of a systolic regurgitant jet within the right atrium is one criter-

ion that has been proposed.[152] No attempt to quantitate the degree of regurgitation has been made thus far. Another Doppler technique examines the jugular venous flow pattern by way of continuous-wave Doppler.[151] With tricuspid regurgitation, there is retrograde systolic flow. In this study, the authors then calculated a ratio of systolic and diastolic flow to semiquantitate the degree of regurgitation.

An occasional case of tricuspid regurgitation can be detected by direct examination of the tricuspid valve. An example of traumatic tricuspid regurgitation producing diastolic fluttering of the septal tricuspid valve leaflet has been reported.[153] Another study felt that a decreased diastolic slope of the tricuspid valve was frequently present in patients with tricuspid regurgitation.[154] However, in view of the nonspecificity of the diastolic slope, it is unlikely that this sign is reliable.

Several echocardiographic reports demonstrate tricuspid valve prolapse.[155–161] Figure 6–71 shows one of the earliest reports on a prolapsing tricuspid valve. A possibly more severe form of tricuspid valve prolapse is

noted in Figure 6–72. This valve had somewhat chaotic motion and wide excursions as
well as late systolic posterior displacement
of the leaflets (P). Tricuspid valve prolapse
has also been demonstrated with two-

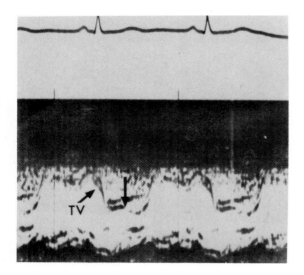

Fig. 6–71. Tricuspid valve echocardiogram (TV)
depicting prolapse of the tricuspid valve *(arrow)*.
(From Chandraratna, P.A.N., et al.: Echocardiographic detection of tricuspid valve prolapse. Circulation, *51*:823, 1975.)

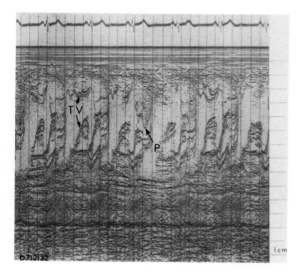

Fig. 6–72. M-mode scan of a tricuspid valve (TV)
in a patient with tricuspid valve prolapse. The excursion and separation of the tricuspid leaflets increase,
and posterior displacement of the valve (P) occurs in
late systole.

dimensional echocardiography.[159,160] The
four-chamber view is the recommended
examination for this diagnosis, although the
examination has been made by way of a subcostal approach.[161] Tricuspid valve prolapse
almost always occurs in patients with associated mitral valve prolapse. In fact, some reports demonstrate a high incidence of the
coexistence of the two abnormalities. The
true incidence is debatable depending on
the criteria used for the diagnosis of tricuspid
valve prolapse.

PULMONARY VALVE DISEASE

The most common pulmonary valve problem is congenital pulmonic stenosis. Since
this problem is a congenital abnormality, the
topic is discussed further in the chapter on
congenital heart disease. There is an occasional acquired form of pulmonary valve disease, the most common of which is pulmonic
insufficiency. This valvular regurgitation
may be secondary to pulmonary hypertension or to iatrogenic causes secondary to
pulmonary valvotomy. Pulmonary regurgitation is another cause for right ventricular
volume overload. Thus the echocardiographic findings of right ventricular volume
overload with a dilated right ventricle and
abnormal septal motion may occur in these
patients. In addition, fluttering of the tricuspid valve may be seen in patients with pulmonic insufficiency. Because the pulmonary
pressures are usually not as high as those
with aortic pressures, the frequency of the
oscillations or fluttering of the tricuspid
valve with pulmonary insufficiency is frequently lower than that noted in the mitral
valve with aortic regurgitation. Figure 6–73
demonstrates a tricuspid valve in a patient
with pulmonic insufficiency. The diastolic
fluttering of the tricuspid valve is not specific
for pulmonic insufficiency. Such fluttering
has also been demonstrated in patients with
various congenital problems with an increased flow across the tricuspid valve.

A rare case of acquired pulmonic stenosis
secondary to carcinoid syndrome has been
reported.[142] The echocardiogram showed a
flat pulmonary valve diastolic slope and no A
wave. The patient also had tricuspid
stenosis; this valvular problem may have in-

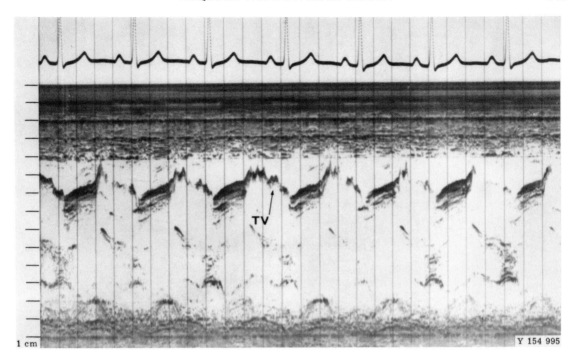

Fig. 6–73.   Coarse diastolic fluttering of the tricuspid valve (TV) in a patient with pulmonic insufficiency.

fluenced pulmonary valve motion more than did the pulmonic stenosis.

ENDOCARDITIS

Echocardiography is proving to be an invaluable diagnostic aid in the management of patients with valvular endocarditis. As already discussed in the cases of mitral and aortic regurgitation, sudden destruction of the valves can produce acute valvular regurgitation that can be detected echocardiographically. In addition to the secondary hemodynamic effects of valvular disruption, echocardiography can also detect the vegetations on the valve leaflets.[161a-f] Figure 6–74 shows one of the original echocardiograms demonstrating a vegetation on a posterior mitral leaflet. The echocardiographic diagnosis consists of a mass of somewhat "shaggy" echoes on the valve leaflet. Differentiating these echoes from those owing to fibrosis is that motion of the leaflet is not impaired. In fact, in cases of valve destruction valve motion may actually be increased. A similar type of echocardiogram with a vegetation on the anterior leaflet is seen in Fig-

ure 6–39. Again, one sees an abnormal mass of echoes on a valve leaflet with totally unobstructed motion. Figure 6–75 shows a slightly more confusing echocardiogram of a patient with a vegetation on the mitral valve. An increased number of echoes in the vicinity of the mitral valve is visible. In addition, valve motion is clearly not restricted. Clearly identifying the origin of these echoes is somewhat more difficult. To complicate matters further, the patient also has mitral valve prolapse. As noted in Figure 6–36, patients with prolapsed mitral valve and myxomatous changes can also show increased echoes of the mitral valve.[83]

Diagnosing a vegetation is somewhat easier when the vegetation is mobile. Figure 6–76 shows a mitral valve vegetation that extends into the left atrium. One cannot totally exclude the possibility that this valve merely represents a flail mitral valve when part of the valve protrudes into the left atrium similar to that seen in Figure 6–40. Since a flail mitral valve frequently is associated with bacterial endocarditis, there is a tendency to call the echoes seen in the left

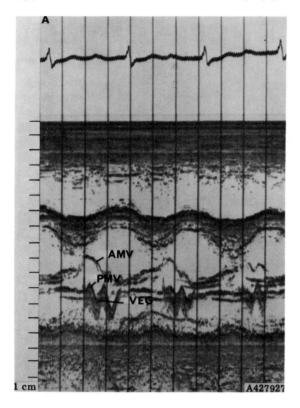

Fig. 6–74. Mitral valve echocardiogram of a patient with bacterial endocarditis and vegetations (VEG) on the posterior mitral valve leaflet (PMV). AMV = anterior mitral valve leaflet. (From Dillon, J.C., et al.: Echocardiographic manifestations of valvular vegetations. Am. Heart J. 86:698, 1973.)

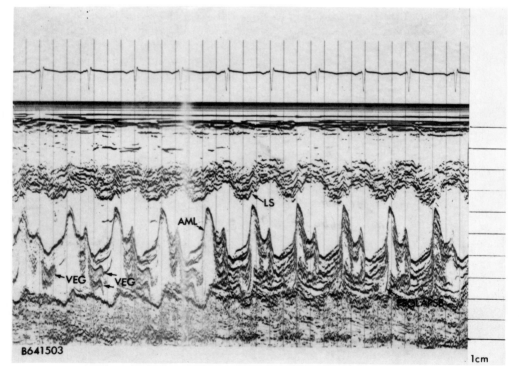

Fig. 6–75. M-mode echocardiogram of a mitral valve with vegetations (VEG) and mitral valve prolapse. LS = left septum; AML = anterior mitral valve leaflet.

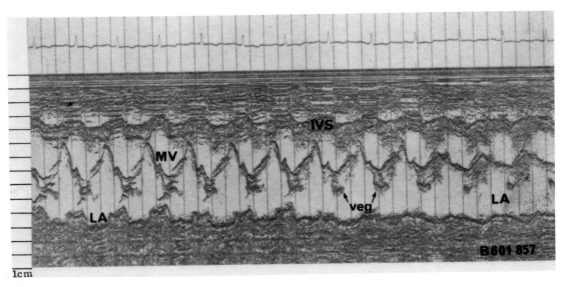

Fig. 6–76.   M-mode scan of a patient with bacterial endocarditis and vegetations on the mitral valve (MV). Echoes from the vegetation (veg) are visible within the left atrial cavity (LA) during systole. IVS = interventricular septum. (From Chang, S.: M-mode Echocardiographic Techniques and Pattern Recognition. Philadelphia, Lea & Febiger, 1976.)

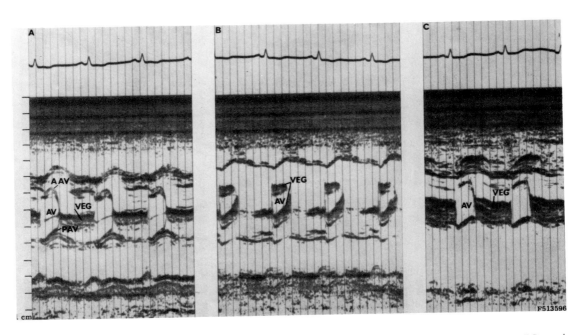

Fig. 6–77.   Aortic valve echocardiograms of a patient with bacterial endocarditis and vegetations (VEG) on the aortic valve (AV). AAV = anterior aortic valve leaflet; PAV = posterior aortic valve leaflet; VEG = vegetation. (From Dillon, J.C., et al.: Echocardiographic manifestations of valvular vegetations. Am. Heart J., *86*:698, 1973.)

atrium vegetations. Subtle differences occasionally exist between a mobile mitral valve vegetation and a flail valve. Vegetations tend to have more echoes and are more eccentric than is the case with a flail valve and no vegetations. However, a noninfected flail valve may have almost the identical echocardiographic appearance, and thus the differentiation is not clear in many situations.

Vegetations on the aortic valve are similar to those on the mitral valve. In some ways, the diagnosis of aortic valve vegetations is easier since multiple echoes from the aortic valve are not as common as they are in the noninfected mitral valve. Figure 6–77 is an early tracing from a patient with aortic valve vegetation. Again one sees increased echoes from the aortic valve leaflets with no restriction of motion. The three views of this patient note the variability that one can record in a patient with an eccentrically located vegetation. The echoes from the vegetation

may be seen best either in systole or in diastole depending on the direction of the ultrasonic beam. As with mitral valve vegetations, a mobile vegetation is more apparent on the M-mode echocardiogram.[116,162,163] Figure 6–78 demonstrates a vegetation on the aortic valve that is recorded as a mass of echoes within the aorta in diastole. In addition, part of the vegetation can be seen in the left ventricular outflow tract above the mitral valve. Recording these abnormal echoes within the left ventricular outflow tract is more convincing than merely finding excess echoes on the aortic valve.[122] Again, as with mitral valve vegetations, it is not totally clear whether the abnormal echoes originate from the vegetation or from part of a flail aortic valve.[122] Thus the echocardiographic diagnosis would be consistent with, but not necessarily diagnostic of, a mobile vegetation on the aortic valve with or without disruption of the valve. Aortic valve vegetations

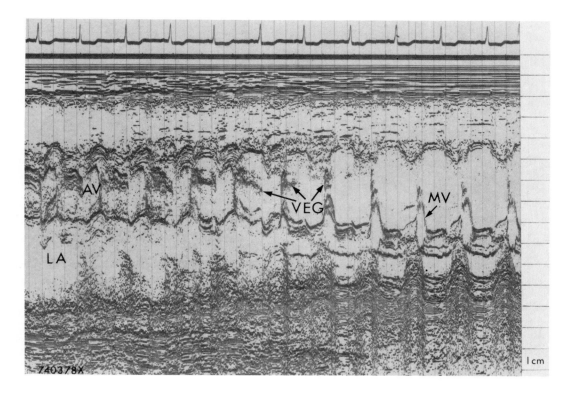

Fig. 6–78.   M-mode scan of a patient with bacterial endocarditis and vegetations on the aortic valve (AV). During diastole, echoes from the vegetations (VEG) extend into the left ventricular outflow tract above the mitral valve (MV). LA = left atrium.

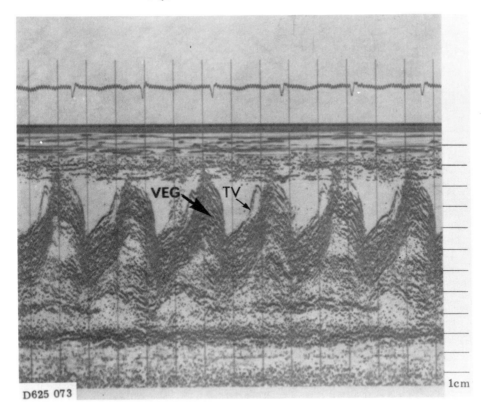

Fig. 6–79.   M-mode echocardiogram demonstrating a massive bacterial vegetation (VEG) on the tricuspid valve (TV).

may be massive.[164] There is a report whereby the vegetation produced lethal obstruction to blood flow into the aorta.[165]

Vegetations involving the tricuspid valve can also be seen echocardiographically.[166-168] Their appearance is similar to that of the mitral valve. Occasionally, one might note an unusually large vegetation. Figure 6–79 shows a large vegetation involving the tricuspid valve. In this case the infected mass is so large that it is difficult to distinguish from a neoplasm. An unusual case whereby a clot was caught in the tricuspid valve and simulated a tricuspid valve vegetation is illustrated in Figure 6–80.[169] Examples of echocardiographically detected pulmonary valve vegetations have also been reported (Fig. 6–81).[170-173]

Two-dimensional echocardiography can also detect vegetative masses on the valves. Figure 6–82 demonstrates a mobile vegetation on a mitral valve. This mobile mass of

tissue (arrow), attached to a probable flail mitral valve, can be seen protruding into the left atrium in systole and into the left ventricular outflow tract in diastole. The real-time examination, or videotape, was clearly striking as this mass flopped about within the heart. A two-dimensional study of an aortic valve vegetation is seen in Figure 6–83. This vegetation was less mobile than that seen in Figure 6–82. However, the irregular mass (VEG) is easily identified, especially in diastole. If the vegetation is more mobile or extends into the left ventricle, then a more dramatic picture is presented, especially in real time (Fig. 6–57). Similar two-dimensional vegetations have been reported with tricuspid valve vegetations.[167]

There is some debate over the role of two-dimensional echocardiography in the diagnosis of valvular vegetations. Some authors feel that one can more reliably detect vegetations by way of this new tech-

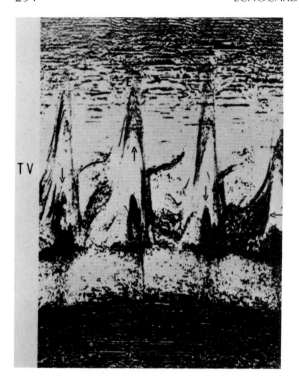

Fig. 6–80.   Tricuspid valve echocardiogram showing multiple "shaggy" echoes *(arrows)* attached to the tricuspid valve (tv). These echoes originated from a clot that was trapped within the tricuspid valve and simulated a vegetation. (From Covarrubias, E.A., Sheikh, M.U., and Fox, L.M.: Echocardiography and pulmonary embolism. Ann. Intern. Med., *87*:720, 1977.)

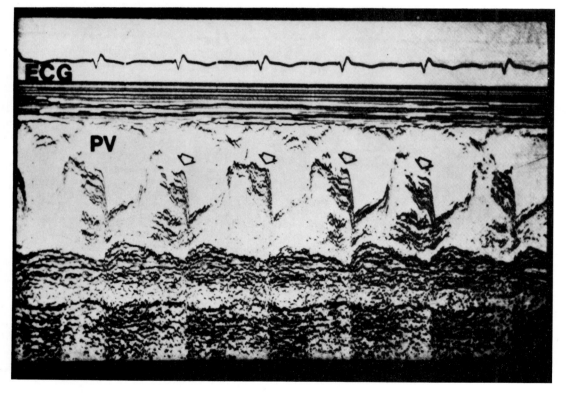

Fig. 6–81.   M-mode echocardiogram of a pulmonary valve (PV) demonstrating vegetation *(arrows)* on that valve. (From Dzindzio, B.S., et al.: Isolated gonococcal pulmonary valve endocarditis: diagnosis by echocardiography. Circulation, *59*:1320, 1979. By permission of the American Heart Association, Inc.)

nique.[174,174a] Others feel that the sensitivity for detecting vegetations echocardiographically is no different with either M-mode or two-dimensional examinations.[175] However, the two-dimensional study better assesses the size, shape, and mobility of the vegetation, and possibly provides more information on complications of the infection.[176,177] In such situations as infected prosthetic valves or right-sided

vegetations, the two-dimensional echocardiographic examination may be clearly superior to the M-mode technique.

The literature varies with regard to the role of echocardiography in managing patients with bacterial endocarditis. In one study, only a third of the patients with clinically proven bacterial endocarditis had echocardiographically detected vegetations.[177a] In other series, as much as 70 per-

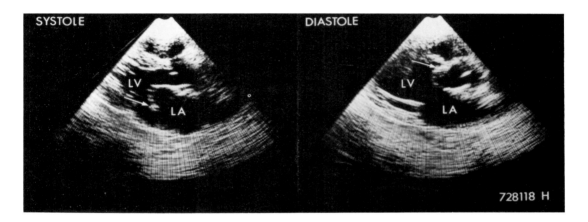

Fig. 6–82. Long-axis echocardiogram demonstrating a mobile vegetation *(arrows)* on the anterior mitral leaflet. In systole the vegetation protrudes into the left atrium, and in diastole the vegetation moves into the left ventricular outflow tract. LV = left ventricle; LA = left atrium.

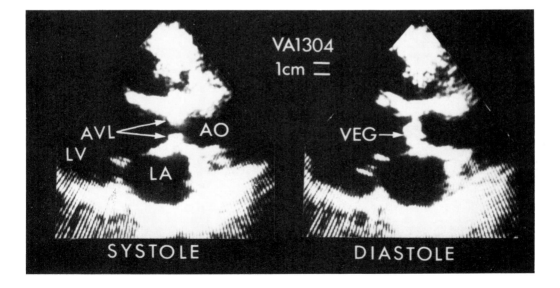

Fig. 6–83. Long-axis two-dimensional echocardiograms of an aortic valve in a patient with vegetations on the valve. The mass of echoes from the vegetations (VEG) is best seen in diastole. AVL = aortic valve leaflet; AO = aorta; LV = left ventricle; LA = left atrium.

cent of all patients with clinical evidence of bacterial endocarditis show echocardiographic vegetations.[178,178a,178b] It has been stated that patients who show vegetations on their echocardiogram usually do poorly clinically and require valvular replacement.[179,180] Although it was initially believed that virtually all patients with echocardiographic vegetations required surgery, more experience has demonstrated that many of these patients do well clinically and that the vegetations may actually regress with time.[181,183-185] Even in those who do not require surgery, patients with vegetations have a higher incidence of valvular regurgitation and other complications such as emboli.[185a] It should also be remembered that echocardiography cannot distinguish between active and healing vegetations.[185,186]

Another controversy concerns the management of patients with large mobile vegetations, such as those seen in Figure 6–81. These masses appear frightening in real time and would certainly seem a likely source of systemic emboli. Although some examples of embolization in patients with mobile vegetations have been reported, the likelihood

of such a complication is unknown, and there is probably no justification for prophylactic surgery in these patients to prevent systemic emboli.

Not all vegetations are due to bacterial infection. Fungal vegetations have also been detected echocardiographically.[187-189] In addition, several forms of noninfectious endocarditis have been reported.[190] Figure 6–84 shows an echo-producing mass involving the mitral valve. Although the specific etiology is not clear from the echocardiogram, the abnormal echoes proved to originate from a nonbacterial thrombotic form of endocarditis.[191] Figure 6–85 shows an M-mode scan of a patient with Libman-Sacks endocarditis. Note the abnormal echoes in the vicinity of the posterior mitral leaflet (white arrow) as well as thickening of the chordae and papillary muscle (black arrow). Figure 6–86 is from another patient with a noninfectious form of endocarditis. This patient had Loeffler's endocarditis, which produced thickening and actual hemodynamic narrowing of the mitral valve.[192] The mass of echoes primarily involved the posterior leaflets and chordae.

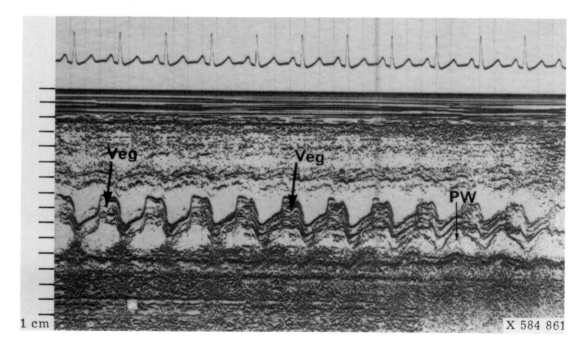

Fig. 6–84. Mitral valve echocardiogram of a patient with a nonbacterial thrombotic mass (Veg) involving the mitral valve. PW = posterior wall.

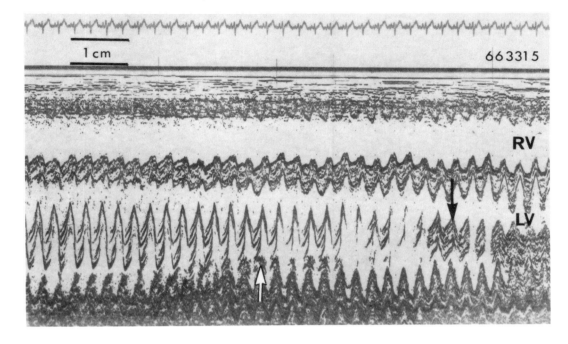

Fig. 6–85. M-mode scan of a patient with Libman-Sacks endocarditis. Note abnormal echoes in the vicinity of the posterior mitral leaflet *(white arrow)* as well as thickening of the chordae and papillary muscle *(black arrow)*. RV = right ventricle; LV = left ventricle.

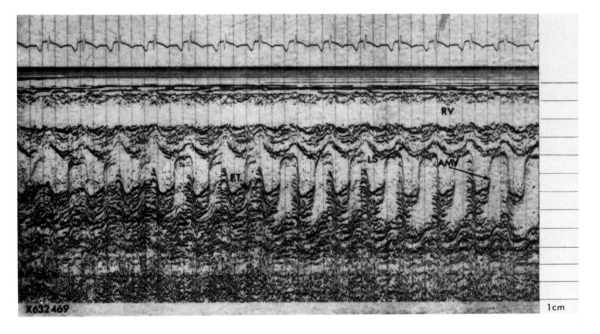

Fig. 6–86. M-mode echocardiogram of the mitral valve in a patient with Löffler's endocarditis. A fibrinous thrombotic mass (FT) was attached to the mitral valve and appeared to be superimposed on the echoes from the left ventricular posterior wall. The left ventricular cavity is diminished. Mitral blood flow was obstructed. RV = right ventricle; AMV = anterior mitral valve leaflet; LS = left septum. (From Weyman, A.E., et al.: Löffler's endocarditis presenting as mitral and tricuspid stenosis. Am. J. Cardiol., *40*:438, 1977.)

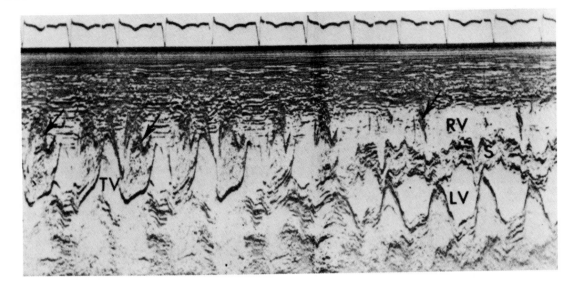

Fig. 6–87. Echocardiogram of a patient with bacterial endocarditis and a ventricular septal defect. Echoes from the vegetations *(arrows)* can be seen anterior to the tricuspid valve (TV) in the right ventricular outflow tract (RV). S = interventricular septum; LV = left ventricle. (From Aziz, K.U., Newfeld, E.A., and Paul, M.H.: Echocardiographic detection of bacterial vegetation in a child with a ventricular septal defect. Chest, *70:*780, 1976.)

Bacterial endocarditis does not always involve the valves. A case of endocarditis with a vegetation on a ventricular septal defect has been seen on an echocardiogram (Fig. 6–87).[193] An aortic ring abscess has also been identified echocardiographically.[194] Another recent report describes the two-dimensional echocardiographic appearance of a myocardial abscess.[195]

PROSTHETIC VALVES

Many papers have been written about the echocardiographic examination of prosthetic valves. Despite these reports, the overall usefulness of echocardiography in determining the status of prosthetic valves is still unclear. A possible reason for this confusion is that there are various types of prosthetic valves being used, and many diverse problems occur with these valves. In addition, because it is difficult for any one institution to accumulate a large number of malfunctioning valves, no single group has established firm echocardiographic criteria for what constitutes an abnormal valve.

The following discussion is basically a review of the literature on this subject. It is hoped that some light will be shed on the areas in which echocardiography might be useful in detecting malfunctioning prosthetic valves.

Normally Functioning Prosthetic Valves

There are four general types of prosthetic valves in use. One is the ball-cage variety, of which the Starr-Edwards type is most common. The second is a disc-cage valve, in which the disc moves parallel to the sewing ring throughout its excursion. A third type of prosthetic valve is the tilting disc variety, of which the Bjork-Shiley valve is most common. A new tilting-disc valve, the St. Jude, is arousing interest. The fourth major category of prosthetic valve is the bioprosthetic valve. Although homograft and fascialata valves were used in the past, the most common bioprosthetic valve in use today is the xenograft, or porcine heterograft, valve. The echocardiographic examination of these various valves differs, as may their potential malfunction. Thus the discussion of prosthetic valves must be subdivided into the various types.

Figure 6–88 diagrammatically demonstrates how ball-cage-type prosthetic valves can be examined. One of the objectives in

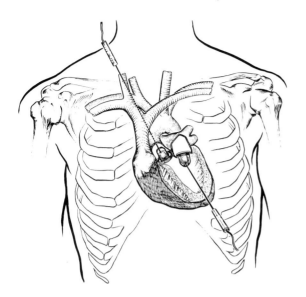

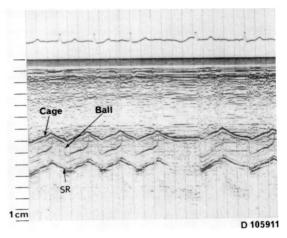

Fig. 6–88. Diagram showing location of the transducer for recording maximum amplitude of excursion of the Starr-Edwards-type ball valve prosthesis. (From Chang, S.: M-mode Echocardiographic Techniques and Pattern Recognition. Philadelphia, Lea & Febiger, 1976.)

Fig. 6–89. Echocardiogram of a mitral valve-ball valve prosthesis with the transducer near the cardiac apex. The most anterior echo originates from the struts of the cage. The leading edge of the ball produces an echo resembling moderate mitral stenosis. The more posterior echo, which is parallel to the anterior cage echo, originates from the posterior portion of the cage or the sewing ring (SR). (From Schuchman, H., et al.: Intracavitary echoes in patients with mitral prosthetic valves. J. Clin. Ultrasound, 3:111, 1975.)

studying such valves is to record the excursion of the ball.[196] Since the ball moves in a basic superior-inferior direction, this type of prosthesis is best examined when the transducer is not located along the left sternal border. Thus, to detect the maximum excursion of a mitral ball valve, the transducer is best placed at the cardiac apex and directed up toward the left atrium (Fig. 6–88). Figure 6–89 shows a recording of a mitral Starr-Edwards ball valve with the transducer located near the cardiac apex. The echo that is closest to the transducer and exhibits motion similar to that of the mitral annulus originates from the tip of the cage. Immediately behind the echo from the cage is a more rapidly moving echo that resembles an echo originating from a mildly or moderately stenotic mitral valve. This echo undoubtedly originates from the leading edge of the ball as it moves between the left atrium and the left ventricle. The findings behind these two echoes may be variable. In this illustration another echo, which exhibits identical motion to that of the cage echo, is visible behind the echo from the ball. The exact identity of

this echo is not clear, but it must originate from a part of the cage, annulus, or sewing ring; most likely it is part of the sewing ring. Theoretically, if the ultrasonic beam were directed exactly parallel to the motion of the ball, the beam might traverse the orifice of the valve and the sewing ring would not be recorded. Because the ultrasonic beam is so wide, and because the sewing ring is such a strong reflector, some echo from the sewing ring or the rear of the cage is invariably recorded.

In order to record the maximum motion of the ball valve in the aortic position, the transducer should be placed in the right supraclavicular fossa and directed toward the ascending aorta (Fig. 6–88).[197,198] Figure 6–90 is an echocardiogram of a patient with an aortic prosthesis. The transducer is in the right supraclavicular fossa, and the recording is similar to that taken from the mitral position except that here the cage motion is reduced. Again, the leading echo most likely originates from the tip of the cage (AC) extending into the aorta. The leading edge of the ball (AB) exhibits an upward motion with ventricular systole and a downward motion with diastole similar to that noted in the anterior leaflet of a normal aortic valve. An almost identical echo is seen posteriorly and most likely occurs from the posterior surface of the ball (PB). Parts of the valve's sewing

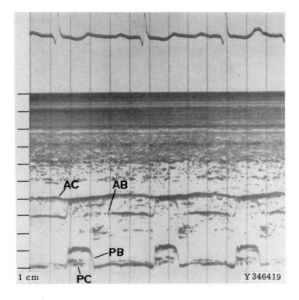

Fig. 6–90. Echocardiogram recorded with the transducer in the right supraclavicular fossa from a patient with an aortic valve prosthesis. AC = anterior cage; AB = anterior ball; PB = posterior ball; PC = posterior cage or sewing ring.

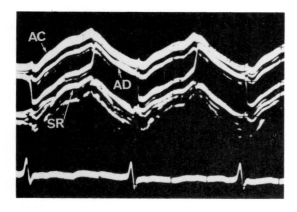

Fig. 6–91. M-mode scan of a patient with a mitral disc prosthesis. AC = anterior cage; AD = anterior disc; SR = sewing ring. (From Johnson, M.L., Holmes, J.H., and Paton, B.C.: Echocardiographic determination of mitral disc valve excursion. Circulation, 47:1274, 1973.)

ring or aortic annulus may also be recorded (PC).

The echocardiographic recording from a parallel-moving disc valve is similar to that of a ball-cage valve, except that the amplitude of excursion of the disc may be less. Figure 6–91 shows a recording of a disc valve in the mitral position that is similar to the recording in Figure 6–89. The principal difference is the location of the posterior sewing ring (SR). Since the echo-reflecting surface of a disc valve is flat, it is even more important to orient the ultrasonic beam as parallel to the excursion of the disc as possible.

The Bjork-Shiley disc valve is very popular. The disc in this valve tilts and thus presents a variety of echocardiographic patterns that depend on the exact relationship of the ultrasonic beam to the tilting disc.[199–201,201a] Figure 6–92 shows some echocardiographic patterns that can be obtained from this valve. As might be expected, the echocardiographic recording can vary somewhat depending on the surgical insertion of the prosthetic valve. Since the pattern can be quite confusing, some experience is necessary to evaluate the function of this particular valve. However, one usually does not encounter all of the various patterns exhibited in this figure. One usually tries to record the maximum excursion of the tilting disc in a recording, such as that in Figure 6–92B. One sees a brisk upward displacement of the disc with gradual closure during diastole. Closure with ventricular systole is again brisk. Thus far, there have been no reports on the echocardiographic examination of the St. Jude split, tilting-disc valve.

The most commonly used bioprosthetic valve is the porcine three-leaflet aortic valve. This valve, inserted in a frame with three stents, may then be inserted in any valvular position. Figure 6–93 demonstrates an M-mode echocardiogram of a normally functioning porcine heterograft inserted in the mitral position. The initial echo recorded with this prosthesis is the anterior stent (ST).[202–205] A parallel-moving posterior stent is visible 2 to 3 cm below the anterior stent. Between the two stents are thin echoes that open in diastole and close in systole. Al-

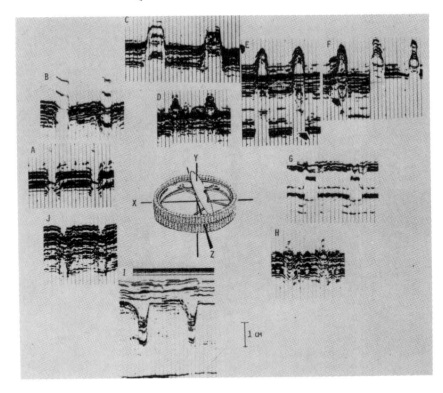

Fig. 6–92. Illustration demonstrating the various echocardiograms one can obtain from a Bjork-Shiley tilting disc valve. (From Douglas, J.E. and Williams, G.D.: Echocardiographic evaluation of the Bjork-Shiley prosthetic valve. Circulation, *50*:52, 1974.)

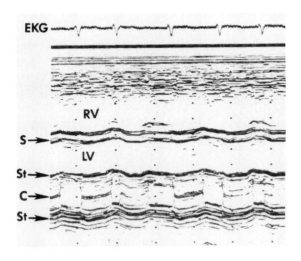

Fig. 6–93. M-mode echocardiogram of a normally functioning porcine heterograft in the mitral position. S = interventricular septum; St = stents; C = cusps; RV = right ventricle; LV = left ventricle. (From Alam, M., et al.: M-mode and two-dimensional echocardiographic features of porcine valve dysfunction. Am. J. Cardiol., *43*:502, 1979.)

though they superficially resemble an aortic valve, they open as the mitral valve does. The valve is mildly to moderately stenotic; thus mid-diastolic closure as usually observed with a normal mitral prosthetic valve is rarely seen. The leaflets are not as easily recorded with a tissue prosthesis as is the disc or ball of a nontissue prosthetic valve. The echoes from the stents are more prominent because they are more echo-reflective. If the stent is directly in front of the leaflets, it is sometimes difficult to record leaflet motion. The best tracings are obtained when the center of the beam passes through two of the three stents.

Figure 6–94 shows a heterograft porcine valve in the aortic position. The leaflets are faintly visible within the aorta between the stents. The motion resembles that of a normal aortic valve. The strong echoes from the stents tend to hide the leaflets and the resultant leaflet echoes are faint.

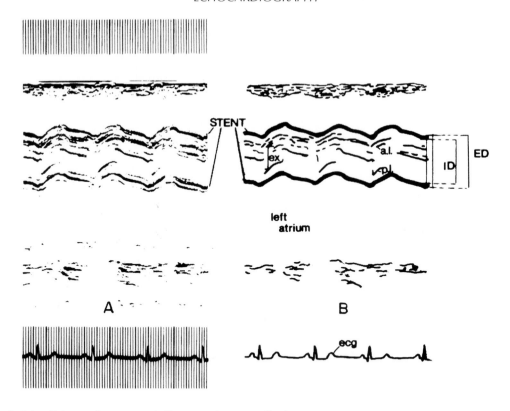

Fig. 6–94.   Echocardiogram and diagram of a normally functioning porcine prosthetic valve in the aortic position. al = anterior leaflet; pl = posterior leaflet; ex = excursion of the leaflets; ID = internal diameter of the prosthesis; ED = external dimension of the prosthesis. (From Harston, W.E., Jr., Robertson, R.M., and Friesinger, G.C.: Echocardiographic evaluation of porcine heterograft in the mitral and aortic positions. Am. Heart J., 96:448, 1978.)

On rare occasion, one may see echoes from a remnant of the excised mitral valve. These echoes exhibit motion similar to a normal mitral valve.[205a]

Malfunctioning Prosthetic Valves

Probably the most common and serious problem involved in the use of prosthetic valves is clot formation. When clot forms around the valve, it frequently interferes with valvular function. A clot can either reduce the effective orifice or impair the motion of the ball, disc, or leaflets. One possible way to use echocardiography to detect clot is to record an echo-producing mass in the vicinity of the prosthetic valve with total absence of any disc or ball motion.[205,206,206a,207–210] Figure 6–95A is an echocardiogram of a patient with an aortic Bjork-Shiley disc valve. Note that only a large mass of echoes with no clearly identifiable disc motion is

recorded. The patient was operated on and the clot was removed. The postoperative echocardiogram showed a striking change. The large mass of echoes encompassing the prosthetic valve is gone, and one can now see normal disc motion (Fig. 6–95B).

Figure 6–96 shows a porcine heterograft in the mitral position with thrombus surrounding both stents. Multiple, dense nonhomogenous echoes can be seen between the valve stents (arrow). Multiple echoes are also visible about the posterior stent. Leaflet motion is not recorded in this patient.

Figure 6–97 shows the difficulty involved in identifying clots surrounding a prosthetic valve. The multiple echoes from the valve in Figure 6–97 certainly suggest clot, although no clot was noted at the time of surgery in this patient. The multiple echoes could represent reverberations, or they may be due to beam-width artifacts that result from the

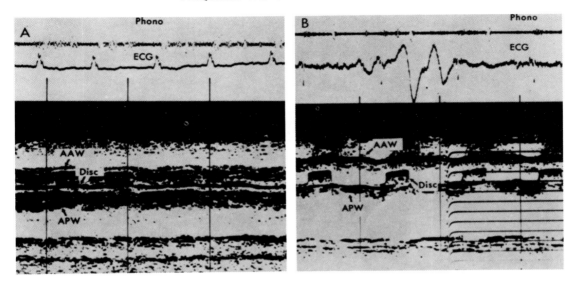

Fig. 6–95.   Echocardiograms of a patient with an aortic Bjork-Shiley disc valve. *A*, Aortic valve is completely occluded by a clot. *B*, Aortic valve after the clot was surgically removed. The space between the anterior (AAW) and posterior (APW) aortic wall echoes is completely filled with echo-producing material, most likely originating from the clot. The post-operative echocardiogram shows the moving disc echoes without echo-producing clots. (From Ben-Zvi, J., et al.: Thrombosis on Bjork-Shiley aortic valve prosthesis: clinical, arteriographic, echocardiographic, and therapeutic observations in seven cases. Am. J. Cardiol., *34*:538, 1974.)

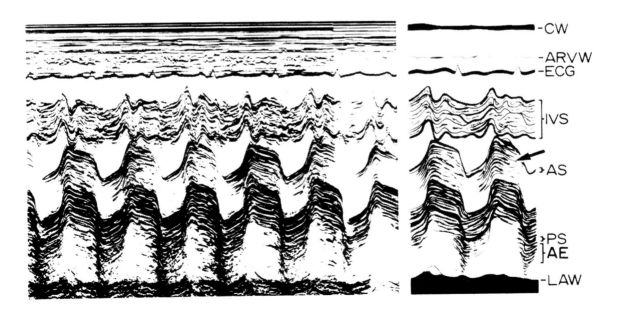

Fig. 6–96.   M-mode echocardiogram of a porcine heterograft in the mitral position with thrombus surrounding both stents. Multiple, dense nonhomogeneous echoes *(arrow)* can be seen attached to the anterior stent (AS) and behind the posterior stent (PS). CW = chest wall; ARVW = anterior right ventricular wall; AE = abnormal echoes. IVS = interventricular septum; LAW = left atrial wall. (From Bloch, W.N., et al.: Echocardiogram of the porcine aortic bioprosthesis in the mitral position. Am. J. Cardiol., *38*:293, 1976.)

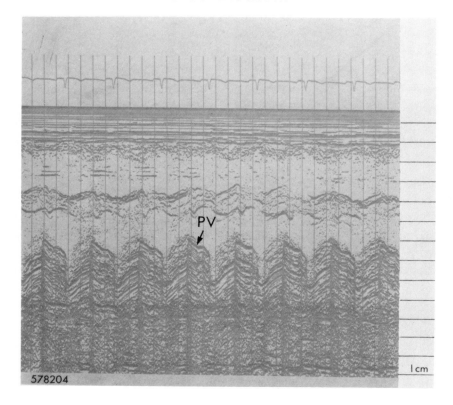

Fig. 6–97.   Multiple echoes surrounding a prosthetic mitral valve (PV). Despite these echoes, no clot was noted at surgery.

beam transecting both the prosthesis and the tissue beside the valve.

The clot usually cannot be clearly identified echocardiographically. Instead one may note alteration in excursion of the disc or ball.[207,209,211–217] In Figure 6–98 a ball valve prosthesis exhibits intermittent abnormal opening.[213] During cardiac complex 2 the ball does not open completely to the cage echo. In subsequent complexes the opening is significantly delayed. Thus the ball is clearly not free and is intermittently impeded in its opening position. The patient proved to have a large ingrowth of thrombus about the rim of the valve. Figure 6–99 shows another example of a malfunctioning ball valve that exhibits delay in opening of the valve.[213,216,217] The opening motion following the second QRS complex is markedly delayed (arrow) compared with the other complexes. When ball motion is intermittently abnormal, then the echocardiogram

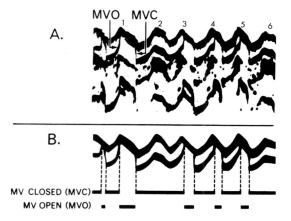

Fig. 6–98.   Echocardiogram, A, and diagram, B, of a patient with intermittent failure or delay in opening of the mitral ball valve. In cardiac complex 1, the mitral valve opening (MVO) and closure (MVC) are normal. In complex 2, there is minimal, if any, opening of the valve, and in complexes 3, 4, and 5, the opening is delayed. (From Pfeifer, J., et al.: Malfunction of mitral ball valve prosthesis due to thrombosis. Am. J. Cardiol., 29:95, 1972.)

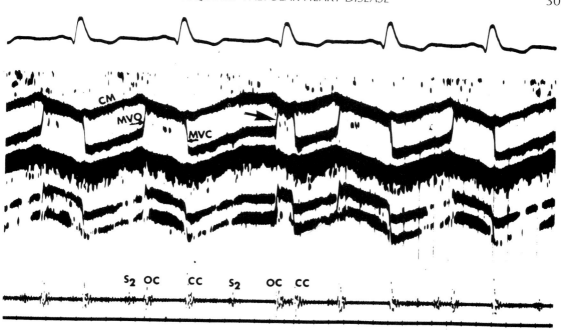

Fig. 6–99.   Echocardiogram from a malfunctioning mitral prosthetic valve, demonstrated by a delayed mitral valve opening (MVO) in the third cardiac complex *(arrow)*. CM = cage of mitral valve; MVC = mitral valve closing; S2 = second heart sound; OC = opening click; CC = closing click. (From Pfeifer, J., et al.: Malfunction of mitral ball valve prosthesis due to thrombosis. Am. J. Cardiol., 29:95, 1972.)

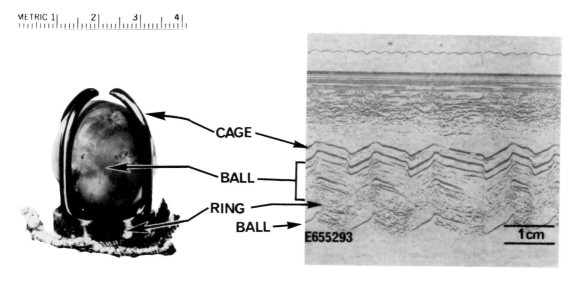

Fig. 6–100.   Photograph and echocardiogram of a patient with ball variance. The silastic ball swelled and became lodged within the cage. The echoes from the ball demonstrate minimal motion, and the leading edge of the ball fails to reach the leading echo from the cage. (From Wann, L.S., et al.: Ball variance in a Harken mitral prosthesis. Echocardiographic and phonocardiographic features. Chest, 72:785, 1977.)

may prove diagnostic if the examination is performed during the malfunction.

Figure 6–100 shows a valve with reduced motion owing to ball variance.[218] Old ball valves had silastic balls that would occasionally swell, thus restricting ball movement within the cage. As noted in this figure, ball motion may be markedly restricted, and the leading echo from the ball may not reach the cage during diastole. Although this example is from a patient with a prosthesis that manifested ball variance, a similar recording might be noted if restriction of the ball was due to clot surrounding the prosthesis.[216] Again, the leading edge of the ball may not reach the leading edge of the cage.

Many investigators believe that the best method for detecting abnormal prosthetic valve function is to combine echocardiography with phonocardiography.[219-223] It has been suggested that the interval between the aortic second sound and the point of opening of the mitral prosthetic valve or disc may be useful in determining abnormally functioning disc or ball prostheses. If the ball is malfunctioning because of clot, then its opening may be delayed (Figs. 6–98, 6–99). With obstructed flow through the prosthesis, either owing to clot or tissue ingrowth, the ball or disc may not be delayed but may actually open earlier than usual. This earlier opening may be a result of the elevated left atrial pressure and is comparable to the early opening snap seen with mitral stenosis. As a result, the interval between the aortic second sound (A2) and the mitral valve opening (MVO), has been considered an indicator of malfunctioning mitral prosthetic valves.[221] A shortened interval would have equal significance as a short A2–OS interval with mitral stenosis. This interval may be short in patients who have obstruction or a paravalvular leak around a mitral valve prosthesis.[220] A similarly shortened A2–MVO interval was noted in patients whose left ventricles were functioning poorly.[220]

One must remember that the normally functioning prosthetic valve may exhibit variations in motion. Figure 6–101 shows a patient with atrial fibrillation. During a long diastolic interval, separation between the ball (AB) and the anterior cage (AC) is not

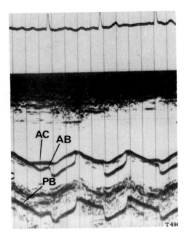

Fig. 6–101. Prosthetic mitral ball valve echocardiogram of a patient with atrial fibrillation. During a long R–R interval there is separation between the anterior cage (AC) and the anterior ball (AB). This separation is a normal finding and does not signify malfunction. PC = posterior cage or sewing ring; PB = posterior ball.

wholly unexpected. The anterior cage and ball echoes are usually in apposition to each other throughout diastole, since one does not see the usual mitral diastolic closure of the ball or disc as one would with a normal mitral valve. The lack of mid-diastolic closure with prosthetic valves may be partially due to the inertia of the ball and to the fact that the valve is at least mildly stenotic, even when functioning normally. Porcine valves, however, may exhibit normal mid-diastolic closure. With a long P-R interval, one may occasionally see premature closure of a prosthetic valve. Figure 6–102 shows such premature closure of a disc-type mitral prosthesis.[221] As best as can be determined, this motion was merely a function of the conduction defect and did not indicate an abnormal prosthetic valve.

Aside from clot formation, fibrin or other tissue may grow into the prosthesis and impair its function. Figure 6–103 illustrates two examples of malfunctioning Bjork-Shiley prostheses. Figure 6–103A shows the excursion of a normally functioning Bjork-Shiley prosthesis in the tricuspid position. Figure 6–103 (B and C) illustrates patients with malfunctioning Bjork-Shiley valves. Both valves

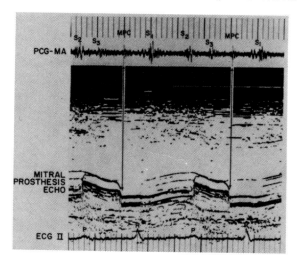

Fig. 6–102. Phonocardiogram and echocardiogram from a mitral disc prosthesis demonstrating premature closure (MPC) in an apparently normally functioning prosthetic valve. The patient has prolonged atrioventricular conduction as demonstrated by a long PR interval on the electrocardiogram. (From Gibson, T.C., et al.: Echocardiographic and phonocardiographic characteristics of the Lillehei-Kaster mitral valve prosthesis. Circulation, *49*:434, 1974.)

were in the tricuspid position, and disc motion was indistinct or absent.

A somewhat more specific abnormality has been noted with the Bjork-Shiley prosthesis. Figure 6–104 notes a rounding of the early diastolic motion of the disc at the E point.[224] The abnormal pattern of motion was apparently because of an ingrowth of fibrous tissue around the sewing ring and hinges of the Bjork-Shiley valve. The valve was hemodynamically obstructed. This rounded motion of the Bjork-Shiley valve has also been noted in a patient whose valve was leaking because of a paravalvular leak.[225] The rounded E point, or "hump," was due to rocking of the prosthesis and not to obstruction.

An example of abnormal valve motion due to valve dehiscence is noted in Figure 6–105. The echo from the anterior ball (AB) exhibits a rapid diastolic motion greater than that seen in the posterior ball echo (PB).

Malfunctioning tissue prosthetic valves may manifest different types of abnormalities on the echocardiogram. One feature

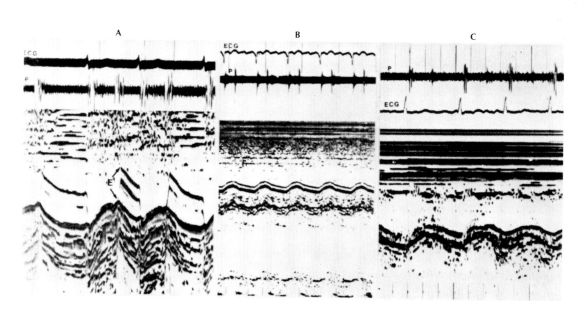

Fig. 6–103.   Echocardiograms from three Bjork-Shiley prostheses in the tricuspid position. *A* demonstrates a normally functioning valve. Disc motion is virtually absent in *B* and *C*, which are recordings from malfunctioning prosthetic valves. (From Bouridillon, P.D.V. and Sharratt, G.P.: Malfunction of Bjork-Shiley valve prosthesis in tricuspid position. Br. Heart J., *38*:1149, 1976.)

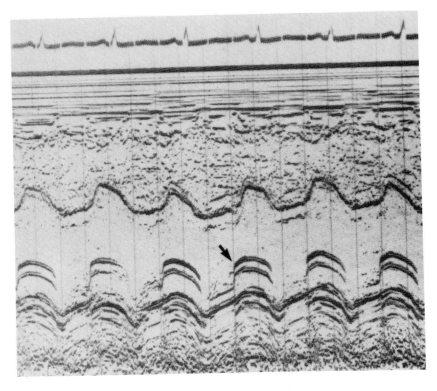

Fig. 6–104.   Echocardiogram from a Bjork-Shiley prosthesis in the mitral position demonstrating rounding of the E point *(arrow)*. There was partial obstruction of the valve due to an ingrowth of fibrous tissue. (From Clements, S.D. and Perkins, J.V.: Malfunction of a Bjork-Shiley prosthetic heart valve in the mitral position producing an abnormal echocardiographic pattern. J. Clin. Ultrasound, 6:334, 1978.)

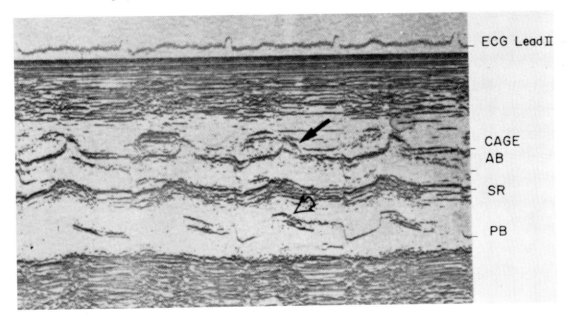

Fig. 6–105.   Echocardiogram of a ball cage prosthetic valve positioned in the mitral valve, which is partially dehisced. Note rocking motion of both cage and ball *(arrows)* in early diastole. AB = anterior ball; PB = posterior ball. (From Berndt, T.B., Goodman, D.J., and Popp, R.L.: Echocardiographic and phonocardiographic confirmation of suspected cage mitral valve malfunction. Chest, 70:221, 1976.)

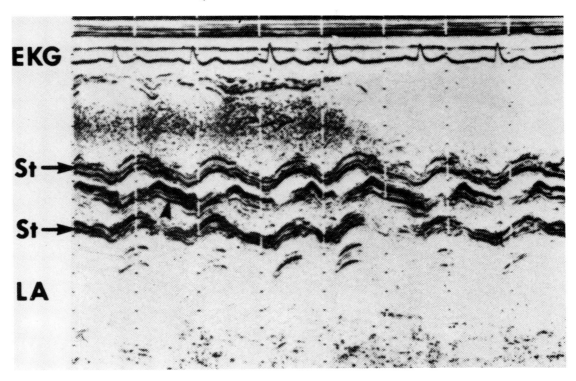

Fig. 6–106.   M-mode echocardiogram of a porcine heterograft in the aortic position with marked thickening and infection of the leaflets. The thickened echoes *(arrow)* are best appreciated in diastole. St = stent; LA = left atrium. (From Alam, M., et al.: M-mode and two-dimensional echocardiographic features of porcine mitral valve dysfunction. Am. J. Cardiol., *43*:502, 1979.)

of possible valve malfunction and/or degeneration is thickening of the leaflets.[226,227] Figure 6–106 shows a porcine valve in the aortic position with marked thickening of the leaflets. Subtle motion changes have also been noted with tissue valves. Fluttering of the valve leaflets may occur in patients with malfunctioning prostheses.[226] Figure 6–107 is an M-mode echocardiogram of a porcine valve in the mitral position in a patient with mitral regurgitation. Note the diastolic fluttering (upper arrowhead) as well as faint systolic fluttering (lower arrowhead). Dehiscence of a porcine valve in the mitral position has also been seen echocardiographically.[226,229] Parts of the prosthesis herniated into the left atrium.

Two-dimensional echocardiography has been used to examine prosthetic valves. The usefulness of this two-dimensional technique with disc or ball valves has not been established. However, there is evidence that the two-dimensional examination can be particularly helpful in examining the heterograft prosthesis.[227] Figure 6–108 shows a two-dimensional examination of a patient with a mass on a porcine valve that is directly posterior to the anterior stent.[227] This clot may have been observed with M-mode echocardiography; however, the spatial orientation inherent in the two-dimensional examination increases the possibility of recognizing such a mass in a markedly echo-producing prosthetic valve.

In Figure 6–109, there is dehiscence of a porcine valve in the aortic position.[227] During diastole the angle of the prosthesis changes, and one can see a separation between the echoes from the prosthesis and the aortic wall.

There have been a few isolated reports of peculiar findings in patients with prosthetic valves. One observation is the presence of tiny echoes apparently coming through a mi-

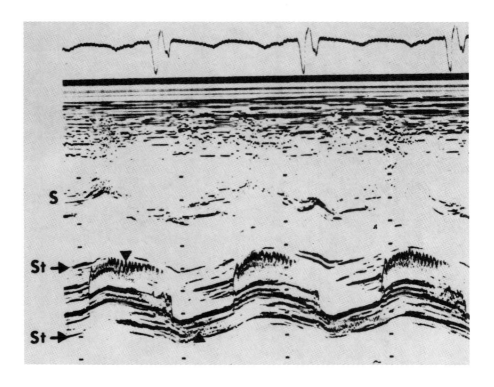

Fig. 6–107.   Diastolic and systolic fluttering of a porcine heterograft in the mitral position in the presence of mitral regurgitation *(upper and lower arrowheads, respectively)*. S = interventricular septum; St = stents. (From Alam, M., et al.: M-mode and two-dimensional echocardiographic features of porcine mitral valve dysfunction. Am. J. Cardiol., *43*:502, 1979.)

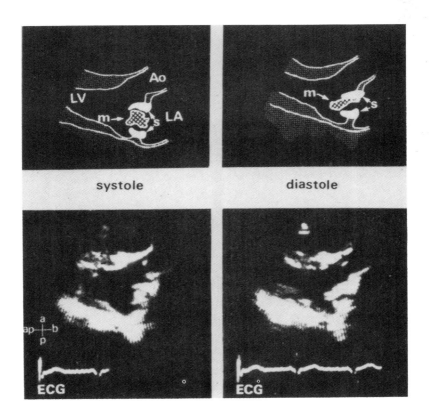

Fig. 6–108. Two-dimensional echocardiogram and diagram of a patient with a mass (m) on a porcine prosthetic valve in the mitral position. AO = aorta; LV = left ventricle; LA = left atrium; s = stents. (From Schapira, J.N., et al.: Two-dimensional echocardiographic assessment of patients with bioprosthetic valves. Am. J. Cardiol., 43:514, 1979.)

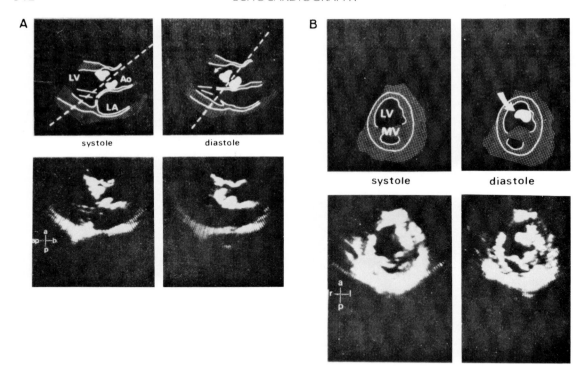

Fig. 6–109.   Two-dimensional echocardiograms and diagrams of the long axis, *A*, and short axis, *B*, of a patient with a porcine heterograft in the aortic position that is detached form the anterior aorta. In diastole the prosthesis tilts into the left ventricular outflow tract *(arrow)*. (From Schapira, J.N., et al.: Two-dimensional echocardiographic assessment of patients with bioprosthetic valves. Am. J. Cardiol., *43*:514, 1979.)

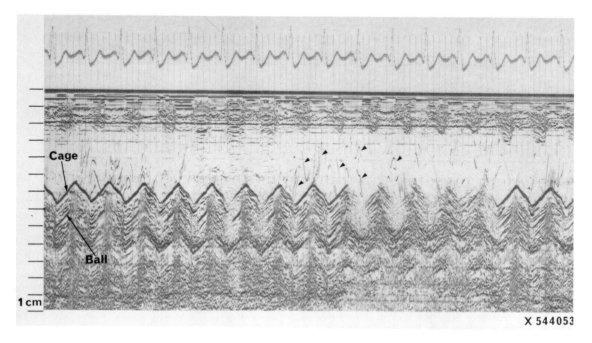

Fig. 6–110.   Intracavitary echoes *(arrowheads)* originating from a mitral valve prosthesis. The transducer was at the cardiac apex, the reject was low, and the gain was high in order to record these fine echoes. (From Schuchman, H., et al.: Intracavitary echoes in patients with mitral prosthetic valves. J. Clin. Ultrasound, *3*:111, 1975.)

tral prosthetic valve.[230,231] Figure 6–110 shows an example of such a situation. The patient has a mitral Starr-Edwards valve. The transducer is at the cardiac apex. One can note rapidly moving echoes (arrowheads) moving from the vicinity of the mitral valve into the more anterior left ventricle during diastole. The echoes are similar to those seen with contrast echocardiography. Moving away from the ball during diastole, they turn around and move away from the transducer, possibly out of the left ventricular outflow tract, during systole. The origin and significance of these echoes are not clear. They often occur with cloth-covered valves. However, Figures 6–111 and 6–112 show similar findings in a patient with a porcine mitral valve. During systole (Fig. 6–111, 6–112A), the left ventricle is free of any intracavitary echoes. However, during diastole (Fig. 6–111, 6–112B), a shower of echoes (arrows) passes through the prosthetic valve (PV). Although the origin of these peculiar echoes is unknown, most pa-tients manifesting this phenomenon have some clinical problem, but these problems are not consistent and all valves are not hemodynamically impaired.

Indirect Signs of Malfunctioning Prosthetic Valves

There are several indirect echocardiographic findings in patients with malfunctioning prosthetic valves. For example, a leaking aortic prosthetic valve may show signs of aortic regurgitation with fluttering of the mitral valve and/or interventricular septum. In addition, one may also note signs of a volume overload of the left ventricle with either a leaking aortic or mitral prosthesis. The left ventricular volume overload may not necessarily produce mere left ventricular dilatation and exaggerated interventricular septal motion. Figure 6–113 shows the usual findings following valve replacement in a patient who had preoperative valvular regurgitation. In the preoperative echocardiogram (Fig. 6–113A), septal motion is exag-

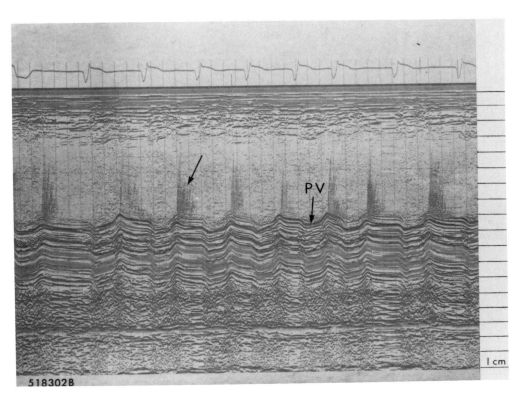

Fig. 6–111.   M-mode echocardiogram of a porcine mitral valve (PV) in the mitral position through which a shower of echoes *(arrow)* passes in diastole.

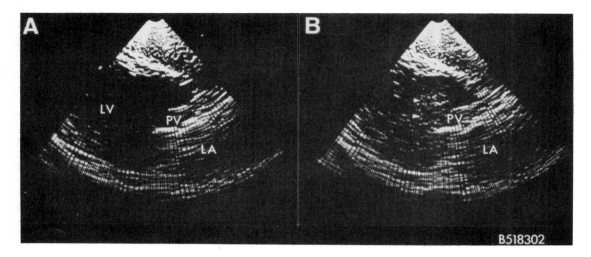

Fig. 6–112.   Long-axis two-dimensional echocardiogram of the patient in Figure 6–111. *A,* During systole, the left ventricular cavity is free of echoes. *B,* In diastole, a shower of echoes *(arrowheads)* passes through the prosthetic (PV) valve into the left ventricle (LV). LA = left atrium.

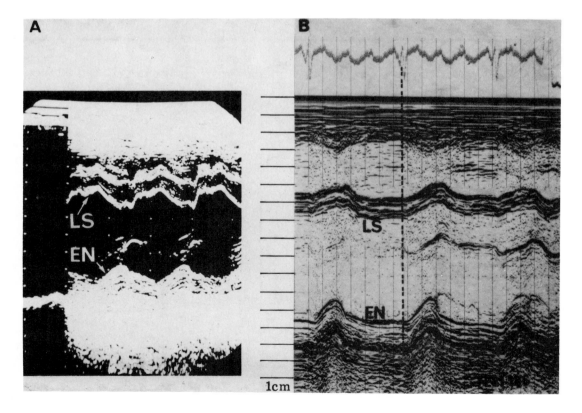

Fig. 6–113.   Preoperative, *A,* and postoperative, *B,* echocardiograms of a patient with mitral regurgitation who had a prosthetic mitral valve inserted. Prior to surgery the septal motion (LS) is exaggerated and moves downward with ventricular systole. Following surgery the septal motion is paradoxical. EN = posterior left ventricular endocardium.

gerated. A peculiar and not totally explained finding is that after surgical correction of the valvular regurgitation, septal motion becomes paradoxical and moves anteriorly during systole (Fig. 6–113B).[137,232-235] This paradoxical septal motion is a fairly characteristic finding in all patients undergoing open heart surgery. The motion may return to normal after several months.[137,232,235,236] The mechanism for this postoperative finding is still unresolved. Several explanations have been proposed, including ischemia of the septum during cardiopulmonary bypass, total displacement of the heart anteriorly during systole secondary to adhesions between the sternum and the heart,[234,236] or changes in cardiac motion secondary to pericardiotomy.[237] Unfortunately, none of these explanations adequately satisfy all observations. A situation in which the paradoxical motion may not occur postoperatively is when a volume overload of the left ventricle is superimposed on this postoperative septal motion. If there is regurgitation through the prosthetic valve, then the septal motion may be normal or in some cases even exaggerated.

Obstruction of flow across a mitral prosthetic valve can be evaluated by observing the left atrial emptying index from the aortic valve echocardiogram (Fig. 6–16). As with mitral stenosis, the atrial emptying index becomes markedly reduced when flow is obstructed through a malfunctioning prosthetic valve.[27] Although most prosthetic valves are mildly obstructive, this echocardiographic index apparently can help identify those that are beyond the obstruction of a normally functioning prosthesis.

Some authors have suggested using the total amplitude of motion of the disc, ball, or prosthesis to judge the presence of obstruction to flow.[202,204,205] Other authors have suggested recording the diastolic E to F slope of the ball, cage, or stent.[238] Most measurements require critical angulation and positioning of the transducer so that the maximum excursion of the valve is recorded. It should also be emphasized that the diastolic slope of the disc, ball, or leaflet is more likely related to the motion of the annulus since the moving part of the prosthesis is

usually completely open throughout diastole. These types of measurements are probably more useful in serial examination of a given patient. It is difficult to use any of these measurements for comparing one individual with another. However, if one gets a baseline echocardiographic examination when the valve is obviously functioning well after surgery, then these measurements may indeed be useful in following the course of the patient to determine whether any distortion of function occurs later on.[238]

CALCIFIED MITRAL ANNULUS

Numerous articles in the literature describe the echocardiographic findings in patients with a calcified mitral annulus.[239,239a-c] The principal observation on the M-mode echocardiogram is a band of dense high-intensity echoes between the mitral valve and the posterior left ventricular wall (Fig. 6–114). This band of echoes is immediately posterior to the posterior mitral valve leaflets. Frequently, these echoes may obscure that leaflet. The echoes from the annulus may also be in direct contact with the posterior left ventricular endocardial echo and may partially obscure those echoes from acoustic shadowing (see Chapter 1). The myocardial echoes posterior to the annulus on the right side of the illustration are far weaker than those on the left side, in which the annulus echoes are absent. Figure 6–115 is a slow M-mode scan showing the extent to which the calcified annulus echoes can appear on the M-mode echocardiogram. The bright echoes (CA) can be seen extending far into the left ventricular cavity and into the left atrium. Because of the highly reflective nature of the calcium, the effective beam width is wide. Thus some apparent echoes may be artifactual. Most of the calcium appears to be posterior to the mitral valve on the left ventricular side of the atrioventricular groove. One group of investigators suggest that "calcified mitral annulus" is a misnomer.[240] The calcification is actually in the submitral region between the mitral valve and the posterior left ventricular wall and not in the annulus.

Figure 6–116 shows a two-dimensional view of a calcified mitral annulus. This pa-

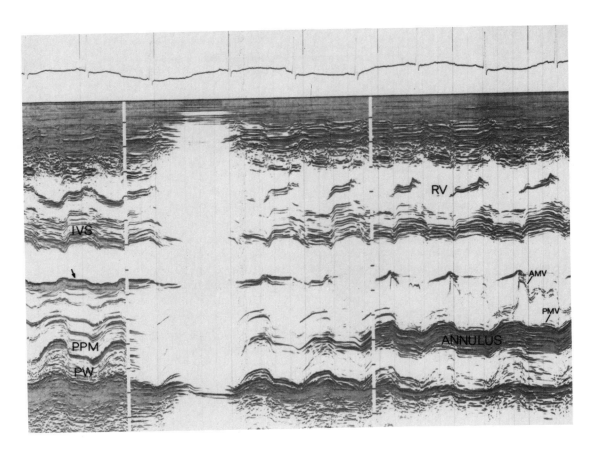

Fig. 6–114.   M-mode echocardiogram of a patient with a calcified mitral annulus. The dense echoes from the annulus are immediately posterior to the posterior mitral valve leaflet (PMV) and partially obscure the echoes from the posterior left ventricular wall (PW). AMV = anterior mitral valve leaflet; RV = right ventricle; IVS = interventricular septum; PPM = posterior papillary muscle.

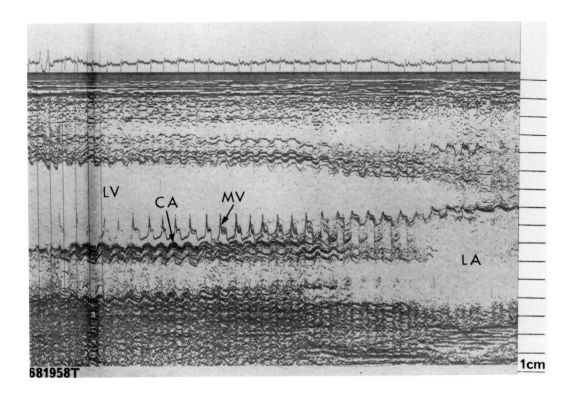

Fig. 6–115.   M-mode scan of a patient with a calcified mitral annulus demonstrating how echoes from the calcified annulus (CA) extend from the left ventricle (LV) to the left atrium (LA). MV = mitral valve.

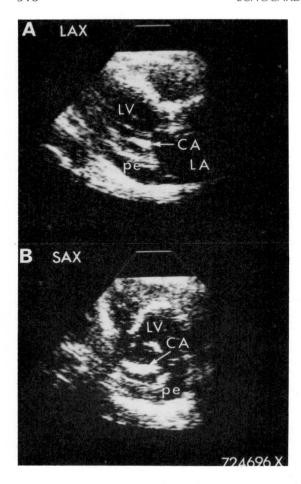

Fig. 6–116. Long-axis (LAX) and short-axis (SAX) two-dimensional echocardiograms of a patient with a calcified mitral annulus (CA) and a posterior pericardial effusion (pe). Note the curved nature of the calcified annulus in the short-axis view (see text for details). LV = left ventricle; LA = left atrium.

tient also has pericardial effusion (pe). The calcified annulus (CA) is visible as a bright, somewhat linear echo between the mitral valve and the posterior left ventricular wall. The long-axis view (LAX) shows the bright calcified echoes (CA) extending into the left ventricular cavity (Fig. 6–116A). The short-axis view (SAX) demonstrates the curved nature of the calcified annulus (CA, Fig. 6–116B). The echoes from the calcification obscure the posterior left ventricular endocardial echo and it cannot be clearly identified in these recordings.

Calcification may not be limited to only the annular or submitral area. Calcification

frequently extends throughout the base of the heart. It may extend into both the mitral and aortic valves.[239] It may involve the root of the aorta and may even extend into the left ventricle.[241] Figure 6–117 shows a two-dimensional echocardiogram of a patient with extensive calcification involving the entire base of the heart. Calcium is seen involving the ventricular wall, the mitral valve, the root of the aorta, and even part of the aortic valve.

There are many reasons for recognizing the echocardiographic features of calcified mitral annulus. First, the echocardiogram can be confusing from an interpretative point of view. An echocardiogram, such as that in Figure 6–114, can mimic pericardial effusion in some situations.[239] The calcification may also produce echoes similar to those produced in mitral stenosis.[239,241,242] In addition, the calcification frequently obscures the posterior mitral leaflet and may prevent an adequate recording of the posterior left ventricular wall echoes.

Many conditions have been reported in association with calcified mitral annulus. Calcific aortic stenosis, mitral valve prolapse,[243] and hypertrophic subaortic stenosis[244] have all been reported in association with mitral annulus calcification.[245] The

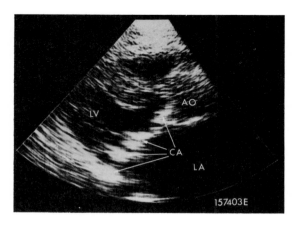

Fig. 6–117. Long-axis two-dimensional echocardiogram of a patient with a calcified annulus. Note extensive calcification (CA) extending from the base of the left ventricular wall through the mitral valve and into the root of the aorta (AO). LV = left ventricle; LA = left atrium.

calcified annulus also impairs normal function of the mitral valve apparatus and frequently produces mitral regurgitation.

REFERENCES

1. Edler, I.: Ultrasound cardiogram in mitral valve disease. Acta Chir. Scand., *111*:230, 1956.
2. Edler, I. and Gustafson, A.: Ultrasonic cardiogram in mitral stenosis. Acta Med. Scand., *159*:85, 1957.
3. Zaky, A., Nasser, W.K., and Feigenbaum, H.: Study of mitral valve action recorded by reflected ultrasound and its application in the diagnosis of mitral stenosis. Circulation, *37*:789, 1968.
4. Effert, S., Erkens, H., and Grossebrockhoff, F.: Ultrasonic echo method in cardiological diagnosis. German Med. Mth., *2*:325, 1957.
5. Gustafson, A.: Correlation between ultrasound-cardiography, haemodynamics and surgical findings in mitral stenosis. Am. J. Cardiol., *19*:32, 1967.
6. Gustafson, A.: Ultrasound cardiography in mitral stenosis. Acta Med. Scand. (Suppl.), *461*:82, 1966.
7. Joyner, C.R., Reid, J.M., and Bond, J.P.: Reflected ultrasound in the assessment of mitral valve disease. Circulation, *27*:506, 1963.
8. Segal, B.L., Likoff, W., and Kingsley, B.: Echocardiography: clinical application in mitral stenosis. J.A.M.A., *193*:161, 1966.
9. Edler, I., Gustafson, A., Karlefors, T., and Christensson, B.: Ultrasound cardiography. Acta Med. Scand. (Suppl.), *370*:68, 1961.
10. Effert, S.: Pre- and post-operative evaluation of mitral stenosis by ultrasound. Am. J. Cardiol., *19*:59, 1967.
11. Silver, W., Rodriguez-Torres, R., and Newfelt, E.: The echocardiogram in a case of mitral stenosis before and after surgery. Am. Heart J., *78*:811, 1969.
12. Duchak, J.M., Jr., Chang, S., and Feigenbaum, H.: The posterior mitral valve echo and the echocardiographic diagnosis of mitral stenosis. Am. J. Cardiol., *29*:628, 1972.
13. Shah, P.M., Gramiak, R., and Kramer, D.H.: Ultrasound localization of left ventricular outflow obstruction in hypertrophic obstructive cardiomyopathy. Circulation, *40*:3, 1969.
14. Nichol, P.M., Gilbert, B.W., and Kisslo, J.A.: Two-dimensional echocardiographic assessment of mitral stenosis. Circulation, *55*:120, 1977.
15. Wann, L.S., Weyman, A.E., Feigenbaum, H., Dillon, J.C., Johnston, K.W., and Eggleton, R.C.: Determination of mitral valve area by cross-sectional echocardiography. Ann. Intern. Med., *88*:337, 1978.
16. Hueter, D., Drew, F., McInerney, K., Flessas, A., and Ryan, T.: Analysis of diastolic motion of the posterior leaflet in mitral stenosis. Circulation (Suppl. II), *54*:99, 1976. (Abstract)
17. Levisman, J.A.: Leaflet motion in mitral stenosis. Chest, *71*:4, 1977. (Editorial)
18. Shiu, M.F., Jenkins, B.S., and Webb-Peploe, M.M.: Echocardiographic analysis of posterior mitral leaflet movement in mitral stenosis. Br. Heart J., *40*:372, 1978.
19. Glasser, S.P. and Faris, J.V.: Posterior leaflet motion in mitral stenosis. Chest, *71*:87, 1977.
20. Thomas, R.D., Mary, D.A.S. and Ionescu, M.I.: Echocardiographic pattern of posterior mitral valve leaflet movement after mitral valve repair. Br. Heart J., *41*:399, 1979.
20a. Berman, N.D., Gilbert, B.W., McLaughlin, P.R., and Morch, J.E.: Mitral stenosis with posterior diastolic movement of posterior leaflet. Can. Med. Assoc. J., *112*:976, 1975.
21. Henry, W.L., Griffith, J.M., Michaelis, L.L., McIntosh, C.L., Morrow, A.G., and Epstein, S.E.: Measurement of mitral orifice area in patients with mitral valve disease by real-time, two-dimensional echocardiography. Circulation, *51*:827, 1975.
22. Martin, R.P., Rakowski, H., Kleiman, J.H., Beaver, W., London, E., and Popp, R.L.: Reliability and reproducibility of two-dimensional echocardiographic measurement of the stenotic mitral valve orifice area. Am. J. Cardiol., *43*:560, 1979.
23. Kastl, D., Henry, W.L., McIntosh, C., Redwood, D.R., Griffith, J.M., Itscoitz, S.B., and Morrow, A.G.: Cross-sectional echocardiographic assessment of mitral commissurotomy: comparison of hemodynamic and echocardiographic data. Circulation (Suppl. II), *54*:99, 1976. (Abstract)
24. Weyman, A.E., Wann, L.S., Rogers, E.W., Godley, R.W., Dillon, J.C., Feigenbaum, H., and Green, D.: Five-year experience in correlating cross-sectional echocardiographic assessment of the mitral valve area with hemodynamic valve area determinations. Am. J. Cardiol., *43*:386, 1979. (Abstract)
25. Shiu, M.F.: Mitral valve closure index: echocardiographic index of severity of mitral stenosis. Br. Heart J., *39*:839, 1977.
26. Shiu, M.F., Crowther, A., Jenkins, B.S., and Webb-Peploe, M.M.: Echocardiographic and exercise evaluation of results of mitral valvotomy operations. Br. Heart J., *41*:139, 1979.
27. Strunk, B.L., London, E.J., Fitzgerald, J., Popp, R.L., and Barry, W.H.: The assessment of mitral stenosis and prosthetic mitral valve obstruction, using the posterior aortic wall echocardiogram. Circulation, *55*:885, 1977.
28. Feigenbaum, H.: Clinical applications of echocardiography. Prog. Cardiovasc. Dis., *14*:531, 1972.
29. Gramiak, R. and Shah, P.M.: Cardiac untrasonography: a review of current applications. Radiol. Clin. North Am., *9*:469, 1971.
30. Nanda, N.C., Gramiak, R., Shah, P.M., and Lipchik, E.O.: Ultrasound evaluation of mitral valve calcification. Circulation (Suppl. II), *46*:46, 1972. (Abstract)
31. Nishimura, K., Sakakibara, T., Hibi, N., Kato, T., Fukui, Y., Arakawa, T., Tatematsu, H., Miwa, A., Tada, H., Kambe, T., and Hisanaga, H.: High-speed ultrasono-cardiotomography: echocardiographic manifestations of papillary muscles and chordae tendineae. J. Cardiogr., *7*:1, 1977.
32. Jinnouchi, J., Sugi, K., Itaya, K., Yoshioka, H., Koga, Y., Toshima, H., Toyomasu, K., Ohishi, K., and Koga, M.: Detection of the structural lesion in the mitral apparatus using real time cross-sectional echocardiography. J. Cardiogr., *8*:1, 1978.
33. Weyman, A.E., Heger, J.J., Kronik, G., Wann, L.S., Dillon, J.C., and Feigenbaum, H.: Mechanism of paradoxical early diastolic septal motion in patients with mitral stenosis: cross-sectional echocardiographic study. Am. J. Cardiol., *40*:691, 1977.
34. Kalmanson, D., Veyrat, C., Bouchareine, F., and Degroote, A.: Non-invasive recording of mitral valve flow velocity patterns using pulsed Doppler

echocardiography: application to diagnosis and evaluation of mitral valve disease. Br. Heart J., 39:517, 1977.

35. Hatle, L., Brubakk, A., Tromsdal, A., and Angelsen, B.: Noninvasive assessment of pressure drop in mitral stenosis by Doppler ultrasound. Br. Heart J., 40:131, 1978.

36. Nichol, P.M., Boughner, D.R., and Persaud, J.A.: Noninvasive assessment of mitral insufficiency by transcutaneous Doppler ultrasound. Circulation, 54:656, 1976.

37. Diebold, B., Theroux, P., Bourassa, M.G., Thuillez, C., Peronneau, P., Guermonprez, J.L., Xhaard, M., and Waters, D.D.: Non-invasive pulsed Doppler study of mitral stenosis and mitral regurgitation: preliminary study. Br. Heart J., 42:168, 1979.

38. Holen, J. and Simonsen, S.: Determination of pressure gradient in mitral stenosis with Doppler echocardiography. Br. Heart J., 41:529, 1979.

38a. Thuillez, C., Theroux, P., Bourassa, M.G., Blanchard, D., Peronneau, P., Guermonprez, J-L., Diebold, B., Waters, D.D., and Maurice, P.: Pulsed Doppler echocardiographic study of mitral stenosis. Circulation, 61:381, 1980.

39. Joyner, C.R. and Reid, J.M.: Application of ultrasound in cardiology and cardiovascular physiology. Prog. Cardiovasc. Dis., 5:482, 1963.

40. Kim, H., Kinoshita, M., Shirahama, Y., Tomonaga, G., and Kusukawa, R.: An attempt to correlate the mitral valve echogram with the hemodynamics of patients with pure mitral insufficiency. Jpn. Circ. J., 37:403, 1973.

41. Segal, B.L., Likoff, W., and Kingsley, B.: Echocardiography: clinical application in mitral regurgitation. Am. J. Cardiol., 19:50, 1967.

42. Edler, I.: Mitral valve function studied by the ultrasound echomethod. In Diagnostic Ultrasound: Proceedings of the First International Conference. Edited by C.C. Grossman, J.H. Holmes, C. Joyner, and E.W. Purnell. New York, Plenum Press, 1966.

43. Winters, W.L., Jr., Hafer, J., Jr., and Soloff, L.A.: Abnormal mitral valve motion as demonstrated by the ultrasound technique in apparent pure mitral insufficiency. Am. Heart J., 77:196, 1969.

43a. Konstantinov, B.A., Zaretskii, V.V., Bobokov, V.V., Sandrikov, V.A., and Likushkina, E.F.: Echocardiographic diagnosis of rheumatic mitral valve insufficiency. Kardiologiia, 17:28, 1977.

44. Burgess, J., Clark, R., Kamingaki, M., and Cohn, K.: Echocardiographic findings in different types of mitral regurgitation. Circulation, 48:97, 1973.

45. Millward, D.K., McLaurin, L.P., and Craige, E.: Echocardiographic studies of the mitral valve in patients with congestive cardiomyopathy and mitral regurgitation. Am. Heart J., 85:413, 1973.

46. Wann, L.S., Feigenbaum, H., Weyman, A.E., and Dillon, J.C.: Cross-sectional echocardiographic detection of rheumatic mitral regurgitation. Am. J. Cardiol., 41:1258, 1978.

47. Nimura, Y., Nagata, S., Beppu, S., Tamai, M., Senda, S., Matsumoto, M., Matsuo, H., Yoshioka, Y., Kawashima, Y., and Sakakibara, H.: Causes of mitral regurgitation and ultrasono-cardiotomographic approaches. J. Cardiogr., 6:237, 1976.

48. Fujino, T., Ito, M., Kanaya, S., Kawamura, T., Kinoshita, R., Fujino, M., Hamanaka, Y., and Mashiba, H.: Echocardiographic abnormal motion of interventricular septum in mitral insufficiency. J. Cardiogr., 6:613, 1976.

49. Ajisaka, R., Iesaka, Y., Takamoto, T., Iiizumi, T., Fujiwara, H., Taniguchi, K., and Takeuchi, J.: Echocardiographic assessment of left ventricular volume overloading in aortic insufficiency and mitral insufficiency. J. Cardiogr., 8:209, 1978.

50. Rosenblatt, A., Clark, R., Burgess, J., and Cohn, K.: Echocardiographic assessment of the level of cardiac compensation in valvular heart disease. Circulation, 54:509, 1976.

51. Fujino, T., Ito, M., Kanaya, S., Kawamura, T., Kinoshita, R., Fujino, M., Hamanaka, Y., and Mashiba, H.: Echocardiographic abnormal motion of interventricular septum in mitral insufficiency. J. Cardiogr., 6:613, 1976.

52. Levisman, J.A.: Echocardiographic diagnosis of mitral regurgitation in congestive cardiomyopathy. Am. Heart J., 93:33, 1977.

53. Sheikh, M.U., Morjaria, M., Covarrubias, E.A., Dejo, J., and Fox, L.M.: Echocardiographic demonstration of premature notching of the interventricular septal motion in aortic incompetence. Clin. Res., 26:271A, 1978. (Abstract)

54. Patton, R., Dragatakis, L., Marpole, D., and Sniderman, A.: The posterior left atrial echocardiogram of mitral regurgitation. Circulation, 57:1134, 1978.

55. Yorozu, T., Matsuzaki, M., Sasada, T., Ehara, K., Ishida, K., Fukagawa, K., Tanikado, O., Shimizu, M., Nomoto, R., and Kusukawa, R.: Echocardiographic estimation of stroke volume and mitral regurgitant volume using new parameter from aortic posterior wall motion. J. Cardiogr., 8:473, 1978.

56. Hall, R.J.C., Clarke, S.E., and Brown, D.: Evaluation of posterior aortic wall echogram in diagnosis of mitral valve disease. Br. Heart J., 41:522, 1979.

57. Reeves, W.C., Nanda, N.C., and Gramiak, R.: The relationship between aortic valve closure and aortic root motion. Radiology, 127:751, 1978.

58. Chandraratna, P.A.N., Vlahovich, G., and Aronow, W.S.: Echocardiographic study of significance of left ventricular minor axis shortening during pre-ejection phase of systole. Br. Heart J., 41:392, 1979.

59. Tei, C., Tanaka, H., Kashima, T., Yoshimura, H., Minagoe, S., and Kanehisa, T.: Real-time cross-sectional echocardiographic evaluation of the interatrial septum by right atrium-interatrial septum-left atrium direction of ultrasound beam. Circulation, 60:539, 1979.

60. Lorch, G., Rubenstein, S., Baker, D., Dooley, T., and Dodge, H.: Doppler echocardiography: use of a graphical display system. Circulation, 56:576, 1977.

61. Stevenson, J.G., Kawabori, I., and Guntheroth, W.G.: Differentiation of ventricular septal defects from mitral regurgitation by pulsed Doppler echocardiography. Circulation, 56:14, 1977.

62. Miyatake, K., Sakakibara, H., Kinoshita, N., Nagata, S., Beppu, S., and Nimura, Y.: Noninvasive recognition of localization and direction of mitral regurgitant flow with a combined use of cross-sectional echocardiography and pulsed Doppler technique. Circulation (Suppl. II), 60:154, 1979. (Abstract)

62a. Abbasi, A.S., Allen, M.W., DeCristofaro, D., and Ungar, I.: Detection and estimation of the degree of mitral regurgitation by range-gated pulsed Doppler echocardiography. Circulation, 61:143, 1980.

62b. Miyatake, K., Kinoshita, N., Nagata, S., Beppu, S.,

Park, Y-D., Sakakibara, H., and Nimura, Y.: Intracardiac flow pattern in mitral regurgitation studied with combined use of the ultrasonic pulsed Doppler technique and cross-sectional echocardiography. Am. J. Cardiol., 45:155, 1980.

63. Higgins, C.B., Reinke, R.T., Gosink, B.B., and Leopold, G.R.: The significance of mitral valve prolapse in middle-aged and elderly men. Am. Heart J., 91:292, 1976.

64. Markiewicz, W., Stoner, J., London, E., Hunt, S.A., and Popp, R.L.: Mitral valve prolapse in one hundred presumably healthy young females. Circulation, 53:464, 1976.

65. Darsee, J.R., Mikolich, R., Nicoloff, N.B., and Lesser, L.E.: Prevalence of mitral valve prolapse in presumably healthy young men. Circulation, 59:619, 1979.

66. Bloch, A., Vignola, P.A., Walker, H., Kaplan, A.D., Chiotellis, P.N., Lees, R.S., and Myers, G.S.: Echocardiographic spectrum of posterior systolic motion of the mitral valve in the general population. J. Clin. Ultrasound, 5:243, 1977.

67. Sahn, D.J., Wood, J., Allen, H.D., Peoples, W., and Goldberg, S.J.: Echocardiographic spectrum of mitral valve motion in children with and without mitral valve prolapse: the nature of false positive diagnosis. Am. J. Cardiol., 39:422, 1977.

68. Terasawa, Y., Tanaka, M., Nitta, K., Kashiwagi, M., Meguro, T., Hikichi, H., Watanabe, S., and Takeda, H.: Production mechanism of systolic click in mid-systolic click-late systolic murmur syndrome. J. Cardiogr., 6:593, 1976.

69. Yokota, Y., Kawanishi, H., Ohmori, K., Oda, A., Inoh, T., and Fukuzaki, H.: Studies on systolic anterior motion (SAM) pattern in idiopathic mitral valve prolapse by echocardiography. J. Cardiogr., 9:259, 1979.

70. Mathews, E., Jr., Henry, W.L., Ronan, J.A., and Griffith, J.M.: Two dimensional echo evaluation of mitral valve prolapse—an explanation of the patterns seen with M-mode echocardiograms. Circulation (Suppl. II), 54:235, 1976. (Abstract)

71. Markiewicz, W., London, E., and Popp, R.L.: Effect of transducer placement on echocardiographic mitral valve motion. Am. Heart J., 96:555, 1978.

72. Cohen, M.V.: Real-time sector scan study of the mitral valve prolapse syndrome. Br. Heart J., 40:964, 1978.

73. Rakowski, H., Martin, R.P., and Popp, R.L.: Two-dimensional echocardiographic findings in mitral valve prolapse. Circulation (Suppl. III), 56:154, 1977. (Abstract)

74. DeMaria, A.N., Bommer, W., Weinnert, L., Neumann, A., and Mason, D.T.: Abnormalities of cardiac structure in mitral prolapse syndrome: evaluation by cross-sectional echocardiography. Circulation (Suppl. III), 56:111, 1977. (Abstract)

75. Lieppe, W., Scallion, R., Behar, V.S., and Kisslo, J.A.: Two-dimensional echocardiographic findings in atrial septal defect. Circulation, 56:447, 1977.

76. Fraker, T.D., Behar, V.S., and Kisslo, J.A.: Coaptation instead of prolapse: refined echo descriptors for balloon mitral valve. Circulation (Suppl. II), 58:233, 1978. (Abstract)

77. Gilbert, B.W., Schatz, R.A., VonRamm, O.T., Behar, V.S., and Kisslo, J.A.: Mitral valve prolapse. Two-dimensional echocardiographic and angiographic correlation. Circulation, 54:716, 1976.

78. Mardelli, T.J., Morganroth, J., Chen, C.C., and Naito, M.: Apical cross-sectional echocardiography: the standard for the diagnosis of mitral valve. Circulation (Suppl. II), 60:154, 1979. (Abstract)

79. D'Cruz, I., Shah, S., Hirsch, L., and Goldberg, A.: Abnormal systolic motion of the posterolateral basal left ventricle in mitral valve prolapse: a new cross-sectional echocardiographic sign. Am. J. Cardiol., 45:434, 1980. (Abstract)

80. Davies, M.J., Moore, B.P., and Braimbridge, M.V.: The floppy mitral valve: study of incidence, pathology, and complications in surgical, necropsy, and forensic material. Br. Heart J., 40:468, 1978.

81. Isner, J.M. and Roberts, W.C.: Morphologic observations on the mitral valve at necropsy in patients with systolic clicks with or without systolic murmurs and/or echocardiographic evidence of mitral valve prolapse. Am. J. Cardiol., 43:368, 1979. (Abstract)

82. Gramiak, R. and Nanda, N.C.: Mitral valve. In Cardiac Ultrasound. Edited by R. Gramiak and R. Waag. St. Louis, C.V. Mosby Co., 1975.

83. Chandraratna, P.A.N. and Langevin, E.: Limitations of the echocardiogram in diagnosing valvular vegetations in patients with mitral valve prolapse. Circulation, 56:436, 1977.

84. Tallury, V.K., DePasquale, N.P., and Burch, G.E.: The echocardiogram in papillary muscle dysfunction. Am. Heart J., 83:12, 1972.

85. Mintz, G.S., Kotler, M.N., Segal, B.L., and Parry, W.R.: Two-dimensional echocardiographic evaluation of patients with mitral insufficiency. Am. J. Cardiol., 44:670, 1979.

86. Godley, R.W., Weyman, A.E., Feigenbaum, H., Rogers, E.W., and Green, D.: Patterns of mitral leaflet motion in patients with probable papillary muscle dysfunction. Am. J. Cardiol., 43:411, 1979. (Abstract)

87. Godley, R.W., Rogers, E.W., Wann, L.S., Dillon, J.C., Feigenbaum, H., and Weyman, A.E.: Relation of incomplete mitral leaflet closure to the site of dyssynergy in patients with papillary muscle dysfunction. Circulation (Suppl. II), 60:204, 1979. (Abstract)

88. Ogawa, S., Dupler, D.A., Pauletto, F.J., Chaudry, K.R., and Drefius, L.S.: Flail mitral valve in rheumatic heart disease. Chest, 74:88, 1978.

89. Ahmad, S., Kleiger, R.E., Connors, J., and Krone, R.: The echocardiographic diagnosis of rupture of a papillary muscle. Chest, 73:232, 1978.

90. Matsukubo, H., Yoshioka, K., Kajita, Y., Katsuki, A., Watanabe, T., Asayama, J., Katsume, H., Kunishige, H., Endo, N., Matsuura, T., and Ijichi, H.: Echocardiographic findings of vegetation and ruptured chordae tendineae: two cases of bacterial endocarditis. Cardiovasc. Sound Bull., 5:717, 1975.

91. Terasawa, Y., Tsuda, K., Ohno, K., Tsugawa, K., Kawakami, A., Yoshida, T., and Takamiya, M.: Ultrasono-cardiotomogram and ultrasound cardiogram of mitral regurgitation due to ruptured chordae tendineae. J. Cardiogr., 8:349, 1978.

92. Humphries, W.C., Hammer, W.J., McDonough, M.T., Lemole, G., McCurdy, R.R., and Spann, J.F., Jr.: Echocardiographic equivalents of a flail mitral leaflet. Am. J. Cardiol., 40:802, 1977.

93. Nishimura, T., Takahashi, M., Osakada, G., Yasunaga, K., Kawai, C., Kotoura, H., Konishi, Y., and Tatsuta, N.: Two-dimensional echocardio-

graphic findings in ruptured chordae tendineae of the mitral valve. J. Cardiogr., 8:589, 1978.

94. Jamal, N., Winters, W., and Nelson, J.: Echocardiographic features of flail mitral valve leaflets: ruptured chordae tendineae versus ruptured papillary muscle. Circulation (Suppl. II), 58:43, 1978. (Abstract)

95. Mintz, G.S., Kotler, M.N., Segal, B.L., and Parry, W.R.: Two-dimensional echocardiographic recognition of ruptured chordae tendineae. Circulation, 57:244, 1978.

95a. Ogawa, S., Mardelli, T.J., and Hubbard, F.E.: The role of cross-sectional echocardiography in the diagnosis of flail mitral leaflet. Clin. Cardiol., 1:85, 1978.

96. Sze, K.C., Nanda, N.C., and Gramiak, R.: Systolic flutter of the mitral valve. Am. Heart J., 96:157, 1978.

97. Meyer, J.F., Frank, M.J., Goldberg, S., and Cheng, T.O.: Systolic mitral flutter, an echocardiographic clue to the diagnosis of ruptured chordae tendineae. Am. Heart J., 94:3, 1977.

98. Child, J.S., Skorton, D.J., Taylor, R.D., Krivokapich, J., Abbasi, A.S., Wong, M., and Shah, P.D.: M-mode and cross-sectional echocardiographic features of flail posterior mitral leaflets. Am. J. Cardiol., 44:1383, 1979.

98a. Mintz, G.S., Kotler, M.N., Parry, W.R., and Segal, B.L.: Statistical comparison of M-mode and two-dimensional echocardiographic diagnosis of flail mitral leaflets. Am. J. Cardiol., 45:253, 1980.

99. Chang, S., Clements, S., and Chang, J.: Aortic stenosis: echocardiographic cusp separation and surgical description of aortic valve in 22 patients. Am. J. Cardiol., 39:499, 1977.

100. Williams, D.E., Sahn, D.J., and Friedman, W.F.: Cross-sectional echocardiographic localization of sites of left ventricular outflow tract obstruction. Am. J. Cardiol., 37:250, 1976.

101. Weyman, A.E., Feigenbaum, H., Hurwitz, R.A., Girod, D.A., and Dillon, J.C.: Cross-sectional echocardiographic assessment of the severity of aortic stenosis in children. Circulation, 55:773, 1977.

102. DeMaria, A.N., Joye, J.A., Bommer, W., Neumann, A., Weinert, L., Lee, G., and Mason, D.T.: Sensitivity and specificity of cross-sectional echocardiography in the diagnosis and quantification of valvular aortic stenosis. Circulation (Suppl. II), 58:232, 1978. (Abstract)

103. Le, L.R., Barrett, M.J., Leddy, C.L., Wolf, N.M., and Frankl, W.S.: Determination of aortic valve area by cross-sectional echocardiography. Circulation (Suppl. II), 60:203, 1979. (Abstract)

104. Schwartz, A., Vignola, P.A., Walker, H.J., King, M.E., and Goldblatt, A.: Echocardiographic estimation of aortic-valve gradient in aortic stenosis. Ann. Intern. Med., 89:329, 1978.

105. Johnson, G.L., Meyer, R.A., Schwartz, D.C., Korfhagen, J., and Kaplan, S.: Echocardiographic evaluation of fixed left ventricular outlet obstruction in children. Circulation, 56:299, 1977.

106. Bass, J.L., Einzig, S., Hong, C.Y., and Moller, J.H.: Echocardiographic screening to assess the severity of congenital aortic valve stenosis in children. Am. J. Cardiol., 44:82, 1979.

107. Johnson, G.L., Meyer, R.A., Schwartz, D.C., Korfhagen, J., and Kaplan, S.: Left ventricular function by echocardiography in children with fixed aortic stenosis. Am. J. Cardiol., 38:611, 1976.

108. Gaasch, W.H.: Left ventricular radius to wall thickness ratio. Am. J. Cardiol., 43:1189, 1979.

109. Mokotoff, D.M., Quinones, M.A., Winters, W.L., and Miller, R.R.: Non-invasive quantification of severity of aortic stenosis by echocardiographic wall thickness-radius ratio. Am. J. Cardiol., 43:406, 1979. (Abstract)

110. Gewitz, M.H., Werner, J.C., Kleinman, C.S., Hellenbrand, W.E., and Talner, N.S.: Role of echocardiography in aortic stenosis: pre- and postoperative studies. Am. J. Cardiol., 43:67, 1979.

111. Aziz, K.U., van Grondelle, A., Paul, M.H., and Muster, A.J.: Echocardiographic assessment of the relation between left ventricular wall and cavity dimensions and peak systolic pressure in children with aortic stenosis. Am. J. Cardiol., 40:775, 1977.

112. Blackwood, R.A., Bloom, K.R., and Williams, C.M.: Aortic stenosis in children. Experience with echocardiographic predictions of severity. Circulation, 57:263, 1978.

113. Sheppard, J.M., Shah, A.A., Sbarbaro, J.A., and Brooks, H.L.: Distinctive echocardiographic pattern of posterior wall endocardial motion in aortic stenosis. Am. Heart J., 96:9, 1978.

114. Young, J.B., Quinones, M.A., Waggoner, A.D., and Miller, R.R.: Diagnosis and quantification of aortic stenosis by pulsed Doppler echocardiography. Circulation (Suppl. II), 58:42, 1978. (Abstract)

115. Estevez, C.N., Dillon, J.C., Walker, P.D., Feigenbaum, H., and Chang, S.: Echocardiographic manifestations of aortic cusp rupture in a case of myxomatous degeneration of the aortic valve. Chest, 69:544, 1976.

116. Ramirez, J., Guardiola, J., and Flowers, N.C.: Echocardiographic diagnosis of ruptured aortic valve leaflet in bacterial endocarditis. Circulation, 57:634, 1978.

117. Rolston, W.A., Hirschfeld, D.S., Emilson, B.B., and Cheitlin, M.D.: Echocardiographic appearance of ruptured aortic cusp. Am. J. Med., 62:133, 1977.

118. Weaver, W.F., Wilson, C.S., Rourke, T., and Caudill, C.C.: Mid-diastolic aortic valve opening in severe acute aortic regurgitation. Circulation, 55:145, 1977.

119. Das, G., Lee, C.C., and Weissler, A.M.: Echocardiographic manifestations of ruptured aortic valvular leaflets in the absence of valvular vegetations. Chest, 72:464, 1977.

120. Whipple, R.L., III, Morris, D.C., Felner, J.M., Merrill, A.J., Jr., and Miller, J.I.: Echocardiographic manifestations of flail aortic valve leaflets. J. Clin. Ultrasound, 5:417, 1977.

121. Srivastava, T.N. and Flowers, N.C.: Echocardiographic features of flail aortic valve. Chest, 73:90, 1978.

122. Chandraratna, P.A.N., Robinson, M.J., Byrd, C., and Pitha, J.V.: Significance of abnormal echoes in left ventricular outflow tract. Br. Heart J., 39:381, 1977.

123. Shiu, M.F., Coltart, D.J., and Braimbridge, M.V.: Echocardiographic findings in prolapsed aortic cusp with vegetation. Br. Heart J., 41:118, 1979.

124. El Shahawy, M., Graybeal, R., Pepine, C.J., and Conti, C.R.: Diagnosis of aortic valvular prolapse by echocardiography. Chest, 69:411, 1976.

125. Mardelli, T.J., Morganroth, J., Naito, M., Chen, C.C., Meixell, L., and Parrotto, C.: Cross-sectional echocardiographic identification of aortic valve prolapse. Circulation (Suppl. II), 60:797, 1979. (Abstract)

126. Koda, J., Nakamura, K., Atsuchi, Y., Nagai, Y., Komatsu, Y., Kondo, M., Shibuya, M., and Hirosawa, K.: Diastolic aortic cusp separation in aortic regurgitation. J. Cardiogr., 7:163, 1977.

127. D'Cruz, I., Cohen, H.C., Prabhu, R., Ayabe, T., and Glick, G.: Flutter of left ventricular structures in patients with aortic regurgitation, with special reference to patients with associated mitral stenosis. Am. Heart J., 9:684, 1976.

128. Henzi, M., Burckhardt, D., Raeder, E.A., and Follath, F.: Echocardiography as a method for the determination of the severity of aortic insufficiency. Schweiz. Med. Wochenschr., 106:1557, 1976.

129. Fujioka, T., Ueda, K., Ohkawa, S., Kamata, C., Kitano, K., Ito, Y., Takahashi, R., Shinagawa, T., Matsushita, S., Sugiura, M., Murakami, M., and Hada, Y.: A clinicopathological study of aortic regurgitation with septal fluttering on echocardiogram. J. Cardiogr., 8:697, 1978.

130. Johnson, A.D. and Gosink, B.B.: Oscillation of left ventricular structures in aortic regurgitation. J. Clin. Ultrasound, 5:21, 1977.

131. Nakao, S., Tanaka, H., Tahara, M., Yoshimura, H., Sakurai, S., and Tei, C.: An experimental study on the mechanism of echocardiographic findings in aortic regurgitation: with special reference to the direction of regurgitant jet. Circulation (Suppl. II), 60:798, 1979. (Abstract)

131a. Pridie, R.B., Beham, R., and Oakley, C.M.: Echocardiography of the mitral valve in aortic valve disease. Br. Heart J., 33:296, 1971.

131b. Oki, T., Matsuhisa, M., Tsuyuguchi, N., Kondo, C., Matsumura, K., Niki, T., Mori, H., and Sawada, S.: Echo patterns of the anterior leaflet of the mitral valve in patients with aortic insufficiency. J. Cardiogr., 6:307, 1976.

131c. Ambrose, J.A., Meller, J., Teichholz, L.E., and Herman, M.V.: Premature closure of the mitral valve: echocardiographic clue for the diagnosis of aortic dissection. Chest, 73:121, 1978.

131d. Mann, T., McLaurin, L., Grossman, W., and Craige, E.: Assessing the hemodynamic severity of acute aortic regurgitation due to infective endocarditis. N. Engl. J. Med., 293:108, 1975.

131e. Fox, S., Kotler, M.N., Segal, B.L., and Parry, W.: Echocardiographic diagnosis of acute aortic valve endocarditis and its complications. Arch. Intern. Med., 137:85, 1977.

132. Pietro, D.A., Parisi, A.F., Harrington, J.J., and Askenazi, J.: Premature opening of the aortic valve: an index of highly advanced aortic regurgitation. J. Clin. Ultrasound, 6:170, 1978.

133. McDonald, I.G.: Echocardiographic assessment of left ventricular function in aortic valve disease. Circulation, 53:860, 1976.

134. Henry, W.L., Bonow, R.O., Borer, J.S., Ware, J.H., Kent, K.M., Redwood, D.R., McIntosh, C.L., Morrow, A.G., and Epstein, S.E.: Observations on the optimum time for operative intervention for aortic regurgitation. I. Evaluation of the results of aortic valve replacement in symptomatic patients. Circulation, 61:471, 1980.

134a. Henry, W.L., Bonow, R.O., Rosing, D.R., and Epstein, S.E.: Observations on the optimum time for operative intervention for aortic regurgitation. II. Serial echocardiographic evaluation of asymptomatic patients. Circulation, 61:484, 1980.

135. Johnson, A.D., Alpert, J.S., Francis, G.S., Vieweg, V.R., Ockene, I., and Hagan, A.D.: Assessment of left ventricular function in severe aortic regurgitation. Circulation, 54:975, 1976.

136. Cunha, C.L.P., Giulinai, E.R., Fuster, V., Seward, J.B., and Brandenburg, R.O.: Surgery for aortic insufficiency: valve of M-mode echocardiography as a prognostic indicator. Am. J. Cardiol., 43:406, 1979. (Abstract)

137. Schuler, G., Peterson, K.L., Johnson, A.D., Francis, G., Ashburn, W., Dennish, G., Daily, P.O., and Ross, J.: Serial noninvasive assessment of left ventricular hypertrophy and function after surgical correction of aortic regurgitation. Am. J. Cardiol., 44:585, 1979.

138. Al-Nouri, M., Hellman, C., and Schmidt, D.H.: Echocardiographic indices predictive of early left ventricular dysfunction in patients with aortic regurgitation. Circulation (Suppl. II), 60:137, 1979. (Abstract)

138a. Abdulla, A.M., Frank, M.J., Canedo, M.I., and Stefadouros, M.A.: Limitations of echocardiography in the assessment of left ventricular size and function in aortic regurgitation. Circulation, 61:148, 1980.

139. Ward, J.M., Baker, D.W., Rubenstein, S.A., and Johnson, S.L.: Detection of aortic insufficiency by pulsed Doppler echocardiography. J. Clin. Ultrasound, 5:5, 1977.

140. Pearlman, A.S., Dooley, T.K., Franklin, D.W., and Weiler, T.: Detection of regurgitant flow using duplex (two-dimensional/Doppler) echocardiography. Circulation (Suppl. II), 60:154, 1979. (Abstract)

141. Joyner, C.R., Hey, B.E., Jr., Johnson, J., and Reid, J.M.: Reflected ultrasound in the diagnosis of tricuspid stenosis. Am. J. Cardiol., 19:66, 1967.

142. Okada, R.D., Ewy, G.A., and Copeland, J.G.: Echocardiography and surgery in tricuspid and pulmonary valve stenosis due to carcinoid syndrome. Cardiovasc. Med., 4:871, 1979.

143. Reference deleted.

144. Gramiak, R. and Shah, P.M.: Cardiac ultrasonography: a review of current applications. Radiol. Clin. North Am., 9:469, 1971.

145. Kessler, K.M., Foianini, J.E., Davia, J.E., Anderson, W.T., Pfuetze, K., Pinder, T., and Cheitlin, M.D.: Tricuspid insufficiency due to nonpenetrating trauma. Am. J. Cardiol., 37:442, 1976.

146. Seides, S.F., DeJoseph, R.L., Brown, A.E., and Damato, A.N.: Echocardiographic findings in isolated, surgically created tricuspid insufficiency. Am. J. Cardiol., 35:679, 1974.

147. Reference deleted.

148. Lieppe, W., Behar, V.S., Scallion, R., and Kisslo, J.A.: Detection of tricuspid regurgitation with two-dimensional echocardiography and peripheral vein injections. Circulation, 57:128, 1978.

149. Nanda, N.C., Shah, P.M., and Gramiak, R.: Echocardiographic evaluation of tricuspid valve incompetence by contrast injections. Clin. Res., 24:233A, 1976.

150. Wise, N.K., Myers, S., Stewart, J.A., Waugh, R., Fraker, T., and Kisslo, J.: Echo inferior venacavography: a technique for the study of right-sided heart disease. Circulation (Suppl. II), 60:202, 1979. (Abstract)

151. Sivaciyan, V. and Ranganathan, N.: Transcutaneous Doppler jugular venous flow velocity recording: clinical and hemodynamic correlates. Circulation, 57:930, 1978.

152. Waggoner, A.D., Quinones, M.A., Verani, M.S., and Miller, R.R.: Pulsed Doppler echocardiographic detection of tricuspid insufficiency: diagnostic sensitivity and correlation with right ventricular hemodynamics. Circulation, 58:150, 1978. (Abstract)

153. Kawaratani, H., Narita, M., Kurihara, T., and Usami, Y.: A case of traumatic tricuspid insufficiency. J. Cardiogr., 7:393, 1977.

154. Nishimura, T., Morioka, S., Kawai, C., and Kotoura, H.: Echocardiographic evaluation of tricuspid regurgitation. J. Cardiogr., 7:177, 1977.

155. Rippe, J.M., Angoff, G., Sloss, L.J., Wynne, J., and Alpert, J.S.: Multiple floppy valves: an echocardiographic syndrome. Am. J. Med., 66:817, 1979.

156. Chandraratna, P.A., Littman, B.B., and Wilson, D.: The association between atrial septal defect and prolapse of the tricuspid valve: an echocardiographic study. Chest, 73:839, 1978.

157. Werner, J.A., Schiller, N.B., and Prasquier, R.: Occurrence and significance of echocardiographically demonstrated tricuspid valve prolapse. Am. Heart J., 96:180, 1978.

158. Sasse, L. and Froelich, C.R.: Echocardiographic tricuspid prolapse and nonejection systolic click. Chest, 73:869, 1978.

159. DeMaria, A.N., Bommer, W., Neumann, A., Weinert, L., Barstwo, T., Kaku, R., and Mason, D.T.: Evaluation of tricuspid valve prolapse by two-dimensional echocardiography. Circulation (Suppl. II), 58:43, 1978. (Abstract)

160. Mardelli, T.J., Morganroth, J., Meixell, L.L., and Vergel, J.: Enhanced diagnosis of tricuspid valve prolapse by cross-sectional echocardiography. Am. J. Cardiol., 43:385, 1979. (Abstract)

161. Inoue, D., Katsume, H., Watanabe, T., Matsukubo, H., Furukawa, K., Torii, Y., Sugihara, H., and Ijichi, H.: Tricuspid valve prolapse detected by subxiphoid two-dimensional echocardiography. J. Cardiogr., 9:387, 1979.

161a. Dillon, J.C., Feigenbaum, H., Konecke, L.L., Davis, R.H., and Chang, S.: Echocardiographic manifestations of valvular vegetations. Am. Heart J., 86:698, 1973.

161b. Spangler, R.D., Johnson, M.D., Holmes, J.H., and Blount, S.G., Jr.: Echocardiographic demonstration of bacterial vegetations in active infective endocarditis. J. Clin. Ultrasound, 1:126, 1973.

161c. Martinez, E.C., Burch, G.E., and Giles, T.D.: Echocardiographic diagnosis of vegetative aortic bacterial endocarditis. Am. J. Cardiol., 34:845, 1974.

161d. Gottlieb, S., Khuddus, S.A., Balooki, H., Dominquez, A.E., and Myerburg, R.J.: Echocardiographic diagnosis of aortic valve vegetations in candida endocarditis. Circulation, 50:826, 1974.

161e. DeMaria, A.N., King, J.F., Salel, A.F., Caudill, C.C., Miller, R.R., and Mason, D.T.: Echography

and phonography of acute aortic regurgitation in bacterial endocarditis. Ann. Intern. Med., 82:329, 1975.

161f. Hirschfeld, D.S. and Schiller, N.: Localization of aortic valve vegetations by echocardiography. Circulation, 53:280, 1976.

162. Yoshikawa, J., Tanaka, K., Owaki, T., and Kato, H.: Cord-like aortic valve vegetation in bacterial endocarditis. Circulation, 53:911, 1976.

163. Kleiner, J.P., Brundage, B.H., Ports, T.A., and Thomas, H.M.: Echocardiographic manifestation of flail right and noncoronary aortic valve leaflets: studies in patients with bacterial endocarditis. Chest, 74:301, 1978.

164. Sternberg, L., Sole, M.J., Joza, P., and Scully, H.E.: Echocardiographic features of an unusual case of aortic valve endocarditis. Can. Med. Assoc. J., 115:1022, 1976.

165. Pease, H.F., Matsumoto, S., Cacchione, R.J., Richards, K.L., and Leach, J.K.: Lethal obstruction by aortic valvular vegetation: echocardiographic studies of endocarditis without apparent aortic regurgitation. Chest, 73:658, 1978.

166. Chandraratna, P.A.N. and Aronow, W.S.: Spectrum of echocardiographic findings in tricuspid valve endocarditis. Br. Heart J., 42:528, 1979.

167. Kisslo, J., VonRamm, O.T., Haney, R., Jones, R., Juk, S.S., and Behar, V.S.: Echocardiographic evaluation of tricuspid valve endocarditis: an M-mode and two-dimensional study. Am. J. Cardiol., 38:502, 1976.

168. Jemsek, J.G., Greenberg, S.B., Gentry, L.O., Welton, D.E., and Mattox, K.L.: Haemophilus parainfluenzae endocarditis. Two cases and review of the literature in the past decade. Am. J. Med., 66:51, 1979.

169. Covarrubias, E.A., Sheikh, M.U., and Fox, L.M.: Echocardiography and pulmonary embolism. Ann. Intern. Med., 87:720, 1977.

170. Kramer, N.E., Gill, S.S., Patel, R., and Towne, W.D.: Pulmonary valve vegetations detected with echocardiography. Am. J. Cardiol., 39:1064, 1977.

171. Dzindzio, B.S., Meyer, L.R., Osterholm, R., Hopeman, A., Woltjen, J., and Forker, A.D.: Isolated gonococcal pulmonary valve endocarditis: diagnosis of echocardiography. Circulation, 59:1319, 1979.

172. Sheikh, M.U., Ali, N., Covarrubias, E., Fox, L.M., Morjaria, M., and Dejo, J.: Right-sided infective endocarditis: an echocardiographic study. Am. J. Med., 66:283, 1979.

173. Okumachi, F., Yoshikawa, J., Takatsuka, K., Owaki, T., Kato, H., Yanagihara, K., Takagi, Y., Shingaki, M., Baba, K., Tomita, Y., Fukaya, T., Tatemichi, K., Shomura, T., and Yoshizumi, M.: Cross-sectional echocardiographic diagnosis of pulmonary valve vegetation. J. Cardiogr., 9:279, 1979.

174. Martin, R.P., Meltzer, R.S., Chia, B.L., and Popp, R.L.: The clinical utility of two-dimensional echocardiography in bacterial endocarditis. Circulation (Suppl. II), 58:187, 1978. (Abstract)

174a. Busch, U.W., Garcia, E., Pechacek, L.W., DeCastro, C.M., Jr., and Hall, R.J.: Cross-sectional echocardiographic findings in vegetative aortic valve endocarditis. Cardiovasc. Dis., 5:328, 1978.

175. Wann, L.S., Hallam, C.C., Dillon, J.C., Weyman,

A.E., and Feigenbaum, H.: Comparison of
M-mode and cross-sectional echocardiography in
infective endocarditis. Circulation, 60:728, 1979.

176. Gilbert, B.W., Haney, R.S., Crawford, F.,
McClellan, J., Gallis, H.A., Johnson, M.L., and
Kisslo, J.A.: Two-dimensional echocardiographic
assessment of vegetative endocarditis. Circulation, 55:346, 1977.

177. Mintz, G.S., Kotler, M.N., Segal, B.L., and Parry,
W.R.: Comparison of two-dimensional and
M-mode echocardiography in the evaluation of patients with infective endocarditis. Am. J. Cardiol.,
43:738, 1979.

177a.Wann, L.S., Dillon, J.C., Weyman, A.E., and
Feigenbaum, H.: Echocardiography in bacterial
endocarditis. N. Engl. J. Med., 295:135, 1976.

178. Andy, J.J., Sheikh, M.U., Ali, N., Barnes, B.O., Fox,
L.M., Curry, C.L., and Roberts, W.C.: Echocardiographic observations in opiate addicts with active
infective endocarditis. Am. J. Cardiol., 40:17,
1977.

178a.Thompson, K.R., Nanda, N.C., and Gramiak, R.:
The reliability of echocardiography in the diagnosis of infective endocarditis. Radiology,
125:373, 1977.

178b.Ibrahim, M.M. and El-Said, G.M.: Echocardiographic findings in bacterial endocarditis. Cardiovasc. Dis., 5:337, 1978.

179. Young, J.B., Welton, D., Quinones, M.A., Ishimori,
T., Alexander, J.K., and Miller, R.R.: Prognostic
significance of valvular vegetations identified by
M-mode echocardiography in infective endocar-
ditis. Circulation (Suppl. II), 58:41, 1978.
(Abstract)

180. Strom, J., Davis, R., Frishman, W., Becker, R.,
Matsumoto, M., and Sonnenblick, E.: The demonstration of vegetations by echocardiography in
bacterial endocarditis: an indication for early surgical intervention. Circulation (Suppl. II), 60:37,
1979. (Abstract)

181. Nomeir, A.M., Watts, E., and Philp, J.R.: Bacterial
endocarditis. Echocardiographic and clinical
evaluation during therapy. J. Clin. Ultrasound,
4:23, 1976.

182. Reference deleted.

183. Silimperi, D., Harris, P., and Kisslo, J.A.: Lesion
fate in endocarditis. Circulation (Suppl. II),
58:236, 1978. (Abstract)

184. Cura, G.M., Tajik, A.J., and Seward, J.B.: Correlation of initial echocardiographic findings with outcome in patients with bacterial endocarditis. Circulation (Suppl. II), 58:232, 1978. (Abstract)

185. Stafford, A., Wann, L.S., Dillon, J.C., Weyman,
A.E., and Feigenbaum, H.: Serial echocardiographic appearance of healing bacterial vegetations. Am. J. Cardiol., 44:754, 1979.

185a.Stewart, J.A., Silimperi, D., Harris, P., Wise, N.K.,
Fraker, T.D., and Kisslo, J.A.: Echocardiographic
documentation of vegetative lesions in infective
endocarditis: clinical implications. Circulation,
61:374, 1980.

186. Roy, P., Tajik, A.J., Giuliani, E.R., Schattenberg,
T.T., Gau, G.T., and Frye, R.L.: Spectrum of echo-
cardiographic findings in bacterial endocarditis.
Circulation, 53:474, 1976.

187. Arvan, S., Cagin, N., Levitt, B., and Kleid, J.J.:
Echocardiographic findings in a patient with candida endocarditis of the aortic valve. Chest,
70:300, 1976.

188. Gomes, J.A., Calderon, J., Lajam, F., et al.: Echocardiographic detection of fungal vegetations in
candida parasilopsis endocarditis. Am. J. Med.,
61:273, 1976.

189. Pasternak, R.C., Cannom, D.S., and Cohen, L.S.:
Echocardiographic diagnosis of large fungal verruca attached to mitral valve. Br. Heart J.,38:1209,
1976.

190. Fitchett, D.H. and Oakley, C.M.: Granulomatous
mitral valve obstruction. Br. Heart J.,38:112, 1976.

191. Estevez, C.M. and Corya, B.C.: Serial echocardiographic abnormalities in nonbacterial thrombotic
endocarditis of the mitral valve. Chest, 69:801,
1976.

192. Weyman, A.E., Rankin, R., and King, H.: Loeffler's
endocarditis presenting as mitral and tricuspid
stenosis. Am. J. Cardiol., 40:438, 1977.

193. Aziz, K.U., Newfeld, E.A., and Paul, M.H.: Echocardiographic detection of bacterial vegetation in a
child with a ventricular septal defect. Chest,
70:780, 1976.

194. Mardelli, T.J., Ogawa, S., Hubbard, F.E., Dreifus,
L.S., and Meixell, L.L.: Cross-sectional echocardiographic detection of aortic ring abscess in
bacterial endocarditis. Chest, 74:576, 1978.

195. Scanlan, J.G., Seward, J.B., and Tajik, A.J.:
Myocardial abscess: direct visualization with
wide-angle two-dimensional sector echocardiography. Circulation (Suppl. II), 60:37, 1979.
(Abstract)

196. Siggers, D.C., Srivongse, S.A., and Deuchar, D.:
Analysis of dynamics of mitral Starr-Edwards
valve prosthesis using reflected ultrasound. Br.
Heart J., 33:401, 1971.

197. Gimenez, J.L., Winters, W.L., Jr., Davila, J.C.,
Connell, J., and Klein, K.S.: Dynamics of the
Starr-Edwards ball valve prosthesis: a cinefluoro-
graphic and ultrasonic study in humans. Am. J.
Med. Sci., 250:652, 1965.

198. Winters, W.L., Gimenez, J.L., and Soloff, L.: Clinical applications of ultrasound in the analysis of
prosthetic ball valve function. Am. J. Cardiol.,
19:97, 1967.

199. Chandraratna, P.A.N., Lopez, J.M., Hildner, F.J.,
Samet, P., Ben-Zvi, J., and Gindlesperger, D.:
Diagnosis of Bjork-Shiley aortic valve dysfunction
by echocardiography. Am. Heart J., 91:318, 1976.

200. Douglas, J.E. and Williams, G.D.: Echocardiographic evaluation of the Bjork-Shiley prosthetic
valve. Circulation, 50:52, 1974.

201. Ellis, J., Phillips, B., Friedewald, V.E., Jr., and
Diethrich, E.B.: The evaluation of the Bjork-
Shiley prosthetic valve by echocardiography. J.
Clin. Ultrasound, 2:228, 1974. (Abstract)

201a.Capella, G., Bomba, M.A., Pandolfini, E., and
Rossi, P.: Use of echocardiography in the study of
the Bjork-Shiley disk valve prosthesis. Boll. Soc.
Ital. Cardiol., 20:1779, 1975.

202. Yamamoto, T., Tanimoto, M., Ohogami, T.,
Yasutomi, N., Ando, H., Iwasaki, T., Yorifuji, S.,
Shimizu, Y., Horiguchi, Y., and Miyamoto, T.:
Evaluation of the porcine aortic bioprosthesis by
M-mode and cross-sectional echocardiography. J.
Cardiogr., 7:267, 1977.

203. Bommer, W., Yoon, D., Grehl, T.M., Mason, D.T.,

Neumann, A., and DeMaria, A.N.: In vitro and in vivo evaluation of porcine bioprostheses by cross-sectional echocardiography. Am. J. Cardiol., 41:405, 1978. (Abstract)

204. Harston, W.E., Jr., Robertson, R.M., and Friesinger, G.C.: Echocardiographic evaluation of porcine heterograft valves in the mitral and aortic positions. Am. Heart J., 96:448, 1978.

205. Bloch, W.N., Felner, J.M., Wiskliffe, C., Symbas, P.N., and Schlant, R.C.: Echocardiogram of the porcine aortic bioprosthesis in the mitral position. Am. J. Cardiol., 38:293, 1976.

205a.Kessler, K.M., Rahim, A., Rodriguez, D., Kaplan, S.R., and Samet, P.: Pseudo-mitral-valve echogram following prosthetic mitral valve replacement. J. Clin. Ultrasound, 8:35, 1980.

206. Ben-Zvi, J., Hildner, F.J., Chandraratna, P.A., and Samet, P.: Thrombosis on Bjork-Shiley aortic valve prosthesis: clinical, arteriographic, echocardiographic, and therapeutic observations in seven cases. Am. J. Cardiol., 34:538, 1974.

206a.Copans, H., Lakier, J.B., Kinsley, R.H., Colsen, P.R., Fritz, V.U., and Barlow, J.B.: Thrombosed Bjork-Shiley mitral prostheses. Circulation, 61:169, 1980.

207. Oliva, P.B., Johnson, M.L., Pomerantz, M., and Levine, A.: Dysfunction of the Beall mitral prosthesis and its detection by cinefluoroscopy and echocardiography. Am. J. Cardiol., 31:393, 1973.

208. Srivastava, T.N., Hussain, M., Gray, L.A., Jr., and Flowers, N.C.: Echocardiographic diagnosis of a stuck Bjork-Shiley aortic valve prosthesis. Chest, 70:94, 1976.

209. Chandraratna, P.A.N., Lopez, J.M., Hildner, F.J., Samet, P., and Ben-Zvi, J. (with technical assistance of D. Gindlesperger): Diagnosis of Bjork-Shiley aortic valve dysfunction by echocardiography. Am. Heart J., 91:318, 1976.

210. Bloch, W.N., Jr., Felner, J.M., Wickliffe, C., and Symbas, P.N.: Echocardiographic diagnosis of thrombus on a heterograft aortic valve in the mitral position. Chest, 70:399, 1976.

211. Johnson, M.L., Holmes, J.H., and Paton, B.C.: Echocardiographic determination of mitral disc valve excursion. Circulation, 47:1274, 1973.

212. Kawai, N., Segal, B.L., and Linhart, J.W.: Delayed opening of Beall mitral prosthetic valve detected by echocardiography. Chest, 67:239, 1975.

213. Pfeifer, J., Goldschlager, N., Sweatman, T., Gerbode, E., and Selzer, A.: Malfunction of mitral ball valve prosthesis due to thrombus. Am. J. Cardiol., 29:95, 1972.

214. Bourdillon, P.D.V. and Sharratt, G.P.: Malfunction of Bjork-Shiley valve prosthesis in tricuspid position. Br. Heart J., 38:1149, 1976.

215. Raj, M.V.J., Srinivas, V., and Evans, D.W.: Thrombotic jamming of a tricuspid prosthesis. Br. Heart J., 38:1355, 1976.

216. Sugiki, K., Kusajima, K., Kitaya, T., Kamata, K., and Komatsu, S.: Echocardiographic analysis for various prosthetic valves and malfunctioning Wada-Cutter valve. Cardiovasc. Sound Bull., 5:727, 1975.

217. Orita, Y., Tanaka, S., Takeshita, A., Nakamura, M., and Hirata, T.: A case with the malfunction of a Starr-Edwards caged-lens mitral prosthetic valve: four episodes of transient malfunction with their clinical, phonocardiographic, and echocardiographic findings. J. Cardiogr., 6:753, 1976.

218. Wann, L.S., Pyhel, H.J., Judson, W.E., Tavel, M.E., and Feigenbaum, H.: Ball variance in a Harken mitral prosthesis: echocardiographic and phonocardiographic features. Chest, 72:785, 1977.

219. Belenkie, I., Carr, M., Schlant, R.C., Nutter, D.O., and Symbas, P.N.: Malfunction of a Cutter-Smeloff mitral ball valve prosthesis: diagnosis by phonocardiography and echocardiography. Am. Heart J., 86:339, 1973.

220. Brodie, B.R., Grossman, W., McLaurin, L., Starek, P.J.K., and Craige, E.: Daignosis of prosthetic mitral valve malfunction with combined echo-phonocardiography. Circulation, 53:93, 1976.

221. Gibson, T.C., Starek, J.K., Moos, S., and Craige, E.: Echocardiographic and phonocardiographic characteristics of the Lillehei-Kaster mitral valve prosthesis. Circulation, 49:434, 1974.

222. Berndt, T.B., Goodman, D.J., and Popp, R.L.: Echocardiographic and phonocardiographic confirmation of suspected cage mitral valve malfunction. Chest, 70:221, 1976.

223. Estevez, R., Mookherjee, S., Potts, J., Fulton, M., and Obeid, A.I.: Phonocardiographic and echocardiographic features of Lillehei-Kaster mitral prosthesis. J. Clin. Ultrasound, 5:153, 1977.

224. Clements, S.D. and Perkins, J.V.: Malfunction of a Bjork-Shiley prosthetic heart valve in the mitral position producing an abnormal echocardiographic pattern. J. Clin. Ultrasound, 6:334, 1978.

225. Bernal-Ramirez, J.A., and Phillips, J.H.: Echocardiographic study of malfunction of the Bjork-Shiley prosthetic heart valve in the mitral position. Am. J. Cardiol., 40:449, 1977.

226. Alam, M., Madrazo, A.C., Magilligan, D.J., and Goldstein, S.: M-mode and two-dimensional echocardiographic features of porcine valve dysfunction. Am. J. Cardiol., 43:502, 1979.

227. Schapira, J.N., Martin, R.P., Fowles, R.E., Rakowski, H., Stinson, E.B., French, J.W., Shumway, N.E., and Popp, R.L.: Two-dimensional echocardiographic assessment of patients with bioprosthetic valves. Am. J. Cardiol., 43:510, 1979.

228. Reference deleted.

229. Brown, J.W., Dunn, J.M., Spooner, E., and Kirsh, M.M.: Late spontaneous disruption of a porcine xenograft mitral valve: clinical, hemodynamic, echocardiographic, and pathological findings. J. Thorac. Cardiovasc. Surg., 75:606, 1978.

230. Schuchman, H., Feigenbaum, H., Dillon, J.C., and Chang, S.: Intracavitary echoes in patients with mitral prosthetic valves. J. Clin. Ultrasound, 3:111, 1975.

231. Preis, L.K., Hess, J.P., Austin, J.L., Craddock, G.B., McGuire, L.B., and Martin, R.P.: Left ventricular microcavitations in patients with Beall valves. Am. J. Cardiol., 45:402, 1980. (Abstract)

232. Yoshikawa, J., Owaki, T., Kato, H., and Tanaka, K.: Abnormal motion of interventricular septum in patients with prosthetic valve. Cardiovasc. Sound Bull., 5:211, 1975.

233. Kerber, R.E. and Doty, D.B.: Abnormalities of interventricular septal motion following cardiac surgery: cross-sectional echocardiographic studies. Am. J. Cardiol. (Suppl. II), 41:96, 1978. (Abstract)

234. Morioka, S., Nagai, Y., Kawai, C., and Kotoura, H.: Echocardiographic evaluation of abnormal interventricular septal motion in patients with cardiac surgery. Cardiovasc. Sound Bull., 5:459, 1975.

235. Yoshikawa, J., Owaki, T., Kato, H., and Tanaka, K.:

Abnormal motion of interventricular septum in patients with prosthetic valve. Cardiovasc. Sound Bull., 5:211, 1976.

236. Jinnouchi, J., Bekki, H., Yoshioka, H., Koga, Y., and Toshima, H.: Two-dimensional echocardiographic study on the mechanism of abnormal septal motion. J. Cardiogr., 7:303, 1977.

237. Matsuhisa, M., Ohki, T., Niki, Y., Taniguchi, T., Niki, T., Mori, H., and Sawada, S.: Abnormal interventricular septal motion after heart surgery: a comparative study with jugular pulse tracing. J. Cardiogr., 6:691, 1976.

238. Popp, R.L. and Carmichael, B.M.: Cardiac echography in the diagnosis of prosthetic mitral valve malfunction. Circulation (Suppl. II), 44:33, 1971. (Abstract)

239. Dashkoff, N., Karacuschansky, M., Come, P.C., and Fortuin, N.J.: Echocardiographic features of mitral annulus calcification. Am. Heart J., 94:585, 1977.

239a.Schott, C.R., Kotler, M.N., Parry, W.R., and Segal, B.L.: Mitral annular calcification: clinical and echocardiographic correlations. Arch. Intern. Med., 137:1143, 1977.

239b.Howard, P.F., Cabizuca, S.V., Desser, K.B., and Benchimol, A.: The echocardiographic diagnosis of calcified mitral annulus. Am. J. Med., 273:267, 1977.

239c.Curati, W.L., Petitclerc, R., and Winsberg, F.: Ultrasonic features of mitral annulus calcification: a report of 21 cases. Radiology, 122:215, 1977.

240. D'Cruz, I., Panetta, F., Cohen, H., and Glick, G.: Submitral calcification or sclerosis in elderly patients: M-mode and two-dimensional echocardiography in "mitral annulus calcification." Am. J. Cardiol., 44:31, 1979.

241. Gabor, G.E., Mohr, B.D., Goel, P.C., and Cohen, B.: Echocardiographic and clinical spectrum of mitral annular calcification. Am. J. Cardiol., 38:836, 1976.

242. D'Cruz, I.A., Cohen, H.C., Prabhu, R., Bisla, V., and Glick, G.: Clinical manifestations of mitral annulus calcification, with emphasis on its echocardiographic features. Am. Heart J., 94:367, 1977.

243. McLean, J., Felner, J.M., Whipple, R., Morris, D., and Schlant, R.C.: The echocardiographic association of mitral valve prolapse and mitral annulus calcification. Clin. Cardiol., 2:220, 1979.

244. Kronzon, I., and Glassman, E.: Mitral ring calcification in idiopathic hypertrophic subaortic stenosis. Am. J. Cardiol., 42:60, 1978.

245. Fulkerson, P.K., Beaver, B.M., Auseon, J.C., and Graber, H.L.: Calcification of the mitral annulus: etiology, clinical associations, complications, and therapy. Am. J. Med., 66:967, 1979.

7

Congenital Heart Disease

Congenital heart disease is predominately but not exclusively a disease of infants and children. The echocardiographic examination of younger patients can be considerably different from that of adults, especially in small children and premature infants.[1,2] Examination of such patients offers advantages and disadvantages.[3,4] The main advantage is that there are few bony structures that distort or impede the ultrasonic examination. The transducer can be placed almost anywhere above the precordium, and one can obtain satisfactory cardiac echoes. Since the heart lies close to the transducer and penetration is not a problem, a high-frequency transducer can and should be used to enhance resolution. Since beam width is less of a problem in these small hearts, small-diameter transducers can be used. The technical disadvantages of examining such patients include the lack of cooperation and the need to conduct examinations at times in nurseries and incubators. There may also be chest deformities that impede the echocardiographic study, in addition to excessively rapid heart rate.

Probably the most challenging aspect of using echocardiography to detect congenital heart disease is the complex abnormalities that one may encounter.[5,6] Echocardiographers, whether physicians or technologists, must be knowledgeable of the many possible malformations. Physicians dealing primarily with adult patients see relatively few truly complex congenital anomalies since many patients with congenital heart disease do not survive to adulthood. However, the pediatric echocardiographer who constantly deals with extremely ill infants early in life must be prepared to analyze complicated and confusing congenital anomalies.

Because of the wide variety and possible combinations of congenital defects, the echocardiographic examination of a patient with congenital heart disease can be complex. The following discussion is not an exhaustive description of all possible uses of echocardiography in patients with congenital heart disease. The approach, rather, is somewhat simplified and intends to assist understanding how a patient with congenital heart disease can be approached echocardiographically. It should also be remembered that although the various congenital anomalies are discussed individually, combinations of abnormalities are the rule rather than the exception.

DEDUCTIVE ECHOCARDIOGRAPHY

One technique for analyzing patients with congenital malformations is the use of deductive echocardiography.[7,8,9] The principle behind this approach is to identify and locate the individual parts of the heart and then to try to reconstruct the total cardiac anatomy. One attempts to identify and locate the individual cardiac chambers within the chest. For example, to determine the location of the atria, one can use a chest roentgenogram. The situs of the atria almost invariably follows that of the lungs and usually the abdominal viscera. If a trilobe lung is on the right, as is normal, or if the abdominal viscera, as located by the stomach bubble and liver shadow, are in their correct positions, then the atria will also be in their proper locations. If the trilobed lung is on the left, then the atria will be reversed.[9]

The atria can also be positively identified by way of two-dimensional echocardiography.[9a] Through the subcostal examination, the inferior vena cava and hepatic veins can be identified. The chamber into which these vessels drain represents the systemic, or right atrium. It is possible to identify the pulmonary veins by way of an apical four-chamber two-dimensional examination. The pulmonary veins drain into the left atrium.

To locate and identify the atrioventricular valve one assumes that the mitral valve is continuous with a semilunar valve, normally the aortic valve.[8,10] There is no intervening tissue or crista between the mitral valve and its corresponding semilunar valve. Thus one scans from an atrioventricular valve toward the base of the heart. If the valve is continuous with a semilunar valve, then it is probably the mitral valve. Since the tricuspid valve is separated from its semilunar valve by a mass of tissue, it is not continuous. Having identified an atrioventricular valve as a mitral valve, one must then know the direction of the ultrasonic beam to determine whether that valve is on its proper left side or is malpositioned to the right.[9]

Two-dimensional echocardiography can also be used to identify the atrioventricular valves. The technique depends on the usual appearance of these valves in their short-axis presentation.[12] During diastole the two-leaflet mitral valve appears as an oval or "fish mouth" (Fig. 7–1). The tricuspid valve is a three-leaflet valve that has a hinge-like motion, with the anterior leaflet resembling a "comma" or "eyebrow." Occasionally, the three commissures can be positively identified (Fig. 7–2).

Another two-dimensional echocardiographic technique for identifying the atrioventricular valves depends on the insertion of the atrioventricular valves on the interventricular septum.[9a,12a] The tricuspid septal leaflet inserts in a more apical or inferior position than does the mitral septal leaflet. This identification is made by way of the apical four-chamber two-dimensional examination.

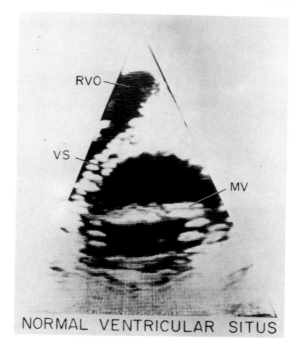

NORMAL VENTRICULAR SITUS

Fig. 7–1. Short-axis two-dimensional echocardiogram of a normal mitral valve (MV). This two-leaflet valve has a "fish-mouth" appearance when open. VS = ventricular septum; RVO = right ventricular outflow tract. (From Henry, W.L., and Griffith, J.M.: Cross-sectional echocardiographic evaluation of the atrioventricular valve in acquired and congenital heart disease. In Echocardiology. Edited by N. Bom. The Hague, Martinus Nijhoff, 1979.)

Locating and identifying the ventricles depend on the corresponding atrioventricular valves.[8] The left ventricle is invariably attached to the mitral valve and the right ventricle to the tricuspid valve. Thus, if the echocardiographer can identify the mitral valve echo, then the corresponding chamber in which it lies is the left ventricle. After identifying the proper chamber, one must again decide whether it is correctly positioned within the chest.

The next phase of this deductive approach is to identify the semilunar valves. Because of the higher resistance in the systemic circulation, the ejection time of the aortic valve is usually shorter than that of the pulmonary valve. Thus one way of differentiating between the aortic and pulmonary valves is to measure the ejection time; the valve with the shorter ejection time is the aortic valve. As

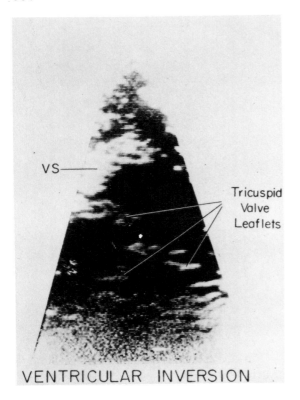

VS

Tricuspid
Valve
Leaflets

VENTRICULAR INVERSION

Fig. 7–2. Short-axis two-dimensional echocardiogram of a patient with ventricular inversion. A
three-leaflet tricuspid valve is in an inverted ventricle, which is in the normal position of the left ventricle. Note the three commissures. VS = ventricular
septum. (From Henry, W.L., and Griffith, J.M.: Cross-
sectional echocardiographic evaluation of the atrioventricular valves in acquired and congenital heart
disease. In Echocardiology. Edited by N. Bom. The
Hague, Martinus Nijhoff, 1977.)

one might expect, the differentiation may be
difficult in patients with severe pulmonary
hypertension, whereby the resistance in the
two circuits might be relatively equal. The
inhalation of oxygen may occasionally drop
the pulmonary vascular resistance sufficiently to make the differentiation. Pediatric echocardiographers who use this approach believe that this problem is not as
common as one might expect.

Having identified the semilunar valves,
the echocardiographer must then note the
direction of the ultrasonic beam as he attempts to position the valves in relation to
the ventricles. The corresponding great artery is identified by its corresponding

semilunar valve. Once the aortic valve is
recognized, then it is known that the artery in
which it lies is the aorta. The same is true for
the pulmonary valve and the pulmonary artery.

As expected, two-dimensional echocardiography assists greatly in the identification
of the semilunar valves and the great arteries.[13,14] When recording the two-
dimensional study, one is not nearly as dependent on the exact direction of the transducer. The two-dimensional technique also
offers a new approach for identifying the
great arteries. It is possible to recognize the
bifurcation of the pulmonary artery into its
right and left branches. Finding a great artery with this type of bifurcation helps establish the identity of the pulmonary artery.[15]
One may also record the arch of the aorta and
its branches to positively identify that great
artery.

Thus deductive echocardiography can
permit one to decipher many complex congenital anomalies. Naturally, the mere detection of the various parts of the heart can be
critical in the management of an individual
patient. Just knowing that a patient has four
cardiac valves can be extremely important. It
cannot be stressed too strongly that this approach requires an echocardiographer who
is familiar with complex congenital problems.

VENTRICULAR OUTFLOW OBSTRUCTION

Echocardiography's ability to record detailed cardiac anatomy enables the differentiation of many problems with similar clinical presentations. It may be difficult at times
to differentiate the various possible obstructions to ventricular outflow at the bedside.
Even hemodynamic and angiographic
studies may be limited in determining the
exact site of obstruction. The echocardiographic literature is filled with examples of
when echocardiography can be significant in
these congenital anomalies.

Valvular Aortic Stenosis

Aortic stenosis was discussed in the preceding chapter on acquired valvular heart
disease. However, because of the important
role of congenital aortic stenosis, this valvu-

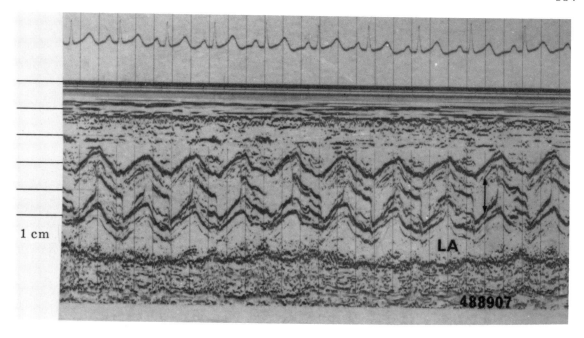

Fig. 7–3. M-mode echocardiogram of the aortic valve in a four-and-a-half-year-old child with severe congenital aortic stenosis. The apparent separation of the aortic valve leaflets *(arrow)* is within normal limits. LA = left atrium. (From Chang, S.: M-mode Echocardiographic Techniques and Pattern Recognition. Philadelphia, Lea & Febiger, 1976.)

lar problem is reviewed at this time. Although M-mode echocardiography is helpful in the qualitative diagnosis of valvular aortic stenosis, there is one important exception. Patients with congenital aortic stenosis and little calcium or thickening of the valve can manifest confusing M-mode echocardiograms. Because of the usual domed configuration of the congenital valve, the M-mode echocardiographic beam may merely record that portion of the valve near its attachment to the aortic annulus. During ventricular systole, this portion of the valve may separate quite adequately and one may see a normal box-like configuration of the aortic valve.[16] Figure 7–3 is an M-mode echocardiogram of a young child with severe congenital aortic stenosis. It would be difficult for one to make the proper diagnosis, and one certainly could not judge the severity of the stenosis from this particular tracing. Thus M-mode echocardiography has limited value in judging congenital valvular aortic stenosis, especially in the young patient without significant thickening of the valve.

Two-dimensional echocardiography plays an important role in the qualitative diagnosis of congenital aortic stenosis. Figure 7–4 demonstrates a two-dimensional examination of a patient with a normal aortic valve. In systole the leaflets open and are parallel to each other and to the walls of the aorta. Figure 7–5 shows a diastolic and systolic two-dimensional examination of a patient with congenital aortic stenosis. During diastole the multiple echoes from the thickened aortic valve are visible with the leaflets in the closed position. More important, during systole the curved, domed nature of the leaflets can be identified. The presence of "doming" is one of the most important two-dimensional criteria for the diagnosis of any stenotic valve.[17] The curved configuration demonstrates that the lack of opening of the orifice is due to anatomic limitations to opening the valve and not merely to a decrease in flow. With reduced flow the leaflets may not open widely, but they remain straight and not curved. Thus two-dimensional echocardiography has vastly improved the ultrasonic

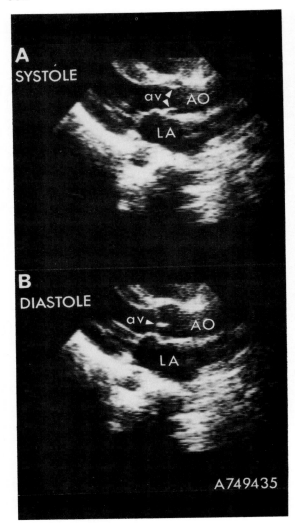

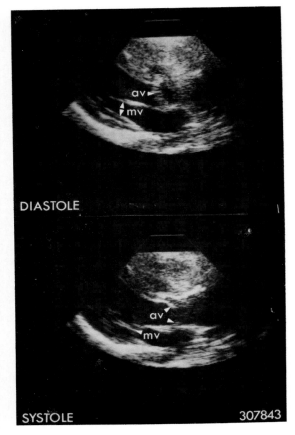

Fig. 7–5.   Long-axis two-dimensional echocardiograms of a patient with congenital aortic stenosis. The thickened aortic leaflets (av) can be seen in the closed position in diastole. In systole the leaflets curve into the aorta or "dome." mv = mitral valve.

Fig. 7–4.   Two-dimensional long-axis echocardiograms of a normal aortic valve. *A,* In systole, two of the aortic valve leaflets (av) open, making them parallel to each other as they lie near the walls of the aorta (AO). *B,* In diastole a bright echo is noted (av) at the point where the commissures of the leaflets meet. Faint echoes can be seen from the body of the leaflets. LA = left atrium.

technique's ability to qualitatively detect congenital valvular aortic stenosis.

Data indicate that the two-dimensional study can provide quantitative information concerning the degree of stenosis.[17] Figure 7–6 demonstrates how the separation of the leaflets at the tip of the orifice can be measured. As one would expect, a relationship exists between the separation of the leaflets and the severity of the stenosis. Figure 7–6 also demonstrates one way in which the leaflet separation or maximum aortic cusp separation (macs) can be corrected for body size. Instead of using body surface area or weight, a ratio of the leaflet separation (macs) and the diameter of the aortic annulus (AOD) is used for judging the severity of the stenosis.[18] The annular dimension gives the maximum potential opening of the leaflets. Theoretically, a normal valve should have a ratio of one. The ratio decreases significantly when the separation of the leaflets is reduced disproportionate to the size of the annulus.

It is apparent that a diameter of an orifice only predicts the cross-sectional area if the configuration of the orifice is a circle. As

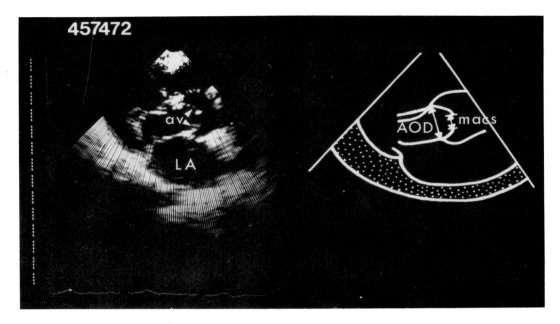

Fig. 7–6. Long-axis two-dimensional echocardiogram and diagram of a patient with a congenitally stenotic aortic valve that demonstrate how to measure the maximum aortic cusp separation (macs). This separation can be compared with the aortic diameter (AOD) in order to correct for body size. Note again the doming of the aortic leaflets (av). LA = left atrium.

noted in Chapter 6, aortic valve separation frequently does not correlate with the severity of the stenosis in calcific aortic stenosis. With a calcified valve the orifice infrequently assumes the shape of a perfect circle. However, with congenital heart disease the leaflets are more pliable, and if the tissue can assume the optimal geometric shape for flow, the stenotic orifice approximates a circle. Figure 7–7 is a short-axis study of a congenitally stenotic aortic valve. The thickened three-leaflet valve can be appreciated in diastole (A). With systole (B), an oval orifice is produced. The oval appearance is due partially to beam width that makes the lateral and medial borders thicker than the anterior and posterior borders of the orifice. The fact that most congenital valves in relatively young patients are sufficiently elastic to permit a somewhat circular orifice probably explains the good relationship between the echocardiographic diameter of valve opening and the severity of the stenosis.[18] Considering the limitations of judging the severity of aortic stenosis by way of hemodynamic or angiographic data, the correlation appears to have good clinical relevance. Unfortunately, as the valve becomes thicker, more fibrotic, and possibly calcified, the same problems that arise with calcific aortic stenosis arise when attempting to quantitate aortic stenosis by way of this technique.

Although a short-axis two-dimensional view of the aortic valve should provide a more accurate assessment of the degree of stenosis, from a technical point of view it is more difficult to examine the valve in this plane. In addition, the short-axis view of the aortic valve has some of the same limitations as the M-mode examination in that the plane of the examination constantly moves, and one cannot be absolutely certain as to when he is examining the tip of the orifice and that portion of the leaflets attached to the annulus. Figure 7–8 shows two aortic valve orifices from the same patient. The larger "orifice" (Fig. 7–8A) is a section through the valve near its attachment to the aorta. Figure 7–8B represents the true flow-restricting orifice.

As already discussed in the chapters on

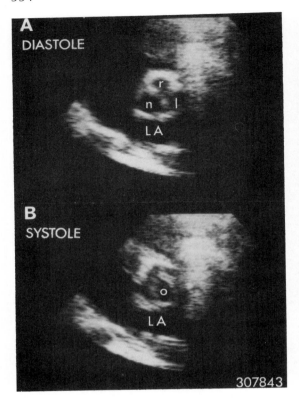

Fig. 7–7.   Short-axis echocardiogram of a congenitally stenotic aortic valve. *A*, In diastole, thickened cusps of the three-leaflet aortic valve can be seen. *B*, In systole, the oval, narrowed aortic orifice (o) can be detected. r = right coronary cusps; n = noncoronary cusps; l = left coronary cusps; LA = left atrium.

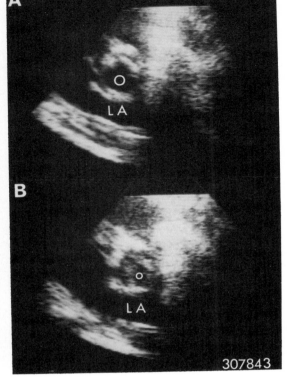

Fig. 7–8.   Short-axis echocardiograms of the aortic valve of the patient in Figure 7–7. The true flow-restricting aortic valve orifice (o) is noted in *B*. However, if the valve is examined closer to its attachment to the aorta, as in *A*, a larger orifice (O) can be recorded. LA = left atrium.

hemodynamics and acquired valvular heart disease (see Chapters 4 and 6), many echocardiographers have attempted to quantitate aortic stenosis by judging the hypertrophy of the left ventricle.[19–23] The most frequently used measurement is a ratio of the left ventricular thickness and the left ventricular cavity dimension at end-systole. Although there are obvious limitations to this approach, many studies demonstrate that this echocardiographic technique is of some value in young patients with valvular aortic stenosis.

Discrete Subaortic Stenosis

Discrete subaortic stenosis is usually divided into two basic subsections.[24–26] Type I is also known as membranous subaortic stenosis. Type II is a more diffuse fibromus-

cular type of stenosis.[26a] A more extreme example is the so-called tunnel aortic stenosis. Echocardiography provides both specific and nonspecific findings in discrete subaortic stenosis. The nonspecific finding common to all types of subaortic obstruction is systolic closure of the aortic valve.[27,28] Figure 7–9 shows an example of a patient with discrete subaortic stenosis. The aortic valve shows brisk opening of the valve in early systole. Immediately after opening, the valve partially closes with a marked downward motion of the anterior leaflet (arrow). As discussed in Chapter 4, this type of aortic valve echocardiogram is highly consistent in but not absolutely diagnostic of subaortic obstruction. Dynamic subvalvular stenosis also produces early systolic closure of the valve. Other abnormalities such as mitral

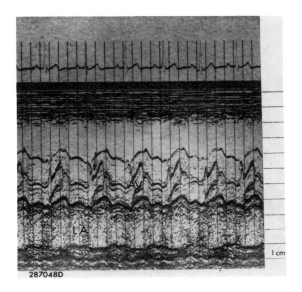

Fig. 7–9. M-mode echocardiogram of an aortic valve (AV) in a patient with discrete subaortic stenosis. In early systole there is rapid partial closure *(arrow)* of the aortic valve leaflets. LA = left atrium.

regurgitation and ventricular septal defect may also cause systolic aortic valve closure (see Chapter 4).

Both M-mode and two-dimensional echocardiography have been used to record the obstructing subvalvular tissue.[25,26,26a,29–33] Figure 7–10 shows an M-mode scan of a patient with diffuse fibromuscular, or Type II, subaortic stenosis.[25,29] The narrow left ventricular outflow tract (LVOT) between the

left ventricle (LV) and the aorta (AO) is demonstrated. The mitral valve also exhibits some systolic anterior motion, suggesting an element of dynamic subaortic stenosis. Another example of discrete subaortic stenosis is noted in Figure 7–11. This patient had a membranous, or Type I, subaortic obstruction, and a band of echo-producing tissue (large arrow) extends downward from the left side of the septum (LS) and nearly touches the mitral valve.[31] There is also an echo (small arrow) above the mitral valve that approaches the interventricular septum during systole. This echo does not resemble the typical systolic anterior motion found with dynamic subaortic obstruction.

Although the M-mode scan can demonstrate the area of narrowing in discrete subaortic stenosis, there is a lack of spatial orientation. In addition, if the M-mode scan is not made properly from the left ventricle into the aorta, one can obtain false-negative and false-positive recordings. Two-dimensional echocardiography is proving to be an important method for the diagnosis of discrete subaortic stenosis. Figure 7–12 shows the narrowed subaortic obstruction (SAO) in a patient with a Type II, or diffuse, obstruction. The narrowed area is produced principally by an anterior displacement of tissue from the junction between the anterior mitral leaflet and the aorta. There is also slight protrusion of tissue from the interventricular septum. Figure 7–13 shows a patient with a

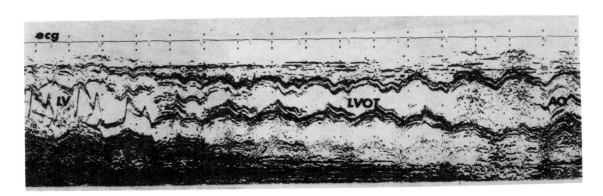

Fig. 7–10. M-mode scan of a patient with diffuse subvalvular aortic stenosis. Note the narrowed left ventricular outflow tract (LVOT) and the widened aorta (AO) at the level of the aortic valve. An element of systolic anterior motion of the mitral valve can be seen in the left ventricle (LV). (From Popp, R.L., et al.: Echocardiographic findings in discrete subvalvular aortic stenosis. Circulation, 49:226, 1974.)

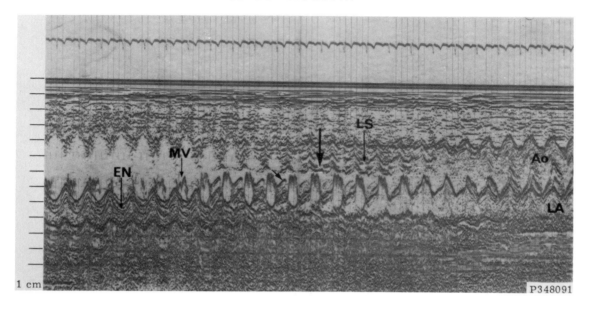

Fig. 7–11.   M-mode scan from the left ventricle to the aorta (AO) in a patient with a membranous, Type I subaortic stenosis. Extra echoes *(large arrow)* can be noted posterior to the left septal echoes (LS). There is also an echo *(small arrow)* attached to the mitral valve (MV) that is fairly prominent during systole. The abnormal echoes produce a significantly narrowed left ventricular outflow tract. EN = posterior left ventricular endocardium; LA = left atrium. (From Chang, S.: M-mode Echocardiographic Techniques and Pattern Recognition. Philadelphia, Lea & Febiger, 1976.)

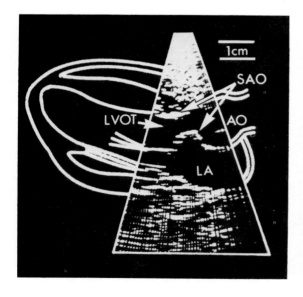

Fig. 7–12.   Two-dimensional long-axis echocardiogram of a patient with discrete subaortic stenosis. Note the subaortic obstruction (SAO) between the left ventricular outflow tract (LVOT) and the aorta (AO). LA = left atrium.

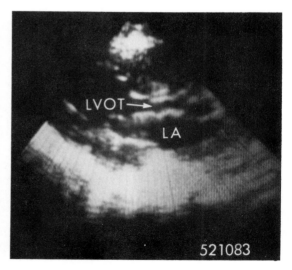

Fig. 7–13.   Long-axis two-dimensional echocardiogram of the left ventricular outflow tract (LVOT) in a patient with a tunnel subaortic obstruction. The subaortic narrowing is long and completely encompasses the left ventricular outflow tract. LA = left atrium.

more extreme form of diffuse subaortic stenosis. The narrowed area (LVOT) is long and is frequently referred to as a "tunnel" subaortic stenosis.[26a,29] These patients can be difficult to manage surgically. Type I, or membranous, subaortic stenosis manifests a different two-dimensional recording. Figure 7–14 shows a two-dimensional study of a patient with a discrete subaortic membranous obstruction. Echoes from the edges of the membrane (DSM) are frequently all that is recorded. Most of the relatively thin membrane is parallel to the ultrasonic beam and is not seen. It is sometimes difficult to identify the exact orifice of the membrane. The obstructing abnormality is considerably thinner than might be expected, judging from the width of the echo. One must remember that beam width makes the echo appear wider than the actual structure. In any case, the relatively narrow area of obstruction produces a strikingly different two-dimensional echocardiogram than does the more diffuse longer obstruction seen in the Type II variety. Thus two-dimensional echocardiography cannot only assist with the positive diagnosis of discrete subaortic

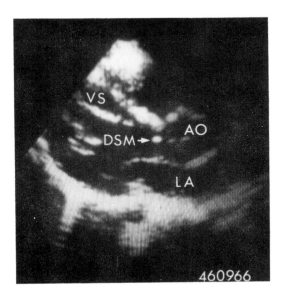

Fig. 7–14. Two-dimensional long-axis echocardiogram of a patient with a discrete, membranous subaortic stenosis. A single, bright echo can be seen originating from the discrete subaortic membrane (DSM) between the ventricular septum (VS) and the aorta (AO). LA = left atrium.

stenosis, but it can be helpful in subdividing the various types of subvalvular obstruction. Attempts at quantitating the degree of obstruction have not been successful thus far. Although one might suspect that the separation of the two sides of the subaortic obstruction might be related to the degree of obstruction, thus far such a measurement has not proved reliable.[32] Others have used wall thickness measurements, as in cases of valvular aortic stenosis, to judge the severity of dicrete subaortic obstruction.[34]

Dynamic Subaortic Obstruction

As noted in Figure 7–10, patients with fixed subaortic or valvular obstruction may also show evidence of dynamic obstruction. The echocardiographic feature for dynamic aortic obstruction is systolic anterior motion of the mitral valve. This topic is discussed more fully in Chapter 9 on cardiomyopathy. It should be remembered that dynamic obstruction is seen in patients with fixed ventricular outflow tract obstructions and should be looked for periodically. It is not easy to diagnose combined fixed and dynamic obstruction with any technique other than echocardiography.

Supravalvular Aortic Stenosis

Figure 7–15 is an M-mode scan of a patient with supravalvular aortic stenosis. The distance between the anterior and posterior walls of the aorta is 2.7 cm in the vicinity of the aortic valve. Immediately beyond the aortic valve, the aorta diminishes to 1.8 cm. As the scan proceeds superiorly, the aorta expands to 2.2 cm. Several investigators have demonstrated similar M-mode echocardiographic recordings.[30,35–38,38a] Such an examination requires constant scanning. If the examiner stops the scan or hesitates, the picture is distorted. In addition, one must constantly direct the beam through the center of the aorta, otherwise one could produce a false-positive narrowing of the aorta as the beam cuts across the wall rather than the center of the aorta.

Figure 7–16 shows a two-dimensional examination of a patient with supravalvular aortic stenosis. Again, the spatial orientation inherent in this examination improves the

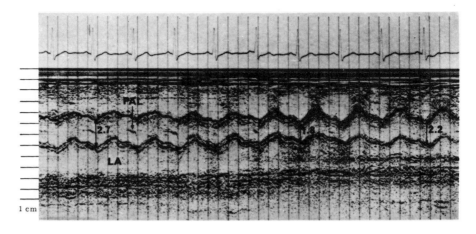

Fig. 7–15.   M-mode scan of a patient with supravalvular aortic stenosis. The aorta measures 2.7 cm at the level of the aortic valve leaflets and then diminishes to 1.8 cm above the aortic valve. As the beam proceeds superiorly, the aorta expands to 2.2 cm. PAL = posterior aortic valve leaflet; LA = left atrium. (From Chang, S.: M-mode Echocardiographic Techniques and Pattern Recognition. Philadelphia, Lea & Febiger, 1976.)

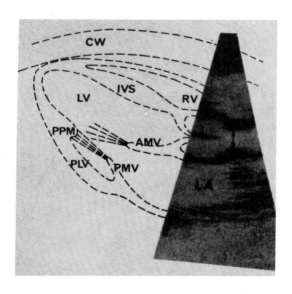

Fig. 7–16.   Cross-sectional echocardiogram of a patient with supravalvular aortic stenosis. Note the narrowed aorta above the aortic valve *(arrows)*. CW = chest wall; RV = right ventricle; LV = left ventricle; PPM = posterior papillary muscle; PMV = posterior mitral valve leaflet; PLV = posterior left ventricular wall; AO = aorta; LA = left atrium. (From Weyman, A.E., et al.: Localization of left ventricular outflow obstruction by cross-sectional echocardiography. Am. J. Med., 60:33, 1976.)

accuracy for this diagnosis.[17,30,39] The supravalvular area of narrowing (arrows) is readily apparent, and quantitation of the degree of obstruction is theoretically possible although such a study has yet to be done.

Hypoplastic Aorta and Aortic Atresia

Figure 7–17 shows an M-mode scan of a patient with a hypoplastic ascending aorta and congenital aortic stenosis. A marked decrease in the diameter of the aortic annulus is readily apparent from this study. A more extreme form of hypoplastic aorta is aortic atresia. Figure 7–18 is an M-mode scan of a patient with aortic atresia. The aorta is smaller than in Figure 7–17 and little, if any, aortic valve echoes can be seen. Figure 7–19 shows a two-dimensional examination of a patient with severe aortic hypoplasia, or atresia. As expected, the root of the aorta is extremely narrow.[17,39]

Aortic atresia is one of the causes of hypoplastic left heart syndrome.[40-44] The principal echocardiographic finding is a markedly underdeveloped left ventricle. Figure 7–20 shows a patient with aortic atresia and a hypoplastic left ventricle. The diagram

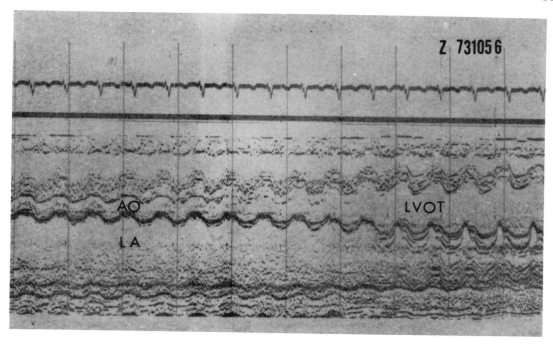

Fig. 7–17. M-mode scan of a patient with congenital aortic stenosis and a hypoplastic ascending aorta (AO). LVOT = left ventricular outflow tract; LA = left atrium.

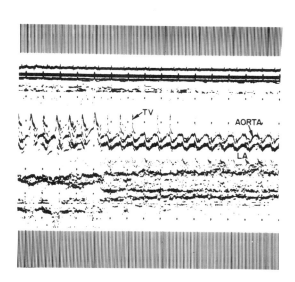

Fig. 7–18. M-mode scan of a patient with aortic atresia. A small aorta is visible as the beam moves from the tricuspid valve (TV) to the left atrium (LA). (From Meyer, R.A.: Pediatric Echocardiography. Philadelphia, Lea & Febiger, 1977.)

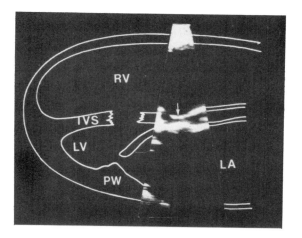

Fig. 7–19. Two-dimensional echocardiogram of a patient with severe hypoplasia of the aortic annulus and ascending aorta. The area of greatest narrowing is indicated by the arrow. RV = right ventricle; IVS = interventricular septum; LV = left ventricle; PW = posterior left ventricular wall; LA = left atrium. (From Weyman, A.E., et al.: Cross-sectional echocardiographic characterization of aortic obstruction. I. Supravalvular aortic stenosis and aortic hypoplasia. Circulation, 57:491, 1978. By permission of the American Heart Association, Inc.)

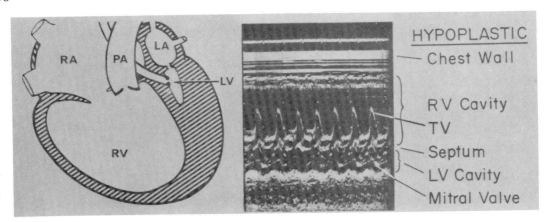

Fig. 7–20. Diagram and M-mode echocardiogram of a patient with aortic atresia and a hypoplastic left ventricle. RA = right atrium; PA = pulmonary artery; RV = right ventricle; LA = left atrium; LV = left ventricle; TV = tricuspid valve. (From Meyer, R.A. and Kaplan, S.: Echocardiography in the diagnosis of hypoplasia of the left or right ventricle in a neonate. Circulation, 45:55, 1972.)

demonstrates the aortic atresia and a very small left ventricular cavity. The echocardiogram shows a large right ventricular cavity, tricuspid valve, and a diminutive left ventricular cavity. A barely perceptible mitral valve can be noted. Probably the most reliable echocardiographic sign for hypoplastic left heart syndrome is an anterior mitral leaflet excursion of 5 mm or less.[44a]

Coarctation of the Aorta

Two-dimensional echocardiography now permits an ultrasonic recording of the arch of the aorta and the descending aorta.[45] Figure 7–21 shows a two-dimensional study of a normal aortic arch. One can frequently identify some branches of the aorta. There may be some artifactual narrowing of the descending aorta (DA) owing to beam width. Figure 7–22 shows a two-dimensional study of a patient with coarctation of the aorta. The carotid and subclavian arteries can be seen. Just distal to the subclavian artery is a marked decrease in the lumen of the aorta. Beyond the obstruction is a widened area corresponding to the poststenotic dilatation that commonly occurs with coarctation. Another prominent finding in the real-time examination of patients with coarctation is marked pulsations of the aorta proximal to the obstruction. Figure 7–23 is another two-dimensional study of the aorta in a pa-

tient with a coarctation. The narrowed area of the coarctation (C) is readily apparent. The poststenotic dilatation is marked and produces an aneurysm (AN) of this portion of the aorta.

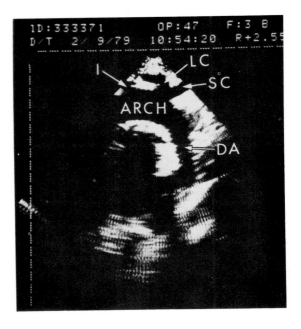

Fig. 7–21. Suprasternal two-dimensional echocardiogram of a normal aortic arch. The descending aorta (DA) may be artifactually narrowed because of beam width. I = innominate artery; LC = left common carotid; SC = subclavian.

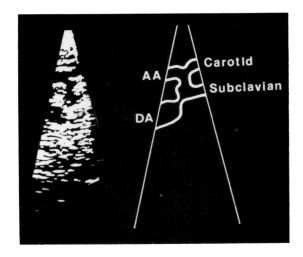

Fig. 7–22. Suprasternal two-dimensional echocardiogram and diagram of the arch of the aorta (AA) and descending aorta (DA) in a patient with coarctation. Note the narrowed area between the subclavian and the descending aorta. (From Weyman, A.E., et al.: Cross-sectional echocardiographic detection of aortic obstruction. II. Coarctation of the aorta. Circulation, 55:498, 1978. By permission of the American Heart Association, Inc.)

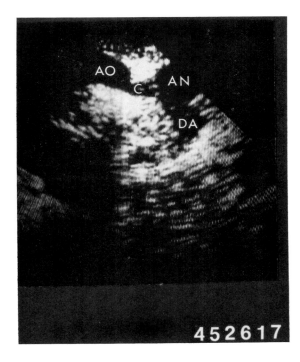

Fig. 7–23. Suprasternal two-dimensional echocardiogram of the aortic arch in a patient with coarctation and aneurysmal dilatation of the poststenotic area. The aneurysm (AN) is visible distal to the area of coarctation (C). AO = aorta; DA = descending aorta.

Pulmonic Stenosis

The M-mode echocardiographic criteria for the diagnosis of pulmonic stenosis depends on an exaggerated pulmonary valve A wave producing presystolic opening of the valve (Fig. 7–24).[46,47] Unfortunately, there are some false positives with this echocardiographic sign. Patients with slow heart rates and large stroke volumes may also have exaggerated A waves. Another limitation of the M-mode findings for pulmonic stenosis is that the sign is insensitive. Patients with mild pulmonic stenosis do not exhibit exaggerated A waves. Although this insensitivity is a limitation, the necessity for the pulmonic obstruction to be at least moderate or severe has introduced some quantitation into the diagnosis. If a patient with pulmonic stenosis has exaggerated A waves, there is a high probability that the obstruction is hemodynamically significant.

Two-dimensional echocardiography probably offers a better method for the qualitative diagnosis of pulmonic stenosis.[48] A normal pulmonary valve opens to its fullest extent and lies against the walls of the pulmonary artery (Fig. 7–25). In fact, it is normally difficult to see the pulmonary valve during systole because it is lost in the echoes from the pulmonary artery. In patients with valvular pulmonic stenosis, one again sees doming, which is a hallmark of all stenotic valves. During systole the stenotic and somewhat thickened valve curves away from the pulmonary artery and extends into the lumen of the vessel (Fig. 7–26). Usually one only sees the posterior pulmonary valve leaflet. On rare occasion one may also see an anterior leaflet curved into the pulmonary artery (Fig. 7–27). Since the anterior leaflet is rarely recorded, attempts at quantitating the degree of pulmonic stenosis is not practical by way of this technique. However, if a patient shows two-dimensional evidence of pulmonic stenosis and the M-mode echocardiogram shows exaggerated A waves, one has good evidence that hemodynamically significant pulmonary stenosis exists. If the two-dimensional echocardiogram is positive and the M-mode study is negative, then there is reasonable assurance that the degree of obstruction is mild.

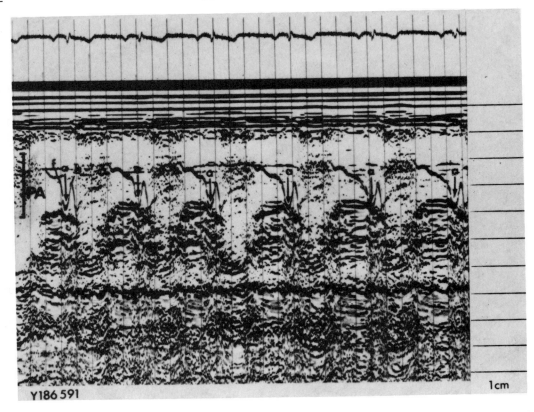

Fig. 7–24. M-mode echocardiogram of a pulmonary valve in a patient with pulmonic stenosis. Markedly accentuated A waves (a) can be noted. PA = pulmonary artery. (From Weyman, A.E.: Pulmonary valve echo motion in clinical practice. Am. J. Med., 62:843, 1977.)

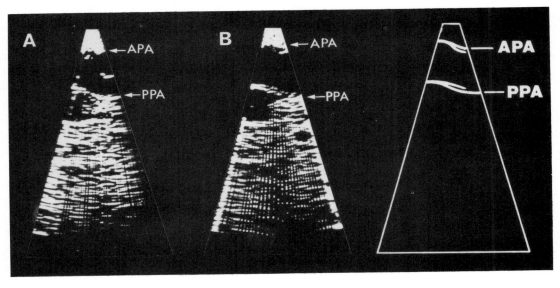

Fig. 7–25. Two-dimensional echocardiogram and diagram of a normal pulmonary valve in diastole, A, and systole, B. The diagram demonstrates the location of the opened leaflets against the walls of the pulmonary artery. APA = anterior wall of the pulmonary artery; PPA = posterior wall of the pulmonary artery. (From Weyman, A.E., et al.: Cross-sectional echocardiographic visualization of the stenotic pulmonary valve. Circulation, 56:769, 1977. By permission of the American Heart Association, Inc.)

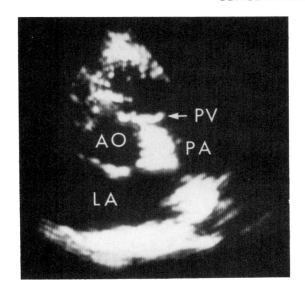

Fig. 7–26. Two-dimensional echocardiogram of a patient with pulmonic stenosis. The domed stenotic pulmonary valve (PV) curves into the pulmonary artery (PA) in this systolic frame. AO = aorta; LA = left atrium.

Doppler echocardiography has been used for the qualitative diagnosis of pulmonic stenosis.[49] The turbulent flow in the pulmonary artery can be detected with the Doppler technique. However, the reliability and sensitivity of this examination is still uncertain.

Subpulmonic Stenosis

Figure 7–28 is a pulmonary valve echocardiogram of a patient with subpulmonic stenosis. The striking observation is a fluttering of the pulmonary valve throughout systole.[50] Unfortunately, this finding may be subtle, since some fluttering can be normal, as it is with the aortic valve. The differentiating feature probably depends on the amplitude of the fluttering rather than on the frequency. In Figure 7–28 the individual fluttering motions are clearly distinct and may be several millimeters in depth. Figure 7–29 is from another patient with subpulmonic stenosis. Again, fluttering of the pulmonary valve can be detected. In this case, the frequency of the fluttering is possibly less rapid than in Figure 7–28. However, the

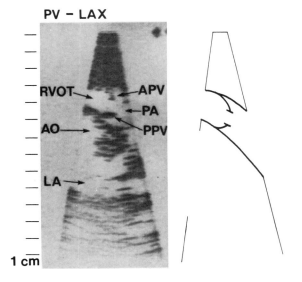

Fig. 7–27. Two-dimensional echocardiogram of a stenotic pulmonary valve demonstrating doming of both the anterior (APV) and posterior (PPV) pulmonary valve leaflets. RVOT = right ventricular outflow tract; PA = pulmonary artery; AO = aorta; LA = left atrium.

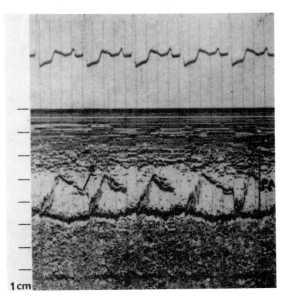

Fig. 7–28. Pulmonary valve M-mode echocardiogram of a patient with mild infundibular pulmonic stenosis. Note the fine fluttering of the valve throughout systole (a). PA = pulmonary artery. (From Weyman, A.E., et al.: Echocardiographic differentiation of infundibular from valvular pulmonic stenosis. Am. J. Cardiol., 36:21, 1975.)

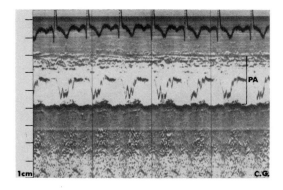

Fig. 7–29. M-mode echocardiogram of a pulmonary valve in a patient with severe infundibular stenosis. Coarse systolic fluttering can be seen throughout systole, continuing into early diastole. In addition, no A wave is detected. PA = pulmonary artery.

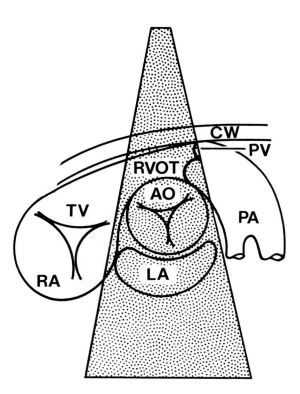

Fig. 7–30. Diagram demonstrating how two-dimensional echocardiography can record the right ventricular outflow tract (RVOT). CW = chest wall; PV = pulmonary valve; AO = aorta; TV = tricuspid valve; RA = right atrium; LA = left atrium; PA = pulmonary artery. (From Caldwell, R.L., et al.: Right ventricular outflow tract assessment by cross-sectional echocardiography in tetralogy of Fallot. Circulation, 59:395, 1979. By permission of the American Heart Association, Inc.)

depth of the fluttering motion is quite striking and is several millimeters in amplitude. This patient had severe subpulmonic obstruction and no A wave is detected. The diastolic slope is also flat. There was no pulmonary hypertension. The tight subvalvular obstruction may have been a factor in eliminating the A wave. Note that in Figure 7–28 the A wave is intact and the subpulmonic obstruction was much less.

Subpulmonic obstruction is a common component of other congenital problems. Tetralogy of Fallot is one of the more common anomalies in which obstruction in the subpulmonic area is frequent. Figure 7–30 shows a diagram of a short-axis examination of the right ventricular outflow tract. This examination can be helpful in judging the size of the right ventricular outflow tract for possible subpulmonic obstruction and has been described principally for judging the severity of the outflow obstruction in patients with tetralogy of Fallot.[51]

VENTRICULAR INFLOW OBSTRUCTION

As is the case in outflow obstructions, there is a variety of congenital abnormalities that impede filling of the ventricles. Many of these conditions manifest themselves in similar clinical fashion. Echocardiography has shown value in being able to differentiate between many of these confusing situations.

Congenital Mitral Stenosis

Congenital mitral stenosis may appear echocardiographically similar to acquired rheumatic mitral stenosis.[52] Aside from the fact that these valves probably do not calcify as often, the same echocardiographic criteria used to describe and quantitate mitral stenosis in adults are used to describe congenital mitral stenosis in children.[53-55] However, there are frequent differences with congenital mitral stenosis, especially in young infants. The valves tend to be more pliable, and attempts at quantitation by way of M-mode echocardiography are even less reliable than in acquired mitral stenosis. Figure 7–31 shows a patient with congenital mitral stenosis. The abnormal posterior mitral leaflet (PML) motion is fairly striking

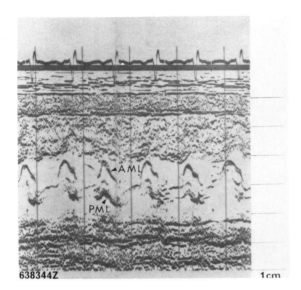

Fig. 7–31. M-mode echocardiogram of a mitral valve in a patient with congenital mitral stenosis. AML = anterior mitral leaflet; PML = posterior mitral leaflet.

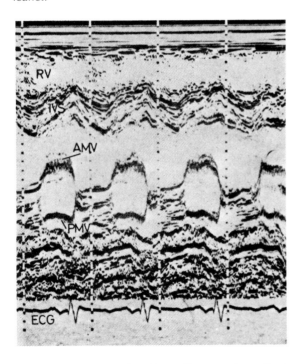

Fig. 7–32. M-mode echocardiogram of a patient with congenital mitral stenosis. The posterior mitral leaflet (PMV) moves downward. Fine diastolic fluttering can be seen in the anterior mitral leaflet (AMV). RV = right ventricle; IVS = interventricular septum. (From Driscoll, D.J., Gutgesell, H.P., and McNamara, D.G.: Echocardiographic features of congenital mitral stenosis. Am. J. Cardiol., 42:259, 1978.)

and is the most obvious sign of mitral stenosis in this patient. In addition, there is a decrease if not a lack of A wave on the mitral valve despite the sinus rhythm. Figure 7–32 shows another patient with congenital mitral stenosis. In this example, the posterior leaflet motion is normal, and only the decreased diastolic slope and decreased A wave provide an opportunity for a correct diagnosis.[55] Figure 7–32 also demonstrates diastolic fluttering of the anterior leaflet (AMV),[55] a finding that is rarely seen in acquired mitral stenosis unless aortic regurgitation is also present.

Parachute Mitral Valve

A parachute mitral valve is another form of congenital mitral stenosis whereby all valve

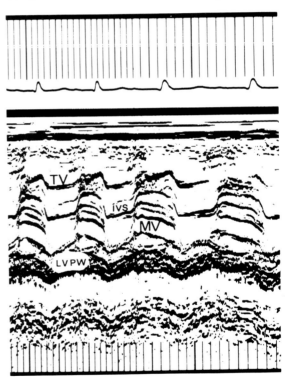

Fig. 7–33. M-mode echocardiogram of a patient with a parachute mitral valve. The principal echocardiographic feature is the presence of multiple echoes from the mitral valve (MV). TV = tricuspid valve; IVS = interventricular septum; LVPW = left ventricular posterior wall. (From LaCorte, M., Havada, K., and Williams, R.G.: Echocardiographic features of congenital left ventricular inflow obstruction. Circulation, 54:562, 1976. By permission of the American Heart Association, Inc.)

chordae insert into a single papillary muscle.[56,57] Figure 7–33 shows an echocardiogram of a patient with a parachute mitral valve. The principal echocardiographic finding is multiple mitral valve echoes. There are at least three different echoes from the anterior leaflet. The posterior leaflet motion is also abnormal, suggesting some element of stenosis.

There are relatively few examples of parachute mitral valve in the echocardiographic literature. Thus the reliability of these echocardiographic findings is unknown. However, there is a case report of a patient with a parachute mitral valve in whom the anterior mitral leaflet produced a left ventricular outflow obstruction that was detected echocardiographically.[58]

Obstructions Within the Left Atrium

Supravalvular mitral stenosis, left atrial membrane, and cor triatriatum are all characterized by an obstructing membrane on the atrial side of the mitral valve.[57,59,60,60a,60b] This obstructing membrane may be close to the mitral valve or may subdivide the left atrial cavity. Figure 7–34 shows a patient with both congenital mitral stenosis and a supravalvular membrane, or ring. The membrane lies immediately posterior to the mitral valve as indicated by the white arrow. The stenotic mitral valve is noted by the black arrow. Figure 7–35 shows a patient with a left atrial membrane (arrow). The membrane can be seen encroaching on the left ventricular inflow tract. A similar echocardiogram is seen in Figure 7–36. This patient had a cor triatriatum. The arrows point to the obstructing membrane in the left atrium. Figure 7–37 illustrates pre- and postoperative M-mode echocardiograms of a patient whose left atrial membrane was removed surgically. The membrane echo (M), noted in the preoperative recording, is absent following surgery.

As might be expected, two-dimensional echocardiography can contribute to the diagnosis of membranes within the left atrium. Figure 7–38 shows a two-dimensional study in which the left atrial membrane is visible within that chamber immediately posterior to the mitral valve.

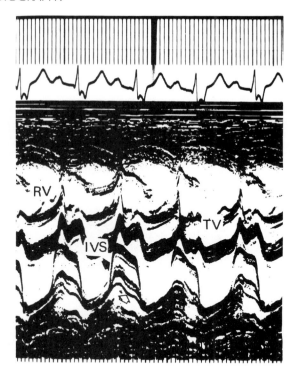

Fig. 7–34. Mitral valve echocardiogram of a patient with a supravalvular membrane or ring and congenital mitral stenosis. Note the echo from the supravalvular ring or left atrial membrane (white arrow). The black arrow indicates the stenotic mitral valve. RV = right ventricle; TV = tricuspid valve; IVS = interventricular septum. (From LaCorte, M. Havada, K., and Williams, R.G.: Echocardiographic features of congenital left ventricular inflow obstruction. Circulation, 54:562, 1976. By permission of the American Heart Association, Inc.)

Mitral Atresia

Figure 7–39 shows an M-mode echocardiogram of a patient with mitral valve atresia. The aorta and tricuspid valve (TV) can be identified. There is no identifiable mitral valve; one can only see some dense echoes coming from the mitral valve region. Another way of diagnosing mitral atresia is to identify a hypoplastic left ventricle (Fig. 7–20).[41–44]

Tricuspid Atresia

Tricuspid atresia may be seen by both adult and pediatric echocardiographers. As expected, tricuspid atresia produces a hypoplastic right ventricle.[40,41,61] Figure 7–40 is an echocardiogram of a patient with

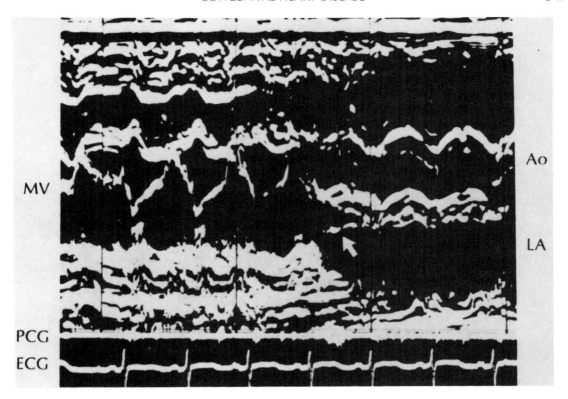

Fig. 7–35.   M-mode scan of a patient with a left atrial membrane. The echo from the membrane *(arrow)* is seen at the junction between the left ventricle and the left atrium. MV = mitral valve; AO = aorta; LA = left atrium; PCG = phonocardiogram; ECG = electrocardiogram. (From Nanda, N.C., and Gramiak, R.: Clinical Echocardiography. St. Louis, C.V. Mosby Co., 1978.)

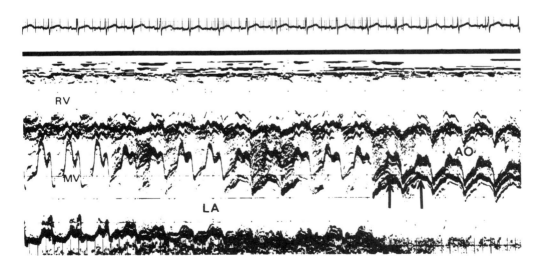

Fig. 7–36.   M-mode scan of a patient with cor triatriatum. The echo from the structure dividing the left atrium into two chambers is indicated by the arrows. RV = right ventricle; LA = left atrium; MV = mitral valve; AO = aorta. (From LaCorte, M., Havada, K., and Williams, R.G.: Echocardiographic features of congenital left ventricular inflow obstruction. Circulation, 54:562, 1976. By permission of the American Heart Association, Inc.)

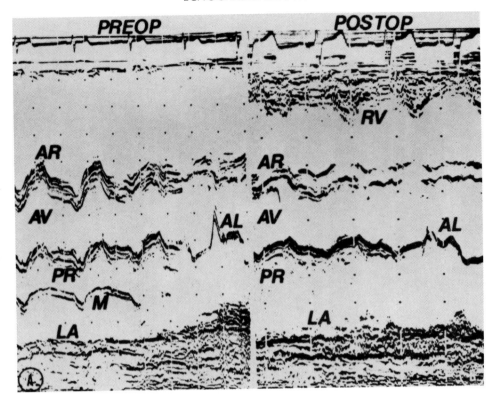

Fig. 7–37.   Pre- and postoperative M-mode echocardiograms of a patient with a left atrial membrane. The echo from the membrane (M) can be seen preoperatively and is no longer present in the postoperative tracing. AR = anterior root of the aorta; AV = aortic valve; AL = anterior leaflet of the mitral valve; PR = posterior root of the aorta; LA = left atrium. (From Ehrich, D.A., et al.: Cor triatriatum: report of case in a young adult with special reference to the echocardiographic features and etiology of the systolic murmur. Am. Heart J., 94:217, 1977.)

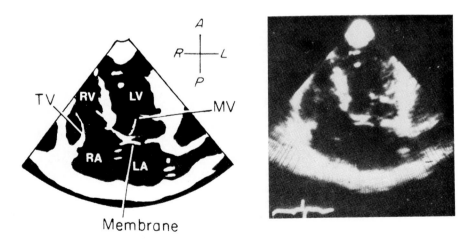

Fig. 7–38.   Apical four-chamber two-dimensional echocardiogram and diagram of a patient with a left atrial membrane. The membrane is visible immediately posterior to the mitral valve (MV) within the left atrium (LA). RV = right ventricle; LV = left ventricle; TV = tricuspid valve; RA = right atrium. (From Roge, Snyder, and Silverman: Echocardiographic evaluation of left ventricular inflow obstruction in children using an 80° two-dimensional sector scanner. In Echocardiology. Edited by C.T. Lancee. The Hague, Martinus Nijhoff, 1979.)

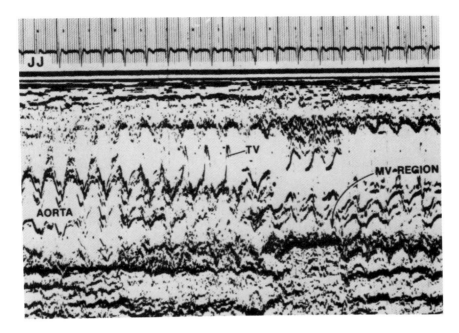

Fig. 7–39. M-mode scan of a neonate with mitral valve atresia and a ventricular septal defect demonstrating the inability to record a mitral valve (MV) echo when scanning in the appropriate area. TV = tricuspid valve. (From Meyer, R.A.: Pediatric Echocardiography. Philadelphia, Lea & Febiger, 1977.)

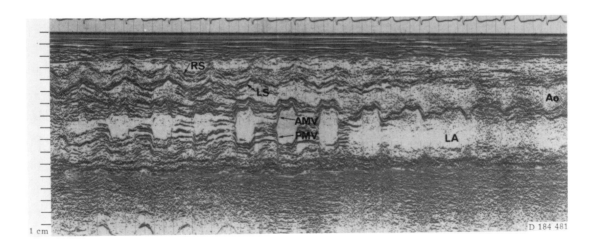

Fig. 7–40. Echocardiogram demonstrating a hypoplastic right ventricle in a patient with tricuspid atresia. There is very little space between the right side of the septum (RS) and the chest wall echoes. LS = left septum; AMV = anterior mitral valve leaflet; PMV = posterior mitral valve leaflet; LA = left atrium; AO = aorta.

tricuspid atresia. The interventricular septal echoes are close to the chest wall with little space for a right ventricular cavity. The mitral valve echoes are quite prominent and open widely since all cardiac output passes through this atrioventricular valve. Occasionally, one may find an echo that simulates a tricuspid valve in a patient with tricuspid atresia.[62]

There have been a few reports of using two-dimensional echocardiography in the diagnosis of tricuspid atresia.[63] Figure 7–41 shows a four-chamber view of a patient with tricuspid atresia. One can identify a large left ventricular cavity (LV) and a small right ventricular chamber (RV). The opened mitral valve (MV) protrudes into the left ventricular cavity. The region of the tricuspid valve, between the right ventricle and right atrium, shows only a dense band of linear echoes. There is no identifiable tricuspid valve. One must be cautious, of course, in making the diagnosis of tricuspid atresia. A band of echoes in the vicinity of the atrioventricular valve is commonly noted. These echoes originate from the atrioventricular annulus.

One must scan the area carefully to ensure that the tricuspid valvular leaflets are not missed and are truly absent.

OTHER CONGENITAL VALVULAR ABNORMALITIES

Bicuspid Aortic Valve

A bicuspid aortic valve is possibly the most common congenital anomaly. Figure 7–42 diagrammatically shows the rationale behind the M-mode echocardiographic criteria for the diagnosis of bicuspid aortic valve. Figure 7–42a illustrates the finding in a normal aortic valve. The principal feature in the normal situation is all three cusps meeting in the midline so that the dominant diastolic echo is approximately equidistant from the anterior and posterior walls of the aorta. Figure 7–42b, c, d depict three types of aortic valve echocardiograms possible with a bicuspid aortic valve. In Figure 7–42b there is a small and a large leaflet. When the valve closes, the commissure between the two cusps is eccentrically located and thus is closer to one of the walls of the aorta. In this

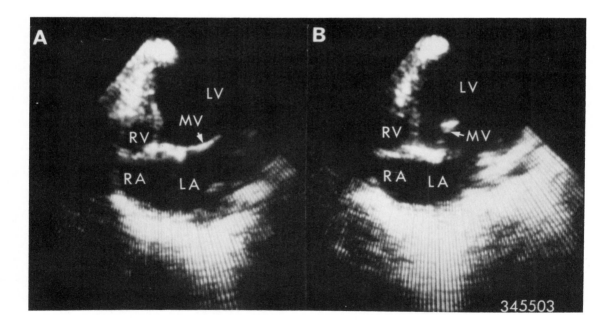

Fig. 7–41. Apical four-chamber two-dimensional echocardiogram of a patient with tricuspid atresia. The mitral valve (MV) can be seen opening into a large left ventricular chamber (LV). The right ventricle (RV) is small and separated from the right atrium (RA) by a dense band of linear echoes. No valvular structure could be identified in the region of the tricuspid valve. LA = left atrium.

illustration the commissure is closer to the anterior wall; in other situations it might be closer to the posterior wall. Thus the finding of eccentricity of the diastolic aortic valve echo is one of the criteria offered as an echocardiographic sign of a bicuspid aortic valve. Figure 7–42c and d show the effect of redundancy of one of the cusps. In one situation, the diastolic echoes may be in one location at the beginning of diastole and then may change position during the rest of diastole. Another variation is multiple diastolic echoes coming from the wavy edge of redundant cusps. Figure 7–43 shows actual echocardiograms of a normal three-leaflet aortic valve (A) and a bicuspid aortic valve (B). Figure 7–43A shows a normal tricuspid valve with the diastolic aortic valve echo between the two aortic valve echoes. Figure 7–43B shows the diastolic echo to be extremely low and immediately above the posterior aortic wall echo.

The echocardiographic finding for bicuspid aortic valve has been confirmed by other investigators.[64] An eccentricity index of 1.3 or more was believed to be a reliable statistic provided there was no associated ventricular septal defect. False-positive indices were obtained with a high membranous ventricular septal defect, possibly the result of a

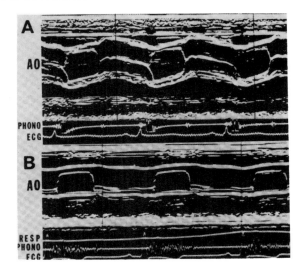

Fig. 7–43. M-mode aortic valve echocardiograms of a normal three-leaflet aortic valve and a bicuspid aortic valve. A, In diastole, the echoes from a normal valve meet in a midposition within the aorta. B, With a bicuspid valve the diastolic echoes are eccentric and much closer to one of the aortic walls. (From Nanda, N.C., et al.: Echocardiographic recognition of the congenital bicuspid aortic valve. Circulation, 49:870, 1974.)

nonsupported aortic cusp. Unfortunately, there have been other false positives and false negatives noted when the eccentricity index alone is used for the diagnosis of bicuspid aortic valve. For example, in Figure 7–4B the closed aortic valve leaflets meet below the midpoint of the aorta and one might suspect a bicuspid valve. Figure 7–44 shows the short-axis two-dimensional examination of this same patient. Three separate leaflets are recorded in this normal aortic valve. Thus the echocardiographic eccentricity index is useful, but it must be placed in its clinical setting because it is not totally reliable.

One group of investigators suggested that one could detect a bicuspid aortic valve with the transducer at the apex.[65] A normal valve would not be seen with this approach since all leaflets would be parallel to the beam. Thus recording the opened aortic valve from this transducer position indicated a possible bicuspid valve.

The two-dimensional echocardiographic examination of bicuspid aortic valve has

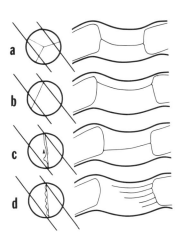

Fig. 7–42. Diagram demonstrating the echocardiographic recording of the normal three-leaflet aortic valve (a) and the various patterns seen with bicuspid aortic valves (b, c, d). (From Nanda, N.C., et al.: Echocardiographic recognition of the congenital bicuspid aortic valve. Circulation, 49:870, 1974.)

been described.[66] As expected, one should see only two aortic cusps in such individuals. Figure 7–45 shows a two-dimensional study of a patient with a bicuspid valve. The commissures are well delineated, and only two cusps are clearly recorded. Unfortunately, the more vertical commissure between the left and noncoronary cusps is not always easy to record echocardiographically (Fig. 7–44). Thus a false-positive diagnosis of bicuspid valve might be a fairly frequent finding. The reliability and sensitivity of two-dimensional echocardiography for the diagnosis of bicuspid aortic valve has not been determined.

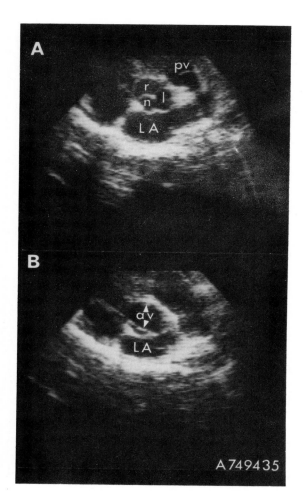

Fig. 7–44. Short-axis two-dimensional echocardiograms of a normal three-leaflet aortic valve (av) in diastole, A, and systole, B. r = right coronary cusps; n = noncoronary cusps; l = left coronary cusps; pv = pulmonary valve; LA = left atrium.

Cleft Mitral Valve

A cleft mitral valve commonly occurs with atrioventricular canal defects. Figure 7–46 shows an example of such an abnormality. This short-axis two-dimensional view of the mitral valve shows a split of the anterior leaflet, so that the usual fish-mouth appearance is not present. The two halves of the split anterior leaflet are readily visible.[67] One must be careful not to confuse a cleft mitral valve with a malpositioned tricuspid valve (Fig. 7–2) or with prominent papillary muscle echoes.

Ebstein's Anomaly

Ebstein's anomaly of the tricuspid valve may produce several echocardiographic changes. Figure 7–47 shows the most consistent M-mode echocardiographic finding in this disease. This echocardiogram recorded simultaneous tricuspid and mitral valve echoes. The most consistent finding is delayed closure of the tricuspid valve, especially when compared with that of the mitral valve.[54,68-73] In the diagram, tricuspid closure, which corresponds with the onset of the tricuspid first sound (T1), is significantly later than mitral valve closure, which occurs with the mitral first sound (M1). If the tricuspid valve closes at least 50 msec after the mitral valve, then the diagnosis of Ebstein's anomaly should be considered.[72] Another study indicated that a tricuspid-mitral closure interval of more than 65 msec was diagnostic for Ebstein's anomaly.[74a] Other investigators have indicated that tricuspid valve intervals of more than 30 msec are compatible with the diagnosis of Ebstein's anomaly.[75] In one case, a patient with Ebstein's anomaly and Type B Wolff-Parkinson-White syndrome had early closure of the tricuspid valve.[76]

Other M-mode echocardiographic criteria for the diagnosis of Ebstein's anomaly have been described.[69,71] Figure 7–47 also demonstrates a decreased diastolic slope that is fairly typical in Ebstein's anomaly.[77] Another tricuspid valve echocardiogram of a patient with Ebstein's anomaly is shown in Figure 7–48 and illustrates that the diastolic slope may be a function of the heart rate. Following a premature ventricular systole and a

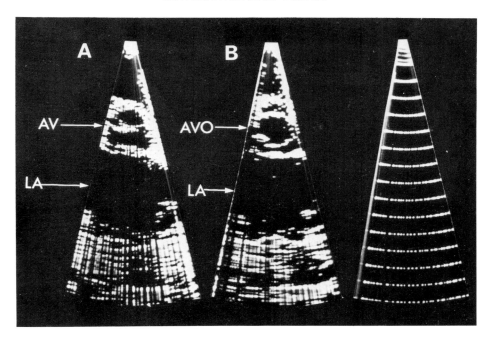

Fig. 7–45.   Short-axis two-dimensional echocardiogram of a bicuspid aortic valve (AV) in diastole, *A*, and systole, *B*. AVO = aortic valve orifice; LA = left atrium.

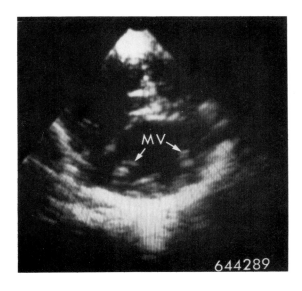

Fig. 7–46.   Short-axis two-dimensional echocardiogram through the left ventricle at the level of the mitral valve in a patient with a cleft mitral valve (MV). The anterior leaflet is split, and the edges of the leaflet are separated in this diastolic frame.

long diastolic interval, a more rapid diastolic slope can be seen. Admittedly, the faster slope occurred late in diastole, and none of the complexes demonstrate a rapid E to F slope. Another echocardiographic finding that has been described in conjunction with this anomaly is increased amplitude of motion of the tricuspid valve leaflet.[69] Figure 7–48 shows this phenomenon; the total excursion of the anterior leaflet is approximately 3 cm. However, it should be remembered that there is significant variability in this congenital problem. Insertions of the leaflets can vary from one patient to another as can the M-mode findings.

Two-dimensional echocardiography can help in the diagnosis of Ebstein's anomaly.[78–80,80a] In some respects, the two-dimensional approach may be more definitive in that this technique provides an opportunity to identify the exact anatomic abnormality. Figure 7–49 shows a two-dimensional echocardiogram and a diagram of a patient with Ebstein's anomaly. This four-chamber view reveals a displaced tricuspid valve in the cavity of the right ventricle.

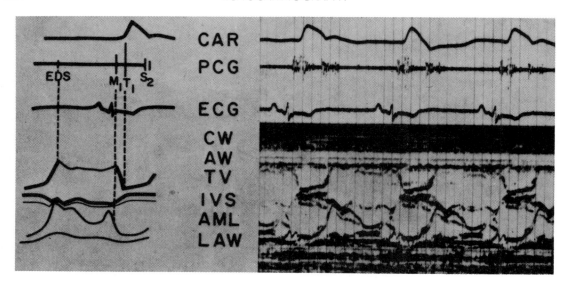

Fig. 7–47.   Diagram and echocardiogram of simultaneous tricuspid and mitral valve recordings of a patient with Ebstein's anomaly. The characteristic finding in this congenital abnormality is delayed closure of the tricuspid valve (TV) at least 50 milliseconds after anterior mitral valve closure (AML). CAR = carotid artery; PCG = phonocardiogram; ECG = electrocardiogram; CW = chest wall; AW = atrial wall; IVS = interventricular septum; LAW = left atrial wall; EDS = early diastolic sound. (From Tajik, A.J., et al.: Echocardiogram in Ebstein's anomaly with Wolff-Parkinson-White pre-excitation syndrome, Type B. Circulation, *47*:813, 1973.)

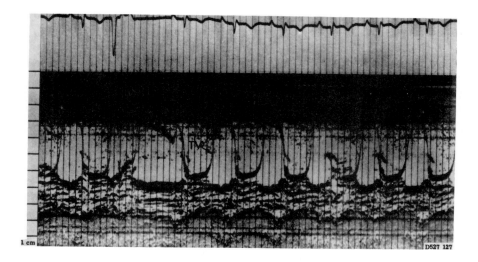

Fig. 7–48.   Tricuspid valve M-mode echocardiogram of a patient with Ebstein's anomaly. The amplitude of motion of the tricuspid valve (TV) is increased, and the diastolic slope is decreased in early diastole. The slope is steeper in late diastole with a long diastolic interval.

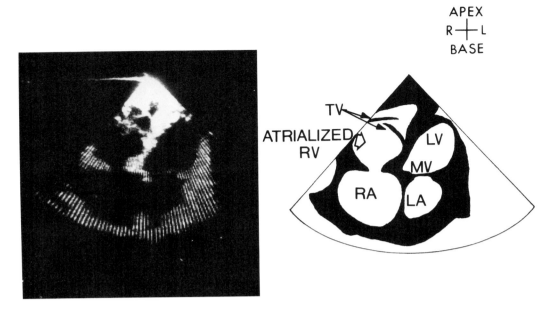

Fig. 7–49.   Apical two-chamber two-dimensional echocardiogram and diagram of a patient with Ebstein's anomaly. The displaced tricuspid valve (TV) is deep within the cavity of the right ventricle, producing a large atrialized right ventricle (RV). RA = right atrium; LA = left atrium; MV = mitral valve; LV = left ventricle. (From Schiller, N.B. and Silverman, N.H.: Two-dimensional ultrasonic cardiac imaging. In Echocardiography: Interpretation and Diagnosis. Edited by J.J. Kleid and S.B. Arvan. New York, Appleton-Century-Crofts, 1978.)

There is still a remnant of the right-sided atrioventricular annulus, but no tricuspid leaflet is recorded in that area. Instead, the tricuspid leaflet was recorded well within the right ventricular cavity, producing an atrialized portion of the right ventricle. In one two-dimensional echocardiographic study of patients with Ebstein's anomaly, the distance between the insertion of the mitral and tricuspid septal leaflets ranged from 1.4 to 3.2 cm.[81] Normally, there is only a few millimeters' separation between the insertion of the two leaflets. Occasionally, echoes from a moderator band can be seen within the right ventricular cavity and must not be confused with a displaced tricuspid valve.

Straddling Tricuspid Valve

A congenital valvular problem that may accompany other abnormalities is a straddling tricuspid valve.[82] This condition invariably accompanies a large ventricular septal defect whereby part of the tricuspid valve apparatus inserts into papillary muscles on the left side of the interventricular septum. Such an abnormality could represent a significant complication when contemplating surgery. The principal echocardiographic criterion with a straddling tricuspid valve is to identify parts of the tricuspid valve posterior to the echoes of the interventricular septum (Fig. 7–50).[83,84] Because of the lack of spatial orientation of the M-mode echocardiogram, such a sign has definite limitations. In patients with an atrioventricular canal defect and no straddling tricuspid valve, the M-mode recording may have a similar appearance. Straddling tricuspid valves can also be seen with two-dimensional echocardiography.[85,86] This condition is best diagnosed in real time. It is difficult to show this anomaly in a single frame. The major two-dimensional criterion is to identify the moving tricuspid leaflet to the left of the interventricular septum.

Straddling of the mitral valve may also occur, but thus far there have not been any echocardiographic recordings of such an abnormality in the literature.

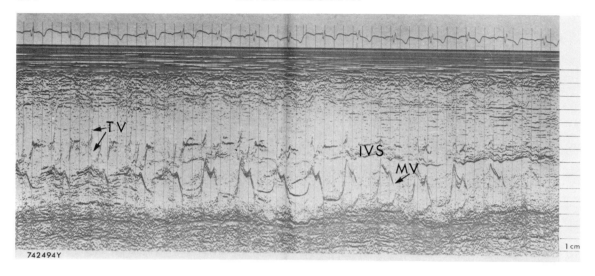

Fig. 7–50. M-mode scan of a patient with a straddling tricuspid valve. Echoes from the tricuspid valve (TV) can be seen above and below the level of the interventricular septal echoes (IVS). MV = mitral valve.

SHUNTS

Patent Ductus Arteriosus

The proper diagnosis of a patent ductus arteriosus is very important, especially in the newborn infant and young child. With a large left-to-right shunt these patients go into severe left heart failure and have a respiratory distress syndrome.[86a,b] The principal echocardiographic technique used to evaluate such patients is the M-mode examination of the left atrium. The shunted blood bypasses the systemic circulation and drains back into the left atrium via the pulmonary circuit. Thus the left atrium must handle both the normal pulmonary venous return and the shunted blood. As a result, dilatation of the left atrium is a common finding in patients with patent ductus arteriosus and a large left-to-right shunt.[87] Several investigators have found that taking the ratio of the left atrial dimension divided by the aortic dimension is a useful way to assess the size of the shunt.[87,88] Normally, this ratio should be between 0.7 and 0.85. In patients with a large patent ductus and a large left-to-right shunt, the left atrium/aorta ratio is approximately 1.2.

The left atrial dimension or the left atrium/aorta ratio has proved useful in following these patients.[89] There can be a dramatic decrease in the size of the left atrium following surgical closure of the defect (Fig. 7–51). Occasionally, spontaneous closure of the ductus may occur, and again the left atrial size shows a marked decrease. Children with respiratory distress syndrome may have severe external retraction with a flattening of the left atrium. In this situation, examination of the left atrium by way of the suprasternal approach may be helpful in obtaining a more accurate left atrial dimension.[87,90]

The increased volume of blood in patients with a patent ductus arteriosus is also handled by the left ventricle. Echocardiographic evidence of left ventricular volume overload with dilatation and excessive motion of the septum and posterior left ventricular wall is also compatible with this diagnosis.[89,91,92] Thus measurements of left ventricular function have been used to evaluate patients with this problem.[87] The echocardiographic measurements of left atrial size and left ventricular function should be able to make the common differential diagnosis of primary lung disease, cardiomyopathy, or patent ductus anteriosus, all of which may produce a respiratory distress syndrome.[89,92]

There are reports demonstrating the two-dimensional echocardiographic visualization of a patent ductus arteriosus.[93,94] Figure 7–52 illustrates such an examination. This

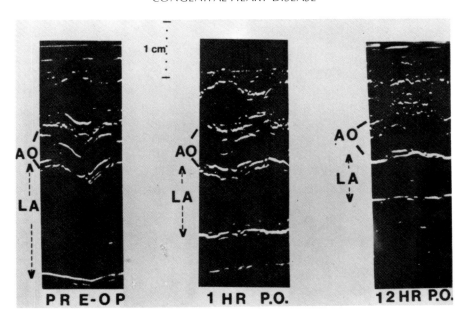

Fig. 7–51.   Serial left atrial echocardiograms of an infant with a patent ductus arteriosus and a large left-to-right shunt. A marked decrease in the size of the left atrium (LA) can be noted within one hour after surgery. The size of the chamber further decreases twelve hours after surgery. AO = aorta. (From Goldberg, S.J., Allen, H.D., and Sahn, D.J.: Pediatric and Adolescent Echocardiography. Chicago, Yearbook Medical Publishers, Inc., 1975.)

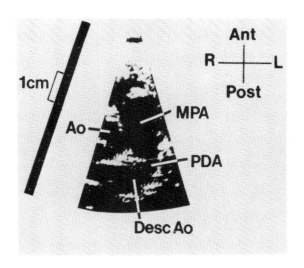

Fig. 7–52.   Two-dimensional echocardiogram of a patient with a patent ductus arteriosus. The patent ductus (PDA) is seen as an echo-free communication between the main pulmonary artery (MPA) and the descending aorta (DescAo). AO = aorta. (From Sahn, D.J.: New techniques for echocardiographic evaluation of cardiac anatomy in congenital heart disease. In Echocardiology. Edited by C.T. Lancee. The Hague, Martinus Nijhoff, 1979.)

30° scan is a short-axis study through the aorta visualizing the length of the main pulmonary artery (MPA). The descending aorta is below the pulmonary artery and an echo-free space from a patent ductus arteriosus (PDA) is visualized. One could easily envision technical difficulties in differentiating a true patent ductus from mere echo dropout. Further experience is necessary to determine the reliability of the two-dimensional technique for visualizing the patent ductus.

Doppler echocardiography has also been suggested as a technique for the detection of patent ductus arteriosus. The flow pattern of the shunted blood from the aorta into the pulmonary artery can be detected by way of this technique. In fact, there is evidence that Doppler echocardiography may be able to detect pulmonary hypertension in patients with a patent ductus arteriosus.[95] If the pulmonary artery pressure is normal, there is pandiastolic flow from the ductus into the pulmonary artery. With an increase in pulmonary artery pressure, the diastolic flow is abbreviated.

Another possible echocardiographic technique for visualizing a patent ductus arteriosus is the use of contrast echocardiography via an umbilical artery catheter.[95a] Such an intra-arterial line is commonly used in these critically ill infants. Contrast injections are made through such a catheter. If it is positioned near the ductus, the contrast echoes traverse the shunt and are visible within the pulmonary artery. This technique is useful in following the patient for spontaneous or drug-induced closure of the ductus.[96]

Ventricular Septal Defect

A ventricular septal defect is one of the most common congenital defects and is frequently found with other abnormalities. Echocardiographers have primarily used the secondary effects of a ventricular septal defect to evaluate these patients. As in the case of a patent ductus arteriosus, the shunted blood must be handled by the left atrium and left ventricle, so that both chambers are dilated. The left atrium/aorta ratio may again be useful in evaluating these patients as it is in patients with a patent ductus arteriosus.[97-99] However, this ratio is not as reliable as it is with a patent ductus arteriosus.[100] Since the right ventricle also handles the large volume, exaggerated septal motion is frequently not present even with a large left-to-right shunt. Thus the echocardiographic examination of the cardiac chambers may be useful in patients with ventricular septal defects, but the findings are not too reliable. The cardiac chambers may be totally normal in a patient with a small ventricular septal defect. Thus this type of echocardiographic evaluation of patients with a ventricular septal defect is insensitive.

There has been increasing interest in directly visualizing the ventricular septal defect echocardiographically. M-mode echocardiography has been proposed as a possible means of detecting a ventricular septal defect. Figure 7–53 demonstrates an M-mode scan of a patient with a large ventricular septal defect. There is discontinuity of the echoes between the interventricular septum and the anterior wall of the aorta. Unfortunately, because of this technique's insensitivity, only patients with a large ventricular septal defect show a consistent discontinuity. In addition, many false positives can occur because of artifactual echo dropout. One can easily record a dropout of the septal echoes when scanning from the ventricle to the aorta (Fig. 7–54). Thus the dis-

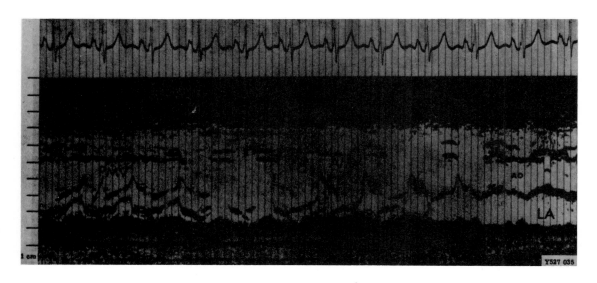

Fig. 7–53.   M-mode scan of a patient with a large ventricular septal defect. During the scan one can appreciate discontinuity of the echoes between the interventricular septum (IVS) and the aorta (AO). PMV = posterior mitral valve leaflet; AMV = anterior mitral valve leaflet; LA = left atrium.

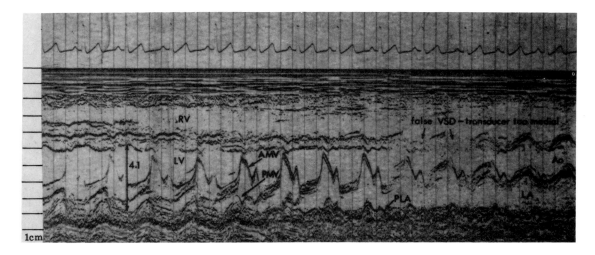

Fig. 7–54. M-mode echocardiographic scan showing a false ventricular septal defect (VSD) owing to the medial direction of the transducer. RV = right ventricle; LV = left ventricle; AMV = anterior mitral valve leaflet; PMV = posterior mitral valve leaflet; PLA = posterior left atrial wall; AO = aorta; LA = left atrium.

appearance of septal echoes on M-mode scans is unreliable for the diagnosis of ventricular septal defects because of the high incidence of false positives and false negatives.

Ventricular septal defects have been demonstrated by way of two-dimensional echocardiography.[101,102] It should be remembered that when examining for ventricular septal defects, one should designate the type of defect since some are easier to detect echocardiographically than others. These types include defects of the membranous septum, the ventricular septal defect associated with atrioventricular canals, the septal abnormality associated with malalignment of the aorta (such as tetralogy of Fallot), the subpulmonic or supracristal ventricular septal defect, and the muscular septal defect.

Figure 7–55 shows a patient with a ventricular septal defect in the area of the membranous septum, as well as a discrete subaortic membrane.[103,104,106] The discontinuity (VSD) between the interventricular septum and the posterior wall of the aorta can be seen in this still frame. The two-dimensional technique shares many of the same limitations with M-mode echocardiography, and factitious echo dropout must be considered as a false positive. Most ventricular septal defects detected with two-dimensional

echocardiography have been in the area of the membranous ventricular septum. Case reports of supracristal defects detected echocardiographically are also in the literature.[103,105] These defects are frequently associated with a prolapsing aortic valve leaflet. Some muscular ventricular septal defects have also been reported, but these are much smaller and more difficult to evaluate.

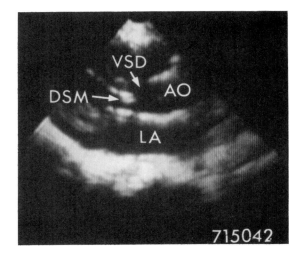

Fig. 7–55. Long-axis two-dimensional echocardiogram of a patient with a membranous ventricular septal defect (VSD) and a discrete subaortic membrane (DSM). AO = aorta; LA = left atrium.

The subcostal examination is advocated as a useful examination for viewing ventricular septal defects.[106a] By making serial sections through the heart from the subcostal view, it is possible to detect the various ventricular septal abnormalities. The muscular defect still has the highest incidence of false positives and false negatives. The other types of septal defects are apparently more easily detected. As a rule, one should use the highest-frequency transducer possible since the defects may be difficult to detect because of their small size and because one needs the best possible axial and lateral resolution. In addition, one should see the ventricular septal defect in more than one view to ensure that one is not dealing with a false positive. The edge of the defect frequently elongates the echo because of beam-width artifact. This type of artifact is useful in delineating the edge of a defect rather than just dropout in echoes. The same finding, which has been called a "T artifact," is helpful in identifying septal defects at the atrial level as well. The same sort of artifact may also be helpful in clearly identifying the orifice of a stenotic valve.

The ventricular septal defect secondary to malalignment is the easiest type of defect to detect echocardiographically. The most common example of such a defect is tetralogy of Fallot. Figure 7–56 shows the lack of continuity between the interventricular septum and the anterior aortic wall (A–Ao). The overriding, or malalignment, of the aorta is quite evident. Following repair of the ventricular septal defect as part of the surgical repair of tetralogy of Fallot, continuity of the echoes from the interventricular septum to the anterior wall of the aorta can be detected.

The membranous ventricular septal defect frequently produces an aneurysm on the right side of the defect as the shunt tends to "repair" itself. Such a membranous aneurysm can be seen both with M-mode and two-dimensional echocardiography.[107, 108,108a] Figure 7–57 shows an M-mode scan of a patient with an aneurysm of the membranous interventricular septum. The echoes from the aneurysm are visible anterior to the junction between the interventricular septum and the anterior aortic wall. The two-dimensional study in Figure 7–58 shows a similar but more obvious aneurysm. The curved aneurysm bulging into the right ventricle (VSA) is clearly apparent.

Contrast echocardiography can be helpful in the detection of ventricular septal defects if the shunt is from right to left.[109–112] Figure 7–59 shows a contrast study in a patient with a right-to-left shunt at the ventricular level.

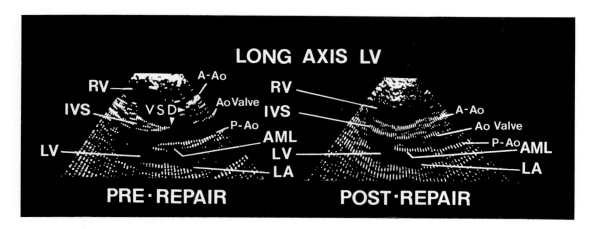

Fig. 7–56.   Pre- and postoperative long-axis two-dimensional echocardiograms of a patient with tetralogy of Fallot. The preoperative recording demonstrates the ventricular septal defect (VSD). The discontinuity between the interventricular septum (IVS) and the anterior wall of the aorta (A–Ao) is no longer present in postrepair. RV = right ventricle; LV = left ventricle; AML = anterior mitral leaflet; LA = left atrium; P–Ao = posterior aortic wall. (From Caldwell, R.L., et al.: Right ventricular outflow tract assessment by cross-sectional echocardiography in tetralogy of Fallot. Circulation, 59:395, 1979. By permission of the American Heart Association, Inc.)

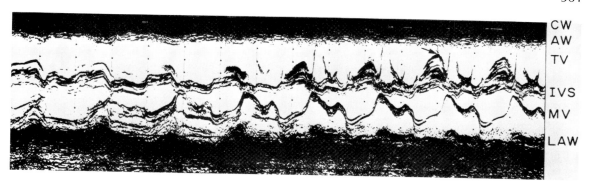

Fig. 7–57. M-mode echocardiographic scan for a patient with an aneurysm *(arrow)* of the membranous interventricular septum (IVS). CW = chest wall; AW = anterior right ventricular wall; TV = tricuspid valve; MV = mitral valve; LAW = left atrial wall. (From Assad-Morell, J.L., Tajik, A.J., and Guiliani, E.R.: Aneurysm of membranous interventricular septum: echocardiographic features. Mayo Clin. Proc., *49*:164, 1974.)

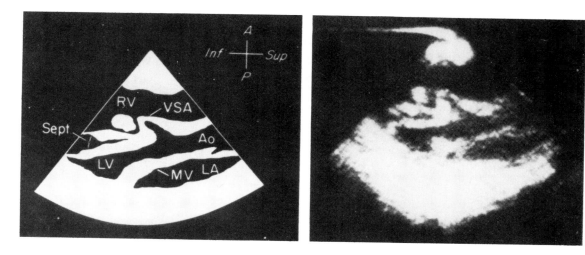

Fig. 7–58. Two-dimensional long-axis echocardiogram and diagram of a patient with a ventricular septal aneurysm. The aneurysm (VSA) can be seen bulging into the right ventricle (RV). LV = left ventricle; AO = aorta; MV = mitral valve; LA = left atrium; SEPT = interventricular septum. (From Snider, A.R., et al.: Echocardiographic evaluation of ventricular septal aneurysm. Circulation, *59*:920, 1979. By permission of the American Heart Association, Inc.)

The contrast echoes initially appear in the right ventricle. With the next cardiac complex (vertical line), contrast is seen below the ventricular septum above the mitral valve in the left ventricular outflow tract. Such a tracing can be distinguished from a right-to-left shunt at the atrial level by the fact that the contrast on the left side goes through the ventricular outflow tract rather than through the inflow tract or the mitral valve.

Contrast echocardiography can also be occasionally helpful in the detection of a left-to-right shunt. If the right ventricular systolic

pressure is more than 50 percent of the systemic pressure, then some right-to-left shunting can be detected.[109,110] The shunt usually occurs during diastole.[110] With an uncomplicated left-to-right shunt, one may produce a negative contrast effect on the right side of the interventricular septum (Fig. 7–60B). In this figure, one sees a small echo-free jet (vsd) on the right side of the ventricular septal defect that is surrounded by multiple echoes from the contrast passing through the right ventricle. Although this technique for negative contrast was initially

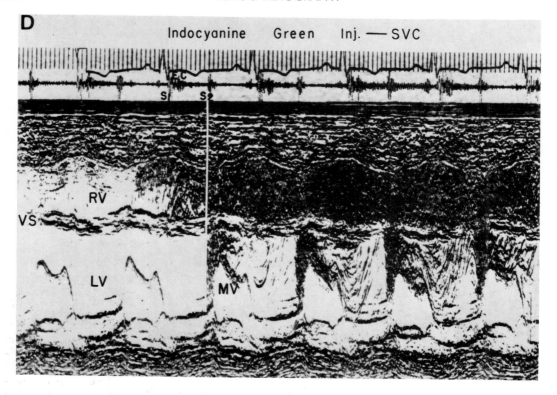

Fig. 7–59.   Contrast M-mode echocardiogram with an injection in the superior vena cava in a patient with a right-to-left shunt at the ventricular level. The contrast echoes initially enter the right ventricle (RV) and later appear in the left ventricle (LV) above the mitral valve (MV). VS = ventricular septum. (From Tajik, A.J. and Seward, J.B.: Contrast echocardiography. Cardiovasc. Clin., 9:2, 1979.)

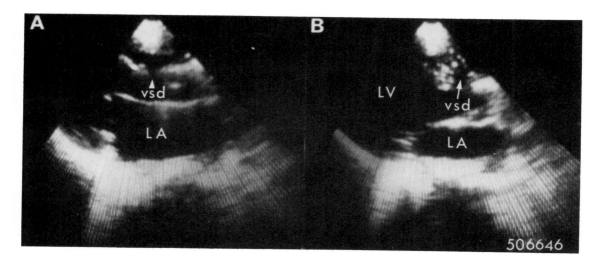

Fig. 7–60.   Two-dimensional long-axis echocardiograms of a patient with a membranous ventricular septal defect. A, The discontinuity of echoes from the ventricular septal defect (vsd) can be seen. B, A peripheral contrast injection fills the right ventricle, but an echo-free jet, i.e., negative contrast, can be seen anterior to the ventricular septal defect. LV = left ventricle; LA = left atrium.

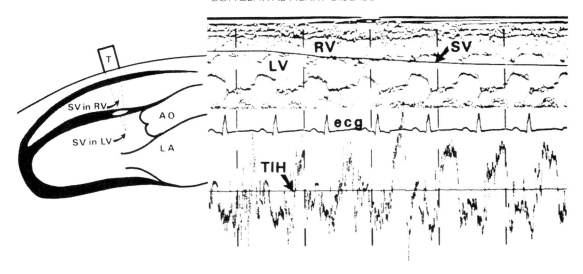

Fig. 7–61. Doppler echocardiographic examination of a patient with a ventricular septal defect. The sample volume (SV) is initially within the right ventricular (RV) side of the septum. Turbulent flow is recorded on the time interval histogram (TIH). As the sample volume passes through the septum to the left ventricle (LV), normal laminar flow is recorded. LA = left atrium; AO = aorta. (From Stevenson, J.G., et al.: Pulsed Doppler echocardiography: applications in pediatric cardiology. *In* Echocardiology. Edited by C.T. Lancee. The Hague, Martinus Nijhoff, 1979.)

described for atrial septal defects and left-to-right shunts, several authors have noted similar findings in patients with ventricular septal defects and left-to-right shunts.

There is increasing interest in using Doppler echocardiography for the detection of ventricular septal defects.[113] Figure 7–61 shows a Doppler study. One attempts to pass the Doppler sample volume through the defect. In this figure, the sample volume is initially within the right ventricle, apparently within the jet flow of the shunted blood. The time-interval histogram (TIH) records chaotic or turbulent flow with multiple echoes both above and below the baseline during systole. As the sample volume passes through the ventricular septum and reaches the left ventricle, one records laminar flow with a smooth signal pattern during systole. As is the case with all Doppler studies, the audible signal is probably more reliable than the graphic recording. Technical skill is also required to ensure that the sample volume passes through the jet of the shunted blood. Experience thus far suggests that Doppler echocardiography may prove to be a reliable technique for the qualitative assessment of certain ventricular septal defects.

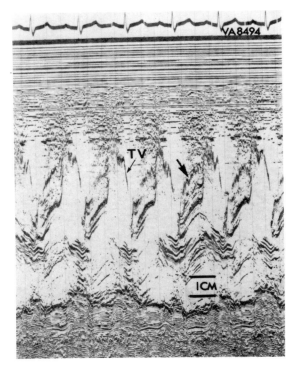

Fig. 7–62. M-mode tricuspid valve echocardiogram (TV) in a patient with a ventricular septal defect and a shunt from the left ventricle into the right atrium. Note fluttering of the tricuspid valve in diastole and systole *(arrow)*.

364 ECHOCARDIOGRAPHY

Occasionally, a ventricular septal defect does not communicate directly with the right ventricle. The shunted blood may pass into the right atrium. Under these circumstances one may see systolic fluttering (arrow) of the tricuspid valve apparatus (Fig. 7–62).[114] There may also be coarse fluttering of the tricuspid valve during diastole. Similar systolic fluttering of the tricuspid valve may occur if the shunt is from the aorta into the right atrium, such as with a ruptured sinus of Valsalva aneurysm.

Atrial Septal Defect

The detection and exclusion of an atrial septal defect has been a major use of echocardiography. The principal M-mode application has utilized the criteria for the diagnosis of a right ventricular volume overload. These criteria require dilatation of the right

ventricular chamber and abnormal septal motion.[115–120] Figure 7–63 shows a characteristic echocardiogram of a patient with an atrial septal defect in whom the right ventricle is dilated, and the interventricular septal echoes move anteriorly with ventricular systole. These echocardiographic findings are not specific for an atrial septal defect. Similar findings are noted in patients with tricuspid insufficiency, pulmonic insufficiency, or anomalous pulmonary venous drainage. There is a crude correlation between the size of the left-to-right shunt in an atrial septal defect and the size of the right ventricular dimension. The pattern of septal motion does not seem to correlate well with the size of the shunt. Some degree of right ventricular dilatation and abnormal septal motion may persist following surgery.[121]

Unfortunately, ventricular septal motion

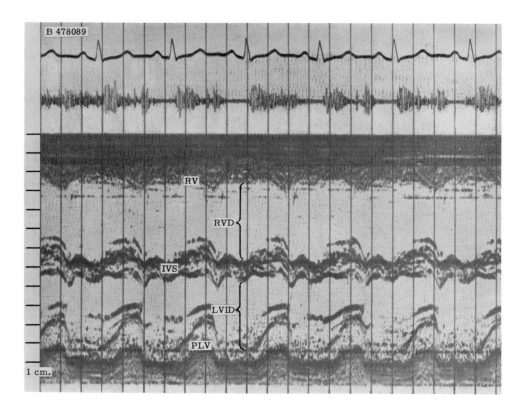

Fig. 7–63. M-mode echocardiogram of a patient with an atrial septal defect. The right ventricular dimension (RVD) is increased, and the right side of the interventricular septum (IVS) moves paradoxically. The left side of the interventricular septum manifests rapid upward motion with the onset of electrical depolarization and then flat motion during ventricular ejection. RV = right ventricle; LVID = left ventricular internal dimension; PLV = posterior left ventricular wall. (From Feigenbaum, H.: Clinical applications of echocardiography. Prog. Cardiovasc. Dis., 14:531, 1972.)

has not been consistent in all patients with an atrial septal defect.[119,122,123] Although most of these patients clearly have abnormal septal motion,[124] there are some patients who may manifest atypical septal motion. Thus ventricular septal motion may not be totally accurate in determining the presence or absence of an atrial septal defect. On the other hand, the right ventricular dimension seems more consistent.[119] As crude as the M-mode echocardiographic right ventricular dimension is, it is extremely unusual for an atrial septal defect with a significant left-to-right shunt to not have some dilatation of the right ventricle. Thus a normal M-mode echocardiogram with a normal right ventricular dimension and normal septal motion is still fairly reliable evidence against the presence of an atrial septal defect with a shunt large enough to be considered for surgical closure. It is conceivable that patients with atrial septal defects and small shunts, less than 1.5:1, may possess normal echocardiograms. On the other hand, these patients probably do not warrant surgical closure, and they should have a normal life expectancy.

Since the interatrial septum can be directly visualized by way of two-dimensional echocardiography, it is not surprising that investigators have attempted to directly record the interatrial septal defect through this ultrasonic technique.[125–129] As noted in previous chapters, the interatrial septum can be seen in the short-axis, the four-chamber, and the subcostal views. Discontinuity of echoes from an interatrial septal defect has been described in all three two-dimensional planes. However, because the ultrasonic beam is essentially parallel to the interatrial septum in both the short-axis and four-chamber views, the subcostal examination is by far the most reliable for examining this cardiac structure.[129] Figure 7–64 shows a subcostal examination in which the interatrial septum (arrow) is clearly visible. The ultrasonic beam is virtually perpendicular to the septum and a high-quality study is obtained. Figure 7–65 shows another subcostal examination of the interatrial septum that used a higher-frequency transducer.[129] Note the finer detail of the interatrial septum. The foramen ovale (arrowheads) can also be appreciated.

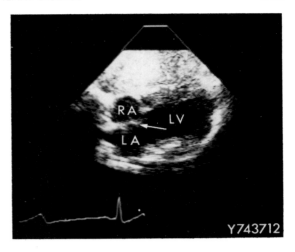

Fig. 7–64. Subcostal two-dimensional echocardiogram demonstrating the interatrial septum *(arrow)*. RA = right atrium; LA = left atrium; LV = left ventricle.

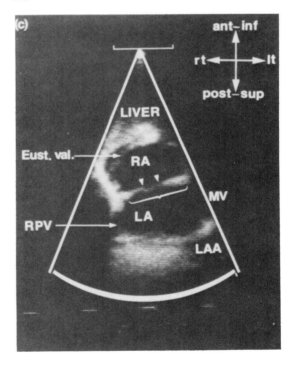

Fig. 7–65. Subcostal two-dimensional echocardiogram of the interatrial septum *(bracket)* using a high-frequency transducer. Note thinning of the septum at the level of the foramen oval *(arrowheads)*. Eust. val. = eustachian valve; RA = right atrium; LA = left atrium; RPV = right pulmonary vein; LAA = left atrial appendage; MV = mitral valve. (From Beirman, F.Z. and Williams, R.G.: Subxiphoid two-dimensional imaging of the interatrial septum in infants and neonates with congenital heart disease. Circulation, 60:80, 1979. By permission of the American Heart Association, Inc.)

Figure 7–66 diagrammatically shows some variations of the interatrial septum that can be detected with a subcostal study. Figure 7–66Ia shows the normal interatrial septum with thinning in the vicinity of the foramen ovale. The small arrow indicates the position of the right pulmonary vein. With a thickened septum primum (Ib), the thin area of the foramen ovale is not seen. Deviations of the septum toward the right atrium can be appreciated, with left atrial dilatation and a left ventricular volume overload (IIa). The septum can be deviated to the left with right atrial dilatation or with right ventricular vol-

ume overload (IIb). With a right atrial volume overload, frequently only the foramen ovale and the thin tissue covering it deviate into the left atrium. Figure 7–66III shows the echocardiographic finding in a secundum-type atrial septal defect. Basically, the thin area of the foramen ovale is missing. Remnants of the septum can be seen at both ends of the defect. Figure 7–66IV shows the echocardiographic finding in an iatrogenically created septal defect following a balloon atrial septostomy. Remnants of the septum can be seen on the left atrial side. A primum-type atrial septal defect is depicted in Figure 7–66V. The location of the defect is closer to the ventricular septum, and there is no remnant of interatrial septum between the defect and the interventricular septum. The lower portion of the interatrial septum is thus bounded by the atrioventricular valves.

Figure 7–67 shows an actual subcostal two-dimensional echocardiogram of a patient with a secundum atrial septal defect. Remnants of the interatrial septum are fairly obvious (ASD). An ostium primum atrial septal defect is shown in Figure 7–68. The location of the defect is different and there is no

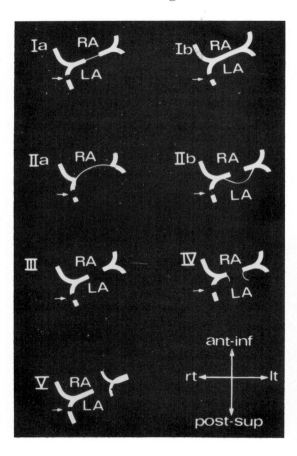

Fig. 7–66. Diagrams illustrating various two-dimensional echocardiograms of the interatrial septum as examined from the subcostal approach using a high-frequency transducer (see text for details). RA = right atrium; LA = left atrium. (From Bierman, F.Z. and Williams, R.G.: Subxiphoid two-dimensional imaging of the interatrial septum in infants and neonates with congenital heart disease. Circulation, 60:80, 1979. By permission of the American Heart Association, Inc.)

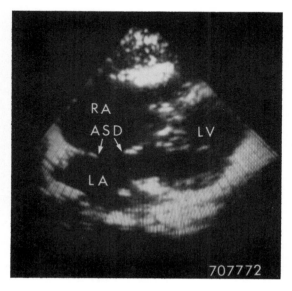

Fig. 7–67. Subcostal two-dimensional echocardiogram of a patient with a secundum atrial septal defect. Remnants of the interatrial septum are visible on both sides of the defect (ASD). RA = right atrium; LA = left atrium; LV = left ventricle.

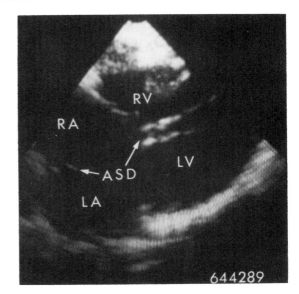

Fig. 7–68. Subcostal two-dimensional echocardiogram of a patient with an ostium primum atrial septal defect. No residual septal tissue can be noted between the defect (ASD) and the interventricular septum. RA = right atrium; LA = left atrium; RV = right ventricle; LV = left ventricle.

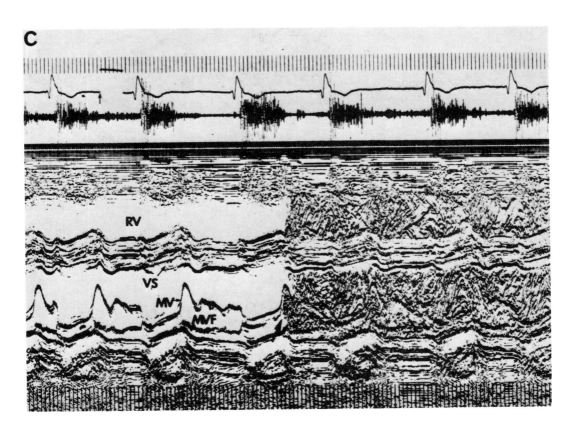

Fig. 7–69. Contrast echocardiogram with a peripheral venous injection in a patient with a right-to-left shunt at the atrial level. The contrast material reaches the right (RV) and left ventricles simultaneously. The contrast echoes *(arrow)* enter the left ventricle through the mitral valve (MV). Thus the contrast comes from the left atrium. VS = ventricular septum; MVF = mitral valve funnel. (From Tajik, A.J. and Seward, J.B.: Contrast echocardiography. Cardiovasc. Clin., 9:2, 1979.)

residual atrial septal tissue in contact with the interventricular septum.

There are reports that identify a primum atrial septal defect by way of the short-axis or four-chamber examinations.[128] The criterion for such a diagnosis is the loss of echoes from the interatrial septum immediately next to the interventricular septum. Attempts at using the short-axis or four-chamber views to detect a secundum-type atrial septal defect is fraught with great error, however. Dropout of echoes in the vicinity of the septal defect is quite common, and one cannot reliably detect or exclude such an abnormality by way of these approaches.

Contrast echocardiography plays an important role in the diagnosis of atrial septal defects. Right-to-left shunting at the atrial level can be detected with a peripheral contrast injection.[110-112] Figure 7–69 shows a patient with a right-to-left shunt at the atrial level. Echoes from the contrast material appear simultaneously within the right and left ventricles. On the left side, contrast echoes appear within the mitral valve (arrow). Thus the contrast-producing echoes enter the left ventricle through the mitral valve from the left atrium. This recording should be compared with that in Figure 7–79 where the right-to-left shunting is at the ventricular level. One can inject contrast material directly into the left atrium through a catheter (Fig. 7–70). Under these circumstances, the dye would first appear within the left ventricle and later in the right ventricle. The contrast echoes would go directly into the left ventricle from the left atrium, whereas the contrast appearing in the right ventricle must pass through the atrial septal defect and then into the right ventricle via the right atrium. Although the invasive use of contrast echocardiography is not widely popular, it does obviate the need for angiography in some of these patients.

Peripheral venous injections of contrast may also be helpful in the detection of left-to-right shunts.[110,130,131] Some investigators indicate that even with a left-to-right shunt

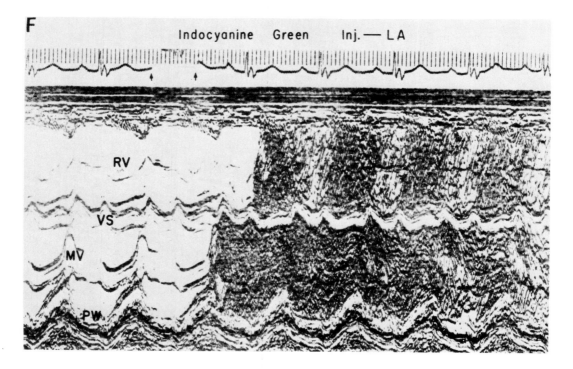

Fig. 7–70. Contrast echocardiogram of a patient with an atrial septal defect and left-to-right shunt in whom injection is made directly into the left atrium using a catheter. The contrast echoes pass through the mitral valve (MV) and fill the left ventricle prior to appearing in the right ventricle (RV). VS = ventricular septum; PW = posterior wall. (From Tajik, A.J. and Seward, J.B.: Contrast echocardiography. Cardiovasc. Clin., 9:2, 1979.)

one may see some passage of contrast from right-to-left in most patients with atrial septal defects. The small right-to-left shunting may be accentuated with a Valsalva maneuver.[131] These studies have primarily used two-dimensional echocardiography utilizing the four-chamber view. Unfortunately, the degree of right-to-left shunting may be so small in some patients that it is difficult to see the few contrast-producing bubbles. Left-to-right shunting at the atrial level can also be detected when looking for a negative contrast effect.[132] Figure 7–71 shows a short-axis examination at the level of the atrial septum and aorta. Only parts of the atrial septum are visualized between the left atrium (LA) and right atrium (RA). The fact that the entire septum is not visualized does not mean the diagnosis of an atrial septal defect, since there could be artifactual dropout of echoes, a common phenomenon. A peripheral contrast injection is made in Figure 7–71B. With the left-to-right atrial shunt, the noncontrast-containing blood from the left atrium produces a negative contrast jet in the right atrium.[132] The contrast echoes fill

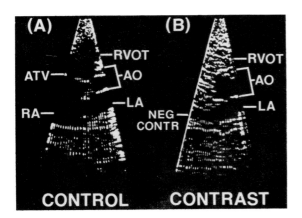

Fig. 7–71. Short-axis two-dimensional contrast echocardiogram in the vicinity of the interatrial septum of a patient with an atrial septal defect and a left-to-right shunt. A, The right atrium (RA) and right ventricular outflow tract (RVOT) are free of any echoes prior to the peripheral injection of contrast. B, With the injection of echo-producing contrast, echoes fill the entire right atrium and right ventricle, except for an echo-free jet (neg. contr.) coming from the left atrium (LA). This echo-free space is due to noncontrast-containing blood shunting from the left to the right atrium. AO = aorta; ATV = anterior tricuspid valve.

the remainder of the right heart, including the right ventricular outflow tract (RVOT). Figure 7–72 shows another example of a negative contrast study in a patient with an atrial septal defect and a large left-to-right shunt. The control tracing is seen in Figure 7–72A. With contrast, the right ventricular outflow tract and part of the right atrium is filled; however, there is a wide echo-free band in the right atrium from the noncontrast-containing shunted blood from the left atrium. This type of negative contrast study can also be performed in the four-chamber or subcostal views. There is the temptation to judge the size of the left-to-right shunt by the width of the echo-free jet in the right atrium. For example, Figure 7–71 shows a much narrower echo-free jet than does Figure 7–72 as well as a smaller shunt. However, no data substantiate this observation.

There are reports on the use of Doppler echocardiography to detect the left-to-right shunt in patients with atrial septal defects.[133,134] The Doppler sample is placed within the right atrium in an attempt to record the blood flow shunting across the defect. This observation requires further confirmation. Thus far, no quantitative information has been demonstrated by way of Doppler techniques.

Secondary effects of atrial septal defect have been reported on the echocardiogram. There is some evidence that the amplitude of atrioventricular valve motion may indicate the degree of shunting. As noted in Chapter 4, the tricuspid and mitral valves may somewhat indicate blood flowing through these orifices. Normally, the amplitude of motion of the tricuspid and mitral valves is essentially equal. In patients with atrial septal defects and left-to-right shunts, one may find the amplitude of opening of the tricuspid valve to exceed that of the mitral valve.[135,136] Unfortunately, this observation has not proved too reliable and has therefore not been popular.

One study emphasized the changes in mitral valve motion in patients with atrial septal defect.[137] A posterior coaptation point was noted in a high percentage of patients with atrial septal defect. It was suggested that a

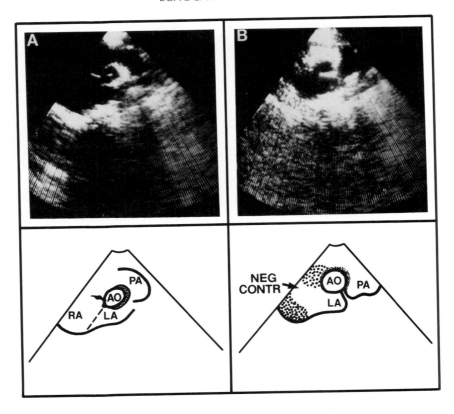

Fig. 7–72.   Two-dimensional contrast echocardiograms and diagrams of a patient with an atrial septal defect and a large left-to-right shunt. A, Short-axis view of the aorta and interatrial septum prior to the injection of contrast. B, With the peripheral injection of echo-producing contrast, the entire right side of the heart fills with echoes except for a negative contrast (neg. contr.) band of echoes communicating with the left atrium (LA). AO = aorta; PA = pulmonary artery; RA = right atrium. (From Weyman, A.E., et al.: Negative contrast echocardiography: a new method for detecting left-to-right shunts. Circulation, 59:498, 1979. By permission of the American Heart Association, Inc.)

high percentage of patients with this congenital anomaly may also have mitral valve prolapse. A more recent investigation indicated that the apparent mitral valve prolapse in patients with atrial septal defect may merely be a function of the distortion of the left ventricular cavity owing to the enlarged right ventricle.[137a] Thus apparent mitral valve prolapse in patients with atrial septal defects may not have the same significance as mitral valve prolapse in patients with myxomatous degeneration of the valves and may merely be a function of a geometric change of the left ventricle.

Angular rotation or displacement of the left ventricle has been noted in patients with atrial septal defect by way of two-dimensional echocardiography.[138] There is a clockwise rotation with systole.

Endocardial Cushion Defect

This congenital anomaly can vary considerably. One common type is the ostium primum atrial septal defect usually seen with a cleft mitral valve. The low-lying ostium primum atrial septal defect has been discussed (see Fig. 7–68). A cleft mitral valve was demonstrated in Figure 7–46. A more extreme version of this anomaly is a complete atrioventricular canal. As one might expect, a spectrum of abnormalities lies between these two extremes.[139] The most common manifestation of an endocardial cushion defect in adults is the ostium primum atrial septal defect. This abnormality shares many of the same echocardiographic findings with a secundum atrial septal defect; both show a dilated right ventricle and abnormal septal motion. Because these

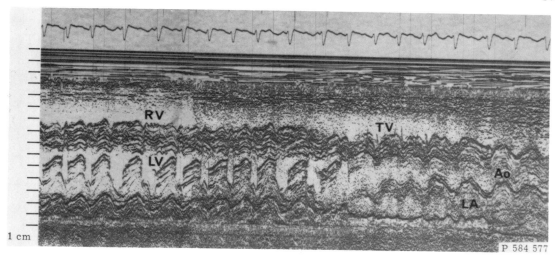

Fig. 7–73. M-mode scan of a patient with an ostium primum atrial septal defect. This tracing shows how the mitral valve echoes seem to attach to the interventricular septum in the left ventricular outflow tract. RV = right ventricle; AO = aorta; LA = left atrium; LV = left ventricle; TV = tricuspid valve.

patients frequently have mitral regurgitation, the abnormal septal motion may be masked. Besides a cleft mitral valve, there is also an abnormal position and insertion of the mitral valve into the interventricular septum. This abnormality may produce fairly characteristic echocardiographic findings.[139-142] In such patients there is close proximity of the anterior mitral leaflet to the interventricular septum, both during systole and diastole.[143,144] Figure 7–73 is an M-mode scan of a patient with an ostium primum atrial septal defect. As the ultrasonic beam scans toward the aorta (AO), the systolic portion of the mitral valve moves closer to the septum. This echocardiographic sign probably corresponds to the abnormal insertion of the mitral valve, which is characteristic of this anomaly.[140,141] Figure 7–74 is another M-mode scan of the same patient. The proximity of the mitral valve to the interventricular septum is again noted. In addition, the tricuspid valve echoes appear to traverse the echoes of the interventricular septum. This is not an uncommon finding in patients with an endocardial cushion defect. Unfortunately, this echocardiographic sign is somewhat confused by a straddling tricuspid valve, as noted in Figure 7–50. The differentiation between these two entities is prob-

ably best done by two-dimensional echocardiography rather than by the M-mode technique.

The endocardial cushion defect can probably be best defined anatomically by way of two-dimensional echocardiography.[67,145,146] Both the atrial and ventricular septal defects commonly present in this anomaly can be detected by way of the apical or subcostal four-chamber views. Figure 7–75 illustrates an apical four-chamber examination of a patient with an endocardial cushion defect. The septal defect (SD) involves the atrial and ventricular septa. This type of examination also permits one to ascertain whether the atrioventricular valves are divided or whether there might be a free-floating common anterior leaflet that may occur with a complete canal.

The M-mode examination may be helpful in detecting associated atrioventricular valve stenosis by noting marked disproportionate size of the ventricles, abnormal tricuspid or mitral valves, or inadequate recording of an atrioventricular valve.[147,148]

Anomalous Pulmonary Venous Return

Anomalous pulmonary veins produce a left-to-right shunt and a right ventricular volume overload that is indistinguishable

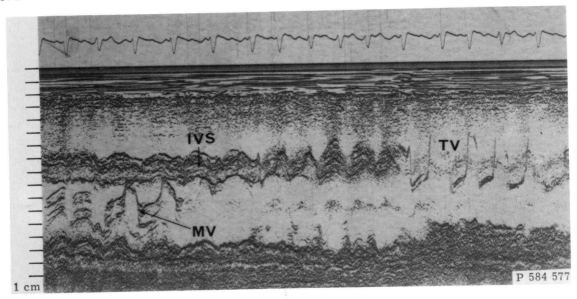

Fig. 7–74.   M-mode scan of a patient with an ostium primum endocardial cushion defect. In the vicinity of the left ventricle, on the left, the right ventricle is dilated, and the interventricular septal echoes (IVS) move abnormally, consistent with a right ventricular volume overload. In addition, the systolic portion of the mitral valve (MV) is abnormally close to the interventricular septum. The tricuspid valve echoes (TV) seem to traverse the interventricular septum; parts of the valve appear within both ventricles.

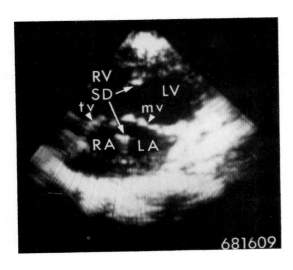

Fig. 7–75.   Apical four-chamber two-dimensional echocardiogram of a patient with an endocardial cushion defect. The septal defect (SD) involves the interventricular and atrial septa. RV = right ventricle; LV = left ventricle; RA = right atrium; LA = left atrium; tv = tricuspid valve; mv = mitral valve.

echocardiographically from an atrial septal defect. One again finds a dilated right ventricle and abnormal septal motion. Most patients with anomalous pulmonary veins have only one or two veins draining into the right side of the heart. A large percentage of these patients also have an associated atrial septal defect. The clinical differentiation between an atrial septal defect and partial anomalous pulmonary venous return is somewhat academic, since in the surgical repair of the anomalous venous return an atrial septal defect is usually created. Whether surgical correction is indicated usually depends on the size of the left-to-right shunt.

When all four veins empty into the right atrium, complete or total anomalous pulmonary venous return may produce a different type of echocardiographic recording. The confluence of these veins produces an extra "chamber" behind the left atrium (Fig. 7–76).[148a] There is an echo-free space behind the left atrium. In Figure 7–77 indocyanine green dye was injected into the chamber that receives all pulmonary veins (CPVC). The dye, initially recorded in this chamber, later

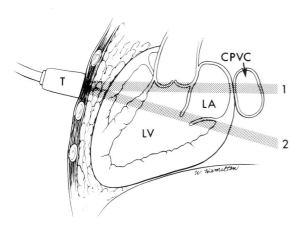

Fig. 7–76. Diagram demonstrating principle of echocardiographic diagnosis of total anomalous pulmonary venous return. The common pulmonary venous chamber (CPVC) lies posterior to the left atrium (LA). LV = left ventricle; T = transducer. (From Paquet, M., and Gutgesell, H.: Echocardiographic features of total anomalous pulmonary venous connection. Circulation, 51:599, 1975.)

appears within the left atrial cavity. There is an atrial septal defect, and some dye appears in the right ventricular outflow tract (RVOT), and somewhat later it appears in the aorta. The illustration in Figure 7–77B shows what happens when dye is injected directly into the left atrial cavity. At this time one sees the echoes in the left atrium and later in the right ventricular outflow tract and aorta. No contrast echoes appear in the common pulmonary venous chamber.

These illustrations demonstrate that one can record such anomalies echocardiographically. However, there are other situations whereby one might find a linear echo running through what appears to be the left atrium. Cor triatriatum, or a left atrial membrane, may produce somewhat similar findings (Figs. 7–36, 7–37). One study indicates that the differential diagnoses of total anomalous pulmonary venous return, cor triatriatum, or left atrial membrane can be

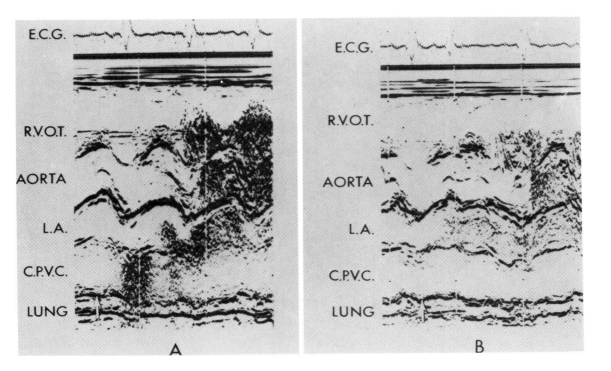

Fig. 7–77. Left atrial echocardiogram of a patient with a total anomalous pulmonary venous return. A, Indocyanine green dye was injected into the common pulmonary venous chamber (CPVC). B, The dye was injected directly into the left atrium (LA). RVOT = right ventricular outflow tract. (From Paquet, M. and Gutgesell, H.: Echocardiographic features of total anomalous pulmonary venous connection. Circulation, 51:599, 1975.)

made by way of pulsed Doppler echocardiography.[149] If the extra echo within the left atrium is due to total anomalous pulmonary venous return, then the flow patterns should be significantly different on either side of the echo. Similar differences are apparently not noted with the other conditions.[149]

A dilated coronary sinus can also produce an echo-free space behind the left atrium. In fact, Figure 7–78 shows an echocardiogram of a patient who had both a prominent coronary sinus and a common pulmonary venous chamber.[150,151] A contrast injection is made directly into the coronary sinus (CS). The dye next appears within the left atrium and the right ventricular outflow tract and then finally in the aorta. Interestingly, there is also late appearance of contrast material in the common pulmonary venous chamber (CPV). Presumably, these contrast echoes were produced by some microbubbles traversing the pulmonary circuit. The anomalous pulmonary veins may drain into the coronary sinus. Thus a dilated coronary sinus is not an uncommon finding with this abnormality.[150]

The descending aorta also produces an echo-free space behind the left atrium (see Chapter 12) that can be superficially confused with a left atrial membrane, common pulmonary venous chamber, or a dilated coronary sinus. An M-mode scan or a two-dimensional study should eliminate any confusion.

There have been descriptions of the common pulmonary venous chamber by way of two-dimensional echocardiography.[152,153] The chamber represents an echo-free space

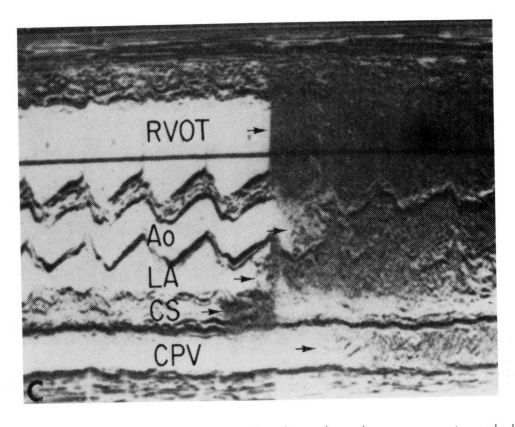

Fig. 7–78. Contrast echocardiogram of a patient with total anomalous pulmonary venous return and a dilated coronary sinus. Contrast is initially injected directly into the coronary sinus (CS). The contrast then appears in the left atrium (LA) and right ventricular outflow tract (RVOT). The dye next appears in the aorta (AO), and a faint amount of contrast traverses the pulmonary vascular bed to appear in the common pulmonary venous chamber (CPV). (From Orsmond, G.S., et al.: Echocardiographic features of total anomalous pulmonary venous connection through the coronary sinus. Am. J. Cardiol., *41*:597, 1978.)

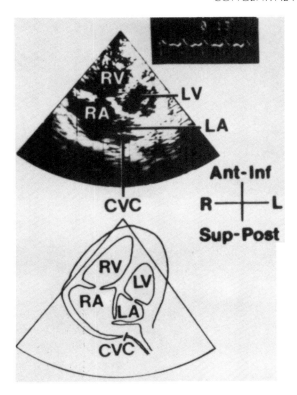

Fig. 7–79. Apical four-chamber two-dimensional echocardiogram and diagram of a patient with total anomalous venous return. The common venous chamber (CVC) is visible behind the left atrium (LA). RV = right ventricle; LV = left ventricle; RA = right atrium. (From Sahn, D.J., et al.: Cross-sectional echocardiographic diagnosis of the site of total anomalous pulmonary venous drainage. Circulation, 60:1317, 1979. By permission of the American Heart Association, Inc.)

behind the left atrium. Figure 7–79 is an apical four-chamber view showing a common venous chamber (CVC) next to the left atrium. Of course, the pulmonary veins need not always enter from behind the left atrium. The anomalous veins may actually insert below the diaphragm, which may offer great difficulty for the echocardiographic diagnosis.[154] In these circumstances, the echocardiogram may be normal.

One study using two-dimensional echocardiography noted that it was usually possible to record one or more pulmonary veins by way of the apical or subcostal examinations. By recording such veins, total anomalous pulmonary venous return can be

excluded. The investigators also believed that two-dimensional echocardiography was more consistent in recording the common pulmonary venous chamber and that the site of drainage of the anomalous veins could be determined.[152]

Single Ventricle

Many reports have noted the echocardiographic findings in patients with single ventricle.[40,82,155–159] This anomaly is also known as common ventricle, primitive ventricle, or univentricular heart. Transposition of the great arteries is commonly associated with this condition, as is straddling of the atrioventricular valves. If there is a small remnant of a ventricle and both atrioventricular valves empty into a single ventricular chamber, then the term double-inlet ventricle is used.[160] The single ventricle is usually classified according to whether there are one or two atrioventricular valves and whether there is an outlet chamber. Figure 7–80 shows a patient with a single ventricle and two atrioventricular valves. The tricuspid (TV) and mitral valves (MV) are clearly visible. There are no interventricular septal echoes between the two valves. Figure 7–81 is an M-mode scan of a patient with a single ventricle and two atrioventricular valves. This patient has an outflow tract chamber and a remnant of an interventricular septum. There is also transposition of the great arteries. At times it is difficult to distinguish the echocardiogram in Figure 7–81 from one showing transposition and only a large ventricular septal defect. Figure 7–82 is a contrast study of a patient with a single ventricle who has only one atrioventricular valve and no outflow tract chamber. The contrast fills the ventricle as it passes above the mitral valve but not through the orifice. Some injections are helpful in judging where the blood is flowing in patients with a single ventricle.[161]

Two-dimensional echocardiography can be helpful in patients with a single ventricle.[157,162] Figure 7–83 shows a four-chamber view of a patient with a single ventricle. The total absence of an interventricular septum is clearly apparent.

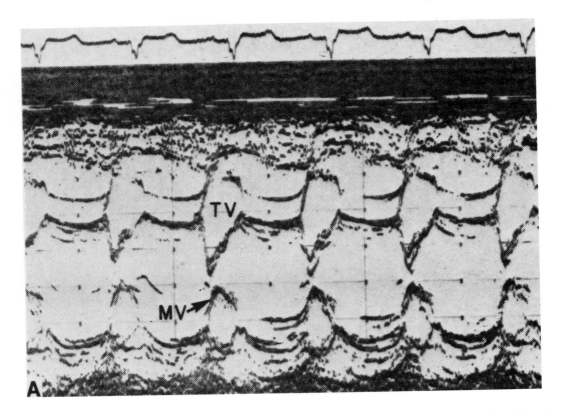

Fig. 7–80.   M-mode echocardiogram of a patient with a single ventricle and two atrioventricular valves. Both tricuspid (TV) and mitral (MV) valves can be recorded with no intervening septal echoes. (From Seward, J.B., et al.: Echocardiogram in common (single) ventricle: angiographic correlation. Am. J. Cardiol., 39:217, 1977.)

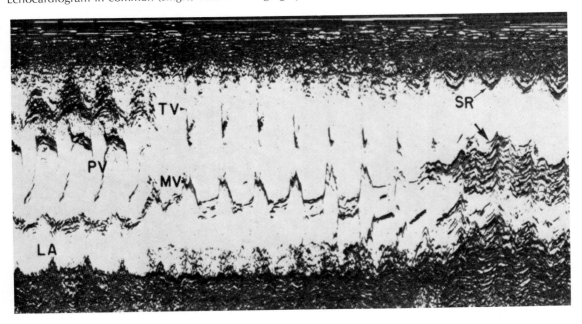

Fig. 7–81.   M-mode scan of a patient with a single ventricle, an outflow tract chamber, and transposition of the great arteries. Both tricuspid (TV) and mitral (MV) valves can be visualized. A septal remnant (SR) moves posteriorly with ventricular systole. The dense band of echoes within the cavity of the left ventricle probably originates from papillary muscle or aberrant muscle bundles. PV = pulmonary valve; LA = left atrium. (From Seward, J.B., et al.: Echocardiogram in common (single) ventricle: angiographic correlation. Am. J. Cardiol., 39:217, 1977.)

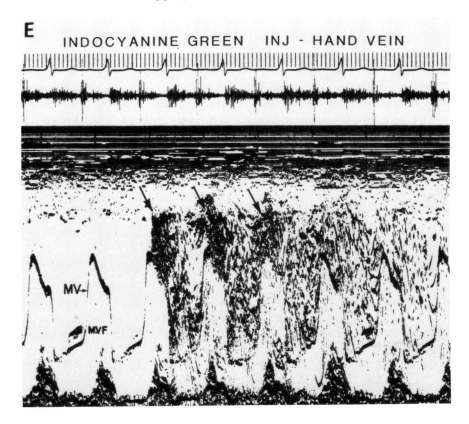

Fig. 7–82.   Contrast M-mode echocardiogram in a patient with a single ventricle and a single atrioventricular valve. The contrast echoes *(arrows)* enter the single ventricle anterior to the mitral valve (MV). MVF = mitral valve funnel. (From Seward, J.B., et al.: Peripheral venous contrast echocardiography. Am. J. Cardiol., *39*:202, 1977.)

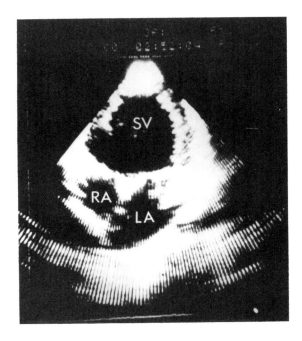

Fig. 7–83.   Apical four-chamber echocardiogram of a patient with a single ventricle (SV). RA = right atrium; LA = left atrium. (From Feigenbaum, H.: Echocardiography. *In* Heart Disease. Edited by E. Braunwald. Philadelphia, W. B. Saunders Co., 1980.)

Pulmonary Arteriovenous Shunt

Shunting of blood through a pulmonary arteriovenous fistula can be detected with contrast echocardiography.[163-165] This technique can make this diagnosis principally because the echo-producing microbubbles are too large to pass through the pulmonary capillaries. Thus the echo-producing bubbles do not appear on the left side of the heart unless there is a right-to-left shunt. Figure 7–84 shows a peripheral venous injection in a patient with a pulmonary arteriovenous shunt. The contrast echoes initially appear in the right ventricle. After several cardiac complexes, contrast begins to appear in the left side of the heart, passing through the mitral valve and the left ventricular outflow tract. Thus the contrast echoes can traverse the pulmonary circulation and appear on the left side of the heart. The time required for the contrast echoes to reach the left side is too long to consider an intracardiac shunt. Thus such a study would be highly indica-

tive if not diagnostic of shunting at the pulmonary arterial level.

It should be pointed out, however, that contrast-producing microbubbles may occasionally traverse the pulmonary capillary bed. Figure 7–78 shows an example of a few microbubbles passing through the pulmonary circuit and appearing in the common pulmonary venous chamber. In addition, recent reports indicate that pressure injections into a catheter in the pulmonary capillary wedge position permits the microbubbles to traverse the capillaries and to appear on the left side of the heart. This technique requires either a right-heart or Swan-Ganz catheter.

Crisscross Atrioventricular Valves

A relatively rare form of intracardiac shunt is a crisscross heart, or crisscross atrioventricular valves. In this situation, blood from the right atrium flows directly into the left ventricle and blood flows from the left atrium to the right ventricle. One of the best

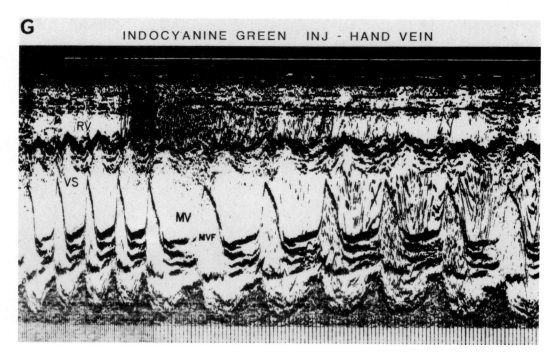

Fig. 7–84.   Contrast echocardiogram with a peripheral venous injection in a patient with a pulmonary arteriovenous shunt. The contrast echoes appear initially in the right ventricle (RV) and after a long delay contrast begins to appear to flow through the mitral valve funnel (MVF) into the left ventricle. Normally all echo-producing micro-bubbles should be filtered out by the pulmonary capillaries, and no contrast should be seen to the left of the septum. VS = ventricular septum; MV = mitral valve. (From Seward, J.B., et al.: Peripheral venous contrast echocardiography. Am. J. Cardiol., 39:202, 1977.)

techniques for making this diagnosis is contrast echocardiography.[166] Figure 7–85 is a subcostal, four-chamber two-dimensional study of a patient with crisscross atrioventricular valves and an atrial septal defect. With a peripheral injection of saline contrast, echoes flow directly from the right atrium through the atrial septal defect into the left ventricle. No contrast echoes appear within the right ventricle or the left atrium.

ABNORMALITIES OF THE GREAT ARTERIES

Malformations of the great arteries include tetralogy of Fallot, truncus arteriosus, double-outlet right ventricle, and transposition of the great arteries. Although there are specific echocardiographic findings in each

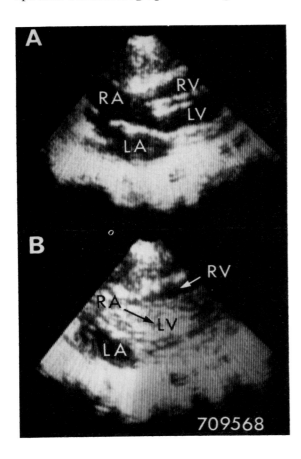

Fig. 7–85. Subcostal two-dimensional contrast echocardiogram in a patient with a crisscross heart. In B, a peripheral venous injection demonstrates how contrast material flows from the right atrium (RA) directly into the left ventricle (LV). No contrast is visible in the right ventricle (RV) or the left atrium (LA).

of these entities, one may approach abnormalities of the great arteries from a deductive echocardiographic approach. A suggested technique is to relate the ventricles with the corresponding great arteries with sequential short-axis two-dimensional sections.[14,15] Superimposing a left ventricular short-axis study and a short-axis examination of the great arteries should provide some indication as to which great artery receives the blood from which ventricle. Normally, the aorta is superimposed on the left ventricle since it receives that chamber's blood supply. With tetralogy of Fallot, the dilated aorta may override the interventricular septum as it receives some of its blood from the right ventricle. With transposition of the great arteries, superimposition of the short-axis two-dimensional examinations of the ventricles of the great vessels shows that the left ventricle communicates with a pulmonary artery. With double-outlet right ventricle both great arteries are continuous with the right ventricle.

Tetralogy of Fallot

Probably the most common cyanotic congenital condition in adults is tetralogy of Fallot. In this abnormality, there is dilatation and dextroposition of the aorta. There is resultant encroachment or narrowing of the right ventricular outflow tract and usually valvular or subvalvular pulmonic stenosis. The malalignment of the aorta also produces a ventricular septal defect, with overriding of the anterior wall of the aorta with respect to the septum. The hemodynamic consequence is a right-to-left shunt through the ventricular septal defect into the overriding aorta. The pressures in the two ventricles are usually equal.

Figure 7–86 shows an M-mode echocardiogram of a patient with tetralogy of Fallot. The principal feature is the large aorta, with the anterior wall closer to the transducer than are the echoes from the interventricular septum.[167-170] In addition, there is usually disruption of continuity between the septum and the aorta (VSD). As mentioned earlier, this ventricular septal defect is probably one of the easiest to detect echocardiographically. The probable reason for this frequent

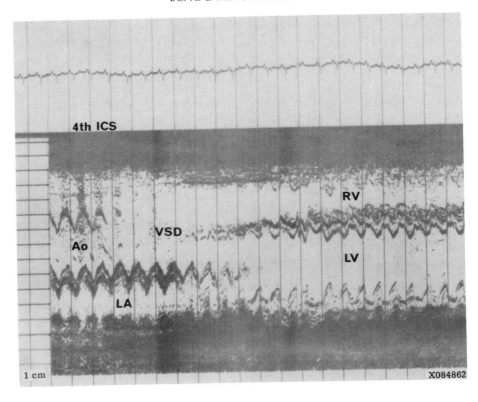

Fig. 7–86. M-mode echocardiogram of a patient with tetralogy of Fallot. The discontinuity of the echoes between the anterior aortic wall and the interventricular septum represents the ventricular septal defect (VSD). The anterior aortic wall is closer to the transducer than is the interventricular septum, a finding consistent with overriding of the aorta (AO). LA = left atrium; RV = right ventricle; LV = left ventricle.

echocardiographic finding is that the ventricular septal defect is more superior and anterior, and the aorta is malaligned. Other echocardiographic features that may be present in this abnormality include thickening of the anterior right ventricular wall, dilatation of the right ventricular chamber, and narrowing of the right ventricular outflow tract. Interventricular septal motion remains normal.[168,169]

The M-mode echocardiographic sign of overriding the aorta can be influenced by the location of the transducer.[171] If the transducer is unusually high, then one can produce artificial aortic overriding (Fig. 7–87, arrow). Because of the high location of the transducer on the chest, the anterior wall of the aorta is naturally closer to the transducer than is the interventricular septum. Figure 7–88 is another echocardiogram of the same patient. Here the transducer is in the usual

midposition of the chest and no "overriding" is recorded. Thus false-positive overriding can be created. On the other hand, if one places the transducer in an unusually low position in a patient wtih tetralogy of Fallot, one may obtain a false-negative tracing (Fig. 7–89). With the transducer in a low position on the chest, the septal echoes are naturally closer to the transducer than are the aortic echoes, and true overriding might be masked. Since most echocardiograms are obtained from a midposition, this distortion is more theoretical than actual; however, it could prove problematic in a given individual. The best safeguard against this potential artifact is to perform multiple scans from several interspaces. Scans from high or low positions are so distorted that they can be recognized by an experienced echocardiographer.

The problem of false-positive or false-

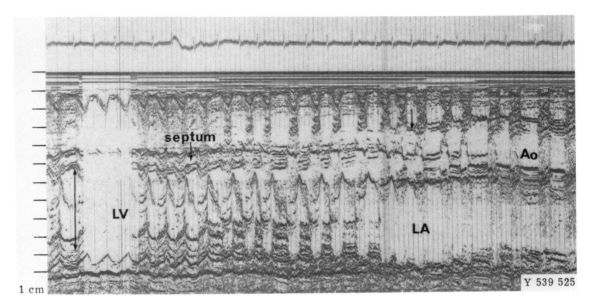

Fig. 7–87. M-mode scan with the transducer placed at a high intercostal space, producing false aortic overriding. The echoes from the anterior aortic wall *(arrow)* are closer to the transducer than are those from the septum, thus giving the appearance of aortic overriding. LV = left ventricle; LA = left atrium; AO = aorta. (From Chang, S.: M-mode Echocardiographic Techniques and Pattern Recognition. Philadelphia, Lea & Febiger, 1976.)

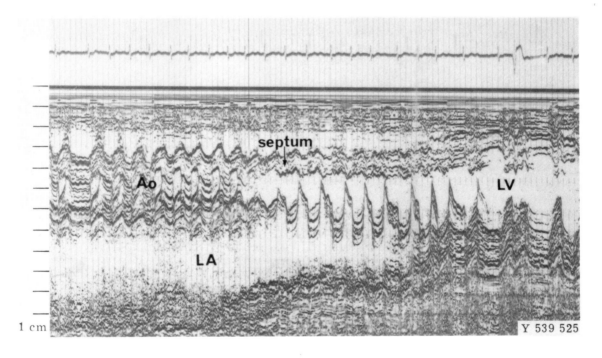

Fig. 7–88. Another M-mode scan from the patient in Figure 7–87, with the transducer in the usual midposition. Note in this tracing how the anterior aortic wall and the septum are equidistant to the transducer and that no apparent overriding is recorded. LA = left atrium; LV = left ventricle; AO = aorta. (From Chang, S.: M-mode Echocardiographic Techniques and Pattern Recognition. Philadelphia, Lea & Febiger, 1976.)

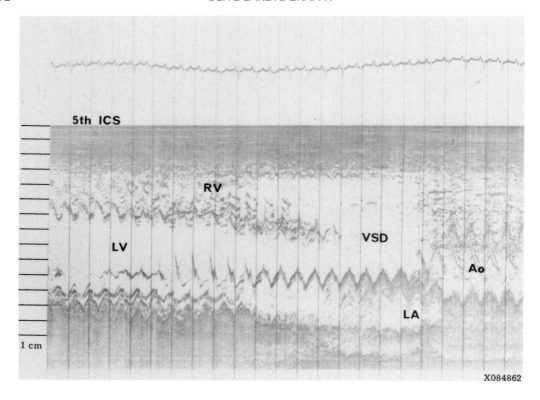

Fig. 7–89.   Another M-mode scan of the patient with tetralogy of Fallot (see Fig. 7–86). The transducer was placed in a lower interspace to demonstrate obliteration of aortic overriding. The dropout in echoes at the level of the ventricular septal defect (VSD) is still present; however, the anterior wall of the aorta (AO) is actually somewhat more apart from the transducer than are the echoes from the interventricular septum. LV = left ventricle; LA = left atrium; RV = right ventricle. (From Chang, S.: M-mode Echocardiographic Techniques and Pattern Recognition. Philadelphia, Lea & Febiger, 1976.)

negative overriding is due to the lack of spatial orientation in M-mode echocardiography and to the distortion produced by displaying a sector scan as a linear recording on strip-chart paper. This problem can be avoided with two-dimensional echocardiography.[172] Figure 7–90 shows a parasternal long-axis examination of a patient with tetralogy of Fallot. The large overriding aorta and ventricular defect are quite apparent. The correct spatial orientation inherent in this system makes this recording more accurate than a similar M-mode examination. Figure 7–56 shows the effect of closure of the ventricular septal defect (VSD) in tetralogy of Fallot. The lack of continuity between the septum and the aorta is corrected following total repair.

Another potential use of two-dimensional echocardiography is the evaluation of the

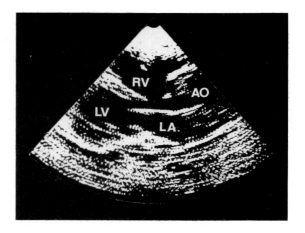

Fig. 7–90.   Long-axis two-dimensional echocardiogram of a patient with tetralogy of Fallot. Overriding of the aorta (AO) is readily apparent, as is dropout of echoes between the interventricular septum and aorta. RV = right ventricle; LV = left ventricle; LA = left atrium.

right ventricular outflow tract in patients with tetralogy of Fallot.[173] Figure 7–30 shows how the outflow tract can be evaluated by way of this two-dimensional technique. A short-axis study at the base of the heart usually provides an excellent evaluation of the right ventricular outflow tract. The severity of the infundibular obstruction is critical in assessing the patient with tetralogy of Fallot. One may also use the two-dimensional technique to assess the size of the pulmonary artery, since the size of this vessel may be an important factor when considering total surgical repair.

The right ventricular outflow tract can also be determined with M-mode echocardiography. However, it is less reliable than the two-dimensional technique.[51] One study suggests assessing the right ventricular outflow tract at surgery with the transducer placed directly on the surface of the heart.[174] Postoperative assessment of the right ventricular outflow tract is important in judging the efficacy of surgical repair. Again, the two-dimensional technique is probably best for that evaluation.

There are other ways of evaluating the postoperative patient following total repair of tetralogy of Fallot. One can judge the relief in obstruction to right ventricular outflow by a ratio of the right and left ventricular dimensions.[175,176] With an adequate relief of the obstruction and no residual shunt, the right ventricular dimension should decrease in size and be about half the size of the left ventricular dimension. If, however, the right ventricular obstruction is not relieved, then the right ventricular dimension is almost equal to the left ventricular dimension.[176] If tricuspid or pulmonic regurgitation becomes significant following surgery, then the right ventricular dimension may again remain large. If the patient develops a large left-to-right shunt postoperatively, then one may expect an increase in the size of the left atrium. Left atrial size has also been suggested as a means of evaluating a palliative shunt procedure, such as a Blalock shunt for patients with tetralogy of Fallot.[177] Such a shunt is functionally similar to a patent ductus arteriosus and can be assessed echocardiographically in a like manner.

Truncus Arteriosus

From an echocardiographic point of view, truncus arteriosus is similar to tetralogy of Fallot. Again, one records a large artery that overrides the septal echoes (Fig. 7–91).[170,178] The degree of overriding should theoretically be more than with tetralogy of Fallot; however, because of the inherent distortion that can be introduced with M-mode scanning techniques, the differentiating features are not reliable.[179] The size of the great artery may be useful in distinguishing between a truncus arteriosus and tetralogy of Fallot. As one might expect, a truncus should probably be larger than the aorta in tetralogy of Fallot. A great vessel measuring 4 cm or more is more likely a truncus than an aorta; however, some degree of overlap exists and this criterion is again not entirely reliable. Probably the best way of eliminating the diagnosis of truncus arteriosus is to locate two semilunar valves. In fact, one group of investigators suggest that the diagnosis of truncus arteriosus can be made by failure to locate more than one semilunar valve.[180] This criterion obviously requires great confidence in one's ability to record a pulmonary valve if present.

Another way of distinguishing truncus arteriosus from tetralogy of Fallot is by two-dimensional echocardiography.[181] In the short-axis examination of tetralogy of Fallot one should see a large aorta and a small pulmonary artery. With truncus arteriosus, only one large great vessel is seen with no pulmonary artery (Fig. 7–92). Again, there are different types of truncal abnormalities and some findings vary significantly. Theoretically, two-dimensional echocardiography should help in differentiating the various types of truncus; however, little in the literature states that the two-dimensional technique can actually distinguish the many types of truncus arteriosus.

Double-Outlet Right Ventricle

The echocardiographic diagnosis of double-outlet right ventricle has been in the literature for a relatively long time.[182] Although there are several varieties of this problem, the basic pathology is that both great arteries come off of the right ventricle.

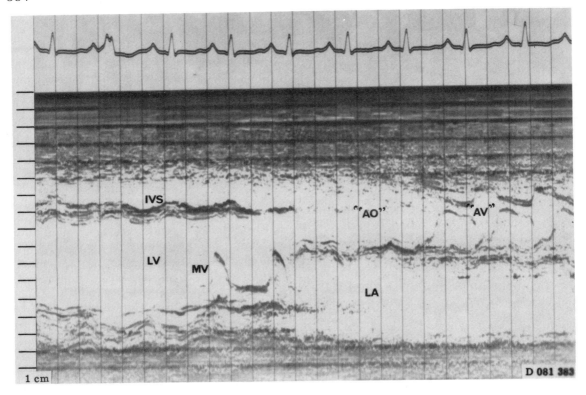

Fig. 7–91.   M-mode echocardiogram of a patient with truncus arteriosus. The apparent "aorta" ("AO") is markedly dilated and clearly overlies the interventricular septal echoes (IVS). "AV" = apparent aortic valve or truncal valve; LV = left ventricle; MV = mitral valve; LA = left atrium.

Clinically, this condition can mimic tetralogy of Fallot; however, the surgical repair is different, a factor that should be considered prior to the operative procedure. The principal M-mode echocardiographic finding is discontinuity between the mitral valve and the aorta. Normally, the mitral valve is in direct contact with the aorta and the aortic valve without any intervening tissue. With double-outlet right ventricle, a ring of tissue is interposed between the mitral valve and the aorta (Fig. 7–93).[183,183a] Although pediatric echocardiographers still find this sign reliable, this criterion has been questioned with the finding of mitral-aortic root discontinuity in patients with a dilated left ventricle.[179] The apparent echocardiographic discontinuity with a dilated ventricle is because of distortion inherent in M-mode scanning.

Double-outlet right ventricle may be more correctly evaluated by way of two-dimensional echocardiography.[184–186] Figure 7–94 is a long-axis two-dimensional study of a patient with double-outlet right ventricle. A mass of echo-producing tissue (conus) lies between the mitral valve and the great vessels. As noted earlier, a deductive two-dimensional technique for the diagnosis of double-outlet right ventricle has been proposed.[187] This examination attempts to relate the great arteries and ventricles in serial short-axis two-dimensional studies. The direct connection between the right ventricle and the two great arteries becomes apparent when short-axis examinations of the ventricle and great arteries are superimposed.[14,184,188]

Transposition of the Great Arteries

Transposition of the great arteries is probably the most common and serious cyanotic condition in the newborn. Correct identification of this entity is crucial in the proper management of these frequently critically ill

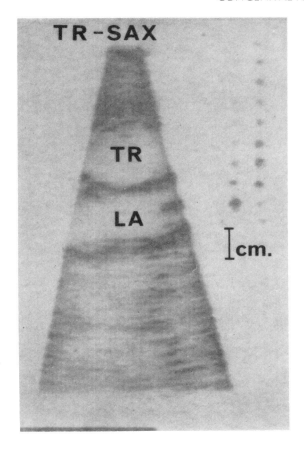

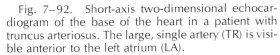

Fig. 7–92. Short-axis two-dimensional echocardiogram of the base of the heart in a patient with truncus arteriosus. The large, single artery (TR) is visible anterior to the left atrium (LA).

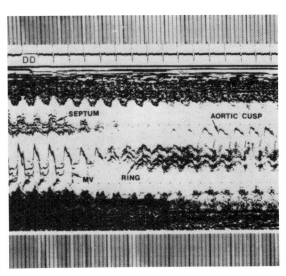

Fig. 7–93. M-mode scan of a patient with a Taussig-Bing-type double outlet right ventricle. Note that the echoes from the mitral valve (MV) and the aortic cusp are discontinuous. The two structures are separated by a band of echoes originating from a muscular rim or ring. (From Meyer, R.A.: Pediatric Echocardiography. Philadelphia, Lea & Febiger, 1977.)

patients. Echocardiography plays an important role in the assessment of these patients. Numerous studies have used both M-mode and two-dimensional echocardiography to help evaluate these patients. The ultrasonic technique is proving helpful in the total management of the patients both before and after surgical therapy.

There are several echocardiographic techniques for the detection of transposition. M-mode echocardiography was first used in the detection of this congenital anomaly. However, the M-mode examination has been superseded by two-dimensional echocardiography. One of the older M-mode techniques relied on recording simultaneous aortic and pulmonary valve echocardiograms.[52,189] Although this application helped

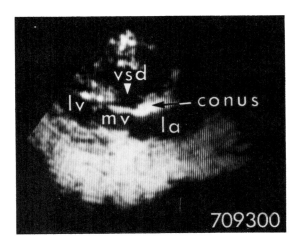

Fig. 7–94. Two-dimensional long-axis echocardiogram of a patient with a double outlet right ventricle. A thick band of tissue originating from the conus separates the mitral valve (mv) from the great artery into which the left ventricle (lv) empties. vsd = ventricular septal defect; la = left atrium.

stimulate interest in examining this type of patient, the M-mode sign was not nearly as reliable as originally hoped.[190] There are many patients, especially young infants, in whom both semilunar valves can be recorded simultaneously without transposition. The other principal M-mode technique was to meticulously identify the location and direction of the ultrasonic beam as each semilunar valve was recorded.[190a] In this way, one could anticipate the malpositioning of the two semilunar valves. One could also use deductive echocardiography to help identify the semilunar valves. The pulmonary valve usually has a longer ejection time and should lie anterior to and on the left of the aortic valve. With transposition, this relationship is altered. Contrast echocardiography, together with M-mode recording of the great arteries, could also be helpful in identifying transposition.[191] A peripheral venous injection normally produces contrast in the more anterior great artery. With transposition, the contrast echoes from a peripheral venous injection appear in the more posterior artery. There is some shunting so the contrast echoes actually appear in both arteries; however, the density of echoes should be greater in the more posterior artery when transposition is present.

Two-dimensional echocardiography is becoming the ultrasonic procedure of choice for evaluating transposition of the great arteries.[181,188,192] Figure 7–95 shows the normal short-axis relationship of the great arteries. The aorta appears as a circular structure, and the right ventricular outflow tract and pulmonary artery curve about the aorta as the two arteries twist around each other. With transposition, the two great vessels are uncoiled and run parallel to each other. Thus a short-axis section through the base of the heart reveals two circular structures that run parallel to each other.

Figure 7–96 shows the most common variety of transposition—the dextro or d-transposition. The more anterior artery is the aorta and is slightly to the patient's right, whereas the pulmonary artery is more posterior and slightly to the left. Both arteries are relatively circular structures in this short-axis examination. The size of the arteries var-

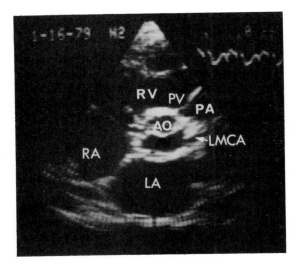

Fig. 7–95. Short-axis two-dimensional echocardiogram through the base of the heart showing how the right ventricle (RV) and pulmonary artery (PA) curve about the aorta (AO). PV = pulmonary valve; RA = right atrium; LA = left atrium; LMCA = left main coronary artery.

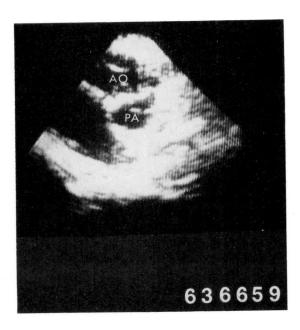

Fig. 7–96. Short-axis two-dimensional echocardiogram of a patient with d-transposition of the great vessels. The aorta (AO) is anterior to and on the right of the pulmonary artery (PA). Both vessels present relatively circular configurations in this view.

ies depending on the amount of flow passing through each vessel. Levo- or l-transposition is less common, and a short-axis section shows the aorta again anterior but on the left and the pulmonary artery as posterior and on the right. Figure 7–97 shows a type of transposition whereby the two arteries are almost side by side. Thus, the anterior-posterior, right-left orientation of the arteries can be appreciated by way of this two-dimensional examination.

A long-axis two-dimensional examination may demonstrate how the two arteries run parallel to each other rather than with transposition (Fig. 7–98). Two-dimensional echocardiography can also identify the great vessels in transposition of the great arteries by noting the course and branches of the arteries. The pulmonary artery divides into right and left pulmonary arteries; the ascending aorta becomes the aortic arch with its respective branches.[192]

The relationship of the ventricles may also alter with transposition. Rather than the ventricles being left and right, a patient with transposition may occasionally have the right ventricle directly anterior to the left. Figure 7–99 shows a patient with transposition whereby the right ventricle is directly anterior to the left ventricle. The ventricles can be identified by the appearance of the atrioventricular valves. The bicuspid mitral valve opens in a fish-mouth appearance (Fig. 7–99B). The tricuspid valve has a more hinge-like motion during diastole. The usual accompanying ventricular septal defect (vsd) can also be appreciated in Figure 7–99 as the two ventricles communicate with each other.

Corrected transposition will have inverted ventricles. Figure 7–100 illustrates such a condition whereby the inverted ventricles are side by side. An accompanying ventricular septal defect can be noted in the more apical short-axis examination (Fig. 7–100B).

Several important features of transposition can be evaluated echocardiographically besides the malposition of the great arteries and possibly that of the ventricles and the ventricular septal defect. Outflow obstruction of the left ventricle, a common and important finding, may be valvular, subvalvular, or dynamic. A ratio of the left ventricular

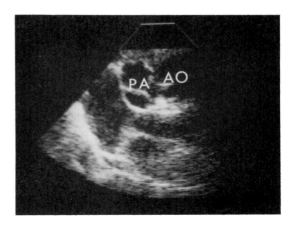

Fig. 7–97. Short-axis two-dimensional echocardiogram of a patient with a form of transposition of the great arteries whereby the great arteries are almost side by side. The aorta (AO) is to the left of and slightly anterior to the pulmonary artery (PA).

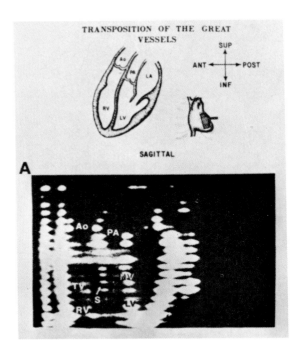

Fig. 7–98. Long-axis two-dimensional echocardiogram and diagram of a patient with transposition of the great vessels using a multi-element transducer. Note how the anterior aorta (AO) and the posterior pulmonary artery (PA) run parallel to rather than crisscross each other. TV = tricuspid valve; S = interventricular septum; MV = mitral valve; LV = left ventricle; RV = right ventricle. (From Sahn, D.J., et al.: Multiple crystal cross-sectional echocardiography in the diagnosis of cyanotic congenital heart disease. Circulation, 50:230, 1974.)

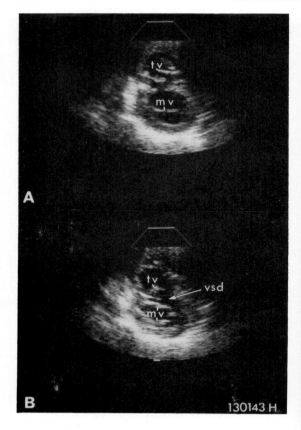

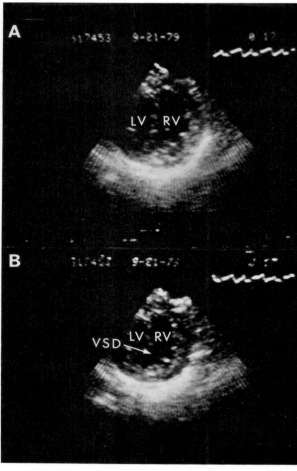

Fig. 7–99.   Short-axis two-dimensional echocardiograms at the level of the mitral valve demonstrating that the right ventricle and tricuspid valve (tv) are directly anterior to the left ventricle and mitral valve (mv). A section closer to the apex of the heart, *B*, shows the discontinuity of echoes from the ventricular septal defect (vsd).

Fig. 7–100.   Short-axis two-dimensional echocardiograms at the level of the ventricles in a patient with corrected transposition. The ventricles are inverted and lie side by side. Note the ventricular septal defect (VSD). *B*, LV = left ventricle; RV = right ventricle.

outflow tract and the pulmonary artery has been used to assess possible obstruction.[193] Systolic anterior motion of the mitral valve may occur in patients with transposition.[194,195] In fact, after a Mustard operation the systolic anterior motion may actually increase.[196] Pulsed Doppler echocardiography has also been used to detect the left ventricular outflow obstruction in patients with transposition of the great arteries.[197] This technique uses the suprasternal approach and may assist in deciding whether or not there is significant obstruction of flow into the pulmonary artery. There are, however, still many technical difficulties with this approach.

Authors have tried to use echocardiographically determined systolic time intervals to assess the pulmonary artery pressure.[198] The pre-ejection period and ejection time of the left ventricle have been shown to correlate roughly with the pulmonary artery diastolic pressure. Unfortunately, the reliability of this technique is not perfect but it apparently has some clinical usefulness. A left ventricular outflow tract obstruction produces systolic closure of the pulmonary valve (Fig. 7–101, arrow) similar to that seen with subaortic obstruction without transposition.[193]

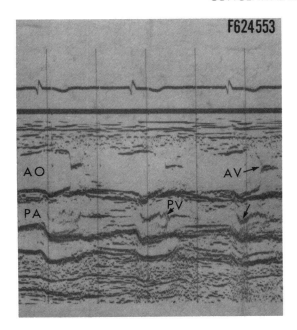

Fig. 7–101. M-mode echocardiogram of a patient with d-transposition of the great vessels and severe subpulmonic stenosis. Early systolic closure *(arrows)* and fluttering of the pulmonary valve (PV) can be noted. AV = aortic valve; AO = aorta; PA = pulmonary artery.

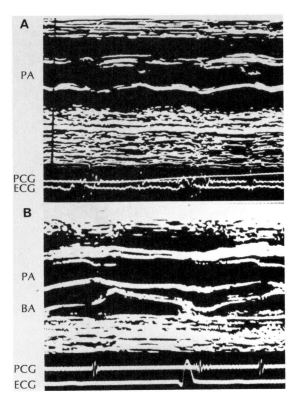

Fig. 7–102. M-mode echocardiograms of a patient with transposition of the great vessels before, *A*, and after, *B*, a baffle is inserted as part of surgical repair. An echo from the baffle (BA) is visible behind the pulmonary artery (PA). ECG = electrocardiogram; PCG = phonocardiogram. (From Nanda, N.C. and Gramiak, R.: Clinical Echocardiography. St. Louis, C.V. Mosby Co., 1978.)

There are two popular forms of treatment for transposition of the great arteries. The first is a palliative atrial septostomy frequently performed through a balloon catheter. The second is a more definitive Mustard procedure whereby an intra-atrial baffle diverts the flow of venous blood into the proper channel. The balloon septostomy can be evaluated with two-dimensional echocardiography. As noted in Figure 7–66, one can actually image the atrial septal defect created by such a technique. The septal fragments may be seen moving from the edges of the defect (Fig. 7–66). Using the subcostal examination and a high-frequency transducer, it is even possible to assess the size of the iatrogenic atrial septal defect.[129,199]

The more definite corrective surgery uses an intra-atrial baffle.[196,200] This structure can be recorded echocardiographically with both M-mode and two-dimensional examinations. Such a baffle represents another possible cause of intra-atrial echoes. Figure 7–102 shows a patient with transposition be-

fore and after a Mustard procedure. The moving baffle echo (BA) can be seen within the left atrium behind the transposed pulmonary artery (PA). Several articles have been written concerning the postoperative echocardiogram following this type of operation. Some findings have included an increased frequency of systolic anterior motion of the mitral valve postoperatively[196,201,202] and fluttering of the mitral valve as a result of the shunting procedure.[201,203] Some studies have indicated a different type of echo from the baffle when it may be obstructing the inflow of systemic venous blood owing to malposition or shrinkage. Two-dimensional studies have attempted to actually image the systemic and pulmonary venous channels postoperatively to assess the functional state. M-mode echocardiographic dimensions of the right and left ventricles have also been helpful in judging the efficacy of the shunt procedure.[202] With an effective operation, the right ventricle should increase and the left ventricle decrease. There has also been an attempt to use Doppler echocardiography to detect obstruction to systemic venous return following repair of transposition.[204]

OTHER CONGENITAL ANOMALIES

Congenital idiopathic dilatation of the pulmonary artery may occur with or without pulmonic insufficiency.[205,205a] Dilatation of the pulmonary artery is easily detected echocardiographically. Figure 7–103 shows an example of a markedly dilated pulmonary artery. A short-axis study through the base of

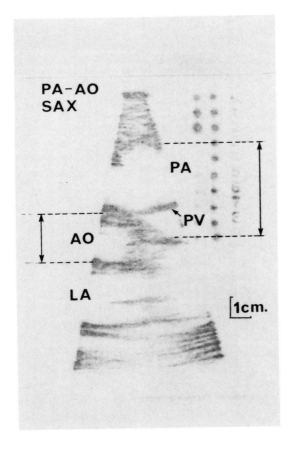

Fig. 7–103. Two-dimensional short-axis (SAX) echocardiogram of a patient with idiopathic dilatation of the pulmonary artery (PA). AO = aorta; LA = left atrium; PV = pulmonary valve.

the heart readily makes this diagnosis. Although the two-dimensional study is more striking, one could also anticipate the proper diagnosis from an M-mode examination of the pulmonary valve in which there is a marked increase in the echo-free space of the pulmonary artery.[205]

Several reports have shown how echocardiography can help diagnose persistent left superior vena cava.[206–209] This anomalous vein usually drains into the coronary sinus and produces coronary sinus dilatation. Thus one of the clues in the echocardiographic diagnosis of persistent left superior vena cava is an unusually large coronary sinus on a two-dimensional examination. A more definite diagnosis can be made by way of a contrast peripheral venous injection in the left upper extremity. Such a contrast injection produces echo-producing microbubbles within the coronary sinus.

Figure 7–104 shows an M-mode examination of a patient with an interatrial septal aneurysm.[210] The aneurysm produces an unusual pulsation of the interatrial septum behind the tricuspid valve. Both echoes are originating from the aneurysm, and a striking feature is separation of the two echoes with atrial systole. During ventricular systole the two echoes approach each other.

There have been some interesting echocardiographic observations in patients with congenital anomalies of the coronary arteries.[211,211a] Figure 7–105 shows a short-axis two-dimensional study of the base of the heart and demonstrates the normal coronary arteries in a young child. The right coronary artery originates from the right coronary sinus of the aorta. The left coronary artery originates from the left coronary sinus. Bifurcation of the left coronary artery into its two major branches can be seen a short distance from the origin of the left main coronary artery (Fig. 7–105B). With anomalous origin of the left coronary artery from the pulmonary artery, one may fail to see a communication between the left coronary artery and the aorta. This finding can be quite subtle since the left coronary artery is otherwise in its normal position. A more dramatic example of an anomalous left coronary artery is seen in Figure 7–106. The left coronary

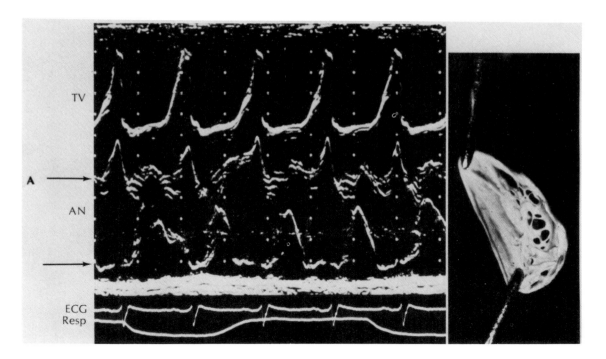

Fig. 7–104. M-mode echocardiogram of a patient with an interatrial septal aneurysm. The undulating echo behind the tricuspid valve (TV) arises from an aneurysm (AN) whose anterior and posterior limits are indicated by the arrows. Phasic differences in motion, as well as changes in wave form related to respiration, suggest the presence of an undulating membrane-like structure rather than a solid mass. The surgical specimen is on the right. (From Nanda, N.C. and Gramiak, R.: Clinical Echocardiography. St. Louis, C.V. Mosby Co., 1978.)

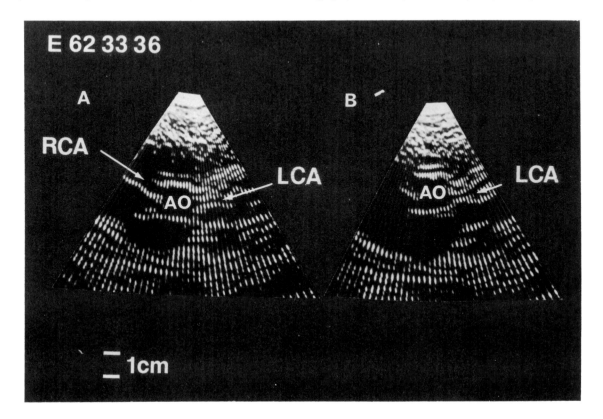

Fig. 7–105. Short-axis two-dimensional echocardiograms through the base of the heart demonstrating the right (RCA) and left (LCA) coronary arteries originating from the aorta (AO).

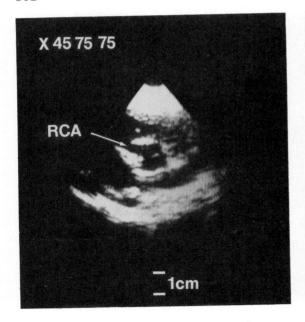

Fig. 7–106. Two-dimensional echocardiogram of a patient with an anomalous left coronary artery that does not communicate with the aorta. Instead one finds a dilated right coronary artery (RCA) that does communicate with the aorta.

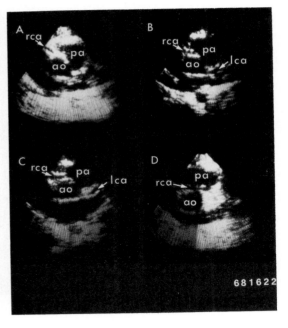

Fig. 7–107. Serial two-dimensional echocardiograms of a patient with an anomalous right coronary artery (rca) that communicates with the pulmonary artery (pa). A, The right coronary artery fails to communicate with the aorta (ao). B and C, The right coronary artery is visible traversing anterior to the aorta. C and D, The right coronary artery appears to communicate with the pulmonary artery. lca = left coronary artery.

artery is not seen; instead a dilated right coronary artery is visualized.

Figure 7–107 shows the echocardiographic findings in a patient with an anomalous right coronary artery. Figure 7–107A shows the right coronary artery (rca) failing to communicate with the aorta (ao). Figure 7–107B shows the course of the right coronary artery as it traverses anterior to the aorta. The normal left coronary artery (lca) can be seen. Figure 7–107C illustrates another view of the right coronary artery anterior to the aorta. Figure 7–107D shows a more distal view of the right coronary artery as it remains anterior to the aorta and communicates with the pulmonary artery (pa).

Anomalous coronary arteries also produce changes in left ventricular function that can be detected echocardiographically. Segmental dyssynergy should be expected in these patients and can help distinguish this entity from a cardiomyopathy.[211] With a cardiomyopathy, diffuse ventricular dysfunction is the rule rather than segmental dyssynergy.

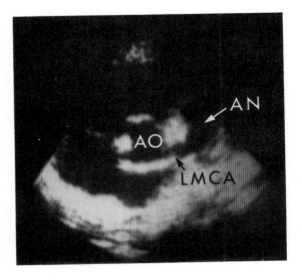

Fig. 7–108. Two-dimensional echocardiogram of a patient with aneurysmal dilatation of the left main coronary artery (lmca). Note that the aneurysm (AN) communicates with that artery. AO = aorta.

Aneurysms of the coronary arteries may also be noted in infants and young children.[212,213] This entity is usually associated with a mucocutaneous lymph node syndrome. Figure 7–108 shows an example of aneurysmal dilatation (AN) of the left coronary artery. These dilatations can be striking and have been reported by several investigators.

A coronary artery fistula in the left ventricle has also been demonstrated in the echocardiographic literature.[214] Figure 7–109 is an M-mode echocardiogram of a patient with a right coronary artery fistula. It must be distinguished from tetralogy of Fallot, since superficially one may incorrectly diagnose overriding of the aorta. The anterior wall of the aorta (AO) is actually at the same level as the septum. The more anterior echoes are coming from the dilated right coronary artery (RCA), which drains into the left ventricle (LV). One may also see fluttering of the left ventricular structures, such as the mitral

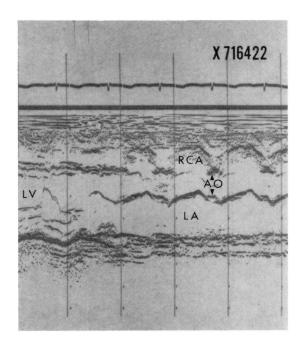

Fig. 7–109. M-mode echocardiogram of a patient with a right coronary artery fistula communicating with the left ventricle (LV). The space anterior to the aorta (AO) is not dilated as this tracing makes superficially apparent. Instead a right coronary artery (RCA) is dilated anterior to the aorta, which has a fistulous connection with the left ventricle. LA = left atrium.

valve or chordae as a result of the anomalous flow of blood into the left ventricle.

Another rare congenital anomaly that may produce characteristic echocardiographic findings is Uhl's anomaly.[215] One usually finds a greatly dilated right ventricle with delayed closure of the tricuspid valve. There may also be paradoxical motion of the interventricular septum.

SUMMARY

Echocardiography has become indispensable in the workup of patients with congenital heart disease. Both M-mode and two-dimensional echocardiography provide information that is not only complementary to other diagnostic techniques but in some patients is definitive and is the best possible information available. Two-dimensional echocardiography has greatly contributed to the value of the ultrasonic examination.[216–219] In many respects, the two-dimensional technique has replaced the M-mode examination in the evaluation of some of these patients. As in all aspects of echocardiography, the echocardiographic diagnosis of congenital heart disease has many potential technical pitfalls and limitations. In addition, it cannot be emphasized too strongly that the person doing the examination must be well versed in the many congenital problems that can exist in these patients. The better the individual understands the complex nature of these anomalies, the more likely he is to anticipate and recognize these problems echocardiographically.

REFERENCES

1. Solinger, R., Elbl, F., and Minhas, K.: Echocardiography in the normal neonate. Circulation, 47:108, 1973.
2. Talner, N.S. and Campbell, A.G.: Recognition and management of cardiologic problems in the newborn infant. Prog. Cardiovasc. Dis., 15:159, 1972.
3. Keutel, J.: Echocardiographic examinations in children. Monatsschr. Kinderheilkd., 121:520, 1973.
4. Lundstrom, N.R.: Clinical applications of echocardiography in infants and children. Acta Paediatr. Scand. (Suppl.), 243:1, 1974.
5. Meyer, R.A., Schwartz, D.C., Covitz, W., and Kaplan, S.: Echocardiographic assessment of cardiac malposition. Am. J. Cardiol., 33:896, 1974.
6. Murphy, K., Kotler, M.N., Reichek, N., and Perloff, J.K.: Ultrasound in the diagnosis of congenital heart disease. Am. Heart J., 89:638, 1975.

7. Nanda, N.C., Gramiak, R., Robinson, T.I., and Shah, P.M.: Echocardiographic evaluation of pulmonary hypertension. Circulation, 50:575, 1974.

8. Solinger, R., Elbl, F., and Minhas, K.: Deductive echocardiographic analysis in infants with congenital heart disease. Circulation, 50:1072, 1974.

9. Kato, H. and Yoshioka, F.: Echocardiographic approach for atrioventricular malalignment and related conditions. J. Cardiogr., 8:521, 1978.

9a.Foale, R.A., Stefanini, L., Rickards, A.F., and Somerville, J.: Two-dimensional echocardiographic features of corrected transposition. Am. J. Cardiol., 45:466, 1980. (Abstract)

10. Nanda, N.C., Gramiak, R., Shah, P.M., DeWeese, J.A., and Mahoney, E.B.: Echocardiographic assessment of left ventricular outflow width in the selection of mitral valve prosthesis. Circulation, 48:1208, 1973.

11. Reference deleted.

12. Henry, W.L., Sahn, D.J., Griffith, J.M., Goldberg, S.J., Maron, B.J., McAllister, H.A., Allen, H.D., and Epstein, S.E.: Evaluation of atrioventricular valve morphology in congenital heart disease by real-time cross-sectional echocardiography. Circulation (Suppl. II), 52:120, 1975. (Abstract)

12a.Hagler, D.J., Tajik, A.J., Seward, J.B., Mair, D.D., and Ritter, D.G.: Wide-angle two-dimensional echocardiographic criteria for ventricular morphology. Am. J. Cardiol., 45:466, 1980. (Abstract)

13. Satomi, G., Shimizu, K., Komatsu, Y., and Takao, A.: Two-dimensional echocardiographic diagnosis of congenital heart disease (segmental approach): spatial interrelationship between the great arteries. J. Cardiogr., 8:557, 1978.

14. Henry, W.L., Maron, B.J., and Griffith, J.M.: Cross-sectional echocardiography in the diagnosis of congenital heart disease: identification of the relation of the ventricles and great arteries. Circulation, 56:267, 1977.

15. Houston, A.V., Gregory, N.L., and Coleman, E.N.: Echocardiographic identification of aorta and main pulmonary artery in complete transposition. Br. Heart J., 40:377, 1978.

16. Weyman, A.E., Feigenbaum, H., Dillon, J.C., and Chang, S.: Cross-sectional echocardiography in assessing the severity of valvular aortic stenosis. Circulation, 52:828, 1975.

17. Weyman, A.E., Feigenbaum, H., Hurwitz, R.A., Girod, D.A., Dillon, J.C., and Chang, S.: Localization of left ventricular outflow by cross-sectional echocardiography. Am. J. Med., 60:33, 1976.

18. Weyman, A.E., Feigenbaum, H., Hurwitz, R.A., Girod, D.A., and Dillon, J.C.: Cross-sectional echocardiographic assessment of the severity of aortic stenosis in children. Circulation, 55:773, 1977.

19. Bass, J.L., Einzig, S., Hong, C.Y., and Moller, J.H.: Echocardiographic screening to assess the severity of congenital aortic valve stenosis in children. Am. J. Cardiol., 44:82, 1979.

20. Gewitz, M.H., Werner, J.C., Kleinman, C.S., Hellenbrand, W.E., and Talner, N.S.: Role of echocardiography in aortic stenosis: pre- and postoperative studies. Am. J. Cardiol., 43:67, 1979.

21. Aziz, K.U., van Grondelle, A., Paul, M.H., and Muster, A.J.: Echocardiographic assessment of the relation between left ventricular wall and cavity dimensions and peak systolic pressure in children with aortic stenosis. Am. J. Cardiol., 40:775, 1977.

22. Bass, J.L., Einzig, S., Hong, C.Y., and Miller, J.H.: Echocardiographic screening to assess the severity of congenital aortic valve stenosis in children. Am. J. Cardiol., 44:82, 1979.

23. Johnson, G.L., Meyer, R.A., Schwartz, D.C., Korfhagen, J., and Kaplan, S.: Echocardiographic evaluation of fixed left ventricular outlet obstruction in children. Circulation, 56:299, 1977.

24. Kelly, D.T., Wulfsberg, E., and Rowe, R.D.: Discrete subaortic stenosis. Circulation, 46:309, 1972.

25. Popp, R.L., Silverman, J.F., French, J.W., Stinson, E.B., and Harrison, D.C.: Echocardiographic findings in discrete subvalvular aortic stenosis. Circulation, 49:226, 1974.

26. Weyman, A.E., Feigenbaum, H., Dillon, J.C., Chang, S., Hurwitz, R.A., and Girod, D.A.: Cross-sectional echocardiography in the diagnosis of discrete subaortic stenosis. Am. J. Cardiol., 37:358, 1976.

26a.Roelandt, J. and vanDorp, W.G.: Long-segment (tunnel) subaortic stenosis. Chest, 72:222, 1977.

27. Davis, R.A., Feigenbaum, H., Chang, S., Konecke, L.L., and Dillon, J.C.: Echocardiographic manifestations of discrete subaortic stenosis. Am. J. Cardiol., 33:277, 1974.

28. Laurenceau, J.L., Guay, J.M., and Gagne, S.: Echocardiography in the diagnosis of subaortic membranous stenosis. Circulation (Suppl. IV), 48:46, 1973. (Abstract)

29. Maron, B.J., Redwood, D.R., Roberts, W.C., Henry, W.L., Morrow, A.G., and Epstein, S.E.: Tunnel subaortic stenosis: left ventricular outflow tract obstruction produced by fibromuscular tubular narrowing. Circulation, 54:404, 1976.

30. Williams, D.E., Sahn, D.J., and Friedman, W.F.: Cross-sectional echocardiographic localization of sites of left ventricular outflow tract obstruction. Am. J. Cardiol., 37:250, 1976.

31. Kronzon, I., Schloss, M., Danilowicz, D., and Singh, S.: Fixed membranous subaortic stenosis. Chest, 67:473, 1975.

32. Krueger, S.K., French, J.W., Forker, A.D., Caudill, C.C., and Popp, R.L.: Echocardiography in discrete subaortic stenosis. Circulation, 59:506, 1979.

33. Ten Cate, F.J., Van Dorp, W.G., Hugenholtz, P.G., and Roelandt, J.: Fixed subaortic stenosis: value of echocardiography for diagnosis and differentiation between various types. Br. Heart J., 41:159, 1979.

34. Berry, T.E., Aziz, K.U., and Paul, M.H.: Echocardiographic assessment of discrete subaortic stenosis in childhood. Am. J. Cardiol., 43:957, 1979.

35. Bolen, J.L., Popp, R.L., and French, J.W.: Echocardiographic features of supravalvular aortic stenosis. Circulation, 52:817, 1975.

36. Nasrallah, A.T. and Nihill, M.: Supravalvular aortic stenosis: echocardiographic features. Br. Heart J., 37:662, 1975.

37. Usher, B.W., Goulden, D., and Murgo, J.P.: Echocardiographic detection of supraventricular aortic stenosis. Circulation, 49:1257, 1974.

38. Mori, Y., Nakano, H., Kamiya, T., and Mori, C.: Echocardiographic and angiocardiographic features of supravalvular aortic atenosis. J. Cardiogr., 7:339, 1977.

38a.Ali, N., Sheikh, M., Mehrotra, P., and Banks, T.: Echocardiographic diagnosis of supravalvular aortic stenosis. South. Med. J., 70:759, 1977.

39. Weyman, A.E., Caldwell, R.L., Hurwitz, R.A., Girod, D.A., Dillon, J.C., Feigenbaum, H., and

Green, D.: Cross-sectional echocardiographic characterization of aortic obstruction. I. Supravalvular aortic stenosis and aortic hypoplasia. Circulation, 57:491, 1978.

40. Chestler, E., Jaffe, H.S., Vecht, R., Beck, W., and Schrire, V.: Ultrasound cardiography in single ventricle and the hypoplastic left and right heart syndromes. Circulation, 42:123, 1970.

41. Meyer, R.A. and Kaplan, S.: Echocardiography in the diagnosis of hypoplasia of the left or right ventricle in the neonate. Circulation, 46:55, 1972.

42. Farooki, Z.Q., Henry, J.G., and Green, E.W.: Echocardiographic spectrum of the hypoplastic left heart syndrome. Am. J. Cardiol., 38:337, 1976.

43. Lange, L., Sahn, D.J., Allen, H., and Goldberg, S.: Cross-sectional echocardiographic diagnosis of hypoplastic left heart syndrome (HLH). Circulation (Suppl. II), 58:51, 1978. (Abstract)

44. Allen, H.D., Sahn, D.J., and Goldberg, S.J.: Caveats in echocardiographic (echo) diagnosis of the hypoplastic left heart (HLH) syndrome. Circulation (Suppl. III), 56:40, 1977. (Abstract)

44a. Bass, J.L., Ben-Shachar, G., and Edwards, J.E.: Comparison of M-mode echocardiography and pathologic findings in the hypoplastic left heart syndrome. Am. J. Cardiol., 45:79, 1980.

45. Weyman, A.E., Caldwell, R.L., Hurwitz, R.A., Girod, D.A., Dillon, J.C., Feigenbaum, H., and Green, D.: Cross-sectional echocardiographic detection of aortic obstruction. II. Coarctation of the aorta. Circulation, 57:498, 1978.

46. Weyman, A.E., Dillon, J.C., Feigenbaum, H., and Chang, S.: Echocardiographic patterns of pulmonic valve motion in pulmonic stenosis. Am. J. Cardiol., 34:644, 1974.

47. Flanagan, W.H. and Shah, P.M.: Echocardiographic correlate of presystolic pulmonary ejection sound in congenital valvular pulmonic stenosis. Am. Heart J., 94:633, 1977.

48. Weyman, A.E., Hurwitz, R.A., Girod, D.A., Dillon, J.C., Feigenbaum, H., and Green, D.: Cross-sectional echocardiographic visualization of the stenotic pulmonary valve. Circulation, 56:769, 1977.

49. Goldberg, S.J., Areias, J.C., Spitaels, S.E.C., and deVilleneuve, V.H.: Echo Doppler detection of pulmonary stenosis by time-interval histogram analysis. J. Clin. Ultrasound, 7:183, 1979.

50. Weyman, A.E., Dillon, J.C., Feigenbaum, H., and Chang, S.: Echocardiographic differentiation of infundibular from valvular pulmonary stenosis. Am. J. Cardiol., 36:21, 1975.

51. Caldwell, R.L., Weyman, A.E., Hurwitz, R.A., Girod, D.A., and Feigenbaum, H.: Right ventricular outflow tract assessment by cross-sectional echocardiography in tetralogy of Fallot. Circulation, 59:395, 1979.

52. Moss, A.J., Gussoni, C.C., and Isabel-Jones, J.: Echocardiography in congenital heart disease. West. J. Med., 124:102, 1976.

53. Lundstrom, N.R.: Ultrasoundcardiographic studies of the mitral valve region in young infants with mitral atresia, mitral stenosis, hypoplasia of the left ventricle and cor triatriatum. Circulation, 45:324, 1972.

54. Lundstrom, N.R.: Echocardiography in the diagnosis of congenital mitral stenosis and an evaluation of the results of mitral valvulotomy. Circulation, 46:44, 1972.

55. Driscoll, D.J., Gutgesell, H.P., and McNamara,

D.G.: Echocardiographic features of congenital mitral stenosis. Am. J. Cardiol., 42:259, 1978.

56. Murphy, K.F., Kotler, M.N., Reichek, N., and Perloff, J.K.: Ultrasound in the diagnosis of congenital heart disease. Am. Heart J., 89:638, 1975.

57. LaCorte, M., Harada, K., and Williams, R.G.: Echocardiographic features of congenital left ventricular inflow obstruction. Circulation, 54:562, 1976.

58. Cooperberg, P., Hazell, S., and Ashmore, P.G.: Parachute accessory anterior mitral valve leaflet causing left ventricular outflow tract obstruction. Circulation, 53:908, 1976.

59. Ehrich, D.A., Vieweg, W.V.R., Alpert, J.S., Folkerth, T.L., and Hagan, A.D.: Cor triatriatum: report of case in a young adult with special reference to the echocardiographic features and etiology of the systolic murmur. Am. Heart J., 94:217, 1977.

60. Canedo, M.I., Stefadouros, M.A., Frank, M.J., Moore, H.V., and Cundey, D.W.: Echocardiographic features of cor triatriatum. Am. J. Cardiol., 40:615, 1977.

60a. Atsuchi, Y., Nagai, Y., Komatsu, Y., Nakamura, K., and Hirosawa, K.: Echocardiographic demonstration of anomalous septum in cor triatriatum. Jpn. Heart J., 18:266, 1977.

60b. Kelley, M.J., Glanz, S., Hellenbrand, W.E., Taunt, K.A., and Berman, M.A.: Diagnosis of cor triatriatum by echocardiography. Radiology, 123:159, 1977.

61. Seward, J.B., Tajik, A.J., Hagler, D.J., and Ritter, D.G.: Echocardiographic spectrum of tricuspid atresia. Mayo Clin. Proc., 53:100, 1978.

62. Silverman, N.H., Payot, M., and Stanger, P.: Simulated tricuspid valve echoes in tricuspid atresia. Am. Heart J., 95:761, 1978.

63. Beppu, S., Nimura, Y., Tamai, M., Nagata, S., Matsuo, H., Kawashima, Y., Kozuka, T., and Sakakibara, H.: Two-dimensional echocardiography in diagnosing tricuspid atresia: differentiation from other hypoplastic right heart syndromes and common atrioventricular canal. Br. Heart J., 40:1174, 1978.

64. Radford, D.J., Bloom, K.R., Izukawa, R., Moes, C.A.F., and Rowe, R.D.: Echocardiographic assessment of bicuspid aortic valves. Circulation, 53:80, 1976.

65. Leech, G., Mills, P., and Leatham, A.: The diagnosis of a non-stenotic bicuspid aortic valve. Br. Heart J., 40:941, 1978.

66. Nanda, N.C. and Gramiak, R.: Evaluation of bicuspid aortic valves by two-dimensional echocardiography. Am. J. Cardiol., 41:372, 1978. (Abstract)

67. Hagler, D.J., Tajik, A.J., Seward, J.B., Mair, D.D., and Ritter, D.G.: Real-time wide-angle sector echocardiography: atrioventricular canal defects. Circulation, 59:140, 1979.

68. Lundstrom, N.R.: Echocardiography in the diagnosis of Ebstein's anomaly of the tricuspid valve. Circulation, 47:597, 1973.

69. Giuliani, E.R., Fuster, V., Brandenburg, R.O., and Mair, D.D.: Ebstein's anomaly: the clinical features and natural history of Ebstein's anomaly of the tricuspid valve. Mayo Clin. Proc., 54:163, 1979.

70. Tajik, A.J., Gau, G.T., Giuliani, E.R., Ritter, D.G., and Schattenberg, T.T.: Echocardiogram in Ebstein's anomaly with Wolff-Parkinson-White

pre-excitation syndrome, Type B. Circulation, 47:813, 1973.

71. Tomonaga, G., Hoshino, T., Shimono, S., Kinoshita, M., and Kusukawa, R.: Echocardiographic findings in Ebstein's anomaly. Cardiovasc. Sound Bull., 5:627, 1975.

72. Milner, S., Meyer, R.A., Venables, A.W., Korfhagen, J., and Kaplan, S.: Mitral and tricuspid valve closure in congenital heart disease. Circulation, 53:513, 1976.

73. Henry, J.G., Gordon, S., and Timmis, G.C.: Corrected transposition of great vessels and Ebstein's anomaly of tricuspid valve. Br. Heart J., 41:249, 1979.

74. Reference omitted.

74a. Daniel, W., Rathsack, P., Walpurger, G., Kahle, A., Gisbertz, R., Schmitz, J., and Lichtlen, P.R.: Value of M-mode echocardiography for non-invasive diagnosis of Ebstein's anomaly. Br. Heart J., 43:38, 1980.

75. Farooki, Z.Q., Henry, J.G., and Green, E.W.: Echocardiographic spectrum of Ebstein's anomaly of the tricuspid valve. Circulation, 53:63, 1976.

76. Koiwaya, Y., Narabayashi, H., Koyanagi, S., Matsuguchi, H., Tanaka, S., Imaizumi, T., Kuroiwa, A., Nakamura, M., and Hirata, T.: Early closure of the tricuspid valve in a case of Ebstein's anomaly with Type B Wolff-Parkinson-White syndrome. Circulation, 60:446, 1979.

77. Lundstrom, N.R. and Edler, I.: Ultrasoundcardiography in infants and children. Acta Paediatr. Scand., 60:117, 1971.

78. Hirschklau, M.J., Sahn, D.J., Hagan, A.D., Williams, D.E., and Friedman, W.F.: Cross-sectional echocardiographic features of Ebstein's anomaly of the tricuspid valve. Am. J. Cardiol., 40:400, 1977.

79. Matsumoto, M., Matsuo, H., Nagata, S., Hamanaka, Y., Fujita, T., Kawashima, Y., Nimura, Y., and Abe, H.: Visualization of Ebstein's anomaly of the tricuspid valve by two-dimensional and standard echocardiography. Circulation, 53:69, 1976.

80. Ports, T.A., Silverman, N.H., and Schiller, N.B.: Two-dimensional echocardiographic assessment of Ebstein's anomaly. Circulation, 58:336, 1978.

80a. Gussenhoven, W.J., Spitaels, S.E.C., Bom, N., and Becker, A.E.: Echocardiographic criteria for Ebstein's anomaly of tricuspid valve. Br. Heart J., 43:31, 1980.

81. Kambe, T., Ichimiya, S., Toguchi, M., Hibi, N., Fukui, Y., Nishimura, K., and Hojo, Y.: Cross-sectional echocardiographic study of Ebstein's anomaly using electronic sector scan. J. Cardiogr., 9:269, 1979.

82. Gibson, D.G. and Traill, T.A.: Echocardiography of atrioventricular valves in patients with univentricular heart. Herz, 4:220, 1979.

83. Seward, J.B., Tajik, A.J., and Ritter, D.G.: Echocardiographic features of straddling tricuspid valve. Mayo Clin. Proc., 50:427, 1975.

84. LaCorte, M.A., Fellows, K.E., and Williams, R.G.: Overriding tricuspid valve: echocardiographic and angiocardiographic features. Am. J. Cardiol., 37:911, 1976.

85. Aziz, K.U., Paul, M.H., Muster, A.J., and Idriss, F.S.: Positional abnormalities of atrioventricular valves in transposition of the great arteries including double outlet right ventricle, atrioventricular valve straddling and malattachment. Am. J. Cardiol., 44:1135, 1979.

86. Seward, J.B., Tajik, A.J., Hagler, D.J. and Mair, D.D.: Straddling atrioventricular valve: diagnostic two-dimensional echocardiographic features. Am. J. Cardiol., 41:354, 1978. (Abstract)

86a. Baylen, B.G., Meyer, R.A., Kaplan, S., Ringenburg, W.E., and Korfhagen, J.: The critically ill premature infant with patent ductus arteriosus and pulmonary disease—an echocardiographic assessment. J. Pediatr., 86:423, 1975.

86b. Halliday, H., Hirschfeld, S., Riggs, T., Liebman, J., Fanaroff, A., and Bormuth, C.: Respiratory distress syndrome: echocardiographic assessment of cardiovascular function and pulmonary vascular resistance. Pediatrics, 60:444, 1977.

87. Goldberg, S.J., Allen, H.D., and Sahn, D.J.: Pediatric and Adolescent Echocardiography. Chicago, Year Book Medical Publishers, Inc., 1975.

88. Laird, W.P. and Fixler, D.E.: Echocardiography of premature infants with pulmonary disease: a noninvasive method for detecting large ductal left-to-right shunts. Radiology, 122:455, 1977.

89. Sahn, D.J., Vaucher, Y., Williams, D.E., Allen, H.D., Goldberg, S.J., and Friedman, W.F.: Echocardiographic detection of large left to right shunts and cardiomyopathies in infants and children. Am. J. Cardiol., 38:73, 1976.

90. Allen, H.D. and Goldberg, S.J.: Usefulness of biaxial left atrial dimension measurements by echocardiography. J. Clin. Ultrasound, 2:222, 1974. (Abstract)

91. Goldberg, S.J., Allen, H.D., Sahn, D.J., Friedman, W.F., and Harris, T.: A prospective 2½ year experience with echocardiographic evaluation of prematures with patent ductus arteriosus (PDA) and respiratory distress syndrome (RDS). Am. J. Cardiol., 35:139, 1975. (Abstract)

92. Baylen, B., Meyer, R.A., Korfhagen, J., Benzing, G., Bubb, M.E., and Kaplan, S.: Left ventricular performance in the critically ill premature infant with patent ductus arteriosus and pulmonary disease. Circulation, 55:182, 1977.

93. Sahn, D.J. and Allen, H.D.: Real-time cross-sectional echocardiographic imaging and measurement of the patent ductus arteriosus in infants and children. Circulation, 58:343, 1978.

94. Baba, K., Kohata, T., Tanimoto, T., Echigo, S., Kaneko, H., Hirose, O., Kamiya, T., Nagata, M., Beppu, S., and Kozuka, T.: Identification of the great artery relations in infants by real-time two-dimensional echocardiography. J. Cardiog., 9:159, 1979.

95. Stevenson, J.G., Kawabori, I., and Guntheroth, W.G.: Noninvasive detection in pulmonary hypertension in patent ductus arteriosus by pulsed Doppler echocardiography. Circulation, 60:355, 1979.

95a. Sahn, D.J., Allen, H.D., Geroge, W., Mason, M., and Goldberg, S.J.: The utility of contrast echocardiographic techniques in the care of critically ill infants with cardiac and pulmonary disease. Circulation, 56:959, 1977.

96. Allen, H.D., Sahn, D.J., and Goldberg, S.J.: New serial contrast technique for assessment of left-to-right shunting patent ductus arteriosus in the neonate. Am. J. Cardiol., 41:288, 1978.

97. Lewis, A.B. and Takahashi, M.: Echocardio-

graphic assessment of left-to-right shunt volume in children with ventricular septal defect. Circulation, *54*:78, 1976.

98. Ahmad, M. and Hallidie-Smith, K.A.: Assessment of left-to-right shunt and left ventricular function in isolated ventricular septal defect. Br. Heart J., *41*:147, 1979.

99. Rees, A.H., Rao, P.S., Rigby, J.J., and Miller, M.D.: Echocardiographic estimation of a left-to-right shunt in isolated ventricular septal defects. Eur. J. Cardiol., 7:25, 1978.

100. Lester, L.A., Vitullo, D., Sodt, P., Hutcheon, N., and Arcilla, R.: An evaluation of the left atrial/aortic root ratio in children with ventricular septal defect. Circulation, *60*:364, 1979.

101. Seward, J.B., Tajik, A.J., Hagler, D.J., and Mair, D.D.: Visualization of isolated ventricular septal defect with wide-angle two-dimensional sector echocardiography. Circulation (Suppl. II), *58*:202, 1978. (Abstract)

102. King, D.L., Steeg, C.N., and Ellis, K.: Visualization of ventricular septal defects by cardiac ultrasonography. Circulation, *48*:1215, 1973.

103. Hada, Y., Umeda, T., Omoto, R., Furuta, S., Machii, K., and Hayashida, N.: Echocardiographic manifestations of supracristal ventricular septal defect. Cardiovasc. Sound Bull., 5:617, 1975.

104. Aziz, K.U., Cole, R.B., and Paul, M.H.: Echocardiographic features of supracristal ventricular septal defect with prolapsed aortic valve leaflet. Am. J. Cardiol., *43*:854, 1979.

105. Glasser, S.P. and Baucum, R.W., Jr.: Pulmonary valve fluttering in subpulmonic ventricular septal defect. Am. Heart J., *94*:3, 1977.

106. Mehta, J., Wang, Y., Lawrence, C.: and Cohn, J.N.: Aortic regurgitation associated with ventricular septal defect. Echocardiographic and hemodynamic observations. Chest, *71*:784, 1977.

106a. Bierman, F.Z. and Williams, R.G.: Prospective diagnosis of ventricular septal defects in infants by subxyphoid two-dimensional echocardiography. Circulation (Suppl. II), *60*:112, 1979. (Abstract)

107. Assad-Morell, J.L., Tajik, A.J., and Giuliani, E.R.: Aneurysm of membranous interventricular septum: echocardiographic features. Mayo Clin. Proc., *49*:164, 1974.

108. Snider, A.R., Silverman, N.H., Schiller, N.B., and Ports, T.A.: Echocardiographic evaluation of ventricular septal aneurysms. Circulation, *59*:920, 1979.

108a. Fast, J.H. and Moene, R.J.: Echocardiographic diagnosis of an aneurysm of the membranous ventricular septum. Acta Paediatr. Scand., *66*:521, 1977.

109. Serwer, G.A., Armstrong, B.E., Anderson, P.A.W., Sherman, D., Benson, D.W., Jr., and Edwards, S.B.: Use of contrast echocardiography for evaluation of right ventricular hemodynamics in the presence of ventricular septal defects. Circulation, *58*:327, 1978.

110. Serruys, P.W., VanDenBrand, M., Hugenholtz, P.G., and Roelandt, J.: Intracardiac right-to-left shunts demonstrated by two-dimensional echocardiography after peripheral vein injection. Br. Heart J., *42*:429, 1979.

111. Valdes-Cruz, L.M., Pieroni, D.R., Roland, J-M.A., and Varghese, P.J.: Echocardiographic detection of intracardiac right-to-left shunts following peripheral vein injections. Circulation, *54*:558, 1976.

112. Seward, J.B., Tajik, A.J., Hagler, D.J., and Ritter, D.G.: Peripheral venous contrast echocardiography. Am. J. Cardiol., *39*:202, 1977.

113. Stevenson, J.G., Kawabori, I., Dooley, T., and Guntheroth, W.G.: Diagnosis of ventricular septal defect by pulsed Doppler echocardiography. Circulation, *58*:322, 1978.

114. Mills, P., McLaurin, L., Smith, C., Murray, G., and Craige, E.: Echocardiographic findings in left ventricular to right atrial shunts. Br. Heart J., *39*:594, 1977.

115. Diamond, M.A., Dillon, J.C., Haine, C.L., Chang, S., and Feigenbaum, H.: Echocardiographic features of atrial septal defect. Circulation, *43*:129, 1971.

116. McCann, W.D., Harbold, N.B., and Giuliani, B.R.: The echocardiogram in right ventricular overload. J.A.M.A., *221*:1243, 1972.

117. Tajik, A.J., Gau, G.T., Ritter, D.G. and Schattenberg, T.T.: Echocardiographic pattern of right ventricular diastolic volume overload in children. Circulation, *46*:36, 1972.

118. Popp, R.L., Wolfe, S.B., Hirata, T., and Feigenbaum, H.: Estimation of right and left ventricular size by ultrasound: a study of the echoes from the interventricular septum. Am. J. Cardiol., *24*:523, 1969.

119. Radtke, W.E., Tajik, A.J., Gau, G.T., Schattenberg, T.T., Giuliani, E.R., and Tancredi, R.G.: Atrial septal defect: echocardiographic observations. Studies in 120 patients. Ann. Intern. Med., *84*:246, 1976.

120. Hayashida, N., Umeda, T., Furuta, S., and Machii, K.: Echocardiographic study on interventricular septal movement in atrial septal defect. J. Cardiogr., 6:349, 1976.

121. Pearlman, A.S., Borer, J.S., Clark, C.E., Redwood, D.R., Morrow, A.G., Epstein, S.E., Burn, C., Cohen, E., and McKay, F.J.: Abnormal right ventricular size and ventricular septal motion after atrial septal defect closure. Am. J. Cardiol., *41*:295, 1978.

122. Hagan, A.D., Francis, G.S., Sahn, D.J., Karliner, J., Friedman, W.F., and O'Rourke, R.: Ultrasound evaluation of systolic anterior septal motion in patients with and without right ventricular volume overload. Circulation, *50*:248, 1974.

123. Tajik, A.J., Gau, G.T., Schattenberg, T.T., and Ritter, D.G.: Normal ventricular septal motion in atrial septal defect. Mayo Clin. Proc., *47*:635, 1972.

124. Radtke, W.E., Tajik, A.J., Gau, G.T., Schattenberg, T.T., Giuliani, E.R., and Tancredi, R.G.: Atrial septal defect: echocardiographic observations. Studies in 120 patients. Ann. Intern. Med., *84*:246, 1976.

125. Fukui, Y., Kato, T., Hibi, N., Arakawa, T., Nishimura, K., Tatematsu, H., Miwa, A., Tada, H., and Kambe, T.: Clinical study on atrial septal defect by means of ultrasono-cardiotomography: with special reference to the backward deviation of interventricular septum. J. Cardiogr., 6:519, 1976.

126. Matsumoto, M.: Ultrasonic features of interatrial septum: its motion analysis and detection of its defect. Jpn. Circ. J., *37*:1382, 1973.

127. Nimura, Y., Matsuo, H., Matsumoto, M., Kitabatake, A., and Abe, H.: Interatrial septum in ultrasonocardiotomogram and ultrasoundcardiogram. Med. Ultrasonics, 9:58, 1971.

128. Dillon, J.C., Weyman, A.E., Feigenbaum, H., Eggleton, R.C., and Johnston, K.: Cross-sectional echocardiographic examination of the interatrial septum. Circulation, 55:115, 1977.

129. Bierman, F.Z. and Williams, R.G.: Subxiphoid two-dimensional imaging of the interatrial septum in infants and neonates with congenital heart disease. Circulation, 60:80, 1979.

130. Fraker, T.D., Harris, P.J., Behar, V.S., and Kisslo, J.A.: Detection and exclusion of interatrial shunts by two-dimensional echocardiography and peripheral venous injection. Circulation, 59:379, 1979.

131. Kronik, G., Slany, J., and Moesslacher, H.: Contrast M-mode echocardiography in diagnosis of atrial septal defect in acyanotic patients. Circulation, 59:372, 1979.

132. Weyman, A.E., Wann, L.S., Caldwell, R.L., Hurwitz, R.A., Dillon, J.C., and Feigenbaum, H.: Negative contrast echocardiography: a new method for detecting left-to-right shunts. Circulation, 59:498, 1979.

133. Goldberg, S.J., Areias, J.C., Spitaels, S.E.C., and DeVilleneuve, V.H.: Use of time interval histographic output from echo-Doppler to detect left-to-right atrial shunts. Circulation, 58:147, 1978.

134. Johnson, S.L., Rubenstein, S., Kawabori, I., Dooley, T.K., and Baker, D.W.: The detection of atrial septal defect by pulse Doppler flowmeter. Circulation (Suppl. II), 54:168, 1976. (Abstract)

135. Chiotellis, P., Lees, R., Goldblatt, A., Liberthson, R., and Myers, G.: New criteria for echocardiographic diagnosis of atrial septal defect. Circulation (Suppl. II), 52:134, 1975. (Abstract)

136. Fujii, J., Morita, K., Watanabe, H., and Kato, K.: Tricuspid valve echograms in various right heart diseases. Cardiovasc. Sound Bull., 5:241, 1975.

137. Lieppe, W., Scallion, R., Behar, V.S., and Kisslo, J.A.: Two-dimensional echocardiographic findings in atrial septal defect. Circulation, 56:447, 1977.

137a. Schreiber, T.L., Feigenbaum, H., and Weyman, A.E.: Effect of atrial septal defect repair on left ventricular geometry and degree of mitral valve prolapse. Circulation, 61:888, 1980.

138. Mirro, M.J., Rogers, E.W., Weyman, A.E., and Feigenbaum, H.: Angular displacement of the papillary muscles during the cardiac cycle. Circulation, 60:327, 1979.

139. Bass, J.L., Bessinger, F.B., Jr., and Lawrence, C.: Echocardiographic differentiation of partial and complete atrioventricular canal. Circulation, 57:1144, 1978.

140. Komatsu, Y., Nagai, Y., Shibuya, M., Takao, A., and Hirosawa, K.: Echocardiographic analysis of intracardiac anatomy in endocardial cushion defect. Am. Heart J., 91:210, 1976.

141. Williams, R.G. and Rudd, M.: Echocardiographic features of endocardial cushion defects. Circulation, 49:418, 1974.

142. Yoshikawa, J., Owaki, T., Kato, H., Tomita, Y., and Baba, K.: Echocardiographic diagnosis of endocardial cushion defects. Jpn. Heart J., 16:1, 1975.

143. Gramiak, R. and Nanda, N.C.: Echocardiographic diagnosis of ostium primum septal defect. Circulation (Suppl. II), 45:46, 1972. (Abstract)

144. Nanda, N.C., Gramiak, R., and Manning, J.A.: Echocardiographic diagnosis of complete atrioventricular canal defect. J. Clin. Ultrasound, 2:261, 1974. (Abstract)

145. Beppu, S., Nimura, Y., Nagata, S., Tamai, M., Matsuo, H., Matsumoto, M., Kawashima, Y., Sakakibara, H., and Abe, H.: Diagnosis of endocardial cushion defect with cross-sectional and M-mode scanning echocardiography: differentiation from secundum atrial septal defect. Br. Heart J., 38:911, 1976.

146. Fisher, D.J., Silverman, N.H., and Schiller, N.B.: Evaluation of endocardial cushion defects by phased array sector scanner. Am. J. Cardiol., 41:353, 1978. (Abstract)

147. Bloom, K.R., Freedom, R.M., Williams, C.M., Trusler, G.A., and Rowe, R.D.: Echocardiographic recognition of atrioventricular valve stenosis associated with endocardial cushion defect: pathologic and surgical correlates. Am. J. Cardiol., 44:1326, 1979.

148. Mehta, S., Hirshfeld, S., Riggs, T., and Liebman, J.: Echocardiographic estimation of ventricular hypoplasia in complete atrioventricular canal. Circulation, 59:888, 1979.

148a. Paquet, M. and Gutgesell, H.: Echocardiographic features of total anomalous pulmonary venous connection. Circulation, 51:599, 1975.

149. Stevenson, J.G., Kawabori, I., and Guntheroth, W.G.: Pulsed Doppler echocardiographic detection of total anomalous pulmonary venous return: resolution of left atrial line. Am. J. Cardiol., 44:1155, 1979.

150. Orsmond, G.S., Ruttenberg, H.D., Bessinger, F.B., and Moller, J.H.: Echocardiographic features of total anomalous pulmonary venous connection to the coronary sinus. Am. J. Cardiol., 41:597, 1978.

151. Aziz, K.U., Paul, M.H., Bharati, S., Lev, M., and Shannon, K.: Echocardiographic features of total anomalous pulmonary venous drainage into the coronary sinus. Am. J. Cardiol., 42:108, 1978.

152. Sahn, D.J., Allen, H.D., Lange, L.W., and Goldberg, S.J.: Cross-sectional echocardiographic diagnosis of the sites of total anomalous pulmonary venous drainage. Circulation, 60:1317, 1979.

153. Bierman, F.Z. and Williams, R.G.: Subxiphoid two-dimensional echocardiographic diagnosis of total anomalous pulmonary venous return in infants. Am. J. Cardiol., 43:401, 1979. (Abstract)

154. Mortera, C., Tynan, M., Goodwin, A.W., and Hunter, S.: Infradiaphragmatic total anomalous pulmonary venous connection to portal vein: diagnostic implications of echocardiography. Br. Heart J., 39:685, 1977.

155. Seward, J.B., Tajik, A.J., Hagler, D.J., Giuliani, E.R., Gau, G.T., and Ritter, D.G.: Echocardiogram in common (single) ventricle: angiographic-anatomic correlation. Am. J. Cardiol., 39:217, 1977.

156. Mortera, C., Hunter, S., Terry, G., and Tynan, M.: Echocardiography of primitive ventricle. Br. Heart J., 39:847, 1977.

157. Seward, J.B., Tajik, A.J., Hagler, D.J., and Mair, D.D.: Cross-sectional echocardiography in common ventricle utilizing 80° phased-array sector scanner. Circulation (Suppl. III), 56:41, 1977. (Abstract)

158. Bini, R.M., Bloom, K.R., Culham, J.A.G., Freedom, R.M., Williams, C.M., and Rowe, R.D.: The reliability and practicality of single crystal echocardiography in the evaluation of single ven-

tricle: angiographic and pathological correlates. Circulation, 57:269, 1978.

159. Felner, J.M., Brewer, D.B., and Franch, R.H.: Echocardiographic manifestations of single ventricle. Am. J. Cardiol., 38:80, 1976.

160. Lamp, L.M. and Bower, P.J.: Echocardiographic diagnosis of double inlet "left" ventricle: indocyanine green contrast studies as an aid to diagnosis. South. Med. J., 71:865, 1978.

161. Seward, J.B., Tajik, A.J., Hagler, D.J., and Ritter, D.G.: Contrast echocardiography in single or common ventricle. Circulation, 55:513, 1977.

162. Ritter, D.G., Seward, J.B., Moodie, D., and Danielson, G.K.: Univentricular heart (common ventricle): preoperative diagnosis. Hemodynamic, angiocardiographic, and echocardiographic features. Herz, 4:198, 1979.

163. McFaul, R.C., Tajik, A.J., Mair, D.D., Danielson, G.K., and Seward, J.B.: Development of pulmonary arteriovenous shunt after auperior vena cava-right pulmonary artery (Glenn) anastomosis. Circulation, 55:212, 1977.

164. Lewis, A.B., Gates, G.F., and Stanley, P.: Echocardiography and perfusion scintigraphy in the diagnosis of pulmonary arteriovenous fistula. Chest, 73:675, 1978.

165. Hernandez, A., Strauss, A.W., McKnight, R., and Hartman, A.F., Jr.: Diagnosis of pulmonary arteriovenous fistula by contrast echocardiography. J. Pediatr. 93:258, 1978.

166. Sieg, K., Hagler, D.J., Ritter, D.G., McGoon, D.C., Maloney, J.D., Seward, J.B., and Davis, G.D.: Straddling right atrioventricular valve in crisscross atrioventricular relationship. Mayo Clin. Proc., 52:561, 1977.

167. Chung, K.J., Nanda, N.C., Manning, J.A., and Gramiak, R.: Echocardiographic findings in tetralogy of Fallot. Am. J. Cardiol., 31:126, 1973.

168. Morris, D.C., Felner, J.M., Schlant, R.C., and Franch, R.H.: Echocardiographic diagnosis of tetralogy of Fallot. Am. J. Cardiol., 36:908, 1975.

169. Tajik, A.J., Gau, G.T., Ritter, D.G., and Schattenberg, T.T.: Echocardiogram in tetralogy of Fallot. Chest, 64:107, 1973.

170. Assad-Morell, J.I., Seward, J.B., Tajik, A.J., Hagler, D.J., Giuliani, E.R., and Ritter, D.G.: Echo-phonocardiographic and contrast studies in conditions associated with systemic arterial trunk overriding the ventricular septum. Circulation, 53:663, 1976.

171. Yoshikawa, J., Owaki, T., Kato, H., Yanagihara, K., Takagi, Y., Okumachi, F., Lee, Y., Kitahara, Y., and Tanaka, K.: Reappraisal of echocardiographic discontinuity in the diagnosis of tetralogy of Fallot and double outlet right ventricle. J. Cardiogr., 6:9, 1976.

172. Hibi, N., Ito, H., Arakawa, T., Nishimura, K., Tatematsu, H., Ishihara, H., Miwa, A., Tada, H., and Kambe, T.: An attempt of diagnosis in tetralogy of Fallot by means of high-speed ultrasonocardiotomography. Cardiovasc. Sound Bull., 5:469, 1975.

173. Sahn, D.J., Terry, R., O'Rourke, R., Leopold, G., and Friedman, W.F.: Multiple crystal cross-sectional echocardiography in the diagnosis of cyanotic congenital heart disease. Circulation, 50:230, 1974.

174. Spotnitz, H.M., Maml, J.R., King, D.L., Pooley, R.W., Bowman, F.G., Jr., Bregman, D., Edie, R.N.,

Reemstsma, K., Korongrad, E., and Hoffman, B.F.: Outflow tract obstruction in tetralogy of Fallot: intraoperative analysis by echocardiography. N.Y. State J. Med., 78:1100, 1978.

175. Oberhansli, I. and Friedli, B.: Echocardiographic study of right and left ventricular dimension and left ventricular function in patients with tetralogy of Fallot before and after surgery. Br. Heart J., 41:40, 1979.

176. Vick, G.W., III and Serwer, G.A.: Echocardiographic evaluation of the postoperative tetralogy of Fallot patient. Circulation, 58:842, 1978.

177. Reitman, M., Goldberg, H., Boris, G., Bakst, A., and Gluck, R.: Echocardiographic assessment of a Blalock-Taussig shunt. J. Clin. Ultrasound, 6:55, 1978.

178. Chandraratna, P.A.N., Bhaduri, U., Littman, B.B., and Hildner, F.J.: Echocardiographic findings in persistent truncus arteriosus in a young adult. Br. Heart J., 36:732, 1974.

179. French, J.W. and Popp, R.L.: Variability of echocardiographic discontinuity in double outlet right ventricle and truncus arteriosus. Circulation, 51:848, 1975.

180. Chung, K.J., Alexson, C.G., Manning, J.A., and Gramiak, R.: Echocardiography in truncus arteriosus: the value of pulmonic valve detection. Circulation, 48:281, 1973.

181. Henry, W.L., Maron, B.J., Griffith, J.M., Redwood, D.R., and Epstein, S.E.: Differential diagnosis of anomalies of the great arteries by real-time, two-dimensional echocardiography. Circulation, 51:283, 1975.

182. Chestler, E., Jaffe, H.S., Beck, W., and Schrire, V.: Echocardiographic recognition of mitral-semilunar valve discontinuity: an aid to the diagnosis of origin of both great vessels from the right ventricle. Circulation, 43:725, 1971.

183. Story, W.E., Felner, J.M., and Schlant, R.C.: Echocardiographic criteria for the diagnosis of mitral-semilunar valve continuity. Am. Heart J., 93:575, 1977.

183a. Yeh, H.C., Wolf, B.S., Steinfield, L., and Baron, M.G.: Echocardiography of double outlet right ventricle: new diagnostic criteria. Radiology, 123:435, 1977.

184. DiSessa, T.G., Hagan, A.D., Pope, C., Samtoy, L., and Friedman, W.F.: Two-dimensional echocardiographic characteristics of double outlet right ventricle. Am. J. Cardiol., 44:1146, 1979.

185. Hojo, Y., Osuga, A., Kato, H., Suzuki, S., Hibi, N., Nishimura, K., Tada, H., and Kanbe, T.: Differential diagnosis between double outlet right ventricle and tetralogy of Fallot by means of high speed ultrasono-cardiotomography and angiocardiography. J. Cardiogr., 6:631, 1976.

186. Hagler, D.J., Tajik, A.J., Seward, J.B., Mair, D.D., and Ritter, D.G.: Wide-angle sector echocardiographic assessment of double-outlet right ventricle. Circulation (Suppl. II), 58:202, 1978. (Abstract)

187. Henry, W.L., Maron, B.J., Griffith, J.M., and Epstein, S.E.: Identification of double outlet right ventricle by two-dimensional echocardiography. Clin. Res., 24:222a, 1976. (Abstract)

188. Houston, A.B., Gregory, N.L., and Coleman, E.N.: Two-dimensional sector scanner echocardiography in cyanotic congenital heart disease. Br. Heart J., 39:1076, 1977.

189. Dillon, J.C., Feigenbaum, H., Konecke, L.L.,

Keutel, J., Hurwitz, R.A., David, R.H. and Chung, S.: Echocardiographic manifestations of d-transposition of the great vessels. Am. J. Cardiol., 32:74, 1973.

190. Bass, N.M., Roche, A.H.G., Brandt, P.W.T., and Neutze, J.M.: Echocardiography in assessment of infants with complete d-transposition of the great arteries. Br. Heart J., 40:1165, 1978.

190a.Gramiak, R., Chung, K.J., Nanda, N., and Manning, J.: Echocardiographic diagnosis of transposition of the great vessels. Radiology, 106:187, 1973.

191. Mortera, C., Hunter, S., and Tynan, M.: Diagnosis of ventriculo-arterial discordance (transposition of the great arteries) by contrast echocardiography. Br. Heart J., 39:844, 1977.

192. Bierman, F.Z. and Williams, R.G.: Prospective diagnosis of d-transposition of the great arteries in neonates by subxiphoid, two-dimensional echocardiography. Circulation, 60:1496, 1979.

193. Aziz, K.U., Paul, M.H., and Muster, A.J.: Echocardiographic assessment of left ventricular outflow tract in d-transposition of the great arteries. Am. J. Cardiol., 41:543, 1978.

194. Aziz, K.U., Paul, M.H., Idriss, F.S., Wilson, A.D., and Muster, A.J.: Clinical manifestations of dynamic left ventricular outflow tract stenosis in infants with d-transposition of the great arteries with intact ventricular septum. Am. J. Cardiol., 44:290, 1979.

195. DiSessa, T.G., Childs, W., Ti, C., and Friedman, W.F.: Systolic anterior motion of the mitral valve in a one day old infant with d-transposition of the great vessels. J. Clin. Ultrasound, 6:186, 1978.

196. Aziz, K.U., Paul, M.H., and Muster, A.J.: Echocardiographic localization of interatrial baffle after Mustard operation for dextrotransposition of the great arteries. Am. J. Cardiol., 38:67, 1976.

197. Areias, J.C., Goldberg, S.J., Spitaels, S.E.C., and deVilleneuve, V.H.: An evaluation of range gated pulsed Doppler echocardiography for detecting pulmonary outflow tract obstruction in d-transposition of the great vessels. Am. Heart J., 96:467, 1978.

198. Gutgesell, H.P.: Echocardiographic estimation of pulmonary artery pressure in transposition of the great arteries. Circulation, 57:1151, 1978.

199. Williams, R.G. and Bierman, F.Z.: Evaluation of balloon atrial septostomy by subxiphoid two dimensional echocardiography. Am. J. Cardiol., 43:401, 1979. (Abstract)

200. Hunter, S., Mortera, C., Terry, G., Goodwin, A., Tynan, M., and Holden, M.: Echocardiographic visualization of the interatrial baffle after Mustard's operation. Br. Heart Jr., 39:954, 1977.

201. Silverman, N.H., Payot, M., Stanger, P., and Rudolph, A.M.: The echocardiographic profile of patients after Mustard's operation. Circulation, 58:1083, 1978.

202. Park, S.C., Neches, W.H., Zuberbuhler, J.R., Mathews, R.A., Lenox, C.C., and Fricker, F.J.: Echocardiographic and hemodynamic correlation in transposition of the great arteries. Circulation, 57:291, 1978.

203. Hagler, D.J., Tajik, A.J., and Ritter, D.G.: Fluttering of atrioventricular valves in patients with d-tranposition of the great arteries after Mustard operation: an echographic observation. Mayo Clin. Proc., 50:69, 1975.

204. Stevenson, J.B., Kawabori, I., Guntheroth, W.G.,

Dooley, T.K., and Dillard, D.: Pulsed Doppler echocardiographic detection of obstruction of systemic venous return after repair of transposition of the great arteries. Circulation, 60:1091, 1979.

205. Bloch, A., Terrapon M. and Bopp, P.: Echocardiographic diagnosis of a pulmonary artery aneurysm. Eur. J. Cardiol., 6:33, 1977.

205a.Weyman, A.E., Feigenbaum, H., Dillon, J.C., Johnson, K.W., and Eggleton, R.C.: Non-invasive visualization of the left main coronary artery by cross-sectional echocardiography. Circulation, 54:169, 1976.

206. Cohen, B.E., Winer, H.E., and Kronzon, I.: Echocardiographic findings in patients with left superior vena cava and dilated coronary sinus. Am. J. Cardiol., 44:158, 1979.

207. Hibi, N., Suzuki, S., Kato, T., Fukui, Y., Arakawa, T., Nishimura, K., Miwa, A., Kambe, T., and Hojo, Y.: Cross-sectional echocardiographic study on persistent left superior vena cava with high speed mechanical sector scanning. J. Cardiogr., 8:391, 1978.

208. Snider, A.R., Ports, T.A., and Silverman, N.H.: Venous anomalies of the coronary sinus: detection by M-mode, two-dimensional and contrast echocardiography. Circulation, 60:721, 1979.

209. Stewart, J.A., Fraker, T.D., Slosky, D.A., Wise, N.K., and Kisslo, J.A.: Detection of persistent left superior vena cava by two-dimensional contrast echocardiography. J. Clin. Ultrasound, 7:357, 1979.

210. Sahn, D.J., Allen, H.D., Anderson, R., and Goldberg, S.J.: Echocardiographic diagnosis of atrial septal aneurysm in an infant with hypoplastic right heart syndrome. Chest, 73:227, 1978.

211. Caldwell, R.L., Weyman, A.E., Girod, D.A., Hurwitz, R.A., and Feigenbaum, H.: Cross-sectional echocardiographic differentiation of anomalous left coronary artery from primary myocardiopathy. Circulation, 58:786, 1978. (Abstract)

211a.Caldwell, R.L., Weyman, A., Hurwitz, R.A., Girod, D.A., and Feigenbaum, H.: Cross-sectional echocardiographic evaluation of coronary artery abnormalities in children. Am. J. Cardiol., 45:467, 1980. (Abstract)

212. Yanagihara, K., Kato, H., Owaki, T., Takagi, Y., Yoshikawa, J., Fukaya, T., Tomita, Y., and Baba, K.: Ultrasonic features of coronary artery dilatation and aneurysm. J. Cardiogr., 8:401, 1978.

213. Hiraishi, S., Yashiro, K., and Kusano, S.: Noninvasive visualization of coronary arterial aneurysm in infants and young children with mucocutaneous lymph node syndrome with two-dimensional echocardiography. Am. J. Cardiol., 43:1225, 1979.

214. Sonotani, N., Nakayama, Y., Chin, N., Takatsu, T., Suwa, M., Kamiuchi, Y., and Hori, K.: A case of right coronary artery fistula to the left ventricle. J. Cardiogr., 6:573, 1976.

215. Aizawa, K., Aoki, T., Aizawa, Y., Shu, T., Sato, H., Tamura, K., and Matsukawa, T.: Echocardiographic findings of Uhl's anomaly: report of a case. J. Cardiogr., 7:233, 1977.

216. Silverman, N.H. and Schiller, N.B.: Apex echocardiography: a two-dimensional technique for evaluating congenital heart disease. Circulation, 57:503, 1978.

217. Lange, L.W., Sahn, D.J., Allen, H.D., and Goldberg, S.J.: Subxiphoid cross-sectional echo-

cardiography in infants and children with congenital heart disease. Circulation, 59:513, 1979.

218. Hibi, N., Nishimura, K., Kambe, T., and Hojo, Y.: Diagnosis of the congenital heart disease with high speed cross-sectional echocardiography. J. Cardiogr., 8:539, 1978.

219. Sahn, D.J., Henry, W.L., Allen, H.D., Griffith, J.M., and Goldberg, S.J.: The comparative utilities of real-time cross-sectional echocardiographic imaging systems for the diagnosis of complex congenital heart disease. Am. J. Med., 63:50, 1977.

8

Coronary Artery Disease

The use of echocardiography in patients with coronary artery disease is indeed a challenge. As a group, these patients can be extremely difficult to examine because of many technical problems. However, these patients represent a sizable percentage of all patients seen by cardiologists. With the advent and widespread use of various surgical procedures for these patients, there is an increasing need for more specific objective data concerning the extent of the disease in these patients. Any assistance that echocardiography can give in the management of these patients is valuable.

There have been many echocardiographic applications described in the literature for patients with coronary artery disease. The principal use of echocardiography is in examining the ischemic left ventricle. Two-dimensional echocardiography has greatly expanded the capability of echocardiography to detect the effect of coronary artery disease on the left ventricle. Aside from a short discussion on the use of echocardiography for examining the coronary arteries, this chapter deals primarily with the way in which echocardiography can detect the effects of coronary artery obstructions on the heart.

DETECTION OF ISCHEMIC MUSCLE

Wall Motion Abnormalities

One of the principal ways of detecting ischemic muscle is by noting abnormal motion of the ischemic segment. Both animal and clinical studies have documented that when the muscle becomes ischemic, its motion is altered almost immediately.[1-9] With

the high sampling rate inherent in M-mode echocardiography, wall motion is recorded extremely well with this technique.[10] Figure 8–1 shows an M-mode echocardiogram

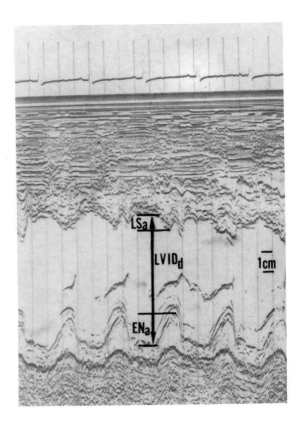

Fig. 8–1. M-mode left ventricular echocardiogram through the midportion of a normal left ventricle demonstrating how one can obtain the diastolic internal dimension (LVID$_d$), and the amplitudes of motion of the left septal echo (LS$_a$) and the posterior left ventricular endocardium (EN$_a$). (From Corya, B.C., et al.: Echocardiography in acute myocardial infarction. Am. J. Cardiol., 36:1, 1975.)

through the midportion of a normal left ventricle just beyond the maximum mitral valve echoes. This is the same examination for which standard left ventricular dimensions are usually obtained (see Chapter 3). The left ventricular diastole dimension (LVID$_d$) is illustrated together with the amplitudes of motion of the left septal echo (LS$_a$) and the posterior left ventricular endocardium (EN$_a$).

Figure 8–2 demonstrates a typical M-mode sector scan and illustrates at least two areas of the left ventricle that can be examined echocardiographically. Figure 8–1 is an example of a "routine" examination of the left ventricle through the body of the chamber just beyond the maximum mitral valve echo. Tilting the transducer toward the "apex" brings the ultrasonic beam into the vicinity of the posterior papillary muscle (PPM) and provides a recording of a different part of the interventricular septum and the posterior left ventricular wall.

The echocardiograms in Figures 8–1 and 8–2 are of normal individuals who exhibited downward systolic motion of the left septum between 3 and 8 mm and an upward anterior systolic motion of the posterior left ventricular endocardium of 8 to 12 mm. In contrast, Figure 8–3 shows markedly reduced or absent motion of the interventricular septum in a patient with coronary artery disease.[10] Although the total amplitude of the posterior left ventricular wall is within normal limits, the minimal motion seen in the interventricular septum is actually paradoxical, if not entirely flat. Figure 8–4 demonstrates another patient with coronary artery disease who has normal or actually exaggerated motion of the interventricular septum. However, the motion exhibited by the posterior left ventricular endocardium is significantly

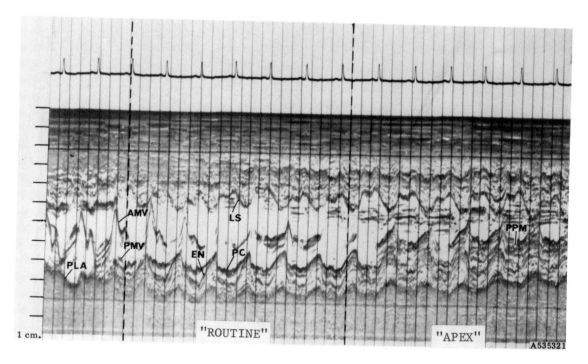

Fig. 8–2. M-mode scan of a normal left ventricle illustrating at least two areas of the left ventricle that can be examined echocardiographically. The usual or "routine" area of the left ventricle is that part of the chamber still containing portions of the mitral valve echoes. When directing the ultrasonic beam toward the "apex," one loses the mitral valve echoes and frequently records the posterior papillary muscle (PPM). LS = left septum; AMV = anterior mitral valve leaflet; PMV = posterior mitral valve leaflet; PLA = posterior left atrial wall; PC = posterior chordae; EN = posterior left ventricular endocardium. (From Jacobs, J.J., et al.: Detection of left ventricular asynergy by echocardiography. Circulation, 48:263, 1963.)

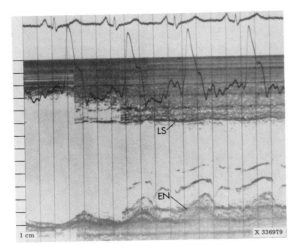

Fig. 8–3.   Left ventricular echocardiogram of a patient with coronary artery disease and obstruction of the proximal portion of the left anterior descending coronary artery. The echo from the left side of the septum (LS) is actually paradoxical if not entirely flat toward the end of systole. Posterior left ventricular wall motion (EN) is reasonably normal.

reduced and would be considered hypokinetic.

Figure 8–5 illustrates the value of M-mode scanning. The left portion of the echocardiogram is taken in the vicinity of the mitral valve, and the posterior left ventricular endocardium (EN) is only slightly hypokinetic. However, in the vicinity of the chordae (C), the endocardial motion is markedly reduced and is virtually flat. In contrast, the motion of the left side of the septum (LS) is normal in both locations. Figure 8–6 shows a similar finding in a patient with ischemic heart disease involving the septum and anterior left ventricular wall. In the region of the mitral valve, the septal motion (LS) is normal; however, beyond the level of the mitral valve the septal motion is completely flat. Unless one scans toward the apex past the mitral valve echoes, the pathologic segment of the left ventricle would be missed in both Figures 8–5 and 8–6.

It is also possible to examine the true anterior left ventricular wall by sliding the transducer in a linear fashion toward the left midclavicular line (Fig. 8–7).[8,11] By moving the transducer to the left, the ultrasonic beam moves off of the interventricular sep-

tum. The anterior wall of the heart now becomes the anterior left ventricular wall. As one might expect, the anterior left ventricular wall moves similar to the interventricular septum, except that there is no intervening

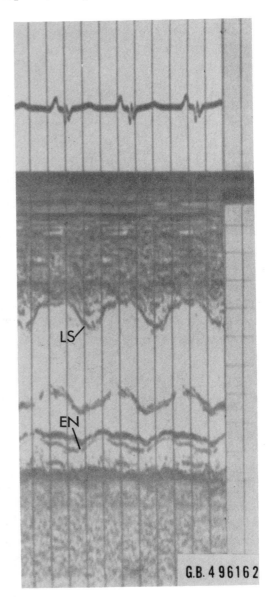

Fig. 8–4.   M-mode echocardiogram through the left ventricle of a patient with an inferior wall myocardial infarction, demonstrating exaggerated motion of the interventricular septum (LS) with hypokinetic motion of the left ventricular endocardial echo (EN). (From Corya, B.C., et al.: Echocardiographic features of congestive cardiomyopathy compared with normal subjects in patients with coronary artery disease. Circulation, 49:1153, 1974.)

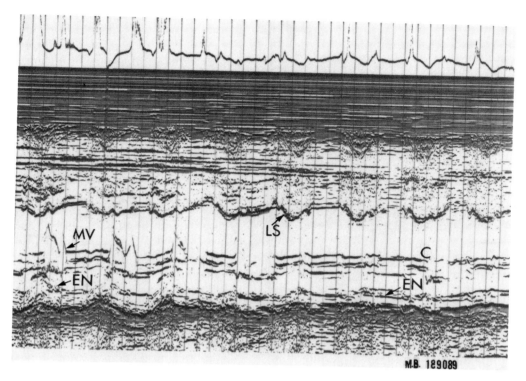

Fig. 8–5.   M-mode scan of a patient with an acute inferior myocardial infarction showing the difference in posterior left ventricular wall motion (EN) in the vicinity of the mitral valve (MV) and at the level of the chordae (C). When the mitral valve is recorded, the posterior ventricular wall motion is slightly hypokinetic, whereas at the chordal area the endocardial motion is flat. LS = left septum. (From Corya, B.C.: Applications of echocardiography in acute myocardial infarction. Cardiovasc. Clin., *II*:113, 1975.)

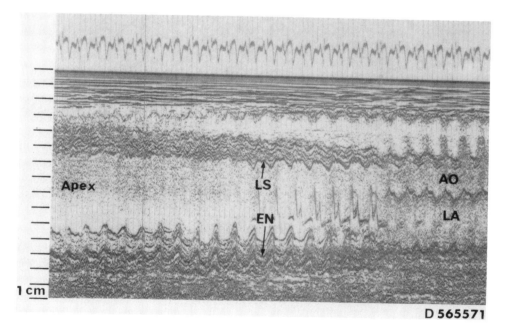

Fig. 8–6.   Slow M-mode scan from the apex to the base of the heart in a patient with an anterior septal infarction and an aneurysm involving the anterior wall. The septal (LS) and posterior endocardial (EN) echoes move normally near the base of the heart and at the level of the mitral valve; however, septal motion abruptly ceases as the ultrasonic beam approaches the apex. AO = aorta; LA = left atrium. (From Dillon, J.C., et al.: M-mode echocardiography in the evaluation of patients for aneurysmectomy. Circulation, *53*:657, 1976.)

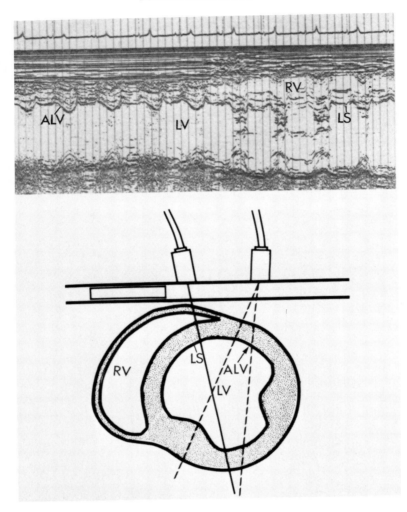

Fig. 8–7.   Echocardiogram and diagram demonstrating how the ultrasonic transducer can be moved laterally to record the anterior left ventricular wall (ALV). The echocardiogram shows that the transducer is actually moved from the level of the anterior left ventricular wall toward the right ventricle (RV) and the interventricular septum (LS). LV = left ventricle.

right ventricle between that structure and the chest wall. This type of examination is not technically easy as one frequently crosses a rib, which interrupts the examination. However, merely placing the transducer laterally and looking at the anterior walls of the heart provides an echocardiographic recording of the anterior left ventricular wall. The echocardiogram in Figure 8–7 was taken from a normal individual. In contrast, Figure 8–8 shows a recording of the anterior left ventricular wall (ALV) in a patient with coronary artery disease and dyskinesis of the anterior left ventricular wall.

With the onset of ventricular systole (arrow), the anterior left ventricular wall moves anteriorly in a paradoxical fashion. As one might expect, the anterior left ventricular wall may exhibit more than one pattern of motion. Figure 8–9 shows two areas of the anterior left ventricular wall, one of which moves normally (ALV') and one that is akinetic (ALV).

The transducer may also be placed directly above the left ventricular apex. Figure 8–10A shows such an M-mode apical study in a normal individual. With systole there is virtual obliteration of the space between the

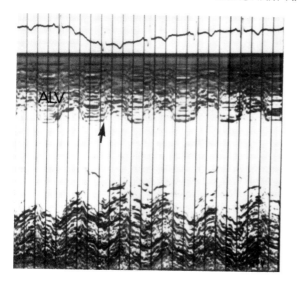

Fig. 8–8. M-mode echocardiogram of the anterior left ventricular wall (ALV) in a patient with coronary artery disease and a dyskinetic anterior wall. At the onset of systole *(arrow)*, the anterior left ventricular wall moves anteriorly or paradoxically.

anterior and posterior walls of the left ventricle. Figure 8–10B is a similar examination in a patient with coronary artery disease. The posterior left ventricular wall (PLV) fails to move anteriorly with systole and actually is dyskinetic (large arrow). One can also perform an M-mode examination from the subcostal, or subxiphoid, area.[8,12] Such an examination actually studies slightly different areas of the interventricular septum and posterior left ventricular wall. Figure 8–11 demonstrates a subcostal M-mode study in a patient with coronary artery disease that demonstrates a marked change in the posterior left ventricular endocardial (EN) motion in the left portion of the recording from that in the right at the level of the mitral valve.

It has been suggested that one might be able to examine the ischemic ventricle with multiple transducer placements on the surface of the precordium.[9,13] Figure 8–12 illustrates this approach. As many as fourteen

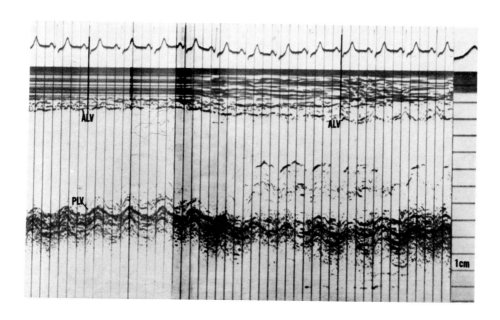

Fig. 8–9. M-mode echocardiogram of an anterior left ventricular wall (ALV) in a patient with coronary artery disease. On the left, the anterior left ventricular wall echoes are hypokinetic and exhibit no motion. On the right, anterior left ventricular wall motion is normal. PLV = posterior left ventricular wall. (From Corya, B.C., et al.: Anterior left ventricular wall echoes in coronary artery disease. Am. J. Cardiol., 34:652, 1974.)

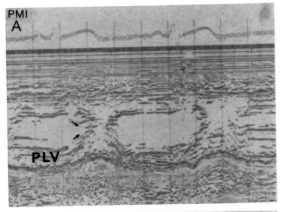

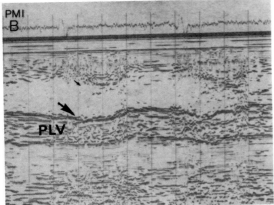

Fig. 8–10. M-mode echocardiograms of the cardiac apex with the transducer placed directly over the apex. *A*, This patient has a normally contracting ventricle. Both walls of the apex move toward each other *(arrows)* and obliterate the cavity in systole. *B*, In this patient with ischemia of the apex, the motion of the posterior left ventricular wall (PLV) is dyskinetic *(large arrow)*. (From Corya, B.C.: Echocardiography. *In* Cardiac Diagnosis and Treatment. 3rd ed. Edited by O. Fowler. Hagerstown, Md., Harper & Row, In press.)

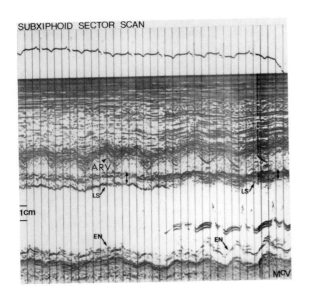

Fig. 8–11. Subcostal or subxiphoid M-mode scan of a patient with coronary artery disease demonstrating absent motion of the posterior left ventricular endocardium (EN) near the apex (on the left). At the level of the mitral valve the posterior left ventricular wall motion is normal (on the right). The anterior right ventricular wall (ARV) motion is exaggerated. LS = left side of the septum. (From Corya, B.C. and Rasmussen, S.: Handbook of Clinical Ultrasound. Edited by M. DeVleiger, et al. New York, John Wiley & Sons, Inc., 1978.)

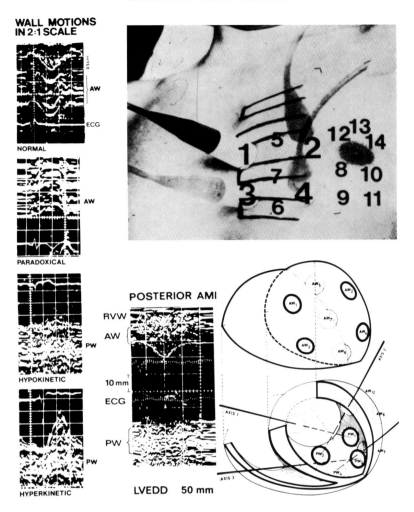

Fig. 8–12. Illustration of the technique of using multiple precordial transducer placement for assessing wall motion of the ischemic heart. AW = anterior wall; PW = posterior wall; RVW = right ventricular wall. (From Heikkila, J. and Nieminen, M.: Rapid monitoring of regional myocardial ischaemia with echocardiography and ST segment shifts in man. Acta Med. Scand. (suppl.), 623:71, 1978.)

M-mode positions have been suggested. With the advent of two-dimensional echocardiography there is decreasing interest in multiple M-mode examinations for visualizing the ischemic left ventricle.

In addition to the direct echocardiographic demonstration of hypokinetic or dyskinetic segments of the left ventricular wall, there is also indirect echocardiographic evidence of segmental left ventricular disease. One may frequently see exaggerated wall motion in the opposing, nonischemic area of the left ventricle.[14,15] In Figure 8–4, for example, although the posterior left ventricular wall is hypokinetic, the septal motion is approximately 1 cm in amplitude, which is beyond the upper limits of normal. Figure 8–13 shows a patient with a hypokinetic septum and exaggerated posterior left ventricular wall motion. Another indirect clue to the presence of a hypokinetic wall segment is the finding of a cloud of intracavitary echoes adjacent to the poorly moving wall.[8] Normally, the cavity of the left ventricle is relatively echo-free and if there are intracavitary echoes, they are uniformly

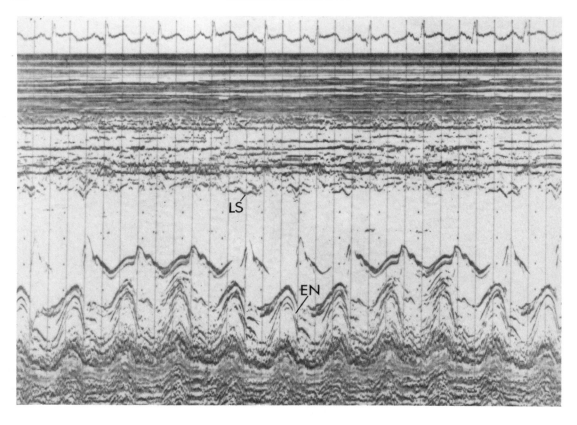

Fig. 8–13. Left ventricular echocardiogram of a patient with coronary artery disease. Note exaggerated motion of the posterior left ventricular endocardium (EN) and hypokinetic motion of the septum (LS).

distributed through the cavity or appear as a series of straight lines. If the gain is relatively high, and/or the reject is low, one may record intracavitary echoes in patients with coronary artery disease. The echoes frequently accumulate next to hypokinetic or dyskinetic segments of the left ventricle. Figure 8–6 shows such a situation whereby a band of fuzzy echoes is visible along the hypokinetic segment of the septum. The explanation for these echoes is unknown. One possibility is that these echoes may be due to stagnant blood next to the hypokinetic wall. Another frequent, indirect sign of ischemic left ventricle is the finding of a prominent, somewhat exaggerated right ventricular wall motion. The anterior right ventricular wall echoes in Figure 8–11 represent a good example of this finding. It is unusual for the amplitude of the right ventricular wall echoes to exceed the amplitude of motion of

the interventricular septum, except in patients with coronary artery disease.

There have been attempts to predict the anatomy of the coronary arteries by segmental wall motion abnormalities on the M-mode echocardiogram.[16–21] Evidence conflicts in the literature as to precisely how well echocardiography can predict the coronary anatomy. Most investigators agree that if the interventricular septal motion is abnormal, it is highly probable that there is a proximal left anterior descending or a left main coronary artery obstruction.[17,19–21] However, normal septal motion in no way precludes the possibility of obstruction in these arteries. One study shows that septal motion correlates better with myocardial perfusion of the septum, rather than with anatomic obstructions of the coronary artery.[19] For example, a tight proximal left anterior descending coronary obstruction with good collateral fill of the vessel may result in normal septal motion. However, if perfusion of the septum is poor or absent, then the likelihood of abnormal septal motion is quite high. The use of posterior ventricular wall motion to predict coronary anatomy is even less reliable.

There are many advantages of the M-mode technique for recording wall motion. The sampling rate is extremely fast, and the motion is accurately recorded. In addition, the axial resolution is usually excellent. However, there are both theoretical and actual limitations to the M-mode examination. Figure 8–14 diagrammatically illustrates the usual M-mode sector scan. This diagram demonstrates that the actual amount of septum (IVS) examined is considerably less than that of the posterior left ventricular wall (PLV) because of angulation of the transducer. Thus it is difficult to attempt to quantitate the amount of abnormally moving wall, especially with respect to the septum since one obtains a distorted impression of the amount of septum actually being examined.

Figure 8–15 shows another common prob-

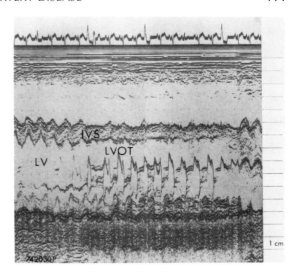

Fig. 8–15. M-mode scan showing the differences in septal motion that can be obtained in a patient without coronary artery disease. The interventricular septum (IVS) moves normally when the ultrasonic beam is directed toward the body of the left ventricular cavity (LV). At the level of the left ventricular outflow tract (LVOT), however, the septal motion is markedly reduced.

lem with the M-mode sector scan. There is frequently a small segment of septum at the attachment to the aorta that may not move vigorously; in this figure it is that portion of the septum above the mitral valve in the left ventricular outflow tract. Although the amount of hypokinetic septum appears great on an M-mode tracing, it actually represents a small segment of muscle. If one only recorded the left ventricle at the level of the mitral valve in the patient illustrated in Figure 8–15, one might suspect a hypokinetic segment. Further scanning of the ultrasonic beam toward the apex shows the true, normal septal motion.

Figure 8–16 illustrates how the angle of the ultrasonic beam, with respect to a moving target, influences the amplitude of motion recorded on the M-mode echocardiogram. If the beam is directly parallel to the direction of the moving echo, then the maximum amplitude of motion is recorded. As the beam becomes less parallel to the motion, the recorded amplitude decreases. Thus examination of echoes in a tangential manner can influence the pattern of motion

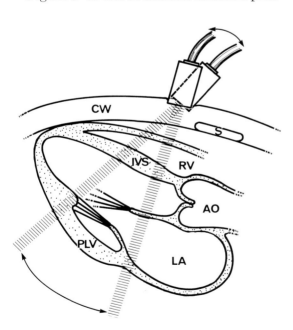

Fig. 8–14. Diagram demonstrating that with a sector M-mode scan the ultrasonic beam traverses more of the posterior left ventricular wall (PLV) than it does the interventricular septum (IVS). CW = chest wall; S = sternum; RV = right ventricle; AO = aorta; LA = left atrium.

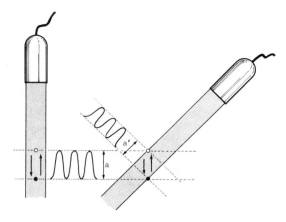

Fig. 8–16.   Drawing illustrating that the amplitude of motion of a moving echo depends on the angle of the ultrasonic beam with respect to the moving target. The maximum amplitude of motion (a) is recorded when the beam is parallel to the direction of the moving echo. If the angle is no longer parallel, then the amplitude of motion will decrease (a').

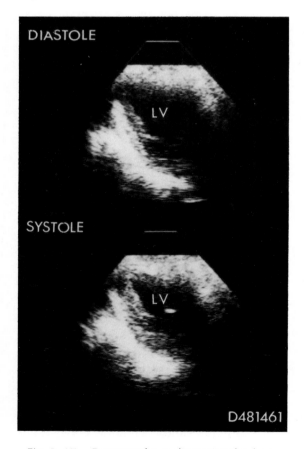

Fig. 8–17.   Parasternal two-dimensional echocardiogram of a normally contracting left ventricular (LV) apex demonstrating the change in wall motion, wall thickness, and cavity size from diastole to systole.

inscribed on the M-mode echocardiogram. The practical aspect of this observation is that if the echoes appear hypokinetic, especially toward the apex, one probably should move the transducer so that the ultrasonic beam is as parallel to the motion of the wall as possible in order to detect the maximum amplitude.

Because of some of the limitations of M-mode echocardiography in examining wall motion and because it is difficult to evaluate the motion of the entire left ventricle, two-dimensional echocardiography plays an increasingly important role in assessing wall motion in the ischemic left ventricle.[22-30]

One of the important areas of the left ventricle that is difficult to examine with M-mode echocardiography is the apex. Although one can occasionally assess this area of the left ventricle with M-mode echocardiography (Fig. 8–10), it is much easier by way of two-dimensional echocardiography. Figure 8–17 demonstrates a parasternal long-axis examination of the left ventricular apex in diastole and systole. Note the tapered appearance of the apex and the significant change in cavity size from diastole to systole. In contrast, Figure 8–18 is a similar parasternal long-axis study of the apex in a patient with coronary artery disease. With systole there is an outward bulge (arrow), or dykinesis, in the posterior aspect of the apex (AP).

The apical four-chamber examination provides another important two-dimensional echocardiographic examination of the ischemic left ventricle. Figure 8–19 shows systolic and diastolic frames of an apical four-chamber study of a normal ventricle. This examination can be compared with Figure 8–20, which shows a patient with coronary artery disease. There is some distortion of shape of the apical half of the left ventricle and there is outward motion of the apical half of the interventricular septum (arrow) in systole. The apical two-chamber view is also used frequently when examining the ischemic heart.

The short-axis studies are also extremely important in judging wall motion in patients with coronary artery disease. Figure 8–21

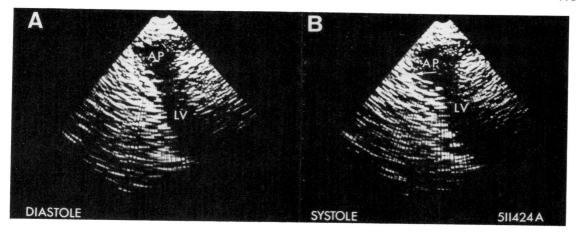

Fig. 8–18.   Two-dimensional echocardiographic examination of the left ventricular apex (AP) in a patient with dyskinesis. During diastole the posterior border of the apex is aligned with the posterior wall of the left ventricle (LV). With systole, the apex bulges outwardly *(arrow)*. (From Feigenbaum, H., et al.: Sensitivity and specificity of M-mode and cross-sectional echocardiographic findings in patients with coronary artery disease. *In* Echocardiology. Edited by C.T. Lancee. The Hague, Martinus Nijhoff, 1979.)

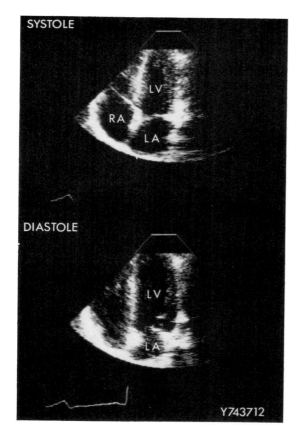

Fig. 8–19.   Apical four-chamber two-dimensional echocardiogram of a normal subject in systole and diastole. LV = left ventricle; RA = right atrium; LA = left atrium.

shows a parasternal short-axis examination of a normal left ventricle. Note the normally contracting walls that make up the circumference of the left ventricle. In contrast, Figure 8–22 demonstrates a parasternal short-axis study of an ischemic ventricle. There are striking motion abnormalities in this particular study. The medial wall actually moves excessively. However, the posterior left ventricular wall motion is paradoxical, moving outward during systole (arrows).

Although wall motion abnormalities cannot be measured with the precision inherent in M-mode echocardiography, the ability of the two-dimensional examination to record the medial, lateral, and apical portions of the left ventricle provides a significant advantage to this technique's assessment of wall motion in the ischemic ventricle. Multiple studies have correlated the two-dimensional examination with angiography[22,30,31] or with nuclear cardiologic tests.[29,32] Although there are significant differences between the radiographic techniques and the ultrasonic examination, there generally is good agreement in most cases. Total agreement actually should not be expected. There are important differences between angiography, nuclear cardiology, and echocardiography. First, the angiographic and nuclear techniques visualize cavity silhouettes. Echocardiography,

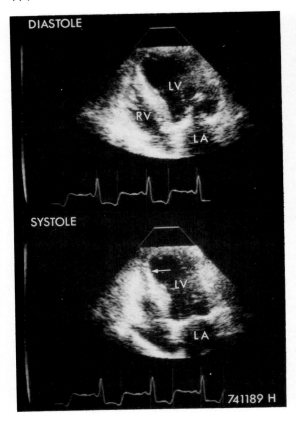

Fig. 8–20.   Apical four-chamber two-dimensional echocardiogram of a patient with coronary artery disease. The apical half of the left ventricle (LV) is dilated, and with systole the apical half of the septum bulges outwardly *(arrow)*. Much dilatation of the diseased ventricle is due to loss in tissue mass of the involved area. RV = right ventricle; LA = left atrium.

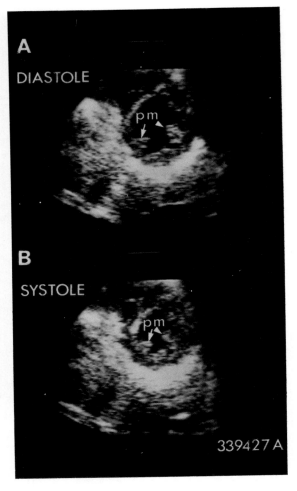

Fig. 8–21.   Short-axis two-dimensional echocardiogram of a normally contracting left ventricle at the level of the papillary muscles (pm).

on the other hand, obtains a slice through the chamber. The standard angiographic and isotopic views do not necessarily correspond with the echocardiographic planes. For example, the right anterior oblique and left anterior oblique views are not exactly equivalent to any of the echocardiographic examinations. With the multiple examinations now available with two-dimensional echocardiography, one can virtually examine every portion of the left ventricle. It is feasible that many areas of the left ventricle that cannot be properly studied with angiography or nuclear techniques can be seen with two-dimensional echocardiography.

Echocardiographic wall motion abnormalities have also been correlated with standard electrocardiographic location of myocardial infarction.[24-26] Again, the correlation has been quite satisfactory. One need not expect 100 percent agreement since the electrocardiogram is not that accurate in locating the exact area of infarction.

Wall Thickening Abnormalities

There are some limitations to using wall motion as the sole criterion for ischemic muscle. The movement of any given segment of the ventricle is influenced by the adjacent muscle to which it is attached. For example, in a chamber with a dyskinetic ischemic segment, some of the adjacent normal tissue may be hypokinetic because its

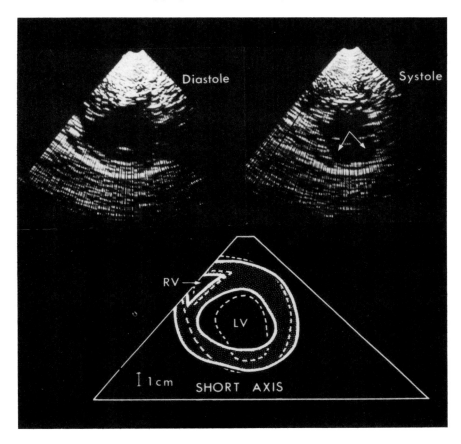

Fig. 8–22.   Diastolic and systolic short-axis two-dimensional echocardiograms and diagram of a patient with an acute inferior myocardial infarction. There is outward bulging and thinning of the posterior wall in systole. The medial wall moves excessively. RV = right ventricle; LV = left ventricle.

motion is influenced by the dyskinetic muscle. The reverse situation may also be true. If vigorously contracting normal muscle is attached to an ischemic area, it may pull the ischemic muscle toward the cavity and may actually mask the abnormal perfusion. In general, one usually overestimates the amount of ischemic muscle when merely looking at motion abnormalities.

Probably a more specific finding for the ischemic muscle is alteration in systolic thickening.[33–39] As noted in Figures 8–1, 8–2, 8–17, 8–19, and 8–21, the normal left ventricular wall is thicker in systole than in diastole. In Figures 8–3 and 8–5 one can appreciate that the ischemic wall segments are not thicker in systole than in diastole. Thus in these two ischemic ventricles the affected areas have diminished or absent thickening. With acute ischemia or infarction, one may actually record systolic thinning, whereby the thickness of the left ventricular wall is greater in diastole than in systole (Fig. 8–23). Thus the affected wall segment not only exhibits paradoxical motion, but also systolic thinning, which is probably more specific for ischemia.

Figure 8–22 shows systolic thinning by way of two-dimensional echocardiography. In this short-axis study note that the posterior left ventricular wall is thicker in diastole than in systole. A similar type of observation is noted in Figure 8–24, which is a two-dimensional examination of an ischemic apex. In this dyskinetic apex there is not only outward motion of the apex in systole, but

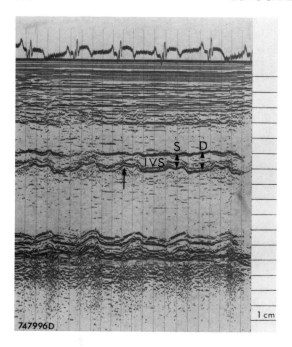

Fig. 8–23. M-mode echocardiogram of a patient with an acute anteroseptal myocardial infarction. The interventricular septum (IVS) is less thick in systole (S) than in diastole (D). In addition, septal motion is abnormal or paradoxical *(arrow)*.

also less wall thickness in systole than in diastole.

Systolic thinning almost always occurs with a dyskinetic segment and is usually associated with acute myocardial infarction. Decreased or no thickening occurs in both chronic and acute ischemia.

Change in Wall Thickness

Whereas alterations in wall thickening usually occur with acute ischemia, chronic ischemia may sometimes produce alterations in wall thickness.[40,41] Figure 8–25 shows an M-mode echocardiogram of a patient with underlying left ventricular hypertrophy and an acute inferior myocardial infarction. The posterior left ventricular wall is thicker than normal and exhibits abnormal motion. There may even be some thinning of the wall with systole. Figure 8–26 demonstrates a follow-up echocardiogram taken two-and-a-half years later. The posterior left ventricular wall thickness is now significantly less than it was during the acute infarction. The wall motion is clearly hypokinetic in keeping with the old inferior

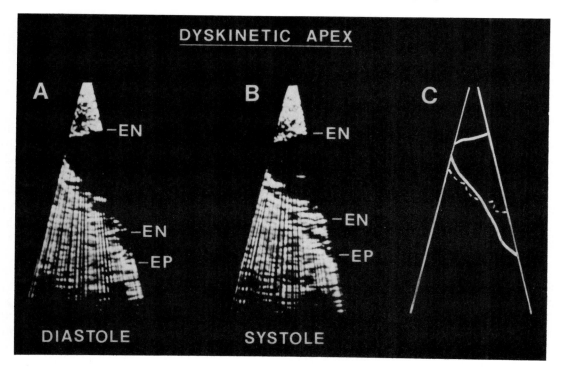

Fig. 8–24. Thirty-degree two-dimensional echocardiograms of the apex in a patient who demonstrates both dyskinesis and thinning of the apex in systole. EN = endocardium; EP = epicardium.

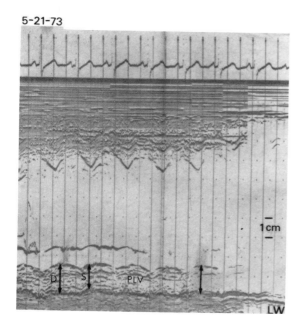

infarction. The interventricular septum remains hypertrophied. A loss in tissue mass of the infarcted posterior wall is evident. In fact, a tracing such as that shown in Figure 8–26 could be misinterpreted as asymmetric septal hypertrophy; however, it is principally due to a decrease in the thickness of chronically ischemic wall segment and is categorized as "disproportionate septal hypertrophy."[40]

Figure 8–27 shows another patient with chronic ischemic heart disease who demonstrates a thin interventricular septum. The thickness of the septum is significantly less than that of the posterior left ventricular wall. Interestingly, some motion still remains in the septum. The recorded motion is probably secondary to adjacent normal muscle.

In some experimental studies, a transient increase in wall thickness has been noted in acute infarction.[42] A similar finding has not been observed in patients thus far.

Change in Acoustic Properties

The healing process of an acute myocardial infarction involves the deposition of collagen and the formation of scar. These changes produce a decrease in thickness of

Fig. 8–25. M-mode echocardiogram of a patient with an acute inferior myocardial infarction whose posterior left ventricular wall (PLV) is thicker in diastole (D) than in systole (S). (From Corya, B.C.: Echocardiography in ischemic heart disease. Am. J. Med., 63:10, 1977.)

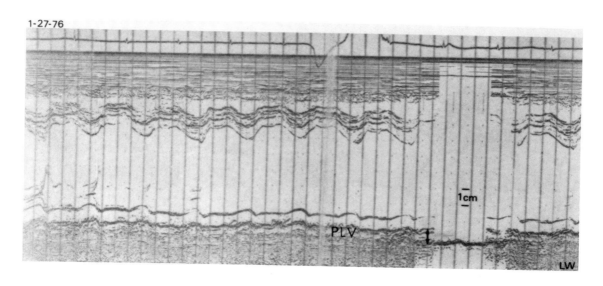

Fig. 8–26. Follow-up M-mode echocardiogram of the patient in Figure 8–25. Two-and-a-half years following myocardial infarction the thickness of the posterior left ventricular wall (PLV) significantly decreases. The motion of the posterior left ventricular wall continues to be abnormal. (From Corya, B.C.: Echocardiography in ischemic heart disease. Am. J. Med., 63:10, 1977.)

the affected wall segment, as demonstrated in Figures 8–26 and 8–27. The second effect of scar formation is a change in the acoustic properties of the segment. Collagen and scar produce a change in the reflective properties of that wall. Fibrosis is a much stronger reflector of ultrasound than is normal myocardium.[43] Figure 8–28 demonstrates an M-mode scan of a patient with a scarred interventricular septum. The normal septal muscle can be seen to the right of the tracing. On the left side of the recording a dense band of echoes appears, which originates from the scarred interventricular septum. The total width of the scarred septum is smaller than that of the normal septum. The commonly noted band of fuzzy echoes adjacent to the hypokinetic septum is also visualized.

Figure 8–29 illustrates another M-mode scan of a patient with a scarred interventricular septum. Motion due to cardiac action is totally absent. There is a respiratory variation in the position of the septum. The total thickness of the septum is markedly diminished, especially when compared to the posterior left ventricular wall. In addition, the intensity of the echoes is somewhat

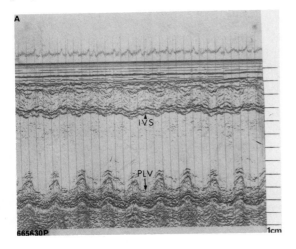

Fig. 8–27. M-mode echocardiogram of a patient with an old anteroseptal myocardial infarction and a thin interventricular septum (IVS). PLV = posterior left ventricular wall.

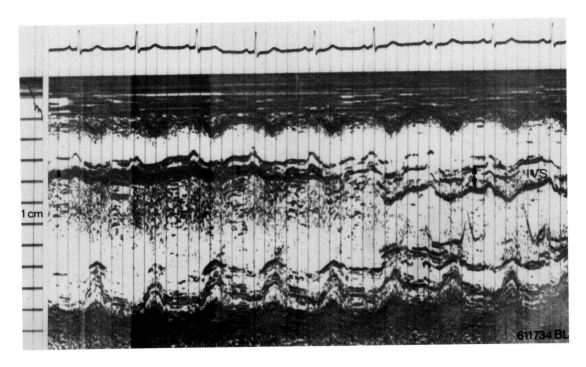

Fig. 8–28. M-mode scan of a patient with a scarred interventricular septum. The interventricular septum (IVS) is normal at the level of the mitral valve. As the ultrasonic beam scans toward the apex (left side of tracing), the septal echoes become thin and dense. A band of fuzzy intracavitary echoes lies next to the scarred septum. (From Rasmussen, S., et al.: Detection of myocardial scar tissue by M-mode echocardiography. Circulation, 57:230, 1978. By permission of the American Heart Association, Inc.)

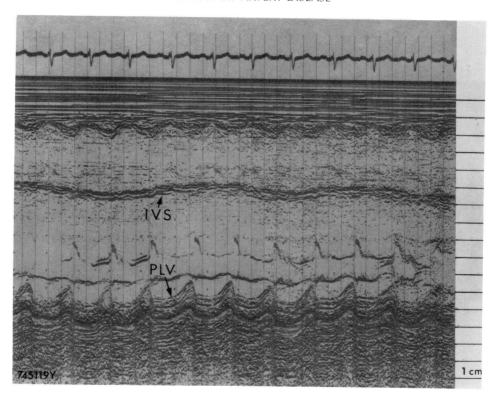

Fig. 8–29. M-mode echocardiogram of a patient with a scarred interventricular septum. The echoes from the interventricular septum (IVS) are thin, immobile and relatively dense. PLV = posterior left ventricular wall.

greater than that of the posterior left ventricular wall. Figure 8–30 demonstrates a two-dimensional echocardiogram of a patient with a scarred interventricular septum. The septal (IVS) echoes again are thin and change minimally from diastole to systole. The intensity of the echoes is also greater than that of the posterior left ventricular wall. Normal thickening of the posterior left ventricular wall can be appreciated in this illustration.

Technical details naturally must be considered when making the echocardiographic diagnosis of scar. The full width of the interventricular septum must be recorded. Any dropout of echoes makes the septum artificially thin. In addition, the intensity of the echoes is relative and can be influenced by the gain setting. However, with practice, the echocardiographic diagnosis of scar should not be difficult.

There has been great interest in studying the acoustic changes of the myocardium with acute myocardial infarction.[44–49] It has been demonstrated that the deposition of collagen is a relatively early finding in the infarcted muscle. This collagen may alter both the attenuation and the reflective properties of the muscle.[47,48,50] Studies using both transmission and backscatter echoes have been performed in the experimental animal, with interesting and encouraging results. Some studies utilize a computer to analyze the subtle differences between the returning echoes from infarcted and normal muscle.[49,51] An interesting technique has been reported that records the area of infarction on a two-dimensional ultrasonic plot of the ventricle.[52] Figure 8–31 shows a recording from such a study. The ischemic area is the light segment on the ultrasonic recording. The pathologic specimen is in the lower half of the illustration. The infarcted segment is stained darker than the normal muscle.

All techniques for examining the changes in acoustic properties in acute ischemia are

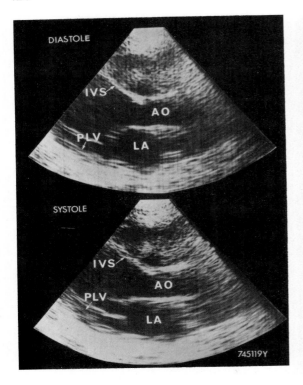

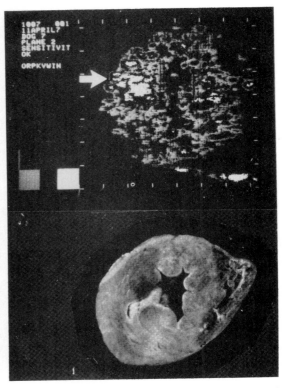

Fig. 8–30. Parasternal two-dimensional echocardiograms of a patient with a scarred interventricular septum. The echoes from the interventricular septum (IVS) are thin and relatively dense. PLV = posterior left ventricular wall; AO = aorta; LA = left atrium.

Fig. 8–31. Illustration demonstrating an investigative ultrasonic technique for displaying an acute myocardial infarction. This 30-minute infarction is detected ultrasonically as light echoes (arrow). The pathologic specimen is in the lower panel, and the perfusion deficit appears black. (From Gramiak, R., et al.: Ultrasonic imaging of experimental myocardial infarctions. In Echocardiology. Edited by C.T. Lancee. The Hague, Martinus Nijhoff, 1979.)

still in the investigative stages; however, the preliminary data are encouraging, and it is hoped that we may be able to clinically detect echocardiographic changes in the acutely infarcted myocardium.

QUANTITATION OF ISCHEMIC MUSCLE

One can grossly estimate the quantity of ischemic muscle with M-mode echocardiography. If virtually all left ventricular segments examined by the M-mode technique move abnormally, one can expect extensive ischemic damage. In contrast, if one fails to record any abnormal muscle, the prospect of extensive damage is considerably less. One investigator used multiple transducer positions for examining the ischemic left ventricle with M-mode echocardiography (Fig. 8–12) and presented data that indicated a correlation between the extent of infarction and the number of abnormal segments.[53]

Despite these observations M-mode echocardiography is a relatively poor method for quantitating the degree of ischemic damage. Two-dimensional echocardiography offers a far better technique.[24,54–58,58a] Because of the inherent spatial orientation in this technique one can determine the actual amount of surface area or muscle mass involved in the ischemia. For example, in Figure 8–32B note that the ventricular muscle below or posterior to the dotted line moves normally in systole. Not only is the wall motion normal, but there is also proper thickening of the muscle posterior and lateral to the dotted line. However, the muscle anterior and medial to the dotted line fails to move with systole, and there is no thickening of the

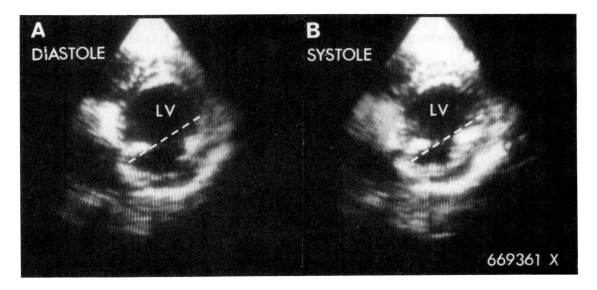

Fig. 8–32.   Short-axis two-dimensional echocardiogram of the left ventricle (LV) in a patient with an anteromedial myocardial infarction. The posterior and lateral walls (below the dotted line) move and thicken normally. The muscle above the dotted line moves and thickens minimally.

walls. Thus one can see how much of the circumference of this chamber is involved in ischemia and how much remains normal.

A variety of techniques have been described in the literature concerning how one can quantitate the degree of ischemic muscle.[54–56,58,59] One possibility is to merely divide the various segments of the left ventricle into appropriate areas (Fig. 8–33). Long-axis views record the anterior and posterior segments together with the cardiac apex. Short-axis examinations visualize the anterior, posterior, medial, and lateral walls. An apical four-chamber view records the apex and the medial and lateral walls. One could assume that each segment is approximately equal in area. By totaling the number of abnormal segments, one could calculate the percent surface area or percent mass of left ventricle that is abnormal.

A somewhat more complicated approach to quantitating the ischemic muscle is demonstrated in Figure 8–34. This technique assumes that the ventricle is a truncated cone. By knowing the length and the radii of each end of the cone, one can calculate the surface area of that object. The apex can be arbitrarily designated as 10 percent of the total surface area of the ventricle. In the illustration,

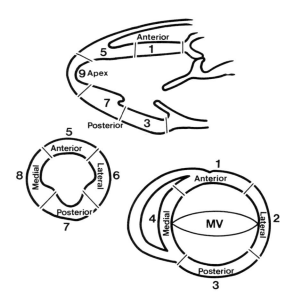

Fig. 8–33.   Diagrams demonstrating how the left ventricle can be divided into segments using two-dimensional echocardiography. (From Heger, J.J., et al.: Cross-sectional echocardiography in acute myocardial infarction: detection and localization of regional left ventricular asynergy. Circulation, 60:531, 1979. By permission of the American Heart Association, Inc.)

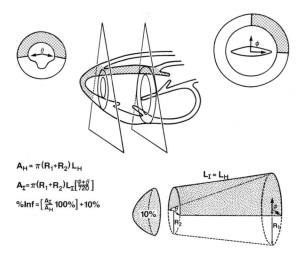

$$A_H = \pi(R_1 + R_2)L_H$$

$$A_I = \pi(R_1 + R_2)L_I[\tfrac{\phi + \theta}{720}]$$

$$\%Inf = [\tfrac{A_I}{A_H} 100\%] + 10\%$$

Fig. 8–34.   Drawing demonstrating how one might be able to calculate infarct size using two-dimensional echocardiography. The technique uses the formula for the surface area of a truncated cone. The left ventricular apex is arbitrarily assigned a value of 10%. In this illustration the darkened area is the presumed infarction. The formula demonstrates how the area of infarction can be calculated.

the gray area represents the ischemic muscle, a frequent distribution for an anterior myocardial infarction.

Figures 8–33 and 8–34 represent only two examples of how the size of an infarcted area can be determined. As a rule, one uses wall motion as the indicator for ischemia. It is technically much more difficult to record changes in thickening. Thus the size of the infarct measured echocardiographically frequently appears to be an overestimate of the true infarct as determined by pathologic studies.[47]

It cannot be overemphasized that the measurements are no better than the raw data. Technically poor recordings give meaningless, or worse, misleading information. Gross estimates of infarct size by way of real-time studies are sometimes more accurate because the eye integrates echo dropout.

ASSESSMENT OF OVERALL PERFORMANCE OF THE ISCHEMIC VENTRICLE

The most common echocardiographic technique for evaluating the left ventricle utilizes M-mode dimensions between the interventricular septum and the posterior left ventricular wall (see Chapter 3). By obtaining diastolic and systolic dimensions, one can measure the size of the left ventricle and assess its overall performance. Investigators have used these dimensions to estimate ventricular volumes and to measure fractional and circumferential shortening (see Chapter 3). Unfortunately, there are well-recognized limitations to this echocardiographic technique that are extremely important in the context of ischemic heart disease. For example, in Figure 8–6 the distance between the left side of the septum (LS) and the posterior left ventricular endocardium (EN) is 5.8 cm, which is slightly above normal; however, the septal and posterior walls move fairly well at the level of the mitral valve apparatus. If the echocardiographic recording were limited to the area immediately beyond the level of the mitral valve (where LS and EN are indicated), one would assume that aside from slight dilatation, overall left ventricular performance was satisfactory. As this scan demonstrates, however, the apical portion of the septum does not move. As one might expect, left ventricular function was actually significantly depressed. In fact, on the left ventricular angiogram, the apical half of the ventricle was aneurysmal, and the overall angiographic ejection fraction was quite poor. Thus it is clear that using M-mode echocardiographic dimensions of the basal half of the ventricle to predict global ventricular function is a limited approach, especially with predicting ejection fraction.

Despite these limitations, M-mode echocardiography can still be used to gain some information concerning overall left ventricular performance. Although the usual echocardiographic dimensions used to estimate left ventricular diastolic volume are inaccurate in patients with segmental disease, there is still some value in this dimension, even in these patients. The diastolic measurement may still provide a rough estimate of the overall size of the left ventricle, especially the basal half. Evidence suggests that the standard echocardiographic measurement may be helpful in judging the extent of ventricular damage, since the basal portion of the left ventricle is usually the last area of the heart to be involved in coronary artery disease. Left ventricular dilatation at the level of the mitral valve is frequently a sign of advanced left ventricular disease. Thus, if one uses the standard echocardiographic left ventricular measurement as a simple dimension and not for volume measurements, it may still be useful in assessing the status of the ischemic ventricle, particularly when the chamber is severely damaged.[60-65]

Unfortunately, this measurement is not a sufficiently sensitive indicator of left ventricular dysfunction, and left ventricular dilatation is obviously nonspecific for coronary artery disease. Several efforts have been made to measure left ventricular volumes by way of two-dimensional echocardiography, many of which are promising.[66-73] The most impressive data thus far are from animal models that provided satisfactory recordings of the entire ventricle. The principal difficulty thus far in making volume measurements from two-dimensional echocardiography is the problem of echo dropout, which may be significant in many patients. Naturally, if volumes can be accurately assessed with two-dimensional echocardiography, then this technique should be able to provide a useful measurement of ejection fraction, which is the clinical standard most physicians use for assessing the function of the ischemic ventricle.

A relatively simple method for estimating ejection fraction from the M-mode echocardiogram is to determine the distance between the mitral valve E point and the left side of the interventricular septum.[74,75] Normally, the mitral valve E point is within 7 or 8 mm of the interventricular septum. However, as noted in Figure 8–6, even though the left ventricle is only mildly dilated and the motion of the walls at the base of the heart is normal, the E point-septal separation is more than 1 cm and is clearly abnormal. This technique's attractiveness is due partly to its simplicity and to the fact that some rational basis exists for this determination. Mitral valve motion is influenced by the amount of blood flowing through that valve and represents left ventricular stroke volume unless there is valvular insufficiency. In addition, when the left ventricle dilates, the interventricular septum is usually displaced ante-

riorly. This measurement does have its limitations, however; false positives and false negatives are to be expected at times.

As indicated in Chapter 4, mitral valve motion may provide hemodynamic information concerning overall left ventricular performance. Patients with coronary artery disease often have a high left ventricular end-diastolic pressure that is primarily a result of an elevated atrial component of ventricular pressure. Such an alteration in left ventricular pressure, and possibly to some extent abnormal ventricular contraction, changes the manner in which the mitral valve closes.[60,76] Figure 8–35 is a mitral valve echocardiogram that demonstrates normal mitral closure. Following the P wave of the electrocardiogram, the mitral valve A wave develops. With atrial relaxation the valve begins to close, and with ventricular systole the valve closes completely at the C point. The interval between the A and C points is quite short, and there is no interruption of valve closure.

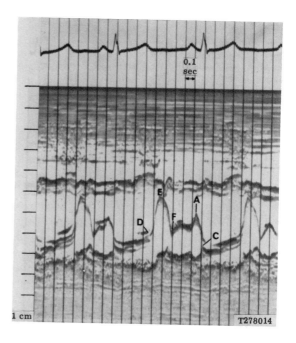

Fig. 8–35. Mitral valve echocardiogram of a patient with normal left ventricular function and normal left ventricular diastolic pressures. (From Konecke, L.L., et al.: Abnormal mitral valve motion in patient with elevated left ventricular end-diastolic pressure. Circulation, 47:989, 1973.)

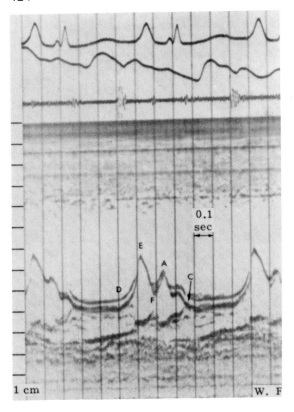

Fig. 8–36. Mitral valve echocardiogram of a patient with coronary artery disease and abnormal left ventricular function. The mitral valve closure between the A and C points is interrupted, and the A to C interval is prolonged.

The mitral valve echocardiogram in Figure 8–36 is considerably different. This patient had an old myocardial infarction and, at cardiac catheterization, had an elevated left ventricular end-diastolic pressure. The most striking finding here is interrupted mitral valve closure between points A and C. Such an interreption has been called a "notch," "plateau," "shoulder," or "B bump." The resultant interval between A and C is prolonged disproportionate to atrioventricular conduction, as indicated by the P–R interval on the electrocardiogram. This finding is not necessarily specific for an elevated left ventricular diastolic pressure and is actually an insensitive sign for such pressure changes. The interrupted closure, or notch, may also be a function of poor contractility of the ventricle. In any case, this finding is indicative of left ventricular dysfunction and can be helpful in assessing the overall global performance of the ischemic ventricle.[60-63]

Several techniques are described that use the mitral valve for estimating mitral valve flow or left ventricular stroke volume in patients with coronary artery disease. One technique utilizes the measurement of the cross-sectional area of the aorta together with the rate of systolic closure of the mitral valve.[77] These two measurements, combined with left ventricular ejection time measured from the aortic valve echocardiogram, provide a formula for measuring cardiac output. Another technique utilizes the mitral valve echocardiogram together with the electrocardiogram to arrive at a formula for assessing mitral valve flow.[78] The echocardiographic measurements include the separation between the anterior and posterior mitral leaflets at the E point and at the D to E slope. The electrocardiographic measurements include heart rate and P–R interval. The derived formula is as follows:

$$\text{Stroke Volume} = \left(\frac{EE}{\text{Heart Rate (HR)}} + \text{P–R}\right) \times 100 +$$

$$2 \times \frac{DE}{\text{Heart Rate (HR)}}$$

Both techniques are relatively new and need further confirmation. There is also report of an effort to use the aortic valve to measure stroke volume (see Chapter 4). One group of investigators correlated the timing of mitral valve opening and the dimensional changes of the left ventricular cavity to judge left ventricular performance.[80-81] Normally, the mitral valve begins to open at about the same time as the left ventricular dimension begins to widen in early diastole. By using a computer, the authors demonstrated that in patients with coronary artery disease there was an outward movement of the left ventricle prior to mitral valve opening. Thus there appeared to be a distortion of the shape of the ventricle during isovolumic relaxation.[81a] The sensitivity and specificity of this technique has not been evaluated. This technique frequently involves a simultaneous M-mode echocardiogram of the left ventricle and apex cardiogram. This same group also attempted to use the duration of isovolumic relaxation to assess overall ventricular function.[80,82] By adding a phonocardiogram, they used the closure of the aortic second sound as the onset of the isovolumic relaxation period and the opening of the mitral valve as its termination. These authors noted that the aortic valve closure was significantly delayed with respect to the minimum left ventricular dimension. In some patients there is also delayed opening of the mitral valve, which prolongs the isovolumic relaxation period. These abnormalities were associated with abnormal wall motion, and the authors speculated that the alterations in diastole were due to incoordinate systolic wall movement in the left ventricle. Dual M-mode echocardiography has also been suggested as a means of measuring isovolumic contraction and relaxation times.[82a]

In summary, despite the significant limitations to echocardiography's ability to assess overall left ventricular performance in patients with coronary artery disease, many of the techniques described can be quite useful. Unfortunately, it is difficult to assess their specificity and sensitivity because the "gold standard" is primarily angiography, and the differences between echocardiography and angiography are significant. Thus considerable research, using animal models to eliminate the inherent differences between angiography and echocardiography, is anticipated. In addition, if one must know the extent or amount of ischemic muscle as compared to the extent and amount of normal muscle, then using the echocardiogram may be significantly better than the usual angiographic ejection fraction.[59] There are many limitations to the use of ejection fraction for assessing overall ventricular function. For example, a patient with a large dyskinetic aneurysm may have a significant amount of normal ventricular muscle. However, the resultant ejection fraction may be so influenced by the aneurysm that the calculated number would not appreciate the amount of normal ventricle.

STRESS ECHOCARDIOGRAPHY

It is well known that under resting conditions left ventricular function may be per-

fectly normal. If there has been no permanent myocardial damage and if the ventricle is not ischemic at the time of the examination, the echocardiographic study of the left ventricle will not reflect the ventricular dysfunction that may be present under ischemic conditions. Thus there has been considerable interest in combining echocardiography with interventions that will produce sufficient stress for ischemia to occur.[83,84] Figure 8–37 demonstrates a patient with coronary artery disease who had normal ventricular function at rest. Following three minutes of handgrip stress the patient developed chest pain and manifested a dramatic change in septal motion. The handgrip was stopped, the pain subsided, and the septal motion returned to normal. Unfortunately, handgrip exercise is an ineffective means of producing ischemia in most patients.[85] Thus other forms of stress have been used.

The form of stress undergoing intensive investigation is isotonic exercise, usually by way of a supine bicycle. Because of movement of the chest, upright exercise has many technical limitations that can be overcome by using a bicycle. Supine exercise decreases some of these difficulties by immobilizing the chest.[84,88] However, many technical difficulties remain despite the use of supine exercise. In one M-mode study using supine exercise, the authors were able to obtain satisfactory echocardiograms that revealed useful information in 24 out of 54 subjects.[83] Thickening and velocities uniformly increased in normal subjects, whereas these measurements uniformly decreased in those patients with exercise-induced ischemia.

There has been interest in using two-dimensional echocardiography for exercise examination of the ischemic ventricle.[84] The availability of the apical window for examining the ischemic ventricle with two-dimensional echocardiography improves the technical ease with which this examination could be done.[84,89] The main technical problem with exercise echocardiography is respiratory interference. Since there is relatively little lung overlying the apex, the respiratory interference is less for apical studies

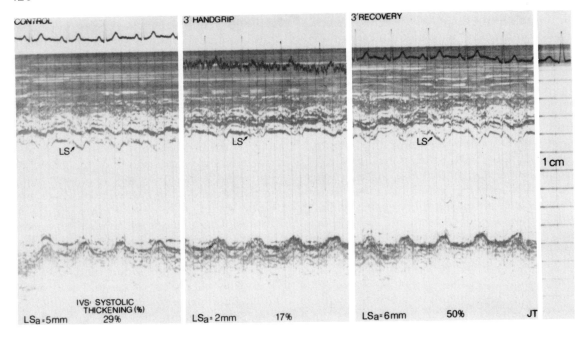

CONTROL   3' HANDGRIP   3'RECOVERY

LS'   LS'   LS'   1 cm

                   IVS' SYSTOLIC
                   THICKENING (%)
LSa=5mm   29%   LSa=2mm   17%   LSa=6mm   50%   JT

Fig. 8–37. M-mode echocardiogram of a patient with obstruction of the left anterior descending coronary artery. During the control period, septal motion (LS) and thickening is normal. Following three minutes of handgrip, the patient developed angina, and septal motion and thickening markedly decreased. Three minutes following recovery the pain disappeared, and septal motion and thickening returned to normal. (From Corya, B.C. and Rasmussen, S.: The clinical usefulness of intervention echocardiography in evaluating regional and global left ventricular function. Cardiovasc. Med. In press.)

than for those done from the left sternal border. Figure 8–38 shows an exercise study of a patient with coronary artery disease. At rest one can appreciate a decrease in the size of the apex from diastole to systole. With exercise the diastolic area becomes somewhat smaller, but there is virtually no change with systole. Thus the apex is akinetic or hypokinetic during exercise compared with the resting situation. Following successful bypass surgery the situation changes (Fig. 8–39). Although the resting state shows some improvement in wall motion, the most dramatic change is with exercise. A sizable increase in wall motion occurs from diastole to systole in the postoperative exercise examination.

Studies using two-dimensional echocardiography still have significant technical limitations. However, using the apical examination, a 70 percent success rate has been reported thus far.[84] It is hoped that with improved techniques and instrumentation the success rate will increase, and stress echocardiography may become a practical examination for patients with coronary artery disease.

SERIAL EXAMINATIONS

One of the principal advantages of echocardiography is that one can obtain frequent examinations to judge the efficacy of therapy or to follow the natural history of the disease.[84,90–92] Figure 8–39 shows an example of how one can judge the benefits of coronary bypass surgery. One may also use echocardiography to note the findings with spontaneous ischemic attacks, such as with Prinzmetal's angina.[7,93] Possibly the most common application of serial echocardiograms is in acute myocardial infarction.[59,60,63,94–97] The value of such studies is demonstrated in the patient whose echocardiograms appear in Figures 8–40 and 8–41. This patient was suspected of having coronary artery disease, but initially had a normal

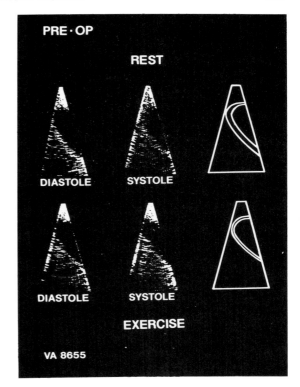

Fig. 8–38. Resting and exercise two-dimensional echocardiograms of the apex in a patient with coronary artery disease. At rest, the inferior wall of the apex moves normally. With exercise, however, the apical walls move minimally. (From Wann, L.S., et al.: Exercise cross-sectional echocardiography in ischemic heart disease. Circulation, *60*:1300, 1979. By permission of the American Heart Association, Inc.)

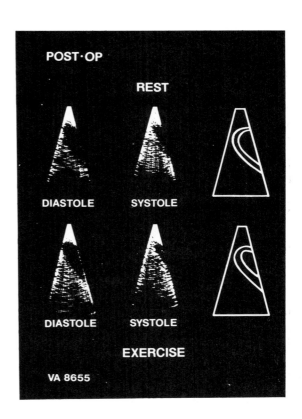

Fig. 8–39. Exercise two-dimensional echocardiographic study following bypass surgery in the patient in Figure 8–38. Following surgery apical motion increases at rest and with exercise increases remarkably. (From Wann, L.S., et al.: Exercise cross-sectional echocardiography in ischemic heart disease. Circulation, *60*:1300, 1979. By permission of the American Heart Association, Inc.)

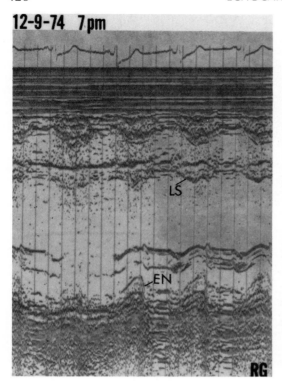
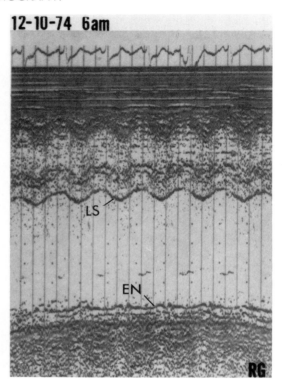

Fig. 8–40.   Serial M-mode echocardiograms of a patient with chest pain who eventually developed an inferior myocardial infarction. On 12/9/74 the echocardiogram demonstrated reasonably normal septal (LS) and endocardial (EN) motion. At 6:00 a.m. on the following day, the patient had severe chest pain and the posterior endocardial echo stopped moving.

left ventricular M-mode echocardiogram (Fig. 8–40, 12/9/74). Approximately 11 hours later, the patient had a bout of chest pain and there was a dramatic change in the motion of the posterior left ventricular endocardial echo (EN, 12/10/74). On the following day (Fig. 8–41, 12/11/74), the posterior left ventricular wall motion improved, although it was definitely hypokinetic. Five days later (12/16/74), the posterior endocardial motion returned to normal and the echocardiogram was not too dissimilar from that seen prior to the infarction (Fig. 8–40, 12/9/74).

These examples demonstrate that echocardiography has the capability to show changes in wall motion, apparently in response to changes in myocardial perfusion. Long-term studies show that some of the affected myocardium will thin, such as in Figures 8–25 and 8–26. Two-dimensional echocardiographic studies can also help determine whether the amount of ischemic mus-

cle changes appreciably.[94,96] Such observations are helpful, not only in judging the possible improvement in myocardial function, but also in determining whether extension or expansion of the ischemic damage occurs.[94]

COMPLICATIONS OF MYOCARDIAL INFARCTION

Ventricular Aneurysm

One of the most common complications of myocardial infarction is aneurysm formation. There are several ways in which echocardiography can give information concerning the existence of left ventricular aneurysms. Figure 8–42 is an M-mode scan taken with a strip-chart recording speed of 10 mm/sec. The transducer is at a relatively low level on the chest, and as the ultrasonic beam approaches the apex, there is a decrease in the distance between the left septum (LS) and the posterior endocardium (EN). Note the

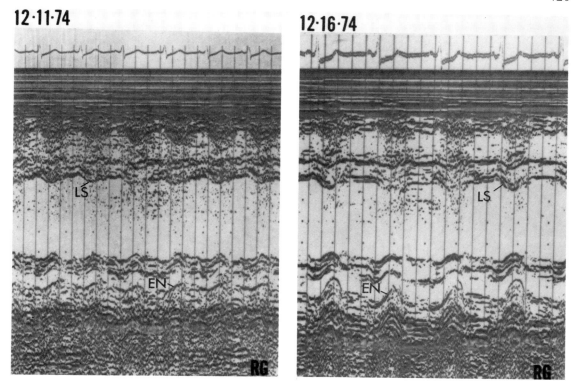

Fig. 8–41.   Serial echocardiogram of the patient in Figure 8–40. On 12/11/74 the motion of the posterior left ventricular endocardium (EN) improved slightly but remained hypokinetic. On 12/16/74 the posterior ventricular endocardial motion was essentially normal. LS = left septum.

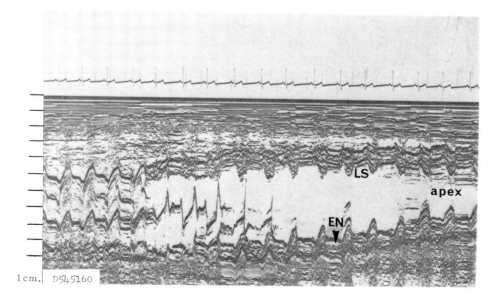

Fig. 8–42.   Slow M-mode scan of a normal left ventricle. Both the septal (LS) and posterior endocardial (EN) echoes move normally throughout the scan, and the distance between the two echoes decreases as the ultrasonic beam approaches the apex. (From Feigenbaum, H.: Use of echocardiography in evaluating left ventricular function. *In* Proceedings of the Second World Congress on Ultrasonics in Medicine. New York, Excerpta Medica, June 1973.)

tapering of the normally shaped left ventricle. The M-mode scan in Figure 8–43 is taken from a patient with a large anterior apical aneurysm. Note the faint echoes from the left septum (LS) in the left ventricular outflow tract. Beyond this point the anterior and septal echoes are relatively indistinct, and they clearly do not continue to move normally and do not exhibit any tapering toward the apex. This examination was taken with the transducer placed above the apex in a low position. A recording of the same patient taken from a slightly higher interspace is shown in Figure 8–6. In this earlier illustration the transducer was in a midposition, and the recording of the septum was much better than when the transducer was in a low position, as in Figure 8–43. The low transducer position was particularly useful in bringing out the aneurysmal dilatation at the apex.

Using the M-mode technique to assess the shape of the left ventricle and particularly to detect ventricular aneurysms[98] requires a knowledge of where the transducer should be placed on the chest. The tapering effect of the apex is seen only when the transducer is

in a low position. If the transducer is relatively high, tapering does not occur.

It is also possible to obtain similar scans with the transducer in the subcostal area.[99-101] Figure 8–44 shows a subcostal M-mode scan of a normally shaped left ventricle that again reveals a decrease in the left ventricular dimension as the ultrasonic beam approaches the apex. In contrast, Figure 8–45 shows a subcostal examination in a patient with an apical aneurysm. Not only does the left ventricular dimension fail to decrease at the level of the apex, but this dimension actually increases. The subcostal examination has the advantage of minimal distortion because of the greater distance between the transducer and the left ventricle and the need for less angulation of the transducer. Thus detection of aneurysmal dilatation of the apex is probably more accurate with the subcostal approach, and one need not be as concerned about the proper location of the transducer.

Unfortunately, the M-mode technique for assessing left ventricular aneurysms is not sufficiently sensitive. The examination can detect large aneurysms and those that in-

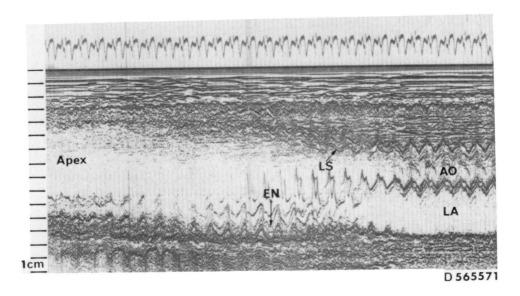

Fig. 8–43. M-mode scan of the patient in Figure 8–6 with the transducer at a lower interspace. This patient had a large aneurysm, and the upward bulging of the septal and anterior wall echoes can be noted as the ultrasonic beam approaches the apex. AO = aorta; LA = left atrium; LS = left septum; EN = posterior left ventricular endocardium. (From Dillon, J.C., et al.: M-mode echocardiography in evaluation of patients for aneurysmectomy. Circulation, 53:657, 1976.)

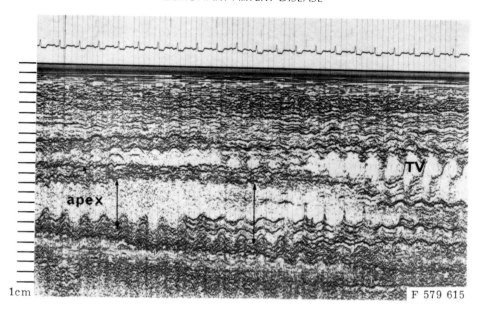

Fig. 8–44.   Slow subcostal scan of the left ventricle of a patient with a normally shaped left ventricle. The left ventricular dimension *(arrows)* is smaller near the apex than in the body of the left ventricle. (From Chang, S.: M-mode Echocardiographic Techniques and Pattern Recognition. Philadelphia, Lea & Febiger, 1976.)

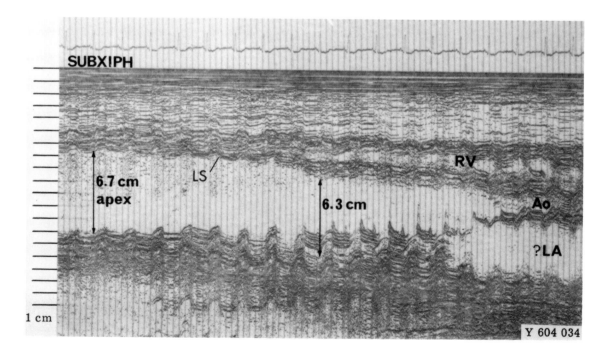

Fig. 8–45.   Subcostal M-mode scan of a patient with a ventricular aneurysm. The apical left ventricular dimension is greater than that through the body of the left ventricle. Note paradoxical motion of the septum (LS). RV = right ventricle; AO = aorta; ?LA = questionable left atrium. (From Chang, S.: M-mode Echocardiographic Techniques and Pattern Recognition. Philadelphia, Lea & Febiger, 1976.)

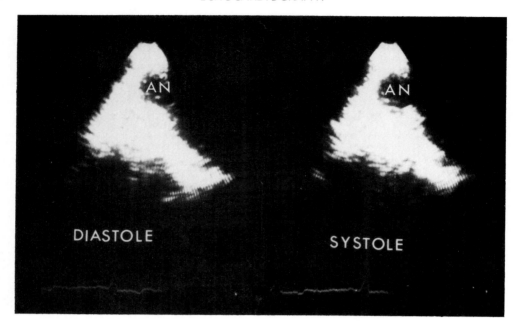

Fig. 8–46.   Parasternal two-dimensional echocardiogram of the cardiac apex of a patient with an apical aneurysm (AN). In diastole, the aneurysmal dilatation can be appreciated, and in systole, the dyskinetic motion of the apex makes the aneurysm even more striking.

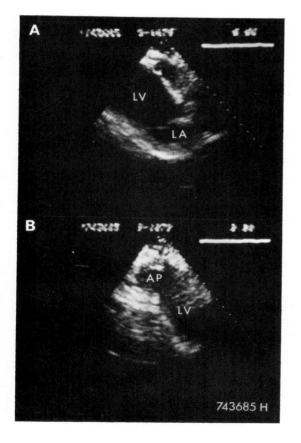

Fig. 8–47.   Parasternal long-axis two-dimensional echocardiograms of a patient with coronary artery disease, a scarred interventricular septum, and an apical aneurysm. A, Body of the left ventricle (LV) and left atrium (LA). Note the thin and relatively echo-dense septum. B, Apical examination reveals the aneurysm (AP).

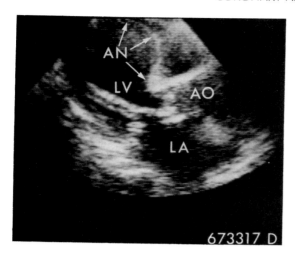

Fig. 8–48. Long-axis parasternal two-dimensional echocardiogram of a patient with coronary artery disease and an anteroseptal aneurysm (AN) of the interventricular septum. AO = aorta; LA = left atrium; LV = left ventricle.

volve the area of the left ventricle at the level of the papillary muscle. Recording satisfactory M-mode tracings below the papillary muscles is rare. Two-dimensional echocardiography, because of its inherent spatial orientation, can vastly improve the echocardiographic determination of ventricular aneurysms.[102–105]

A common site for aneurysms is the apex. Figure 8–46 shows a two-dimensional parasternal examination of the cardiac apex in a patient with an apical aneurysm. The aneurysmal dilatation can be appreciated in diastole. The distortion of the dyskinetic apex becomes even greater with systole. This type of aneurysm is difficult to detect with M-mode echocardiography. Figure 8–47 shows two parasternal long-axis echocardiograms of a patient with an apical aneurysm (AP) as well as a scarred anterior interventricular septum. The parasternal long-axis study through the body of the ventricle (A) demonstrates that the septum is thin and scarred except near the base of the heart. The aneurysmal distortion of the apex is visible when the transducer is placed directly over the apex (B).[102]

Aneurysmal dilatation may occur in almost any part of the ventricle. Figure 8–48 shows an aneurysmal bulge of the interventricular

septum (AN) as seen in the parasternal long-axis view. Figure 8–49 is a long-axis parasternal examination of the left ventricle in a patient with a posterior basal aneurysm (AN). The aneurysmal dilatation is near the junction of the left atrium. A larger posterior aneurysm is illustrated in Figure 8–50. The apical two-chamber view is frequently best for detecting posterior aneurysms.

Figure 8–51 demonstrates one of the most common varieties of aneurysms seen with echocardiography. In this apical four-chamber view one sees aneurysmal dilatation (AN) of the apical two-thirds of the interventricular septum. This abnormality gives an "hourglass," "figure-eight," or "light-bulb" appearance to the left ventricular cavity. This echocardiogram should be compared with the normal apical four-chamber recording noted in Figure 8–19. Another example of an aneurysm depicted in the apical four-chamber examination is shown in Figure 8–20.

The short-axis examination may also detect aneurysm formation. Figure 8–52 shows a patient with a massive anterolateral aneurysm. The left ventricular chamber is relatively small and can be seen in the lower left of the echocardiogram. The anterior (AMV) and posterior (PMV) mitral leaflets are noted within the left ventricular cavity. A

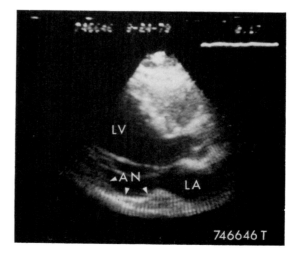

Fig. 8–49. Long-axis parasternal two-dimensional echocardiogram of a patient with a posterior basal aneurysm (AN). LV = left ventricle; LA = left atrium.

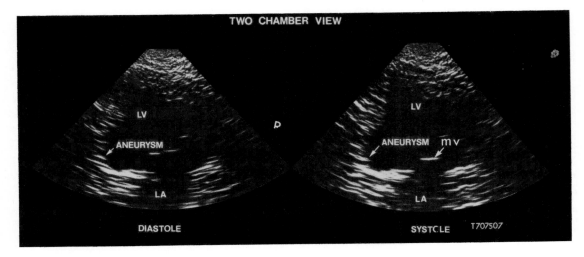

Fig. 8–50. Apical two-chamber echocardiogram during diastole and systole of a patient with a large posterior aneurysm. There is also incomplete closure of the mitral valve (mv) in systole. LV = left ventricle; LA = left atrium.

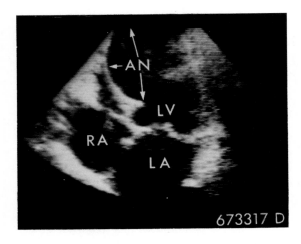

Fig. 8–51. Apical four-chamber two-dimensional echocardiogram of a patient with an aneurysm (AN) of the apical two-thirds of the interventricular septum. LV = left ventricle; LA = left atrium; RA = right atrium.

large aneurysm comes off of the anterior lateral wall of the ventricle. The aneurysm is actually larger than the residual cavity of the left ventricle. Examining this patient in real time permits the examiner to move the probe over the various areas of the aneurysm, indeed a dramatic study. The entire aneurysm could not be visualized at any one time with this 30° scan.

These examples should demonstrate that two-dimensional echocardiography can detect a variety of ventricular aneurysms. In this regard, the examination is proving quite sensitive and reliable. In fact, a technically satisfactory two-dimensional study is probably the definitive examination for excluding or detecting ventricular aneurysms. Figure 8–20 notes that some aneurysms are principally the result of a loss of myocardial tissue rather than any significant outward bulge of the entire thickness of the ventricular wall. Since echocardiography can record myocardial thickness, the differentiation can be readily appreciated. Other techniques that only visualize the cavity cannot depict how much of the aneurysm is a function of thinning of the wall.

In addition to establishing the existence and size of a ventricular aneurysm, echocardiography is proving particularly helpful in assessing the remaining ventricular muscle not involved in the aneurysm formation. Early data demonstrated that the M-mode dimension of the left ventricle at the base of the heart could predict those patients who would survive aneurysmectomy.[62] Another M-mode sign used to evaluate the remaining muscle was normal wall motion of both the septal and posterior ventricular walls. If one could not see normal motion of both walls,

LV – SAX

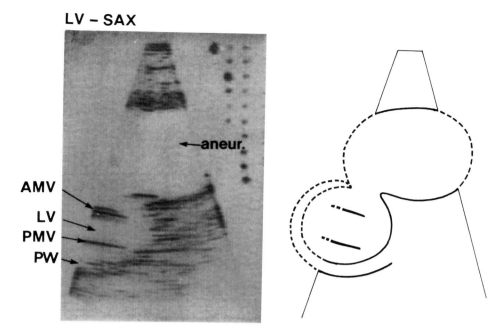

Fig. 8–52. Short-axis (SAX) two-dimensional echocardiogram and diagram of a patient with an unusual ventricular aneurysm involving the anterolateral portion of the ventricle. The anterior (AMV) and posterior (PMV) mitral valve leaflets can be noted within the left ventricle (LV). The aneurysm comes off of the anterolateral wall of the chamber and is actually larger than the left ventricular cavity. PW = pulmonary wall. (From Weyman, A.E., et al.: Detection of left ventricular aneurysms by cross-sectional echocardiography. Circulation, 54:936, 1976. By permission of the American Heart Association, Inc.)

then the probability of successful surgery was much less.

Two-dimensional echocardiography provides a more quantitative basis for judging the amount of normal muscle in patients with aneurysms.[103,104] Several studies now demonstrate that this newer echocardiographic technique can assess the amount of remaining, normally functioning muscle and can well predict the surgical outcome of aneurysmectomy. Thus two-dimensional echocardiography is proving to be an extremely important diagnostic tool for both the detection and the overall evaluation of patients with ventricular aneurysms.

Pseudoaneurysm

Several reports have demonstrated the use of echocardiography for the diagnosis of pseudoaneurysm.[106–111,111a] Such a condition occurs when there is rupture of the free wall of the left ventricle. Blood is trapped within the pericardium, and an aneurysm develops

with the outside wall being pericardium and clot rather than muscle. The M-mode echocardiogram in Figure 8–53 is taken from such a patient. The pseudoaneurysm (PA) is illustrated by a large, relatively echo-free space beyond the posterior left ventricular epicardium (epi). Pseudoaneurysms have also been detected echocardiographically in which the rupture is in the anteroseptal area with perforation into the pericardial sac. Actual discontinuity of the interventricular septum has been detected on the echocardiogram.[108]

There have been several reports of using two-dimensional echocardiography for the detection of pseudoaneurysm.[105,109–111] Figure 8–54 shows an example of a two-dimensional study in a patient with a pseudoaneurysm. The aneurysm (PAn) is seen as a large, echo-free space posterior to the left ventricle. In addition, the actual perforation (arrow) can be detected. When cardiac rupture occurs and the defect is not

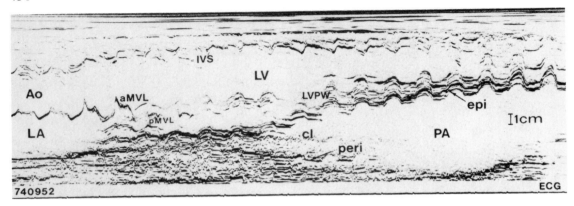

Fig. 8–53.   M-mode scan of a patient with a pseudoaneurysm of the left ventricle following myocardial infarction. The large echo-free space posterior to the left ventricular epicardium (epi) is produced by the large pseudoaneurysm (PA). AO = aorta; IVS = interventricular septum; LV = left ventricle; MVL = anterior mitral valve leaflet; pMVL = posterior mitral valve leaflet; LA = left atrium; cl = clot; peri = pericardium; LVPW = left ventricular posterior wall. (From Roelandt, J., et al.: Echocardiographic diagnosis of pseudoaneurysm of the left ventricle. Circulation, 52:466, 1975.)

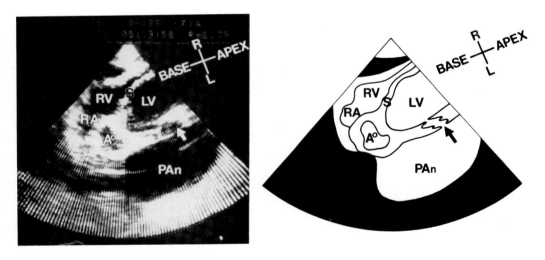

Fig. 8–54.   Two-dimensional echocardiogram and diagram of a patient with a pseudoaneurysm. This modified four-chamber view demonstrates the rupture *(arrow)* in the free wall of the left ventricle. The left ventricular cavity (LV) communicates with the pseudoaneurysm (PAn). RV = right ventricle; RA = right atrium; Ao = aorta. (From Katz, R.J., et al.: Non-invasive diagnosis of left ventricular pseudoaneurysm. Role of two-dimensional echocardiography and radionuclide gated pool imaging. Am. J. Cardiol., 44:372, 1979.)

sealed off with clot, then usually fatal acute hemopericardium results. Such a complication has been detected with two-dimensional echocardiography.[111a,b]

Left Ventricular Thrombi

A relatively common complication of the myocardial infarction is mural thrombi. These thrombi usually occur adjacent to a dyskinetic area, which is frequently aneurysmally dilated. It is difficult to see these usually immobile clots by way of M-mode echocardiography. One may be able to direct the M-mode ultrasonic beam through the thrombus,[112–114] but it is difficult to be certain of the origin of these echoes. On the other hand, two-dimensional echocardiography has proven to be an extremely useful tool for this diagnosis.[114-117] Figure 8–55 shows the most common way two-dimensional echocardiography is used for the detection of mural thrombi. This apical four-chamber view shows dilatation and akinesis of the apical half of the left ventricle. In addition, there is a mass of intracavitary echoes adherent to the apex that originate from a large apical clot (CL). These clots may be immobile or at times may exhibit motion in real time.

Although the apical four-chamber and two-chamber views are usually most successful in detecting thrombi, the clots may also be seen in other two-dimensional studies. Figure 8–56 shows a patient with a smaller apical clot recorded in parasternal long-axis and short-axis views. The clot produces relatively bright echoes that adhere to the akinetic apex.

The sensitivity and reliability of echocardiography in detecting clot is under current study by several investigators. Some false negatives and false positives have been reported. However, the overall success rate has been quite satisfactory. Small thrombi will undoubtedly be missed. However, it is unlikely that this technique will fail to record large thrombi. A number of potential artifacts, especially reverberations, must be recognized to avoid overdiagnosing possible thrombi. (The problem of reverberations was

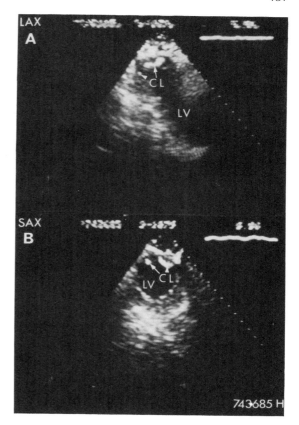

Fig. 8–56. Long-axis (LAX) and short-axis (SAX) parasternal views of a left ventricular apex in which clot (CL) is present. Two clots, one larger than the other, appear to be present. LV = left ventricle.

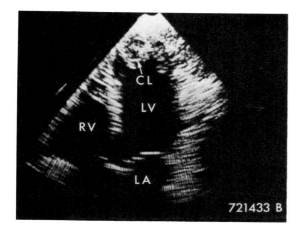

Fig. 8–55. Apical four-chamber two-dimensional echocardiogram of a patient with an apical clot (CL). LV = left ventricle; RV = right ventricle; LA = left atrium.

discussed in Chapter 1.) The appearance of these clots can be menacing at times. One is concerned over whether the thrombi will produce systemic emboli. Thus far no data support the use of surgical intervention for echocardiographically detected thrombi. One may use anticoagulants once the clots are detected.

Ventricular Septal Defect

A less common complication of myocardial infarction is rupture of the ventricular septum. Such a rupture may extend into the pericardium and produce a pseudo-aneurysm.[108] A more usual result of a ruptured septum is communication of blood from the left ventricle into the right ventricle. There have been a few reports using M-mode echocardiography to help in the

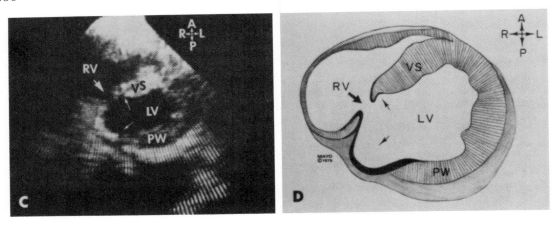

Fig. 8–57.   Short-axis two-dimensional echocardiogram and diagram of a patient with a ruptured interventricular septum secondary to a myocardial infarction. Note the aneurysmal bulging *(arrows)* of the ventricular septum (VS). In addition, echoes are discontinuous with communication between the right ventricle (RV) and the left ventricle (LV) at the site of the defect *(large arrow)*. PW = posterior wall. (From Scanlan, J.G., Seward, J.B., and Tajik, A.J.: Visualization of ventricular septal rupture utilizing wide-angle, two-dimensional echocardiography. Mayo Clin. Proc., *54*:383, 1979.)

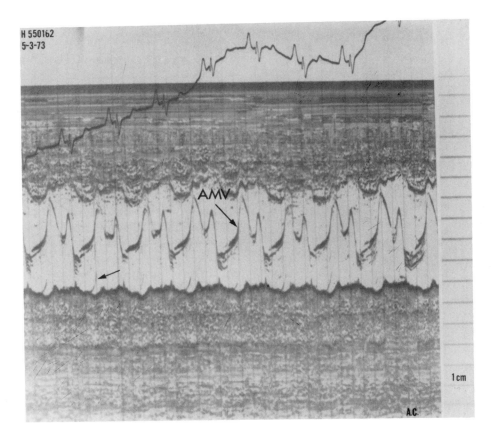

Fig. 8–58.   Mitral valve echocardiogram of a patient with an acute myocardial infarction and severe mitral insufficiency. Note the marked posterior displacement of the mitral valve *(arrow)* during systole. The rest of the mitral valve appears essentially normal. AMV = anterior mitral valve leaflet.

identification of ventricular septal rupture.[118-121] Dilatation of the right ventricle, decreased mitral valve diastolic slope, paradoxical septal motion, and increased excursion of the tricuspid valve have all been reported with this complication. Two-dimensional echocardiography is probably far more effective in detecting ventricular septal rupture secondary to myocardial infarction.[122-124] Figure 8–57 shows a two-dimensional study of a patient with a septal rupture. The defect in the ventricular septum (VS) is indicated by the large white arrow. The communication between the two ventricles is apparent. In addition, there is aneurysmal bulging of the posterior medial portion of the left ventricle in this short-axis parasternal examination.

Frequently, one cannot see the actual communication where the rupture occurred. Instead, one may merely see the aneurysmal bulging of the interventricular septum.[124] Thus far the septal bulge has been uniformly associated with the septal defect; thus, one can probably diagnose ventricular septal rupture by noting the bulging septum. One need not necessarily detect the actual break in the septal continuity.

Mitral Valve Abnormalities

A patient may occasionally develop a flail mitral valve secondary to myocardial infarction. The M-mode echocardiogram may show the findings of a left ventricular volume overload. In addition, the mitral valve may exhibit abnormal motion consistent with a flail valve. Figure 8–58 shows a patient who had marked mitral regurgitation, presumably due to coronary artery disease. The marked posterior displacement of the mitral valve during systole (arrow) can be noted at the junction of the left atrium.

A more common mitral valve complication secondary to myocardial infarction is papillary muscle dysfunction. Early investigators noted a decreased mitral E to F slope in patients with papillary muscle dysfunction.[125] However, this finding is so nonspecific that it is unreliable. There has been a recent description of a two-dimensional technique for the detection of papillary muscle dysfunction.[126] The echocardiographic

finding is incomplete closure of the mitral valve. Figure 8–59 shows diastolic and systolic apical four-chamber frames of a patient with chronic coronary artery disease and aneurysmal dilatation of the apical half of the left ventricle. With systole the closed mitral leaflets do not approach the plane of the atrioventricular groove (dotted line). A possible explanation for the incomplete closure and the resultant mitral regurgitation is that the papillary muscles and/or the adjacent ventricular wall is scarred, which in turn foreshortens the total mitral valve apparatus. Thus the leaflets are unable to close completely. This echocardiographic finding is noted best in the apical four-chamber view. It is also demonstrated in the apical two-chamber examination (Fig. 8–50). Thus far this observation has not been confirmed, hence its reliability and sensitivity are unknown.

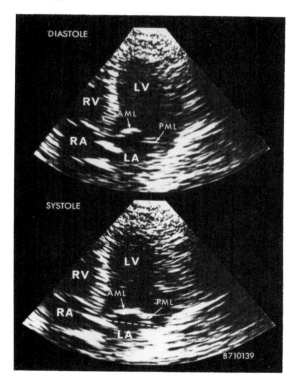

Fig. 8–59. Apical four-chamber two-dimensional echocardiograms of a patient with chronic coronary artery disease and papillary muscle dysfunction. In systole, closure of the mitral leaflets (AML and PML) is incomplete; they fail to reach the plane of the mitral annulus (dotted line). LV = left ventricle; RV = right ventricle; RA = right atrium; LA = left atrium.

Pericarditis

Postmyocardial infarction pericarditis and pericardial effusion are not uncommon problems, and echocardiography should be helpful in assessing these complications.[127] Figure 8–60 is taken from a patient with a recent myocardial infarction who developed a marked fibrinous pericarditis. The patient eventually died and the pericarditis was confirmed pathologically. The echocardiogram is somewhat unusual and shows an excessive number of echoes in the vicinity of the posterior pericardium. Although the exact identity of all of the echoes is not certain, they are excessive. They all move with the epicardium and undoubtedly arise, at least in part, from the markedly thickened pericardium.

Pericardial effusion is probably a more common occurrence and the usual findings for pericardial effusion are detected. The echocardiographic signs for pericardial effusion are discussed in more detail in the chapter on pericardial disease.

Right Ventricular Infarction

Although the chamber that principally suffers the damage of coronary artery disease is the left ventricle, there is increasing evidence that right ventricular infarction may occur and have devastating hemodynamic consequences. Several studies have reported the echocardiographic findings in patients with proven right ventricular infarction.[128-132] The principal abnormality is dilatation of the right ventricular chamber.

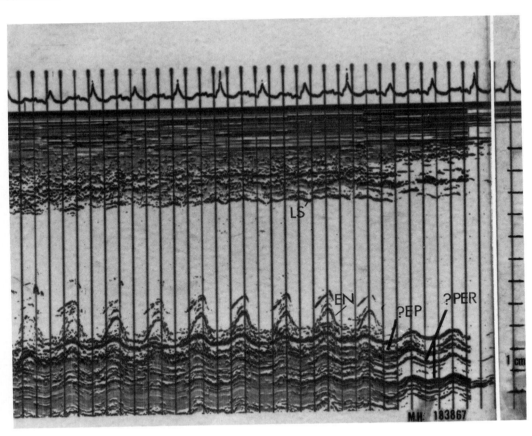

Fig. 8–60. M-mode echocardiogram of a patient with an acute anteroseptal myocardial infarction who developed pericarditis. Multiple echoes are recorded posterior to the left ventricular wall. Although the exact identity of these echoes is unclear, some appear to originate from a thickened pericardium, probably secondary to pericarditis. ?EP = questionable epicardial echoes; ?PER = questionable pericardial echoes; LS = left septum; EN = posterior left ventricular endocardium. (From Corya, B.C.: Applications of echocardiography in acute myocardial infarction. Cardiovasc. Clin., *II*:113, 1975.)

This dilatation can be detected with M-mode or two-dimensional echocardiography. One approach is to take the ratio of the right and left ventricular M-mode dimensions.[131] With right ventricular infarction the ratio increases. The two-dimensional examinations can show the right ventricular enlargement from several views. In addition, one can appreciate right ventricular segmental wall abnormalities by way of the two-dimensional studies. Decreased right ventricular wall motion with right ventricular infarction is in sharp contrast to the usually prominent or exaggerated motion of the right ventricular free wall in patients with ischemic damage of the left ventricle (Fig. 8–11).

Right ventricular infarction is frequently complicated by tricuspid regurgitation. Contrast echocardiographic studies have been helpful in detecting the tricuspid regurgitation.[130] The examination used usually depends on the reflux of contrast into the inferior vena cava and hepatic veins with the presence of tricuspid regurgitation.

EXAMINATION OF THE CORONARY ARTERIES

Two-dimensional echocardiography has the capability of recording the proximal coronary arteries.[133–138,138a,139] Figure 8–61 is a parasternal short-axis examination through the aorta demonstrating the origin of the right coronary artery (RCA) and left coronary artery (LCA). The right coronary artery is more difficult to record. Much of the artery lies directly under the sternum and is thus hidden from view. In addition, the tricuspid valve is in the same general area, and at times it is not easy to distinguish between the right coronary artery and echoes originating from the tricuspid valve annulus. Figure 8–62 shows an early 30° scan of the right coronary artery coming off of the anterior or right coronary sinus of the aorta.

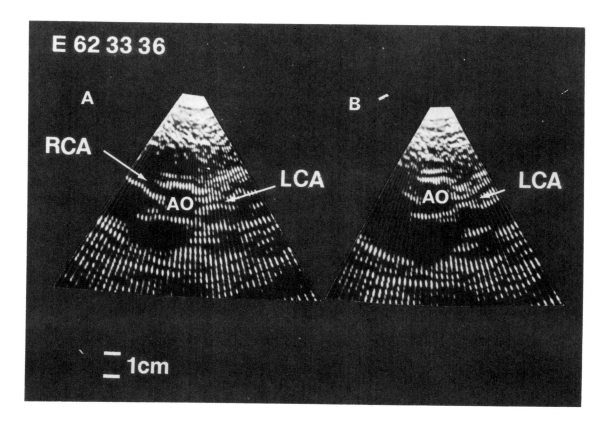

Fig. 8–61.   Short-axis two-dimensional echocardiogram demonstrating the origin of the coronary arteries from the aorta. RCA = right coronary artery; AO = aorta; LCA = left coronary artery.

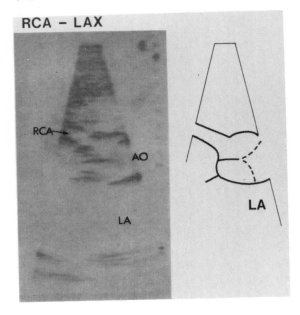

Fig. 8–62. Two-dimensional echocardiogram and diagram through the base of the heart and aorta (AO) demonstrating the origin of the right coronary artery (RCA). LA = left atrium.

The left coronary artery is much easier to detect echocardiographically. Confirmation of the validity of the echocardiographic technique was initially made with the assistance of contrast echocardiography.[133] Figure 8–63 shows an echocardiogram of a patient with a normal left main coronary artery who is undergoing coronary angiography. Prior to the injection of contrast into the coronary artery (A), the echoes from the left coronary artery (arrows) can be seen. With the injection of contrast through the left coronary catheter (B), the left main coronary artery is filled with echoes.

Figure 8–64 shows a left main coronary artery examination of a patient with obstruction (large arrow) near the origin of this artery. The echocardiogram shows a decrease in the lumen due to the increase of echoes in the posterior wall of the artery. Beyond the obstruction (small arrows), the distance between the two walls of the artery is wider. The coronary angiogram in Figure 8–65 shows the ostial lesion (arrow) in this left coronary artery. Aneurysmal dilatation of the coronary arteries has also been detected

Fig. 8–63. Short-axis two-dimensional echocardiogram demonstrating the left main coronary artery before and after direct injection of contrast into the left coronary artery. A, The echoes originating from the walls of the coronary arteries are visible before injection (arrows). B, Following contrast injection the artery fills with echoes. AO = aorta; LA = left atrium. (From Weyman, A.E., et al.: Non-invasive visualization of the left main coronary artery by cross-sectional echocardiography. Circulation, 54:169, 1976.)

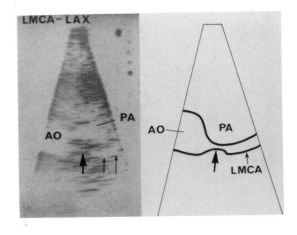

Fig. 8–64. Two-dimensional echocardiogram and diagram of the left main coronary artery in a patient with a proximal lesion of this artery. Instead of the parallel, uninterrupted echoes seen in Figure 8–63, a group of echoes (large arrow) partially occluded this vessel immediately past its origin in the aorta (AO). The more distal portion of the left main coronary artery (LMCA) is apparently normal (small arrows). PA = pulmonary artery. (From Weyman, A.E., et al.: Non-invasive visualization of the left main coronary artery by cross-sectional echocardiography. Circulation, 54:169, 1976.)

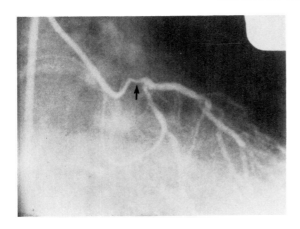

Fig. 8–65. Coronary cineangiogram of the left coronary artery of the patient in Figure 8–64. Note the proximal lesion of the left main coronary artery *(arrow)*. (From Weyman, A.E., et al.: Non-invasive visualization of the left main coronary artery by cross-sectional echocardiography. Circulation, *54*:169, 1976.)

echocardiographically.[133,139] The aneurysms may be secondary to coronary atherosclerotic disease[133] or they may also be a result of the mucocutaneous lymph node syndrome.[139] This condition primarily occurs in children and is discussed in the chapter on congenital heart disease. The angiogram in Figure 8–66 shows aneurysmal dilatation of the left main coronary artery at the junction between the left anterior descending coronary artery and the circumflex coronary artery secondary to atherosclerotic disease. Figure 8–67 is the two-dimensional echocardiographic examination and line drawing of the left main coronary artery in the same patient. A small segment of relatively normal left main coronary artery (LMCA) can be seen coming from the aorta (AO). The artery then leads into a large, echo-free area, which represents the aneurysmal dilatation.

The echocardiographic examination of the coronary arteries is technically difficult. The arteries are constantly moving in and out of the plane of the examination. In addition, attempts to analyze the lumen require frame-by-frame analysis, which is tedious and can be confusing, especially when the plane of the examination cuts tangentially across the wall of the coronary artery. Several improvements have been suggested for the

echocardiographic examination of the coronary arteries. One group noted an improvement when examining the coronary arteries from the apical approach.[135,136] The examination starts with the apical four-chamber view. The examining plane is then adjusted to cut across the aorta and to detect the left main coronary artery coming from the lumen of that vessel.

Another improvement in the technique has been the detection of high-intensity echoes from the region of the left coronary artery in patients with atherosclerotic disease.[136,137,138a,140] Since patients with coronary artery disease frequently have atherosclerotic plaques in the proximal portion of the arteries, it is not surprising to note that diseased arteries have a high incidence of high-intensity echoes originating from the proximal left coronary artery. These high-intensity echoes may be originating from obstructing lesions, or they may come from antherosclerotic plaque that may or may not be obstructing the flow of blood. In any case, such high-intensity echoes occur frequently in patients with obstructing disease of the left coronary artery.[137,140] The instrument must have good gray scale to distinguish the high-intensity echoes from the surrounding

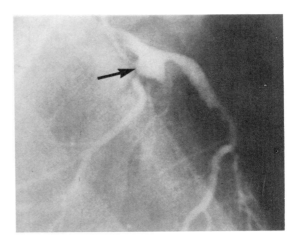

Fig. 8–66. Coronary cineangiogram of a patient with aneurysmal dilatation *(arrow)* of the left main coronary artery at the bifurcation of the left anterior descending coronary artery and the circumflex artery. (From Weyman, A.E., et al.: Non-invasive visualization of the left main coronary artery by cross-sectional echocardiography. Circulation, *54*:169, 1976.)

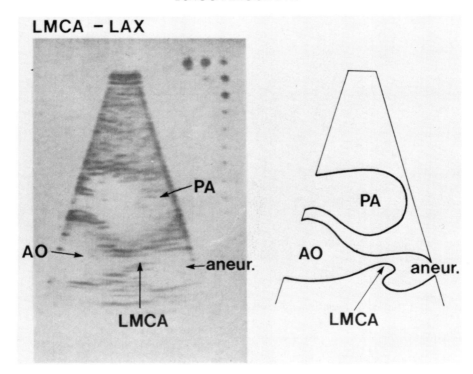

Fig. 8–67.   Two-dimensional echocardiogram of the left main coronary artery of the patient whose angiogram is shown in Figure 8–66. The parallel echoes that comprise the left main coronary artery (LMCA) can be seen originating from the aorta (AO). The echoes lead into a large echo-free space thought to originate from the saccular aneurysm (ANEUR). PA = pulmonary artery. (From Weyman, A.E., et al.: Non-invasive visualization of the left main coronary artery by cross-sectional echocardiography. Circulation, 54:169, 1976.)

echoes. Initially, an image processing technique was used to highlight only the bright echoes to facilitate the recording and visualization of these abnormal echoes.[140] Newer echocardiographs that have a wide dynamic range with log preamplification can differentiate the higher-intensity echoes by using the lowest possible gain. With a low gain setting only the high-intensity echoes are seen. It is much easier to detect high-intensity echoes in real time than it is to detect luminal irregularities.

The high-intensity echoes probably originate from the calcium in the atherosclerotic plaques. As anticipated, there is a strong correlation between the findings of high-intensity echoes and calcium in the coronary artery in fluoroscopy.[140] However, there are many patients with obstructive coronary disease who have high-intensity echoes but do not reveal calcium fluoroscopically. Thus it is possible that echocardiography may be

a more sensitive calcium indicator than fluoroscopy. There is also evidence that the cholesterol crystals have high echogenicity,[140a] and the cholesterol in the atherosclerotic plaque could be contributing to the high-intensity echoes.

Another development in the echocardiographic technique of examining the coronary arteries is the use of a strobe freeze-frame capability.[138] By gating on diastole, one has a better chance of recording the coronary artery. The strobe freeze-frame feature operates so that only that segment of the cardiac cycle indicated on the gate is recorded. Each recording is updated when the next cardiac cycle occurs. Thus one sees diastole repeatedly, and systole is never visualized. This application is helpful since the extraneous echoes recorded in systole do not obstruct and confuse the examination of the coronary artery. One has the opportunity to obtain repeated views of the coronary ar-

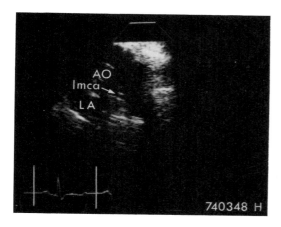

Fig. 8–68. Two-dimensional echocardiogram of the left main coronary artery (lmca) using the strobe freeze-frame technique. The vertical line on the electrocardiogram indicates at what point in the cardiac cycle this recording was obtained. AO = aorta; LA = left atrium.

nary arteries and with the introduction of new videotape and videodisc recorders for better analysis, it is expected that this technique will be clinically useful both in detecting the presence of obstructions of the left main coronary artery and in noting the existence of atherosclerotic disease in the coronary system. The latter finding could repre-

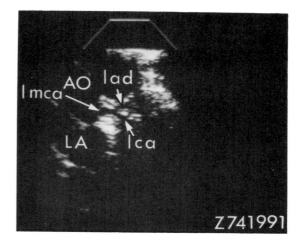

Fig. 8–69. Two-dimensional echocardiogram of the left main coronary artery (lmca), left anterior descending coronary artery (lad), and left circumflex coronary artery (lca). AO = aorta; LA = left atrium.

tery in real time. By making minor adjustments in the angulation of the transducer and in the timing of the gate, one can obtain a fairly extensive examination of the left coronary artery.

Figure 8–68 is an example of a normal left main coronary artery (lmca) obtained by way of the strobe freeze-frame technique. The vertical line on the electrocardiogram indicates the timing of the freeze frame. The left main coronary artery is detected as two thin, relatively bright echoes originating from the aorta (AO). With appropriate angulation of the transducer, one can detect the bifurcation of the left main coronary artery into the left anterior descending (lad) and circumflex (lca) coronary arteries (Fig. 8–69). Figure 8–70 demonstrates a strobe freeze-frame examination of a patient with a left main coronary artery obstruction. The left main coronary artery (lmca) can be seen originating from the aorta (AO). The obstructing lesion is indicated by a bright mass of echoes (O) between the left main coronary artery and the left anterior descending (lad) coronary artery. This obstruction was clearly seen in real time by the repeated strobe freeze-frame technique.

Because of the increased interest in the echocardiographic examination of the coro-

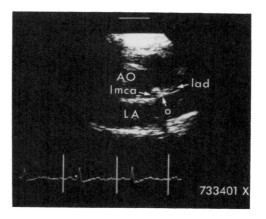

Fig. 8–70. Two-dimensional echocardiogram of a patient with obstruction of the left main coronary artery (lmca), using the strobe freeze-frame technique. The vertical line on the echocardiogram indicates at what point in the cardiac cycle this recording was obtained. The echo-producing mass (o) from the obstructing lesion is repeatedly visible in the real-time examination. lad = left anterior descending coronary artery; AO = aorta; LA = left atrium.

sent an independent risk factor that might be useful in determining whether a patient has coronary atherosclerotic disease. It is also possible that with more research and improved techniques one may be able to detect disease in the proximal left anterior descending or possibly the left circumflex arteries. In addition, the proximal portion of the right coronary artery may also be available for examination. The technical difficulties should not be underestimated. For example, left main obstructions in patients with long left main coronary arteries and lesions at the bifurcation have been consistently missed by the echocardiographic technique.[134] Thus further experience is required before the false positives and false negatives are minimized or eliminated.

An M-mode technique for examining the coronary artery has also been described.[141] Attempting to record the motion of the artery, the authors noted systolic expansion of the normal coronary artery with lack of expansion in the diseased artery. Unfortunately, because it is difficult to obtain an M-mode recording of the left main coronary artery in systole, this technique has limited applications.

Doppler echocardiography has also been used to examine the coronary system. One technique utilizes a Doppler probe at the tip of a coronary catheter.[142,143] The examination of the phasic flow velocities can be recorded with this technique. Different patterns were recorded in arteries that were obstructed downstream versus those that were patent. The principal difference is that in a normal coronary system, flow is principally in diastole. As obstructions occur, the flow assumes more of the characteristics of aortic flow, which is a systolic phenomenon. There has also been a report of using pulsed Doppler echocardiography for the assessment of patency of aortocoronary bypass grafts.[144] The authors reported a fairly high success rate in detecting patency. This technique has not been independently confirmed so that its reliability is still uncertain.

SUMMARY

How echocardiography is used in the management of patients with coronary artery disease depends largely on one's approach to these patients. If one believes that all patients with known or suspected coronary artery disease warrant angiographic study and that angiography is the standard by which to manage patients, then one could argue that echocardiography is superfluous and that few individuals with coronary artery disease warrant echocardiographic study. However, if one recognizes that there are inherent differences between the echocardiographic and angiographic examinations and that some areas visible on the echocardiogram are hidden from view on the angiogram, then echocardiography should be useful, especially in the markedly diseased ventricle. The angiogram may miss areas of well-contracting left ventricle. If the clinician is willing to exclude the possibility of surgery if the ventricle is severely diseased, then an echocardiogram can make this assessment prior to angiographic study, and these individuals can be saved from unnecessary catheterization. On the other hand, if surgery is seriously considered, irrespective of how poor the ventricular function may be, then echocardiography could be redundant.

If the primary indication for consideration of surgery is the possibility of an aneurysm, then echocardiography can be a definitive examination. The data thus far indicate that echocardiography should be able to reliably find or exclude an aneurysm and should be able to assess the function of the remaining ventricle.

Possibly the most useful application of echocardiography is in acute myocardial infarction. If one needs to assess ventricular performance and infarct size, then echocardiography could be the diagnostic tool of choice. Serial examinations are practical and can detect many complications that may occur.

The echocardiographic examination of the coronary arteries is exciting, but because of insufficient data, what its proper role will be in the management of patients with coronary artery disease is still unknown.

REFERENCES

1. Stefan, G. and Bing, R.J.: Echocardiographic findings in experimental myocardial infarction of the posterior left ventricular wall. Am. J. Cardiol., 30:629, 1972.
2. Kerber, R.E., Marcus, M.L., Ehrhardt, J., Wilson,

R., and Abboud, F.M.: Correlation between echocardiographically demonstrated segmental dyskinesis and regional myocardial perfusion. Circulation, 52:1097, 1975.
3. Kerber, R.E. and Abboud, F.M.: Echocardiographic detection of regional myocardial infarction. Circulation, 47:997, 1973.
4. Kerber, R.E., Marcus, M.L., Wilson, R., Ehrhardt, J., and Abboud, F.M.: Effects of acute coronary occlusion on the motion and perfusion of the normal and ischemic interventricular septum. Circulation, 54:928, 1976.
5. Kerber, R.E. and Abboud, F.M.: Effect of alterations of arterial blood pressure and heart rate on segmental dyskinesis during acute myocardial ischemia and following coronary reperfusion. Circ. Res., 36:145, 1975.
6. Kerber, R.E., Marcus, M.L., and Abboud, F.M.: Echocardiography in experimentally induced myocardial ischemia. Am. J. Med., 63:21, 1977.
7. Widlansky, S., McHenry, P.L., Corya, B.C., and Phillips, J.F.: Coronary angiography, echocardiographic, and electrocardiographic studies on a patient with variant angina due to coronary artery spasm. Am. Heart J., 90:631, 1975.
8. Feigenbaum, H., Corya, B.C., Dillon, J.C., Weyman, A.E., Rasmussen, S., Black, M.J., and Chang, S.: Role of echocardiography in patients with coronary artery disease. Am. J. Cardiol., 37:775, 1976.
9. Heikkila, J. and Nieminen, M.: Echoventriculographic detection, localization, and quantification of left ventricular asynergy in acute myocardial infarction: a correlative echo and electrocardiographic study. Br. Heart J., 37:46, 1975.
10. Jacobs, J.J., Feigenbaum, H., Corya, B.C., and Phillips, J.F.: Detection of left ventricular asynergy by echocardiography. Circulation, 48:263, 1973.
11. Corya, B.C., Feigenbaum, H., Rasmussen, S., and Black, M.J.: Anterior left ventricular wall echoes in coronary artery disease. Linear scanning with a single element transducer. Am. J. Cardiol., 34:652, 1974.
12. Chang, S. and Feigenbaum, H.: Subxiphoid echocardiography. J. Clin. Ultrasound, 1:14, 1973.
13. Nieminen, M.S.: Echoventriculography in chronic coronary heart disease: correlation with single plane cineangiography of the left ventricle. Eur. J. Cardiol., 5:343, 1977.
14. Corya, B.C., Feigenbaum, H., Rasmussen, S., and Black, M.J.: Echocardiographic features of congestive cardiomyopathy compared with normal subjects and patients with coronary artery disease. Circulation, 49:1153, 1974.
15. Owaki, T., Kato, H., Yanagihara, K., Takagi, Y., Okumachi, F., Ishihara, T., Kushiro, H., Katagami, H., and Yoshikawa, J.: Diagnostic role of interventricular septal motion in patients with inferior wall infarction. J. Cardiogr., 8:125, 1978.
16. Gordon, M.J. and Kerber, R.E.: Interventricular septal motion in patients with proximal and distal left anterior descending coronary artery lesions. Circulation, 55:338, 1977.
17. Dortimer, A.C., DeJoseph, R.L., Shiroff, R.A., Liedtke, A.J., and Zelis, R.: Distribution of coronary artery disease: prediction by echocardiography. Circulation, 54:724, 1976.
18. Brown, O.R., Popp, R.L., and Harrison, D.C.: Abnormal interventricular septal motion in patients

with significant disease of the left anterior descending coronary artery or other conditions of septal failure. Am. J. Cardiol., 31:123, 1973. (Abstract)
19. Kolibash, A.J., Beaver, B.M., Fulkerson, P.K., Khullar, S., and Leighton, R.F.: The relationship between abnormal echocardiographic septal motion and myocardial perfusion in patients with significant obstruction of the left anterior descending artery. Circulation, 56:780, 1977.
20. Joffe, C.D., Brik, H., Teichholz, L.E., Herman, M.V., and Gorlin, R.: Echocardiographic diagnosis of left anterior descending coronary artery disease. Am. J. Cardiol., 40:11, 1977.
21. Tanaka, K., Yoshikawa, J., Kato, H., Owaki, T., Yanagihara, K., Okumachi, F., Takagi, Y., Lee, Y., and Kitahara, Y.: Reappraisal of the diagnostic significance of posterior left ventricular wall motion in patients with acute myocardial infarction. J. Cardiogr., 6:25, 1976.
22. Kisslo, J.A., Robertson, D., Gilbert, B.W., vonRamm, O., and Behar, V.S.: A comparison of real-time, two-dimensional echocardiography and cineangiography in detecting left ventricular asynergy. Circulation, 55:134, 1977.
23. Yoshikawa, J., Suzuki, T., Kato, H., Owaki, T., Yanagihara, K., Okumachi, F., and Takagi, Y.: Two-dimensional echocardiographic detection of left ventricular asynergy. J. Cardiogr., 7:15, 1977.
24. Heger, J.J., Weyman, A.E., Wann, L.S., Dillon, J.C., and Feigenbaum, H.: Cross-sectional echocardiography in acute myocardial infarction: detection and localization of regional left ventricular asynergy. Circulation, 60:531, 1979.
25. Bloch, A., Morard, J-D., Mayor, C., and Perrenoud, J-J.: Cross-sectional echocardiography in acute myocardial infarction. Am. J. Cardiol., 43:387, 1979. (Abstract)
26. Birnholz, J., Wynne, J., Finberg, H., and Alpert, J.S.: Two-dimensional echocardiography in acute myocardial infarction. Circulation (Suppl. III), 56:82, 1977. (Abstract)
27. Kisslo, J.A., vonRamm, O.T., and Behar, V.S.: Echocardiographic evaluation of ischemia: descriptors of the ventricular short-axis. Circulation (Suppl. II), 58:40, 1978. (Abstract)
28. Davidson, R., Charuzi, Y., Davidson, S., Heng, M.K., Meerbaum, S., and Corday, E.: Differentiation between localized and diffuse left ventricular dysfunction by 2-dimensional echocardiography. Circulation (Suppl. III), 56:152, 1977. (Abstract)
29. Hecht, H.S., Taylor, R.D., Wong, M., Hopkins, J.M., and Shah, P.M.: Evaluation of segmental left ventricular wall motion: comparison of radionuclide angiography and cross-sectional echocardiography. Circulation (Suppl. II), 60:134, 1979. (Abstract)
30. Lengyel, M., Tajik, A.J., Seward, J.B., and Smith, H.C.: Correlation of two-dimensional echocardiographic and angiographic segmental wall motion abnormalities in patients with prior transmural myocardial infarction: a prospective double-blind study. Circulation (Suppl. II), 60:153, 1979. (Abstract)
31. Morrison, C.A., Bodenheimer, M.M., Feldman, M.S., Banks, V.S., and Helfant, R.H.: Ventriculographic-echocardiographic correlation in patients with asynergy. J.A.M.A., 239:1855, 1978.
32. Wynne, J., Birnholz, J.C., Holman, L., Finberg, H., and Alpert, J.S.: Radionuclide ventriculography

and two-dimensional echocardiography in coronary artery disease. Am. J. Cardiol., 41:406, 1978. (Abstract)

33. Dumesnil, J.G., Laurenceau, J.L., Labatut, A., and Gagne, S.: Echocardiographic study of changes in regional ventricular function following nitroglycerine and surgical correlation. Circulation (Suppl. II), 52:134, 1975. (Abstract)

34. Goldstein, S. and Willem de Jong, J.: Changes in left ventricular wall dimension during regional myocardial ischemia. Am. J. Cardiol., 34:56, 1974.

35. Motta, J.A., Valdez, R.S., and Popp, R.L.: Septal motion and thickening in significant left anterior descending coronary artery disease. Circulation (Suppl. II), 54:84, 1976. (Abstract)

36. Arnett, E.N., Weiss, J.L., Garrison, J.B., and Fortuin, N.J.: Quantitative evaluation of regional left ventricular thickening in man by two-dimensional echocardiography. Am. J. Cardiol., 43:377, 1979. (Abstract)

37. Komer, R.R., Edalji, A., and Hood, W.B.: Effects of nitroglycerin on echocardiographic measurement of left ventricular wall thickness and regional myocardial performance during acute coronary ischemia. Circulation, 59:926, 1979.

38. Kerber, R.E., Martins, J.B., and Marcus, M.L.: Effect of acute ischemia, nitroglycerin, and nitroprusside on regional myocardial thickening, stress, and perfusion. Circulation, 60:121, 1979.

39. Theroux, P., Franklin, D., Ross, J., and Kemper, W.S.: Regional myocardial function during acute coronary artery occlusion and its modification by pharmacologic agents in the dog. Circ. Res., 35:986, 1974.

40. Maron, B.J., Savage, D.D., Clark, C.E., Vlodaver, Z., Edwards, J.E., and Epstein, S.E.: Prevalence and characteristics of disproportionate ventricular septal thickening in patients with coronary artery disease. Circulation, 57:250, 1978.

41. Corya, B.C.: Echocardiography in ischemic heart disease. Am. J. Med., 63:10, 1977.

42. Gaasch, W.H. and Bernard, S.A.: The effect of acute changes in coronary blood flow on left ventricular end-diastolic wall thickness: an echocardiographic study. Circulation, 56:593, 1977.

43. Rasmussen, S., Corya, B.C., Feigenbaum, H., and Knoebel, S.B.: Detection of myocardial scar tissue by M-mode echocardiography. Circulation, 57:230, 1978.

44. O'Brien, W.D.: The relationships between collagen and ultrasonic attenuation and velocity in tissue. In Proceedings Ultrasonics International '77. Guilford, England, IPC Science and Technology Press, 1977.

45. Mimbs, J.W., O'Donnell, M., Miller, J.G., and Sobel, B.E.: Changes in ultrasonic attenuation indicative of early myocardial ischemic injury. Am. J. Physiol., 236:H340, 1979.

46. Mimbs, J.W., Yuhas, D.E., Miller, J.G., Weiss, A.N., and Sobel, B.E.: Detection of myocardial infarction in vitro based on altered attenuation of ultrasound. Circ. Res., 41:192, 1977.

47. O'Donnell, M., Mimbs, J.W., Sobel, B.E., and Miller, J.G.: Collagen as a determinant of ultrasonic attenuation in myocardial infarcts. In Ultrasound in Medicine, Vol. 4. Edited by D. White. New York, Plenum Press, 1978.

48. Bauwens, D., O'Donnell, M., Miller, J.G., and Mimbs, J.W.: Detection of acute myocardial ischemia in vivo with quantitative ultrasonic backscatter. Am. J. Cardiol., 45:436, 1980. (Abstract)

49. Dines, K.A., Weyman, A.E., Franklin, Jr., T.D., Cuddeback, J.K., Sanghvi, N.T., Avery, K.S., Baird, A.I., and Fry, F.J.: Quantitation of changes in myocardial fiber bundle spacing with acute infarction, using pulse-echo ultrasound signals. Circulation (Suppl. II), 60:17, 1979. (Abstract)

50. Mimbs, J.W., O'Donnell, M., Bauwens, D., Miller, J.G., and Sobel, B.E.: Characterization of the evolution of myocardial infarction by ultrasonic backscatter. Circulation (Suppl. II), 60:17, 1979. (Abstract)

51. Franklin, Jr., T.D., Cuddeback, J.K., Sanghvi, N.T., Weyman, A.E., Avery, K.S., and Fry, F.J.: Differentiation of A-mode ultrasound signals from normal and ischemic myocardium by multivariate discriminant analysis of waveform parameters. Am. J. Cardiol., 45:403, 1980. (Abstract)

52. Gramiak, R., Waag, R.C., Schenk, E.A., Lee, P.P.K., Thomason, K., and Macintosh, P.: Ultrasonic imaging of experimental myocardial infarcts. In Echocardiography. Edited by C.T. Lancee. The Hague, Martinus Nijhoff, 1979.

53. Heikkila, J. and Nieminen, M.S.: Rapid monitoring of regional myocardial ischaemia with echocardiography and ST segment shifts in man: modification of "infarct size" and hemodynamics by dopamine and beta blockade. Acta Med. Scand., 623:71, 1978.

54. Weyman, A.E., Franklin, T.D., Egenes, K.M., and Green, D.: Correlation between extent of abnormal regional wall motion and myocardial infarct size in chronically infarcted dogs. Circulation (Suppl. III), 56:72, 1977. (Abstract)

55. Heng, M.K., Lang, T-W., Toshimitsu, T., Meerbaum, S., Wyatt, H.L., Lee, S-S., Davidson, R., and Corday, E.: Quantification of myocardial ischemic damage by 2-dimensional echocardiography. Circulation (Suppl. III), 56:125, 1977. (Abstract)

56. Weiss, J.L., Bulkley, B.H., and Mason, S.J.: Two-dimensional echocardiographic quantification of myocardial injury in man: comparison with post mortem studies. Circulation (Suppl. II), 58:153, 1978. (Abstract)

57. Charuzi, Y., Davidson, R., Barrett, M., Shah, P., Berman, D., Waxman, A., Pichler, M., Maddahi, J., Corday, E., and Swan, H.J.C.: A quantitative comparison of cross-sectional echocardiography and radionuclide angiography in acute myocardial infarction. Circulation (Suppl. II), 58:52, 1978. (Abstract)

58. Meltzer, R.S., Woythaler, J.N., Buda, A.J., Griffin, J.C., Harrison, W.D., Martin, R.P., Harrison, D.C., and Popp, R.L.: Two-dimensional echocardiographic quantification of infarct size alteration by pharmacologic agents. Am. J. Cardiol., 44:257, 1979.

58a.Fujii, J., Watanabe, H., and Kato, K.: Detection of the site and extent of the left ventricular asynergy in myocardial infarction by echocardiography and B-scan imaging. Jpn. Heart J., 17:630, 1976.

59. Rogers, E.W., Weyman, A.E., Feigenbaum, H., Heger, J.J., and Dillon, J.C.: Predicting survival after myocardial infarction by cross-sectional echo. Circulation (Suppl. II), 58:233, 1978. (Abstract)

60. Corya, B.C., Rasmussen, S., Knoebel, S.B., and Feigenbaum, H.: Echocardiography in acute myocardial infarction. Am. J. Cardiol., 36:1, 1975.

61. Corya, B.C., Rasmussen, S., Knoebel, S.B., and Feigenbaum, H.: M-mode echocardiography in evaluating left ventricular function and surgical risk in patients with coronary artery disease. Chest, 72:181, 1977.

62. Dillon, J.C., Feigenbaum, H., Weyman, A.E., Corya, B.C., Peskoe, S., and Chang, S.: M-mode echocardiography in the evaluation of patients for aneurysmectomy. Circulation, 53:657, 1976.

63. Shiotani, K., Sagara, T., Sugihara, M., Yamashita, K., Nawata, Y., Torii, S., Nishimoto, S., and Kawahira, K.: Echocardiographic evaluation of the prognosis during acute phase of myocardial infarction: comparison with Tc pyrophosphate and Tl chloride myocardial imagings. J. Cardiogr., 9:285, 1979.

64. Righetti, A., Crawford, M.H., O'Rourke, R.A., Daily, P.O., and Ross, J., Jr.: Echocardiographic and roentgenographic determination of left ventricular size after coronary arterial bypass graft surgery. Chest, 72:455, 1977.

65. Chandraratna, P.A.N., Rashid, A., Tolentino, A., Hildner, F.J., Fester, A., Samet, P., Littman, B.B., and Sabharwal, S. (with technical assistance of Gindlesperger, D.): Echocardiographic assessment of left ventricular function in coronary arterial disease. Br. Heart J., 39:139, 1977.

66. Folland, E.D., Parisi, A.F., Moynihan, P.F., Jones, D.R., Feldman, C.L., and Tow, D.E.: Assessment of left ventricular ejection fraction and volumes by real-time, two-dimensional echocardiography: a comparison of cineangiographic and radionuclide techniques. Circulation, 60:760, 1979.

67. Carr, K.W., Engler, R.L., Forsythe, J.R., Johnson, A.D., and Gosink, B.: Measurement of left ventricular ejection fraction by mechanical cross-sectional echocardiography. Circulation, 59:1196, 1979.

68. Eaton, L.W., Maughan, W.L., Shoukas, A.D., and Weiss, J.L.: Accurate volume determination in the isolated ejecting canine left ventricle by two-dimensional echocardiography. Circulation, 60:320, 1979.

69. Schiller, N.B., Acquatella, H., Ports, T.A., Drew, D., Goerke, J., Ringertz, H., Silverman, N.H., Brundage, B., Botvinick, E.H., Boswell, R., Carlsson, E., and Parmley, W.W.: Left ventricular volume from paired biplane two-dimensional echocardiography. Circulation, 60:547, 1979.

70. Fukaya, T., Tomita, Y., Baba, K., Owaki, T., and Yoshikawa, J.: Computer-aided system analyzing left ventricular volume by real time cross-sectional echocardiograms. J. Cardiogr., 8:431, 1978.

71. Bommer, W., Chun, T., Kwan, O.L., Neumann, A., Mason, D.T., and DeMaria, A.N.: Biplane apex echocardiography versus biplane ventricular volume and function: validation by direct measurements. Am. J. Cardiol., 45:471, 1980. (Abstract)

72. Wyatt, H.L., Heng, M., Meerbaum, S., Davidson, R., Lee, S–S., and Corday, E.: Quantificative left ventricular analysis in dogs with the phased array sector scan. Circulation (Suppl. III), 56:152, 1977. (Abstract)

73. Wyatt, H.L., Heng, M.K., Meerbaum, S., Hestenes, J., Davidson, R., and Corday, E.: Quan-

tification of volumes in asymmetric left ventricles by 2–D echocardiography. Circulation (Suppl. II), 58:188, 1978. (Abstract)

74. Massie, B.M., Schiller, N.B., Ratshin, R.A., and Parmley, W.W.: Mitral-septal separation: new echocardiographic index of left ventricular function. Am. J. Cardiol., 39:1008, 1977.

75. D'Cruz, I.A., Lalmalani, G.G., Sambasivan, V., Cohen, H.C., and Glick, G.: The superiority of mitral E point–ventricular septum separation to other echocardiographic indicators of left ventricular performance. Clin. Cardiol., 2:140, 1979.

76. Konecke, L.L., Feigenbaum, H., Chang, S., Corya, B.C., and Fischer, J.C.: Abnormal mitral valve motion in patients with elevated left ventricular diastolic pressures. Circulation, 47:989, 1973,

77. Lalani, A.V., and Lee, S.J.K.: Echocardiographic measurement of cardiac output using the mitral valve and aortic root echo. Circulation, 54:738, 1976.

78. Corya, B.C.: Echocardiography in ischemic heart disease. Am. J. Med., 63:10, 1977.

79. Reference omitted.

80. Gibson, D.G., Doran, J.H., Traill, T.A., and Brown, D.J.: Regional abnormalities of left ventricular wall movements during isovolumic relaxation in patients with ischemic heart disease. Eur. J. Cardiol., 7:251, 1978.

81. Chen, W. and Gibson, D.: Relation of isovolumic relaxation to left ventricular wall movement in man. Br. Heart J., 42:51, 1979.

81a. Doran, J.H., Traill, T.A., Brown, D.J., and Gibson, D.G.: Detection of abnormal left ventricular wall movement during isovolumic contraction and early relaxation: comparison of echo- and angiocardiography. Br. Heart J., 40:367, 1978.

82. Upton, M.T., Gibson, D.G., and Brown, D.: Echocardiographic assessment of abnormal left ventricular relaxation in man. Br. Heart J., 38:1001, 1976.

82a. Kurata, E., Fujino, T., Kanaya, S., Ito, M., Fujino, M., Yamada, K., Hamanaka, Y., Kinoshita, R., and Ueno, T.: Isometric contraction and relaxation times of the left ventricle in patients with myocardial infarction measured by bi-directional echocardiography. J. Cardiogr., 9:65, 1979.

83. Mason, S.J., Weiss, J.L., Weisfeldt, M.L., Garrison, J.B., and Fortuin, N.J.: Exercise echocardiography: detection of wall motion abnormalities during ischemia. Circulation, 59:50, 1979.

84. Wann, L.S., Faris, J.V., Childress, R.H., Dillon, J.C., Weyman, A.E., and Feigenbaum, H.: Exercise cross-sectional echocardiography in ischemic heart disease. Circulation, 60:1300, 1979.

85. Paulsen, W.J., Boughner, D.R., Friesen, A., and Persaud, J.A.: Ventricular response to isometric and isotonic exercise: echocardiographic assessment. Br. Heart J., 42:521, 1979.

86. Amon, K.W., and Crawford, M.H.: Upright exercise echocardiography. J. Clin. Ultrasound, 7:373, 1979.

87. Goldstein, R.E., Bennett, E.D., and Leech, G.L.: Effect of glyceryl trinitrate on echocardiographic left ventricular dimensions during exercise in the upright position. Br. Heart J., 42:245, 1979.

88. Sugishita, Y. and Koseki, S.: Dynamic exercise echocardiography. Circulation, 60:743, 1979.

89. Hickman, H.O., Weyman, A.E., Wann, L.S., Phillips, J.F., Dillon, J.C., Feigenbaum, H., and

Marshall, J.: Cross-sectional echocardiography of the cardiac apex. Circulation (Suppl. III), 56:153, 1977. (Abstract)

90. Morrison, C.A., Bodenheimer, M.M., Feldman, M.S., Banka, V.S., and Helfant, R.H.: The use of echocardiography in determination of reversible posterior wall asynergy. Am. Heart J., 94:140, 1977.

91. Hardarson, T. and Wright, K.E.: Effect of sublingual nitroglycerin on cardiac performance in patients with coronary artery disease and nondyskinetic left ventricular contraction. Br. Heart J., 38:1272, 1976.

92. Righetti, A., Crawford, M.H., O'Rourke, R.A., Schelbert, H., Daily, P.O., and Ross, J.: Interventricular septal motion and left ventricular function after coronary bypass surgery: evaluation with echocardiography and radionuclide angiography. Am. J. Cardiol., 39:372, 1977.

93. Gerson, M.C., Noble, R.J., Wann, L.S., Faris, J.V., and Morris, S.N.: Noninvasive documentation of Prinzmetal's angina. Am. J. Cardiol., 43:329, 1979.

94. Eaton, L.W., Weiss, J.L., Bulkley, B.H., et al.: Regional cardiac dilatation after acute myocardial infarction: recognition by two-dimensional echocardiography. N. Engl. J. Med., 300:57, 1979.

95. Nieminen, M.S. and Heikkila, J.: Echoventriculography in acute myocardial infarction. II. Monitoring of left ventricular performance. Br. Heart J., 38:271, 1976.

96. Kisslo, J., Ideker, R., Harrison, L., Scallion, R., vonRamm, O., and Pilkington, T.: Serial wall changes after acute myocardial infarction by two-dimensional echo. Circulation (Suppl. II), 60:151, 1979. (Abstract)

97. Prakash, R. and Aronow, W.S.: Spontaneous changes in hemodynamics in uncomplicated acute myocardial infarction: a prospective echocardiographic study. Angiology, 28:677, 1977.

98. Kreamer, R., Kerber, R.E., and Abboud, F.M.: Ventricular aneurysm: use of echocardiography. J. Clin. Ultrasound, 1:60, 1973.

99. Chang, S., Feigenbaum, H., and Dillon, J.C.: Subxiphoid echocardiography: a review. Chest, 68:233, 1975.

100. Feigenbaum, H.: Use of echocardiography to evaluate cardiac performance. In Cardiac Mechanics. Edited by I. Mirsky, D.N. Ghista, and H. Sandler. New York, John Wiley & Sons, 1974.

101. Feigenbaum, H.: Echocardiographic examination of the left ventricle. Circulation, 51:1, 1975.

102. Weyman, A.E., Peskoe, S.M., Williams, E.S., Dillon, J.C., and Feigenbaum, H.: Detection of left ventricular aneurysms by cross-sectional echocardiography. Circulation, 54:936, 1976.

103. Barrett, M., Charuzi, Y., Davidson, R.M., Silverberg, R., Heng, M.K., Swan, H.J.C., and Corday, E.: Two-dimensional echo assessment of residual myocardial function in left ventricular aneurysm. Am. J. Cardol., 41:406, 1978. (Abstract)

104. Rakowski, H., Martin, R.P., Schapira, J.N., Wexler, L., Silverman, J.F., Cipriano, P.R., Guthaner, D.F., and Popp, R.L.: Left ventricular aneurysm: detection and determination of resectability by two-dimensional ultrasound. Circulation (Suppl. III), 56:153, 1977. (Abstract)

105. Kambe, T., Nishimura, K., Hibi, N., Fukui, Y., Miwa, A., and Murase, M: Real time observation of left ventricular aneurysm by B mode echocardiography. J. Clin. Ultrasound, 6:405, 1978.

106. Roelandt, J., Van Den Brand, M., Vletter, W.B., Nauta, J., and Hugenholtz, P.G.: Echocardiographic diagnosis of pseudoaneurysm of the left ventricle. Circulation, 52:466, 1975.

107. Mills, P.G., Rose, J.D., Brodie, B.R., Delaney, D.J., and Craige, E.: Echocardiographic diagnosis of left ventricular pseudoaneurysm. Chest, 72:365, 1977.

108. Davidson, K.H., Parisi, A.F., Harrington, J.J., Barsamian, E.M., and Fishbein, M.C.: Pseudoaneurysm of the left ventricle: an unusual echocardiographic presentation. Ann. Intern. Med., 86:430, 1977.

109. Sears, T.D., Ong, Y.S., Starke, H., and Forker, A.D.: Left ventricular pseudoaneurysm identified by cross-sectional echocardiography. Ann. Intern. Med., 90:935, 1979.

110. Nanda, N.C. and Gatewood, R.P.: Differentiation of left ventricular pseudoaneurysms from true aneurysms by two-dimensional echocardiography. Circulation (Suppl. II), 60:144, 1979. (Abstract)

111. Katz, R.J., Simpson, A., DiBianco, R., Fletcher, R.D., Bates, H.R., and Sauerbrunn, B.J.L.: Noninvasive diagnosis of left ventricular pseudoaneurysm: role of two-dimensional echocardiography and radionuclide gated pool imaging. Am. J. Cardiol., 44:372, 1979.

111a. Morcerf, F.P., Duarte, E.P., Salcedo, E.E., et al.: Echocardiographic findings in false aneurysm of the left ventricle. Cleve. Clin. Q., 43:71, 1976.

111b. Hagemeijer, F., Verbaan, C.J., Sonke, P.C.F., and De Rooij, C.H.: Echocardiography and rupture of the heart. Br. Heart J., 43:45, 1980.

112. Horgan, J.H., O'M Shiel, F., and Goodman, A.C.: Demonstration of left ventricular thrombus by conventional echocardiography. J. Clin. Ultrasound, 4:287, 1976.

113. DeJoseph, R.L., Shiroff, R.A., Levenson, L.W., Martin, C.E., and Zelis, R.F.: Echocardiographic diagnosis of intraventricular clot. Chest, 71:417, 1977.

114. van den Bos, A.A., Bletter, W.B., and Hagemeijer, F.: Progressive development of a left ventricular thrombus: detection and evolution studied with echocardiographic techniques. Chest, 74:307, 1978.

115. DeMaria, A.N., Bommer, W., Neumann, A., Grehl, T., Weinart, L., DeNardo, S., Amsterdam, E.A., and Mason, D.T.: Left ventricular thrombi identified by cross-sectional echocardiography. Ann. Intern. Med., 90:14, 1979.

116. Meltzer, R.S., Guthaner, D., Rakowski, H., Popp, R.L., and Martin, R.P.: Diagnosis of left ventricular thrombi by two-dimensional echocardiography. Br. Heart J., 42:261, 1979.

117. Mikell, F., Asinger, R., Rourke, T., Hodges, M., Sharma, B., and Francis, G.: Detection of intracardiac thrombi by two-dimensional echocardiography (2DE). Circulation (Suppl. II), 58:43, 1978. (Abstract)

118. DeJoseph, R.L., Seides, S.F., Lindner, A., and Demato, A.N.: Echocardiographic findings of ventricular septal rupture in acute myocardial infarction. Am. J. Cardiol., 36:346, 1975.

119. Chandraratna, P.A.N., Balachandran, P.K., Shah, P.M., and Hodges, M.: Echocardiographic observations on ventricular septal rupture complicating myocardial infarction. Circulation, 51:506, 1975.

120. Silverman, B., Kozma, G., Silverman, M., and

King, S.: Echocardiographic manifestations of post-infarction ventricular septal defect. Chest, 68:778, 1975.

121. Kerin, N.Z., Edelstein, J., and De Rue, R.G.: Ventricular septal defect complicating acute myocardial infarction: echocardiographic demonstration confirmed by angiocardiograms and surgery. Chest, 70:560, 1976.

122. Scanlan, J.G., Seward, J.B., and Tajik, A.J.: Visualization of ventricular septal rupture utilizing wide-angle two-dimensional echocardiography. Mayo Clin. Proc., 54:381, 1979.

123. Drobac, M., Morgan, C.D., Gilbert, B.W., Baigrie, R.S., and Rakowski, H.: Complicated acute myocardial infarction: the importance of two-dimensional echocardiography. Am. J. Cardiol., 43:387, 1979. (Abstract)

124. Rogers, E.W., Glassman, R.D., Feigenbaum, H., Weyman, A.E., and Godley, R.W.: Cross-sectional echocardiographic identification of aneurysms of the posterior interventricular septum with post-infarction ventricular septal defect. Chest, in press.

125. Tallury, V.K., DePasquale, N.P., and Burch, G.E.: The echocardiogram in papillary muscle dysfunction. Am. Heart J., 83:12, 1972.

126. Godley, R.W., Weyman, A.E., Feigenbaum, H., Rogers, E.W., and Green, D.: Patterns of mitral leaflet motion in patients with probable papillary muscle dysfunction. Am. J. Cardiol., 43:411, 1979. (Abstract)

127. Corya, B.C.: Applications of echocardiography in acute myocardial infarction. Cardiovasc. Clin., 11:113, 1975.

128. Matsuhisa, M., Uehara, S., Haze, K., Ohe, T., Saito, M., Nakajima, K., Hiramori, K., and Shimomura, Y.: Right ventricular infarction: graphic studies of three cases. J. Cardiogr., 9:375, 1979.

129. Nosaka, H., Goto, M., Kato, T., Mitsudo, K., Mishima, N., Kohchi, K., Wano, Y., Tsubota, W., Ito, Y., and Nobuyoshi, M.: Hemodynamics and interventricular septal motion on echocardiography in acute right ventricular infarction. J. Cardiogr., 9:19, 1979.

130. D'Arcy, B.J., Gondi, B., Nanda, N.C., Gatewood, R.P., and Biddle, T.: Real-time two-dimensional echocardiography in right ventricular infarction. Am. J. Cardiol., 45:436, 1980. (Abstract)

131. Sharpe, D.N., Botvinick, E.H., Shames, D.M., Schiller, N.B., Massie, B.M., Chatterjee, K., and Parmley, W.W.: The noninvasive diagnosis of right ventricular infarction. Circulation, 57:483, 1978.

132. Lorell, B., Leinbach, R.C., Pohost, G.M., Gold, H.K., Dinsmore, R.E., Hutter, A.M., Pastore, J.O., and Desanctis, R.W.: Right ventricular infarction. Am. J. Cardiol., 43:465, 1979.

133. Weyman, A.E., Feigenbaum, H., Dillon, J.C., Johnston, K.W., and Eggleton, R.C.: Noninvasive visualization of the left main coronary artery by cross-sectional echocardiography. Circulation, 54:169, 1976.

134. Arnow, W.S., Chandraratna, P.A.N., Murdock, K., and Milholland, H.: Left main coronary artery patency assessed by cross-sectional echocardiog-

raphy and coronary arteriography. Circulation (Suppl. II), 60:145, 1979. (Abstract)

135. Ogawa, S., Chen, C.C., Hubbard, F.E., Pauletto, F.J., Mardelli, T.J., Morganroth, J., Dreifus, L.S., Akaishi, M., and Nakamura, Y.: A new approach to visualize the left main coronary artery using apical cross-sectional echocardiography. Am. J. Cardiol., 45:301, 1980.

136. Chen, C.C., Morganroth, J., Mardelli, J., Ogawa, S., and Meixell, L.L.: Differential density and luminal irregularities as criteria to detect disease in the left main coronary artery by apex phased array cross-sectional echocardiography. Am. J. Cardiol., 43:386, 1979. (Abstract)

137. Friedman, M.J., Sahn, D.J., Goldman, S., Eisner, D.R., Gittinger, N.C., Lederman, F.L., Puckette, C.M., and Tiemann, J.J.: High frequency, high resolution cross-sectional (2D) echo for evaluation of left main coronary artery disease (LMCAD): Is resolution alone enough? Circulation (Suppl. II), 60:153, 1979. (Abstract)

138. Rink, L.D., Feigenbaum, H., Marshall, J.E., Godley, R.W., Doty, D., Dillon, J.C., and Weyman, A.E.: Improved echocardiographic technique for examining the left main coronary artery. Am. J. Cardiol., 45:435, 1980. (Abstract)

138a. Rogers, E.W., Feigenbaum, H., Weyman, A.E., Godley, R.W., Wills, E.R., and Vakili, S.T.: Evaluation of coronary artery anatomy in vitro by cross-sectional echocardiography. Am. J. Cardiol., 43:386, 1979. (Abstract)

139. Yoshikawa, J., Yanagihara, K., Owaki, T., Kato, H., Takagi, Y., Okumachi, F., Fukaya, T., Tomita, Y., and Baba, K.: Cross-sectional echocardiographic diagnosis of coronary artery aneurysms in patients with the mucocutaneous lymph node syndrome. Circulation, 59:133, 1979.

140. Rogers, E.W., Feigenbaum, H., Weyman, A.E., Dillon, J.C., Wann, L.S., Eggleton, R.C., and Johnston, K.W.: Possible detection of coronary atherosclerosis by cross-sectional echocardiography. Circulation (Suppl. II), 58:56, 1978. (Abstract)

140a. Glancy, J.J., Goddard, J., and Pearson, D.E.: In vitro demonstration of cholesterol crystals' high echogenicity relative to protein particles. J. Clin. Ultrasound, 8:27, 1980.

141. Inoue, K., Kuwaki, K., Ueda, K., Shirai, T., and Utsunomiya, T.: M-mode echocardiogram of the coronary artery. Am. J. Cardiol., 41:391, 1978. (Abstract)

142. Benchimol, A., Stegall, H.F., and Gartlan, J.L.: New method to measure phasic coronary blood velocity in man. Am. Heart J., 81:93, 1971.

143. Cole, J.S. and Hartley, C.J.: The pulsed Doppler coronary artery catheter: preliminary report of a new technique for measuring rapid changes in coronary artery flow velocity in man. Circulation, 56:18, 1977.

144. Diebold, B., Theroux, P., Bourassa, M.D., Peronneau, P., and Guermonprez, J-L.: Noninvasive assessment of aortocoronary bypass graft patency using pulsed Doppler echocardiography. Am. J. Cardiol., 43:10, 1979.

Cardiomyopathy

HYPERTROPHIC CARDIOMYOPATHY

Echocardiography has not only become an important means of detecting hypertrophic cardiomyopathy, but it has also provided many new facts and has raised numerous questions concerning the pathogenesis and pathophysiology of this cardiomyopathy. Because of echocardiography's unique ability to measure wall thickness, this technique is most likely the procedure of choice for the diagnosis of hypertrophic cardiomyopathy.

Asymmetric Septal Hypertrophy

A characteristic feature of hypertrophic cardiomyopathy is hypertrophy of the interventricular septum disproportionate to the free wall of the left ventricle.[1-3,3a,4-6, 6a] Figure 9-1 demonstrates a patient with a mark-

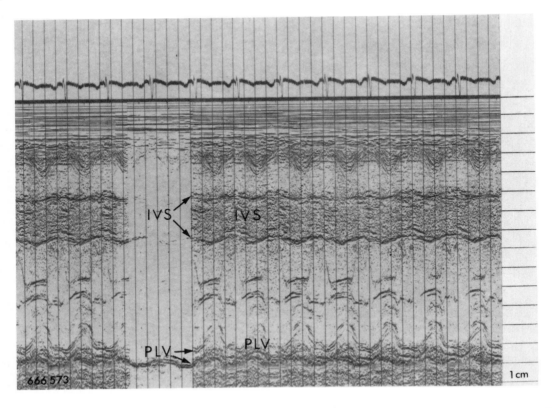

Fig. 9–1. M-mode echocardiogram of a patient with asymmetric septal hypertrophy. The interventricular septum (IVS) is much thicker than the posterior left ventricular wall (PLV). The echoes from the interventricular septum also have a different appearance than those from the myocardium of the posterior left ventricular wall. (From Feigenbaum, H.: Echocardiography. In Heart Disease. Edited by E. Braunwald. Philadelphia, W. B. Saunders Co., 1980.)

edly thickened interventricular septum that is significantly thicker than the posterior left ventricular wall. Figure 9–2 shows an M-mode scan of another patient with asymmetric septal hypertrophy. Again, the disproportionate hypertrophy of the interventricular septum compared to that of the posterior left ventricular wall is striking. One can also appreciate how the hypertrophied septum appears to encroach on the left ventricular outflow tract so that the aorta actually tends to override the hypertrophied septum.

The echocardiograhic diagnosis of asymmetric septal hypertrophy has proved to be an extremely important finding in hypertrophic cardiomyopathy.[1,3,3a,4] This sign has been used as a genetic marker in patients with this disease.[7,8] The abnormal septal hypertrophy may represent the basic defect in this genetically determined cardiomyopathy. As noted in Figures 9–1 and 9–2, the septal motion and thickening is reduced.[8–10] This reduction in contractility may reflect the fiber disarray that is seen histologically in these hypertrophied septa.[11,11a]

There are many problems with both the concept and the echocardiographic diagno-sis of asymmetric septal hypertrophy.[8,9, 12,12a] At times the measurement of the thickness of the interventricular septum can be confusing.[8] The right side of the interventricular septum is frequently trabeculated, and multiple echoes from the tricuspid valve apparatus lie adjacent to the septum. In Figure 9–3, a fairly distinct echo from the left septum (LS) can be identified. In addition, one can identify an echo that probably originates from the right septum (RS). Another echo (?) is anterior to the apparent septum. Clinically, this patient had mild mitral regurgitation. There was no clinical or echocardiographic evidence suggestive of hypertrophic cardiomyopathy. The exact etiology of the echo within the right ventricle is uncertain. Echoes similar to these are frequently part of the tricuspid valve apparatus. One usually can see some tricuspid valve motion within these echoes as the ultrasonic beam is moved toward the tricuspid valve.

Figure 9–4 is another confusing echocardiogram of an interventricular septum. The left side of the septum (LS) is again readily apparent. There are two linear echoes that could represent the right side of the septum.

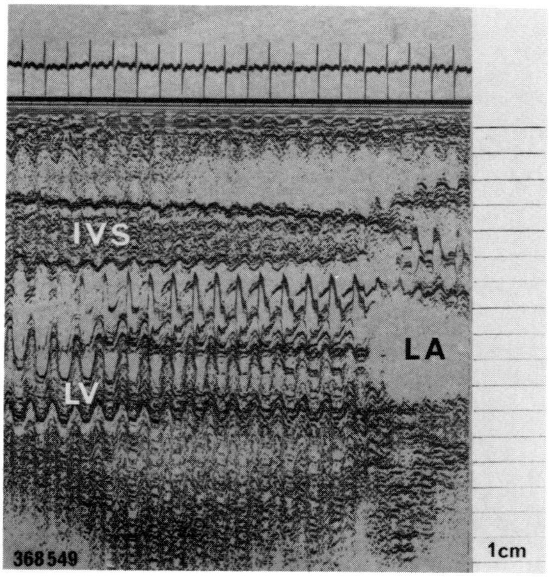

Fig. 9–2. M-mode scan of a patient with asymmetric septal hypertrophy. The interventricular septum (IVS) is much thicker than the posterior left ventricular wall (LV). The left atrium (LA) is dilated.

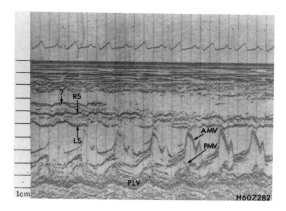

Fig. 9–3. M-mode echocardiogram showing the difficulty in identifying the right side of the septum. A dominant echo, most likely originating from the right septum (RS), is indicated in this patient with mild mitral regurgitation. An additional echo (?) within the right ventricular cavity could easily be interpreted as originating from the right side of the septum. The identity of this additional echo is unclear, but it could originate from such a structure as a right-sided papillary muscle. LS = left septum; AMV = anterior mitral valve; PMV = posterior mitral valve; PLV = posterior left ventricular wall.

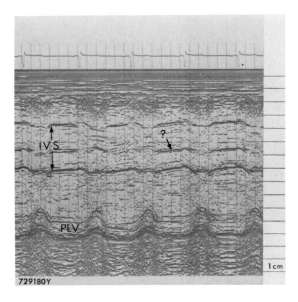

Fig. 9–4. M-mode echocardiogram of a patient with asymmetric septal hypertrophy with a massively hypertrophied interventricular septum (IVS). An echo of unknown origin (?) runs through the center of the interventricular septum. PLV = posterior left ventricular wall.

If one chooses the more anterior echo, the septum is approximately 3 cm thick. If one uses the more posterior echo (?), the patient has a septum barely more than 1 cm thick. This patient proved to have asymmetric septal hypertrophy; the more anterior echo did indeed represent the true right side of the septum, which was encroaching on the right ventricular cavity. The origin of the echo within the substance of the septum is not clear. However, the hypertrophy was not uniform throughout the entire septum, and the beam width may have produced some apparent intramuscular echoes.

Figure 9–5 is an M-mode scan that shows the multiple echoes that can be recorded between the chest wall and the interventricular septum. Echoes similar to those in Figure 9–3 can be recorded within the right ventricular cavity. In this patient, the true right septal echoes (RS) can be identified toward the left portion of the recording. Although the posterior left ventricular wall is not well visualized, the width of the interventricular

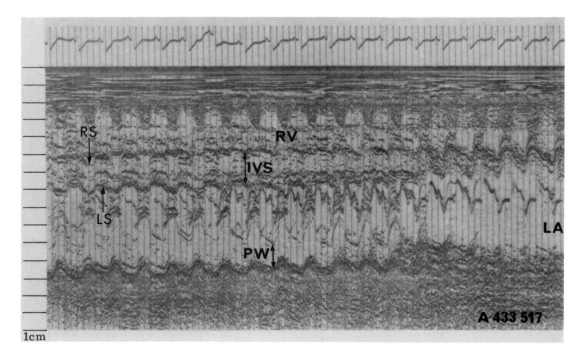

Fig. 9–5. M-mode echocardiographic scan demonstrating the difficulty in identifying the right septal echoes. Multiple echoes within the right ventricular cavity can be recorded. A faint echo thought to represent the true right side of the septum (RS) is indicated. Note the hypertrophied interventricular septum (IVS) in this patient with hypertrophic subaortic stenosis. RV = right ventricle; LS = left side of septum; PW = posterior left ventricular wall; LA = left atrium.

septum (IVS) is somewhat larger than the posterior ventricular wall, a finding that is compatible with asymmetric septal hypertrophy. The patient did indeed have hypertrophic obstructive cardiomyopathy, or hypertrophic subaortic stenosis.

As might be expected, two-dimensional echocardiography can assist in the echocardiographic assessment of septal thickness and asymmetric septal hypertrophy.[13,15, 15a,16-18] Figure 9–6 is a long-axis parasternal sector scan of a patient with septal hypertrophy that primarily involves the basal portion of the septum (IVS). Figure 9–7 shows two parasternal long-axis examinations of a patient with asymmetric septal hypertrophy. The septal hypertrophy was greatest in the basal and apical portions of the interventricular septum in this patient. The width of the septum actually exceeds the diameter of the left ventricular cavity in the apical half of that chamber. Figure 9–8 shows an apical four-chamber view of the same patient. The

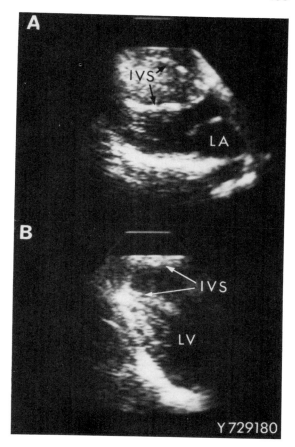

Fig. 9–7. Parasternal long-axis two-dimensional echocardiograms of a patient with asymmetric septal hypertrophy. Marked hypertrophy can be seen in the basal, A, and apical, B, parts of the interventricular septum (IVS). LA = left atrium; LV = left ventricle.

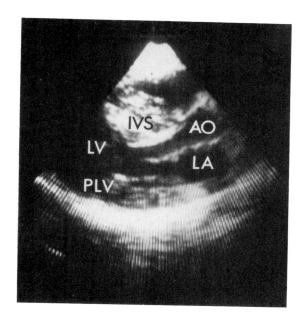

Fig. 9–6. Long-axis two-dimensional echocardiogram of a patient with hypertrophic cardiomyopathy. Note the marked hypertrophy of the interventricular septum (IVS). The maximum septal hypertrophy is located at the left ventricular outflow tract. LV = left ventricle; PLV = posterior left ventricular wall; AO = aorta; LA = left atrium. (From Feigenbaum, H.: Echocardiography. In Heart Disease. Edited by E. Braunwald. Philadelphia, W. B. Saunders Co., 1980.)

hypertrophied septum (arrows) can again be appreciated. The maximum thickness is in the basal and apical portion of the septum.

Some investigators using two-dimensional echocardiography have emphasized the variability of shape of the hypertrophied septum.[13,14] As in Figure 9–6, the hypertrophy may be principally at the basal portion of the interventricular septum. Or, as noted in Figures 9–7 and 9–8, the hypertrophy may be greatest toward the apex. Other patients may have a more diffuse form of septal hypertrophy uniformly distributed throughout the septum.

In addition to measuring the thickness of the interventricular septum, several echocardiographers have noticed a change in the

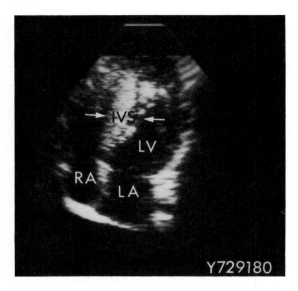

Fig. 9–8.　Apical four-chamber view of the patient in Figure 9–7. Note that the markedly hypertrophied interventricular septum (IVS) is thickest in the apical half of the septum. LV = left ventricle; RA = right atrium; LA = left atrium.

acoustic properties of the septal echoes in patients with hypertrophic cardiomyopathy.[13,17] This finding is most distinct in the intramyocardial echoes from the septum and posterior ventricular wall in Figures 9–1, 9–6, and 9–7. These intramyocardial echoes are sometimes labeled as "speckling."[17] The pathologic or histologic significance of this finding is uncertain. It is tempting to correlate the peculiar echo pattern with the histologic findings of myocardial fiber disarray.[7] However, there is no proof that the two observations are related. It would certainly be convenient if one could reliably distinguish asymmetric septal hypertrophy by the acoustic properties of the intraseptal echoes, because there is an increasing number of entities other than genetically determined hypertrophic cardiomyopathy that can produce septal thickness that exceeds the posterior ventricular wall thickness.[19–26] In the original study, a septal posterior wall ratio in excess of 1.3:1 was believed diagnostic for asymmetric septal hypertrophy.[4] A wide variety of conditions have been reported that give a similar septal-free wall ratio. Inferior myocardial infarction may produce such a

ratio because of thinning of the posterior left ventricular wall.[23,24] Even the developing normal human heart may have disproportionate septal thickening.[19] A variety of acquired or congenital abnormalities with right ventricular hypertrophy may produce disproportionate ventricular septal hypertrophy.[22,27] Patients with long-standing hypertension,[25] especially those on long-term hemodialysis,[28] have been noted to have septal thickness disproportionate to the posterior left ventricular wall thickness. Patients with concentric hypertrophy due to pressure overload may occasionally hypertrophy their septum more than their posterior left ventricular wall.[21] Even a rare intracardiac tumor may produce disproportionate septal hypertrophy if the tumor involves the septum more than the posterior left ventricular wall.[20] Thus the mere finding of septal thickness greater than posterior left ventricular wall thickness is by no means pathognomonic of asymmetric septal hypertrophy or hypertrophic cardiomyopathy.[11a,12a] One would certainly like another parameter for the differential diagnosis. It is hoped that the intramyocardial septal "speckling" might provide such a sign. However, no data substantiate this possibility.

Two-dimensional echocardiography has some value besides assessing the size and shape of the interventricular septum. This ultrasonic technique has been noted as able to identify the site of myotomy and myectomy and to evaluate the amount of septal tissue removed at surgery.[17,29] In addition, the two-dimensional study can survey the papillary muscles since they may be involved in the hypertrophic state.[18] Some investigators reported using a small M-mode transducer in the operating room to assist the surgeon in measuring septal thickness and in assessing the effectiveness of the myectomy.[30]

The septal hypertrophy and abnormal contractility may produce abnormal overall ventricular function.[31] The hypertrophy reduces the left ventricular compliance, and the relaxation and filling patterns in hypertrophic cardiomyopathy are abnormal.[32–34] Delay in mitral valve opening has been noted, and disturbances in the rate, duration and co-ordination of wall motion during filling have been reported.[32] One group of investigators emphasized that the nonhypertrophied free wall of the ventricle frequently overcompensates for the abnormal septal function, making overall left ventricular performance normal.[31] It was suggested that the abnormal septal function was because the hypertrophied wall assumed the shape of the "catenoid."[35] This geometric object would supposedly have equal forces so that no contraction could occur. Unfortunately, there is little support for this otherwise interesting concept.[36]

A relatively rare form of hypertrophic cardiomyopathy principally involves the apical half of the left ventricle. Asymmetric septal hypertrophy is rare in this form of hypertrophic myopathy.[37,37a]

Left Ventricular Outflow Obstruction

A common accompaniment to hypertrophic cardiomyopathy is a dynamic obstruction to left ventricular outflow. When such a hemodynamic alteration occurs, the term used to describe this entity is hypertrophic obstructive cardiomyopathy, or idiopathic hypertrophic subaortic stenosis. Echocardiography has played an important role in both the management and understanding of this obstruction. The initial echocardiographic abnormality in patients with obstructive cardiomyopathy was a systolic anterior motion, or SAM, of the anterior mitral valve leaflet (Fig. 9–9, arrow).[11a,38,39,39a,40–42] The anterior mitral leaflet apparently moves anteriorly toward the interventricular septum shortly after the onset of systole and then returns to its normal position just before the onset of ventricular diastole. This echocardiographic observation not only provides another diagnostic tool for this important clinical abnormality, but helps establish at least one possible mechanism for the obstruction of the left ventricular outflow tract. This echocardiographic finding gives evidence that the mitral valve apparatus might play a role in obliterating the left ventricular outflow tract and might contribute to the pressure gradient found below the aortic valve.[43,43a]

One group of investigators has indicated that the pattern of systolic anterior motion, or SAM, can predict the degree of obstruction.[44] These authors found that the closer the leaflet comes to the septum and the longer the leaflet is in apposition to the septum, the greater the severity of obstruction. They even attempted to measure the area under

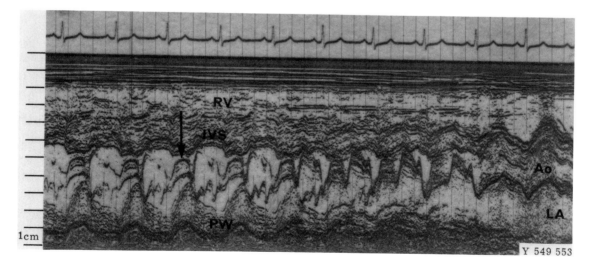

Fig. 9–9. M-mode echocardiographic scan of a patient with hypertrophic subaortic stenosis demonstrating systolic anterior motion (arrow) of the mitral valve. RV = right ventricle; IVS = interventricular septum; PW = posterior left ventricular wall; AO = aorta; LA = left atrium. (From Chang, S.: M-mode Echocardiographic Techniques and Pattern Recognition. Philadelphia, Lea & Febiger, 1976.)

this SAM for a rough indication of the degree of obstruction. Although other echocardiographers have taken issue with the quantitative aspect of this observation,[9,45,46] it is generally known that when the SAM does indeed touch the interventricular septum to a point that it becomes flat, one can be reasonably sure that a high degree of obstruction exists.[43a] However, if the leaflet merely moves upward and may or may not come close to the septum and then drops backward without reaching a plateau, then a lesser degree of obstruction probably exists,[44] and a pressure gradient may not even be present.[9] Whether the echocardiographic appearance of the mitral valve can predict the severity of obstruction, the echocardiogram certainly can be useful in following the effectiveness of therapy for the disease.[39,47–49] Figure 9–10 shows a patient with hypertrophic obstructive cardiomyopathy and severe obstruction as noted by an SAM that is totally flat and in

apposition to the septum (arrow). This elderly patient had excellent results with propranolol, and one can see a total absence of the SAM (X). Figure 9–11 shows a similar finding in a patient who underwent surgical myectomy and myotomy. In the preoperative echocardiogram in Figure 9–11A, one again sees an SAM that approaches and maintains contact with the septum throughout most of systole. In addition, the distance between the mitral valve and the septum is small. Following surgery (Fig. 9–11B), the SAM is no longer present (arrow). In addition, the distance between the mitral valve and septum (LS) is significantly increased.

As is the case with other echocardiographic techniques, certain technical details must be observed when attempting to record the abnormal motion in obstructive cardiomyopathy. Figure 9–12 is an echocardiogram of a patient with hypertrophic obstructive cardiomyopathy, or IHSS. In this scan

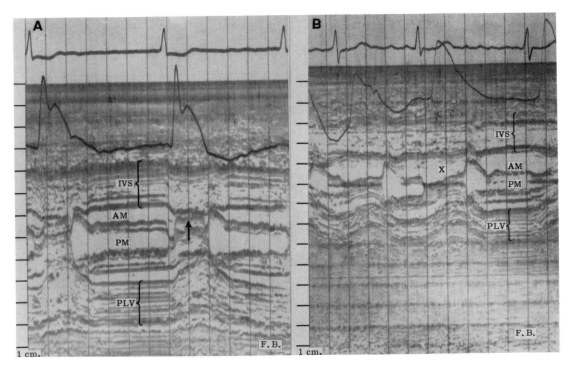

Fig. 9–10. M-mode echocardiograms of a patient with hypertrophic subaortic stenosis before, A, and after, B, treatment with propranolol. The marked anterior systolic motion of the mitral valve (arrow) disappears after treatment with propranolol (X). The hypertrophied interventricular septum (IVS) and posterior left ventricular wall (PLV) are also present. AM = anterior mitral valve; PM = posterior mitral valve. (From Feigenbaum, H.: Clinical applications of echocardiography. Prog. Cardiovasc. Dis., 14:531, 1972.)

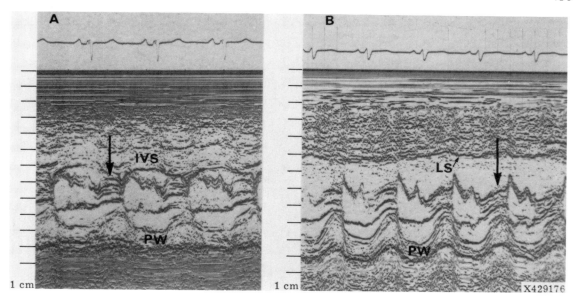

Fig. 9–11.   M-mode echocardiogram of a patient with hypertrophic subaortic stenosis before, *A*, and after, *B*, surgical myectomy and myotomy. Following surgery, preoperative systolic anterior motion *(arrow)* is absent, and the distance between the mitral valve and the left side of the septum (LS) is increased. IVS = interventricular septum; PW = posterior left ventricular wall; LS = left septum. (From Chang, S.: M-mode Echocardiographic Techniques and Pattern Recognition. Philadelphia, Lea & Febiger, 1976.)

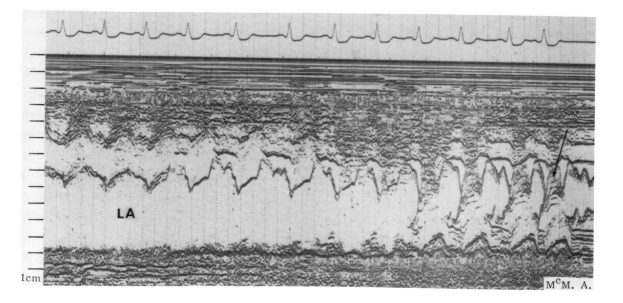

Fig. 9–12.   M-mode scan of a patient with hypertrophic subaortic stenosis. Systolic anterior motion *(arrow)* is best recorded deep within the left ventricle simultaneously with the recording of the posterior and anterior mitral valve leaflet. Abnormal motion is frequently absent in the left ventricular outflow tract. LA = left atrium.

from the base of the heart to the left ventricle, one records several mitral valve echoes near the aorta; little evidence of any abnormality is recorded. Only as the ultrasonic beam is directed deeper into the left ventricle does one see the typical abnormal systolic motion of the mitral valve (arrow). As a rule, the best location for seeing abnormal mitral valve echoes in IHSS is at the edge of the mitral leaflet, usually where one can record both the posterior and anterior mitral leaflets. It is somewhat unusual to be able to record a good SAM with only the anterior leaflet in view. In addition, one usually finds this abnormality when the ultrasonic beam is directed into the left ventricle so that the left ventricular wall should be the posterior cardiac structure rather than the left atrial wall.

The outflow obstruction in patients with hypertrophic cardiomyopathy is classically dynamic and may not always be present at rest.[41,42] This feature is one of the hallmarks of this abnormality. Figure 9–13 demonstrates that the SAM (arrow) may only occur after the compensatory pause following a premature ventricular systole.[50] During the regular sinus beat, the mitral motion during systole is grossly normal. The production of a subaortic pressure gradient after a compensatory pause has been one of the well-recognized features of IHSS. Thus efforts to bring out the abnormal mitral valve motion are occasionally necessary to identify patients with the disease. Provocation, such as Valsalva maneuver, amyl nitrite, intravenous isoproterenol, or even a noninvasively induced premature ventricular systole,[50] brings out systolic anterior motion of the mitral valve when it may be absent at rest.

It must also be remembered that the mitral valve is attached to the mitral annulus, which is an integral part of the left ventricle. Motion exhibited by the mitral valve is in part due to any motion of the mitral annulus and/or left ventricular wall. For example, in any condition where posterior ventricular wall motion is exaggerated, there is exaggerated motion of the systolic component of the mitral valve echoes. This phenomenon may occur in any situation where paradoxical septal motion is present. When the septum is moving abnormally, one frequently finds a "compensa-

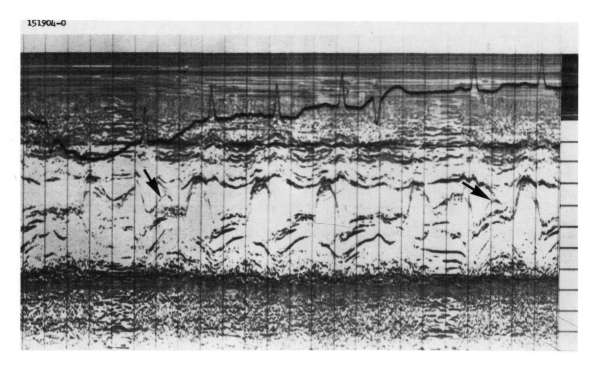

151904–0

Fig. 9–13.   Mitral valve echocardiogram of a patient with hypertrophic subaortic stenosis in whom the systolic anterior motion *(arrows)* only occurs following a premature ventricular systole.

tory" exaggerated motion of the opposing left ventricular wall. Such exaggerated left ventricular wall motion is commonly noted in patients with right ventricular volume overload,[51] and even possibly with a ventricular aneurysm and anterior wall dyskinesis.[52] One must also be careful not to misinterpret aortic wall motion superimposed on mitral valve motion as SAM. A true SAM should return to the baseline prior to the onset of ventricular diastole. If one is recording parts of the aorta, then the false SAM remains in an anterior position when the mitral valve opens.

Dynamic outflow obstruction need not only occur with asymmetric septal hypertrophy, as noted in Figure 9–9. The M-mode echocardiogram in Figure 9–14 again shows systolic anterior mitral motion (arrow); however, the interventricular septum (IVS) and posterior left ventricular wall (PW) are both hypertrophied. Thus dynamic left ventricular outflow obstruction may occur with concentric hypertrophy.[53] Figure 9–15 shows another example of subaortic obstruction and SAM in a patient with concentric left

ventricular hypertrophy. In addition, the patient has pericardial effusion. This patient proves that other accompanying problems frequently bring out the subaortic obstruction. Pericardial effusion seems to be one condition that is associated with hypertrophic subaortic stenosis.[54,55] Anemia and hypovolemia are other entities noted with this condition.[54] Correcting the secondary problem may relieve the obstruction. Another entity commonly associated with hypertrophic subaortic stenosis is mitral annulus calcification. The relationship between these two abnormalities is not understood.[56]

There are increasing reports of patients who show systolic anterior motion of the mitral valve with no evidence of hypertrophic cardiomyopathy.[12a,55,57–59,59a,60] Figure 9–16 shows a patient with catheterization-proven aortic stenosis and aortic insufficiency with predominant insufficiency. Marked fluttering of the anterior leaflet during diastole (FL) is seen in this echocardiogram. Although the interventricular septum is not well recorded, there is no evidence of

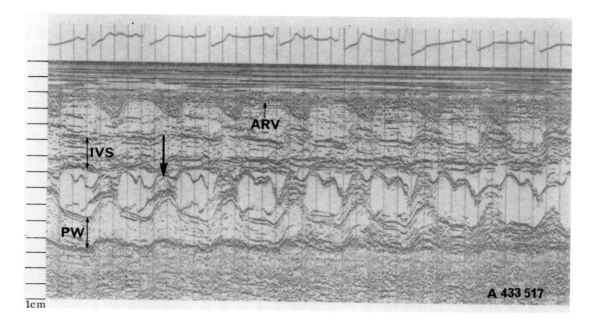

Fig. 9–14. M-mode echocardiogram of a patient with obstructive cardiomyopathy and concentric left ventricular hypertrophy. Systolic anterior motion of the mitral valve (arrow) can be seen obstructing the left ventricular outflow tract. The thickness of the interventricular septum (IVS) and posterior left ventricular wall (PW) are approximately equal. ARV = anterior right ventricular wall.

asymmetric hypertrophy; however, the posterior ventricular wall and the septum were thicker than normal, and there was generalized ventricular hypertrophy secondary to the aortic valve disease. Some anterior motion of the mitral valve can be noted in early systole. Even with provocation, no evidence of subaortic obstruction was identified at cardiac catheterization. In addition, the surgeon could not find any evidence of hypertrophic subaortic stenosis at the time of the operation. Figure 9–17 shows two other illustrations from the same patient. Figure 9–17A is another preoperative echocardiogram that shows a better recording of the interventricular septum. Figure 9–17B shows the postoperative echocardiogram. The left ventricle is considerably smaller, and there is abnormal septal motion that is commonly seen following any surgical procedure. However, the abnormal systolic motion of the mitral valve (arrow) is still present and may even be exaggerated post-operatively.[60a]

The finding of SAM in patients without the clinical syndrome of asymmetric septal hypertrophy makes one wonder whether the mitral motion might be a nonspecific reaction to ventricular hypertrophy or to any distortion of the ventricular cavity.[55,61] The coexistence of dynamic subaortic obstruction is well recognized with fixed outflow obstruction[27,62–64,64a] and in such conditions as transposition of the great arteries.[65,66] There is even an element of systolic anterior motion in patients with mitral valve prolapse (see Chapter 6).[67] One group of authors suggests a hypercontractile state that may simulate hypertrophic cardiomyopathy, including systolic anterior motion of the mitral valve.[68] Newborn infants of diabetic mothers may exhibit transient clinical and echocardiographic findings that are indistinguishable from obstructive hypertrophic cardiomyopathy.[68a]

The abnormal mitral valve motion can be seen on two-dimensional echocardiography,[13,17] although it is still easier to record

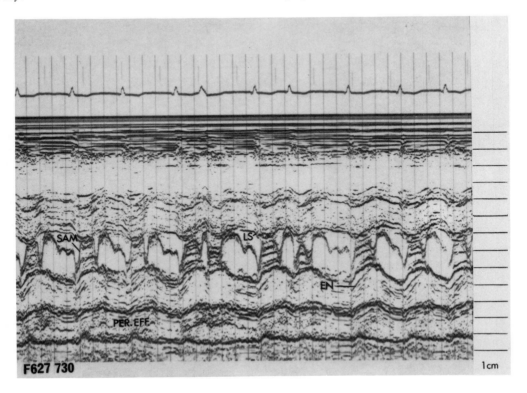

Fig. 9–15. M-mode echocardiogram of a patient with concentric left ventricular hypertrophy and systolic anterior motion (SAM) of the mitral valve producing outflow obstruction. The patient also has significant pericardial effusion (PER. EFF.). LS = left side of septum; EN = posterior left ventricular endocardium.

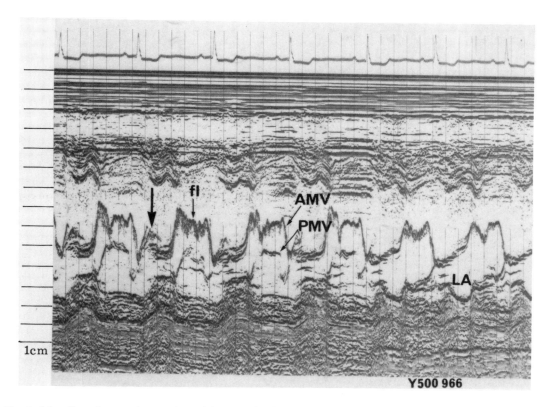

Fig. 9–16. Systolic anterior motion of the mitral valve *(arrow)* in a patient with aortic regurgitation and no hemodynamic evidence of hypertrophic subaortic stenosis. Fluttering (fl) of the mitral valve can be noted. AMV = anterior mitral valve leaflet; PMV = posterior mitral valve leaflet; LA = left atrial wall.

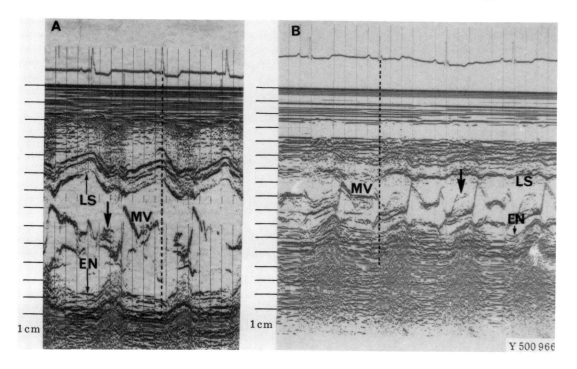

Fig. 9–17. Echocardiograms of the patient with aortic regurgitation shown in Figure 9–16 before and after aortic valve replacement. *A*, Preoperative view of systolic anterior motion *(arrow)*. *B*, Postoperative view of even more striking systolic anterior motion *(arrow)*. Hypertrophic subaortic stenosis was not evident prior to or at the time of surgery. LS = left septum; MV = mitral valve; EN = posterior left ventricular endocardium.

this phenomenon with the M-mode technique. The two-dimensional examination has provided some evidence as to the site of the abnormal mitral motion. Apparently the part of the valve apparatus that moves toward the septum varies from patient to patient. In one subject the body of the leaflet may move anteriorly, whereas in others the chordae may be principally involved. These observations have led to a number of theories regarding the mechanism for the SAM and the subaortic obstruction;[69-71] however, no explanation for the peculiar mitral motion is universally accepted.

The aortic valve also indicates an alteration in blood flow in the aorta in patients with dynamic subaortic obstruction.[39a,42,72,73] Figure 9–18 shows the aortic valve echocardiogram of a patient with IHSS. Midsystolic closure (arrow) of the anterior leaflet can be easily identified. Following relief of the obstruction with the use of propranolol (Fig. 9–18B), the systolic closure is no longer present. Although such conditions as discrete subaortic stenosis or mitral regurgitation can also produce systolic closure of the aortic valve, the closure in hypertrophic subaortic stenosis frequently occurs somewhat later in systole, and the valve tends to reopen in the latter half of systole. However, this rule is not universal. Figure 9–19 is another aortic valve echocardiogram of a patient with hypertrophic subaortic stenosis. Early systolic closure of the valve is again noted (arrow). It would be difficult to distinguish this aortic valve echocardiogram from one showing discrete subaortic stenosis. As a rule, midsystolic aortic valve closure is more reliable for determining the existence of a pressure gradient in patients with obstructive hypertrophic cardiomyopathy than is systolic anterior motion of the mitral valve.

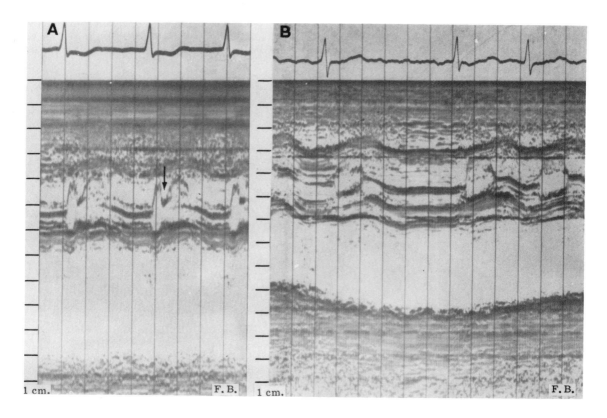

Fig. 9–18. Aortic valve echocardiogram of a patient with hypertrophic subaortic stenosis. During mid-systole the aortic valve closes (arrow) secondary to the subvalvular obstruction and reopens before diastole begins. Following the use of propranolol, the systolic closure of the aortic valve is not apparent, B. (From Feigenbaum, H.: Clinical applications of echocardiography. Prog. Cardiovasc. Dis., 14:531, 1972.)

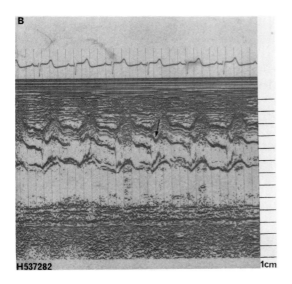

H537282   1cm

Fig. 9–19.   Aortic valve echocardiogram of a patient with obstructive cardiomyopathy. Early systolic closure of the aortic valve *(arrow)* can be seen. This echocardiogram is indistinguishable from that seen with discrete subaortic stenosis. Note also fine systolic fluttering on the aortic leaflets.

Doppler echocardiography also shows an abnormal flow pattern in the aorta in patients with dynamic subaortic obstruction.[75-77] A reduction of flow velocity in midsystole is characteristically noted.

Hypertrophic obstructive cardiomyopathy occasionally manifests obstruction to right ventricular outflow. The echocardiogram may show evidence of right ventricular hypertrophy with increased anterior right ventricular wall thickness.[78,79] Systolic anterior motion of the tricuspid valve and midsystolic closure of the pulmonary valve have been reported.

CONGESTIVE CARDIOMYOPATHY

Patients with congestive cardiomyopathy manifest dilated, poorly contracting left ventricles. They exhibit echocardiographic signs of decreased cardiac output with a poorly moving aorta, decreased mitral valve opening, and gradual closure of the aortic valve. The left atrium is usually dilated, and there frequently is abnormal closure of the mitral valve indicative of an elevated left ventricular diastolic pressure. Most important, the left ventricle is dilated and the walls

move poorly.[80-83] Figure 9–20 is a typical left ventricular M-mode echocardiogram of a patient with congestive cardiomyopathy. Although the left ventricle is dilated and both the septal and posterior ventricular walls move poorly, the wall thickness is within normal limits. Following a premature atrial systole and a prolonged diastolic pause, abnormal closure of the mitral valve can be noted (arrow).

The etiology of the myopathy cannot be determined echocardiographically. Usually in patients with severe coronary artery disease, which is the important differential diagnosis, at least one portion of the left ventricular echocardiogram, usually the posterior wall, continues to exhibit normal motion.[80] However, there are patients with severe forms of ischemic cardiomyopathy who do not show any normal wall motion. In addition, as patients with cardiomyopathy develop mitral regurgitation, septal motion may increase as a result of the left ventricular volume overload and possible afterload reduction. Figure 9–21 shows an M-mode scan of a fifteen-year-old patient with congestive cardiomyopathy. The left ventricle and left atrium are markedly dilated. There is also abnormal closure of the mitral valve (arrow). Both the septal and posterior ventricular walls move poorly; however, the motion of the posterior wall is less than that of the septum. The dissimilar wall motion might prompt one to diagnose segmental rather than diffuse myocardial involvement. However, it is not unusual for the septal motion to exceed the posterior wall motion in some patients with congestive cardiomyopathy, especially when mitral regurgitation complicates the problem.

The etiology of congestive cardiomyopathy is varied. The causes include alcoholic cardiomyopathy, postpartum cardiomyopathy, idiopathic cardiomyopathy, and myocarditis.[81] Some of these problems fluctuate in severity. Echocardiography is an ideal tool for following the natural history or the efficacy of therapy. Figure 9–22 shows serial M-mode left ventricular echocardiograms of a patient with postpartum cardiomyopathy. Figure 9–22A shows poor posterior ventricular wall motion and left ventricular dilatation. Two weeks later the left ventricular dilatation decreased, and the posterior left ventricular wall motion markedly improved (Fig. 9–22B).

One can use any of the M-mode criteria for the evaluation of left ventricular function in patients with diffuse congestive cardiomyopathy.[84] Fractional shortening, mean velocity of circumferential shortening, posterior left ventricular wall velocity, ventricular wall thickening, and even ejection fraction are all useful in attempting to quantitate the degree of ventricular dysfunction in these patients. Usually the abnormalities are so gross that these measurements are unnecessary; however, one may make such calculations in serial examinations to detect subtle changes in ventricular function.

M-mode echocardiography is usually sufficient for the diagnosis of congestive cardiomyopathy. Some features, such as abnormal motion of the mitral valve, aortic valve, or aorta are better appreciated on the M-mode recording. Two-dimensional echocardiography can also detect the dilated, poorly contracting left ventricle in these patients. Figure 9–23 demonstrates a long-axis parasternal examination of a left ventricle that is contracting well. The diameter of the left ventricular cavity is much smaller in systole than in diastole. In contrast, the long-axis parasternal examination in Figure 9–24 is of a patient with congestive cardiomyopathy. The left ventricular diameter varies little from diastole (A) to systole (B). The dilated left atrium and the decreased opening of the mitral valve can also be appreciated on the two-dimensional study. The short-axis

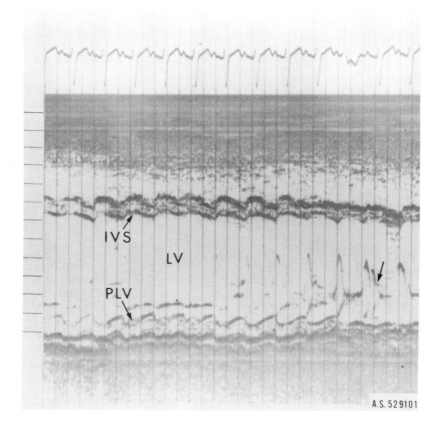

A.S. 529101

Fig. 9–20.   M-mode echocardiogram of the left ventricle in a patient with congestive cardiomyopathy. The left ventricle (LV) is dilated, and the motion of the interventricular septum (IVS) and posterior left ventricular wall (PLV) is markedly reduced. Following a premature atrial systole and a prolonged diastolic pause, abnormal closure of the mitral valve (arrow) can be noted.

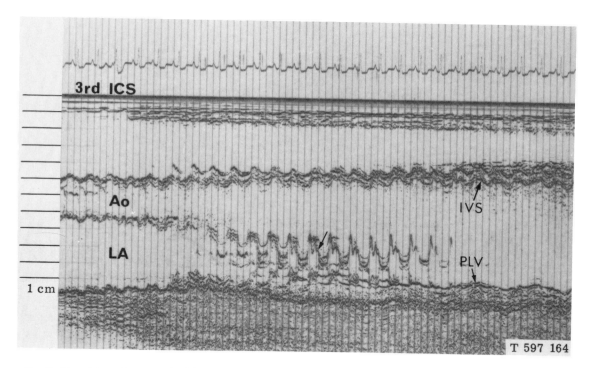

Fig. 9–21. M-mode scan of a fifteen-year-old patient with congestive cardiomyopathy. The left ventricle is dilated, and motion of the posterior left ventricular wall (PLV) is virtually absent. Somewhat better motion of the interventricular septum (IVS) can be appreciated. The left atrium (LA) is dilated, the aortic walls move poorly, and closure of the mitral valve is abnormal *(arrow)*. (From Feigenbaum, H.: Echocardiography. *In* Heart Disease. Edited by E. Braunwald. Philadelphia, W.B. Saunders Co., 1980.)

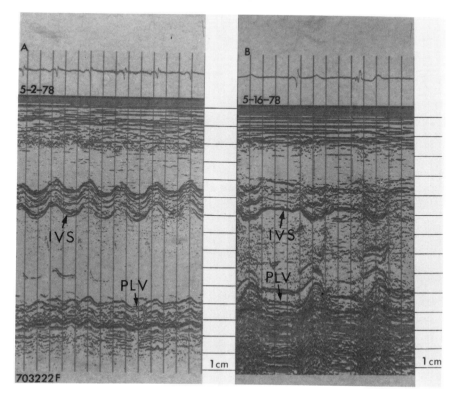

Fig. 9–22. Serial M-mode echocardiograms of the left ventricle in a patient with postpartum cardiomyopathy. *A*, On 5/2/78 the left ventricle was dilated with poor motion of the posterior left ventricular wall (PLV). *B*, Two weeks later the left ventricle decreased in size, and motion of the posterior left ventricular wall (PLV) markedly improved. IVS = interventricular septum.

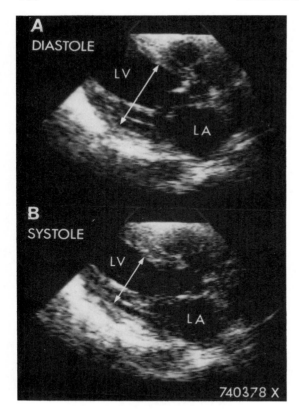

Fig. 9–23.   Long-axis parasternal two-dimensional echocardiogram of a patient whose left ventricle is contracting vigorously. A marked difference in the left ventricular diameter can be detected from diastole, *A*, to systole, *B*. LV = left ventricle; LA = left atrium.

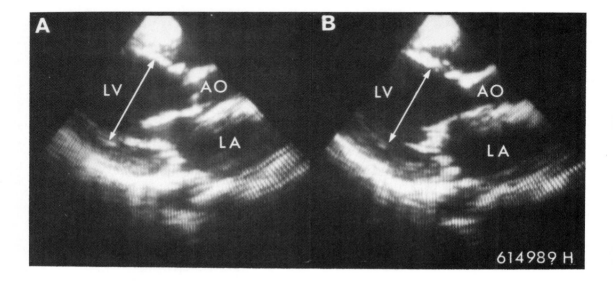

Fig. 9–24.   Long-axis parasternal two-dimensional echocardiogram in diastole, *A*, and systole, *B*, of a patient with congestive cardiomyopathy. Little difference in the left ventricular diameter exists between the two recordings. The mitral valve opening in *A* is also markedly reduced. LV = left ventricle; AO = aorta; LA = left atrium.

examination can provide similar information. Figure 9–25 shows a short-axis parasternal echocardiogram at the level of the papillary muscles in a normally contracting left ventricle. The overall decrease in left ventricular cavity in systole is obvious. In contrast, Figure 9–26 shows a short-axis examination of the left ventricle at the level of the papillary muscles in a patient with congestive cardiomyopathy. The cavity is grossly dilated, and left ventricular cavity size decreases minimally from diastole to systole.

The apical four-chamber view can also provide diagnostic information in patients with congestive cardiomyopathy. In addi-

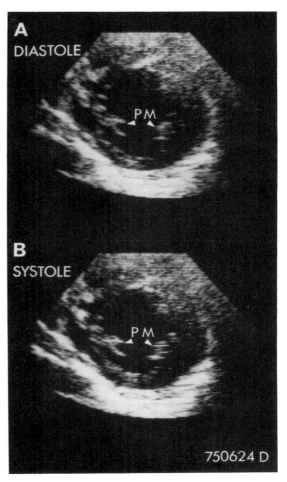

Fig. 9–26. Diastolic and systolic short-axis two-dimensional echocardiogram of the left ventricle at the level of the papillary muscles (PM) in a patient with congestive cardiomyopathy. The ventricular cavity is grossly dilated, and its size decreases minimally from diastole, *A*, to systole, *B*.

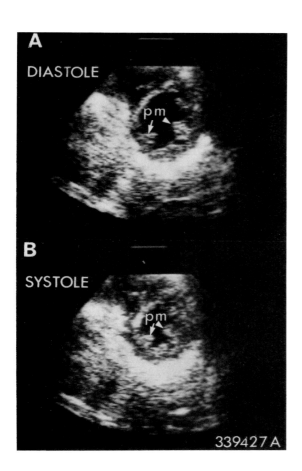

Fig. 9–25. Short-axis parasternal two-dimensional echocardiogram at the level of the papillary muscles (pm) in a normally contracting left ventricle. Note the change in size of the left ventricular cavity from diastole *A*, to systole, *B*.

tion to noting diffuse hypokinesis of the entire ventricle (Fig. 9–27), the apical four-chamber view can also detect papillary muscle dysfunction, which is frequently seen in these patients.[84a] The papillary muscle dysfunction is revealed echocardiographically by incomplete closure of the mitral valve in systole (Fig. 9–27B). The closed mitral valve fails to meet the plane of the mitral annulus (dotted line). Another potential value of the apical two-dimensional studies is the finding of mural thrombi in these patients with congestive cardiomyopathy.

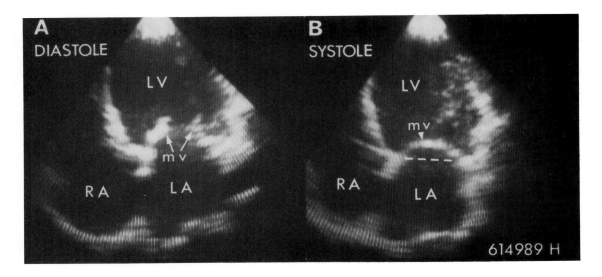

Fig. 9–27. Apical four-chamber two-dimensional echocardiogram of a patient with congestive cardiomyopathy. The size of the left ventricle (LV) changes little from diastole, *A*, to systole, *B*. In addition, there is incomplete closure of the mitral valve (mv) in systole. The closed leaflets fail to reach the plane of the mitral annulus (dotted line). RA = right atrium; LA = left atrium.

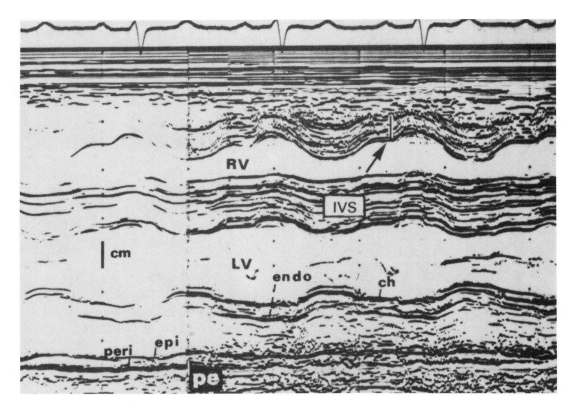

Fig. 9–28. M-mode echocardiogram of a patient with amyloid cardiomyopathy. The thickened anterior right ventricular wall (RV) measures 10 mm in diastole *(arrow)*. The interventricular septum (IVS) and the posterior left ventricular wall between the endocardium (endo) and epicardium (epi) are hypertrophied. The motion of both ventricular walls is reduced, and the overall cavity size is normal. There is a small pericardial effusion (pe). LV = left ventricle; Ch = chordae. (From Child, J.S., Krivokapich, J., and Abbasi, A.S.: Increased right ventricular wall thickness on echocardiography in amyloid infiltrative cardiomyopathy. Am. J. Cardiol., *44*:1391, 1979.)

INFILTRATIVE CARDIOMYOPATHY

Infiltrative cardiomyopathy is a disease of the cardiac muscle secondary to some other disorder that produces histologic changes within the cardiac musculature. The disorders reported to produce myocardial changes on the echocardiogram include amyloidosis,[85-88,88a] collagen diseases such as scleroderma or progressive systemic sclerosis,[89-93] iron overload from multiple transfusions,[94,95] idiopathic hypereosinophilia, sarcoidosis,[96] glycogen storage disease (or Pompe's disease),[97] and acromegaly.[98,99] There are also a number of neuromuscular diseases, such as progressive muscular dystrophy[100] and Friedreich's ataxia,[101] that may show echocardiographic changes. The muscular diseases produce primary rather than truly infiltrative cardiomyopathies. Most patients in the literature having infiltrative cardiomyopathy have amyloid heart disease.[85-88] The principal M-mode echocardiographic features of this disease are hypertrophy of the posterior left ventricular wall, the right ventricular wall, and the interventricular septum, decreased cardiac motion of all walls, and small ventricular cavities. Figure 9–28 demonstrates an M-mode echocardiogram of a patient with amyloid cardiomyopathy. The left ventricular cavity is small. The posterior left ventricular wall, the interventricular septum, and the right ventricular wall are all hypertrophied. The motion of the interventricular septum and posterior ventricular wall is decreased. Unfortunately, the findings in Figure 9–28 are fairly nonspecific and must be interpreted within the clinical setting.

Two-dimensional echocardiography can also be helpful in the diagnosis of amyloid heart disease and may provide more specific findings. Figure 9–29 demonstrates four-chamber and subcostal two-dimensional echocardiograms of a patient with hereditary amyloidosis. Many striking features appear on these echocardiograms. The echoes returning from the myocardium have been described as "patchy, amorphous, high-intensity echoes."[88a] Another characteristic finding on the two-dimensional echocardiogram in these patients is hypertrophy of the interatrial septum. The subcostal examina-

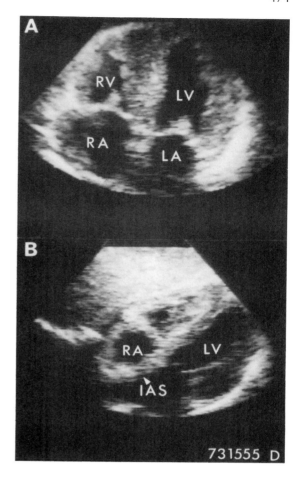

Fig. 9–29. Four-chamber, A, and subcostal, B, two-dimensional echocardiograms of a patient with hereditary amyloidosis. The four-chamber view demonstrates markedly hypertrophied cardiac walls, especially the interventricular septum and the free wall of the right ventricle. The tricuspid and mitral valve leaflets are also thickened. The left ventricular (LV) and right ventricular (RV) cavities are small. The subcostal examination demonstrates the thickened interatrial septum (IAS), which is a characteristic finding in amyloid heart disease. RA = right atrium; LA = left atrium.

tion (Fig. 9–29B) is probably best for detecting the thickness of the interatrial septum. Figure 9–29A also demonstrates the marked hypertrophy of the interventricular septum and the right ventricular and left ventricular free walls. In addition, there is thickening of both the tricuspid and mitral valve leaflets.

Figure 9–30 shows an M-mode echocardiogram of the left ventricle in a four-month-old infant with Pompe's disease.

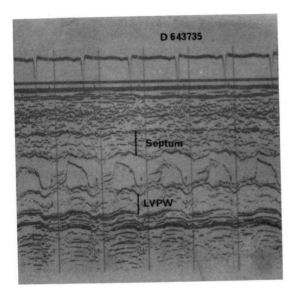

Fig. 9–30.   M-mode echocardiogram of the left ventricle of a four-month-old infant with Pompe's disease. The septum and posterior left ventricular wall (LVPW) are hypertrophied and move poorly. The left ventricular cavity is small.

Again, one sees a hypertrophied septum and posterior left ventricular wall, diminished wall motion, and a relatively small left ventricular cavity. As in the case of amyloidosis, these findings are somewhat nonspecific. Other causes for hypertrophy must be considered. Although cardiac wall hypertrophy, decreased wall motion, and lack of dilatation can be seen with other disease states, these signs can certainly exclude the diagnoses of other clinically confusing entities, such as constrictive pericarditis or congestive cardiomyopathy.

ENDOMYOCARDIAL FIBROSIS

There have been a few reports, principally in the British literature, demonstrating the echocardiographic findings with endomyocardial fibrosis.[102,103] These patients may manifest a primary congestive cardiomyopathy or a restrictive form of cardiomyopathy with abnormal filling characteristics. Pathologically, a layer of fibrosis surrounds the endocardium. Figure 9–31

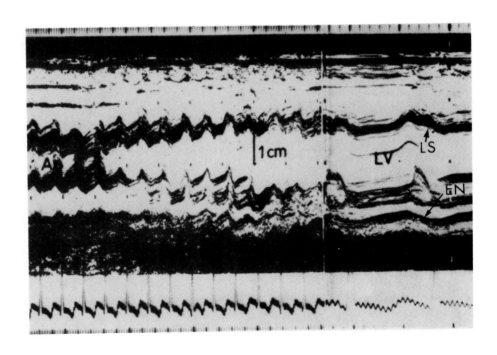

Fig. 9–31.   M-mode echocardiogram of a patient with endomyocardial fibrosis. The echoes from the left side of the septum (LS) and the posterior left ventricular endocardium (EN) are very dense. LV = left ventricle. (From Schmaltz, A.A., et al.: Echocardiographic findings and function analysis in infants with endocardial fibroelastosis. *In* Echocardiology. Edited by C.T. Lancee. The Hague, Martinus Nijhoff, 1979.)

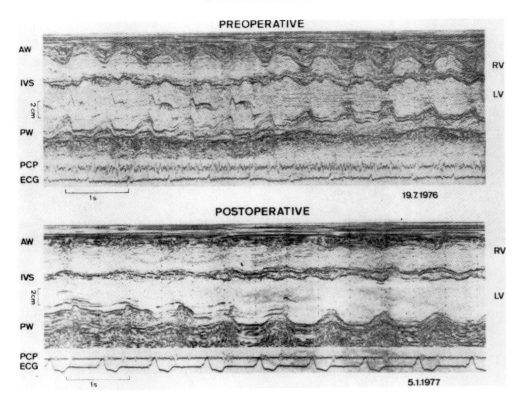

Fig. 9–32.   Pre- and postoperative M-mode echocardiograms in a patient with biventricular endomyocardial fibrosis. Endocardial thickening of the right ventricular anterior wall with systolic obliteration of the right ventricular cavity toward the apex can be seen in the preoperative echocardiogram. Endocardial fibrosis of the left ventricular posterior wall is found toward the left ventricular apex. The postoperative recording shows diminution of the right anterior wall and left posterior endocardial thickening. The systolic obliteration of the right ventricular cavity is no longer present following surgery. AW = anterior wall; IVS = interventricular septum; PW = posterior wall; PCP = phonocardiogram; ECG = electrocardiogram; RV = right ventricle; LV = left ventricle. (From Hess, O.M., et al.: Pre- and postoperative findings in patients with endomyocardial fibrosis. Br. Heart J., 40:406, 1978.)

shows an M-mode recording of such a patient. The dense echoes from the left side of the septum (LS) and from the posterior left ventricular endocardium (EN) are compatible with the existence of fibrosis over these cardiac surfaces. Figure 9–32 demonstrates a pre- and postoperative M-mode echocardiogram of a patient with biventricular endomyocardial fibrosis. In this tracing there is thickening of the anterior right ventricular wall as well as dense echoes along the posterior left ventricular endocardial wall. The thick right ventricular echoes obliterate the right ventricular cavity near the apex. Following surgical removal of the fibrous tissue, the right ventricular wall thickness is markedly reduced, and the size of the right ventricular cavity is increased. Note also an increase in the size of the left ventricular cavity with removal of some of the echoes on the surface of the left ventricular endocardium.

The distribution of the fibrous tissue need not be uniform throughout the heart. The fibrosis may be localized in one area of the heart. Figure 9–33 demonstrates a young adult with an obliterative restrictive form of endomyocardial fibrosis.[104] The fibrotic tissue (arrow) obliterated the apical half of the left ventricle. There was marked restriction of left ventricular filling as indicated by the dilated left atrium. Surgery successfully removed most of the fibrosis.[104]

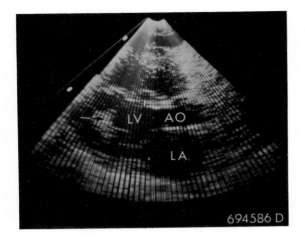

Fig. 9–33. Long-axis parasternal two-dimensional echocardiogram of a patient with an obliterative restrictive form of endomyocardial fibrosis. A mass of fibrous tissue *(arrow)* fills the apical half of the left ventricle (LV). AO = aorta; LA = left atrium.

REFERENCES

1. Abbasi, A.S., MacAlpin, R.N., Eber, L.M., and Pearce, M.L.: Echocardiographic diagnosis of idiopathic hypertrophic cardiomyopathy without outflow obstruction. Circulation, 46:897, 1972.
2. Henry, W.L., Clark, C.E., Roberts, W.C., Morrow, A.G., and Epstein, S.E.: Difference in distribution of myocardial abnormalities in patients with obstructive and non-obstructive asymmetric septal hypertrophy (ASH): echocardiographic and gross anatomic findings. Circulation, 50:447, 1974.
3. Henry, W.L., Clark, C.E., and Epstein, S.E.: Asymmetric septal hypertrophy: the unifying link in the IHSS disease spectrum: observations regarding its pathogenesis, pathophysiology, and course. Circulation, 47:827, 1973.
3a. vanDorp, W.G., tenCate, F.J., Vletter, W.B., Dohmen, H., and Roelandt, J.: Familial prevalence of asymmetric septal hypertrophy. Eur. J. Cardiol., 4/3:349, 1976.
4. Henry, W.L., Clark, C.E., and Epstein, S.E.: Asymmetric septal hypertrophy (ASH): echocardiographic identification of the pathognomonic anatomic abnormality of IHSS. Circulation, 47:225, 1973.
5. Sayaya, J., Longo, M.R., and Schlant, R.C.: Echocardiographic interventricular septal wall motion and thickness: a study in health and disease. Am. Heart J., 87:681, 1974.
6. Maron, B.J., Henry, W.L., Clark, C.E., Redwood, D.R., Roberts, W.C., and Epstein, S.E.: Asymmetric septal hypertrophy in childhood. Circulation, 53:9, 1976.
6a. Schweizer, P., Hanrath, P., Bleifeld, W., and Effert, S.: Echocardiographic criteria of asymmetrical hypertrophy of the ventricular septum without outflow tract obstruction. Dtsch. Med. Wochensch., 100:2189, 1975.
7. Clark, C.E., Henry, W.L., and Epstein, S.E.: Familial prevalence and genetic transmission of idiopathic hypertrophic subaortic stenosis. N. Engl. J. Med., 289:709, 1973.
8. tenCate, F.J., Hugenholtz, P.G., vanDorp, W.G., and Roelandt, J.: Prevalence of diagnostic abnormalities in patients with genetically transmitted asymmetric septal hypertrophy. Am. J. Cardiol., 43:731, 1979.
9. Rossen, R.M., Goodman, D.J., Ingham, R.E., and Popp, R.L.: Echocardiographic criteria in the diagnosis of idiopathic hypertrophic subaortic stenosis. Circulation, 50:747, 1974.
10. Maron, B.J., Henry, W.L., Roberts, W.C., and Epstein, S.E.: Comparison of echocardiographic and necropsy measurements of ventricular wall thickness in patients with and without disproportionate septal thickening. Circulation, 55:341, 1977.
11. Bulkley, B.H., Weisfeldt, M.L., and Hutchins, G.M.: Asymmetric septal hypertrophy and myocardial fiber disarray: features of normal, developing, and malformed hearts. Circulation, 56:292, 1977.
11a. Maron, B.J. and Epstein, S.E.: Hypertrophic cardiomyopathy. Recent observations regarding the specificity of three hallmarks of the disease: asymmetric septal hypertrophy, septal disorganization and systolic anterior motion of the anterior mitral leaflet. Am. J. Cardiol., 45:141, 1980.
12. Fowles, R.E., Martin, R.P., and Popp, R.L.: Erroneous diagnosis of asymmetric septal hypertrophy due to angled interventricular septum. Am. J. Cardiol., 43:348, 1979. (Abstract)
12a. Wei, J.Y., Weiss, J.L., and Bulkley, B.H.: The heterogeneity of hypertrophic cardiomyopathy: an autopsy and one-dimensional echocardiographic study. Am. J. Cardiol., 45:24, 1980.
13. Tajik, A.J., Seward, J.B., and Hagler, D.J.: Detailed analysis of hypertrophic obstructive cardiomyopathy by wide-angle two-dimensional sector echocardiography. Am. J. Cardiol., 43:348, 1979. (Abstract)
14. Taylor, R.D., Child, J.S., and Shah, P.M.: Variations in septal hypertrophy in hypertrophic obstructive cardiomyopathy (HOCM). Am. J. Cardiol., 43:348, 1979. (Abstract)
15. Roelandt, J., Kloster, F.E., tenCate, F.J., vanDorp, W.G., Honkoop, J., Bom, N., and Hugenholtz, P.G.: Multidimensional echocardiography: an appraisal of its clinical usefulness. Br. Heart J., 36:29, 1974.
15a. Brun, P., Beraldo, E., Kulas, A., and Laurent, F.: The value of dynamic echocardiography in the diagnosis of obstructive hypertrophic cardiomyopathies. Ann. Radiol. (Paris), 20:413, 1977. (Author's translation)
16. Cohen, M.V., Teichholz, L.E., and Gorlin, R.: B-scan ultrasonography in idiopathic hypertrophic subaortic stenosis: study of left ventricular outflow tract and mechanism of obstruction. Br. Heart J., 38:595, 1976.
17. Martin, R.P., Rakowski, H., French, J., and Popp, R.L.: Idiopathic hypertrophic subaortic stenosis viewed by wide-angle, phased-array echocardiography. Circulation, 59:1206, 1979.
18. Isshiki, T., Umeda, T., and Machii, K.: Cross-sectional echocardiographic study on the papillary muscles in hypertrophic cardiomyopathy. J. Cardiogr., 8:631, 1978.
19. Maron, B.J., Verter, J., and Kapur, S.: Dispropor-

tionate ventricular septal thickening in the developing normal human heart. Circulation, 57:520, 1978.

20. Isner, J.M., Falcone, M.W., Virmani, R., and Roberts, W.C.: Cardiac sarcoma causing "ASH" and simulating coronary heart disease. Am. J. Med., 66:1025, 1979.

21. Gibson, D.G., Traill, T.A., Hall, R.J.C., and Brown, D.J.: Echocardiographic features of secondary left ventricular hypertrophy, Br. Heart J., 41:54, 1979.

22. Maron, B.J., Clark, C.E., Henry, W.L., Fukuda, T., Edwards, J.E., Mathews, E.C., Jr., Redwood, D.R., and Epstein, S.E.: Prevalence and characteristics of disproportionate ventricular septal thickening in patients with acquired or congenital heart disease. Circulation, 55:489, 1977.

23. Maron, B.J., Savage, D.D., Clark, C.E., Henry, W.L., Vlodaver, Z., Edwards, J.E., and Epstein, S.E.: Prevalence and characteristics of disproportionate ventricular septal thickening in patients with coronary artery disease. Circulation, 57:250, 1978.

24. Stern, A., Kessler, K.M., Hammer, W.J., Kreulen, T.H., and Spann, J.F.: Septal-free wall disproportion in inferior infarction: the echocardiographic differentiation from hypertrophic cardiomyopathy. Circulation, 58:700, 1978.

25. Kansal, S., Roitman, D., and Sheffield, L.T.: Interventricular septal thickness and left ventricular hypertrophy: an echocardiographic study. Circulation, 60:1058, 1979.

26. Henning, H., Roeske, W., Karliner, J., Crawford, M., and O'Rourke, R.: Inferior myocardial infarction (IMI): A common cause of asymmetric septal hypertrophy (ASH). Circulation (Suppl. II), 54:191, 1976. (Abstract)

27. Maron, B.J., Gottdiener, J.S., Roberts, W.C., Hammer, W.J., and Epstein, S.E.: Nongenetically transmitted disproportionate ventricular septal thickening associated with left ventricular outflow obstruction. Br. Heart J., 41:345, 1979.

28. Abbasi, A.S., Slaughter, J.C., and Allen, M.W.: Asymmetric septal hypertrophy in patients on long-term hemodialysis. Chest, 74:548, 1978.

29. Schapira, J.N., Stemple, D.R., Martin, R.P., Rakowski, H., Stinson, E.B., and Popp, R.L.: Single and two-dimensional echocardiographic visualization of the effects of septal myectomy in idiopathic hypertrophic subaortic stenosis. Circulation, 58:850, 1978.

30. Syracuse, D.C., Gaudiani, V.A., Kasti, D.G., Henry, W.L., and Morrow, A.G.: Intraoperative, intracardiac echocardiography during left ventriculomyotomy and myectomy for hypertrophic subaortic stenosis. Circulation (Suppl. II), 58:I23, 1978.

31. tenCate, F.J., Hugenholtz, P.G., and Roelandt, J.: Ultrasound study of dynamic behaviour of left ventricle in genetic asymmetric septal hypertrophy. Br. Heart J., 39:627, 1977.

32. Sanderson, J.E., Traill, T.A., St. John Sutton, M.G., Brown, D.J., Gibson, D.G., and Goodwin, J.F.: Left ventricular relaxation and filling in hypertrophic cardiomyopathy: an echocardiographic study. Br. Heart J., 40:596, 1978.

33. St. John Sutton, M.G., Tajik, A.J., Gibson, D.G., Brown, D.J., Seward, J.B., and Giuliani, E.R.: Echocardiographic assessment of left ventricular filling and septal and posterior wall dynamics in idiopathic hypertrophic subaortic stenosis. Circulation, 57:512, 1978.

34. Dale, H.T., Popio, K.A., and Shah, P.M.: Left ventricular emptying in obstructive and nonobstructive idiopathic hypertrophic subaortic stenosis. Circulation (Suppl. II), 58:121, 1978. (Abstract)

35. Hutchins, G.M., and Bulkley, B.H.: Catenoid shape of the interventricular septum: possible cause of idiopathic hypertrophic subaortic stenosis. Circulation, 58:392, 1978.

36. Bommer, W., Neumann, A., Mason, D.T., and DeMaria, A.N.: In vivo evaluation of the catenoid shape of the interventricular septum in idiopathic hypertrophic subaortic stenosis with two-dimensional echocardiography. Am. J. Cardiol., 43:347, 1979. (Abstract)

37. Nichiyama, S., Yamaguchi, H., Ishimura, T., Nagasaki, F., Takatsu, F., Umeda, T., and Machii, K.: Echocardiographic features of apical hypertrophic cardiomyopathy. J. Cardiogr., 8:177, 1978.

37a. Yamaguchi, H., Ishimura, T., Nishiyama, S., Nagasaki, F., Nakanishi, S., Takatsu, F., Nishijo, T., Umeda, T., and Machii, K.: Hypertrophic nonobstructive cardiomyopathy with giant negative T waves (apical hypertrophy): ventriculographic and echocardiographic features in 30 patients. Am. J. Cardiol., 44:401, 1979.

38. King, J.F., DeMaria, A.N., Reis, R.L., Bolton, M.R., Dunn, M.I., and Mason, D.T.: Echocardiographic assessment of idiopathic hypertrophic subaortic stenosis. Chest, 64:723, 1973.

39. Popp, R.L. and Harrison, D.C.: Ultrasound in the diagnosis and evaluation of therapy of idiopathic hypertrophic subaortic stenosis. Circulation, 40:905, 1969.

39a. Doi, Y.L., McKenna, W.J., Gehrke, J., Oakley, C.M., and Goodwin, J.F.: M-mode echocardiography in hypertrophic cardiomyopathy: diagnostic criteria and prediction of obstruction. Am. J. Cardiol., 45:6, 1980.

40. Pridie, R.B. and Oakley, C.M.: Mechanism of mitral regurgitation in hypertrophic obstructive cardiomyopathy. Br. Heart J., 32:203, 1970.

41. Shah, P.M., Gramiak, R., and Kramer, D.H.: Ultrasound localization of left ventricular outflow obstruction in hypertrophic obstructive cardiomyopathy. Circulation, 40:3, 1969.

42. Shah, P.M., Gramiak, R., Adelman, A.G., and Wigle, E.D.: Role of echocardiography in diagnostic and hemodynamic assessment of hypertrophic subaortic stenosis. Circulation, 44:891, 1971.

43. Henry, W.L., Clark, C.E., Griffith, J.M., and Epstein, S.E.: Mechanism of left ventricular outflow obstruction in patients with obstructive asymmetric septal hypertrophy (idiopathic hypertrophic subaortic stenosis). Am. J. Cardiol., 35:337, 1975.

43a. Gustavson, A., Liedholm, H., and Tylen, U.: Hypertrophic cardiomyopathy: a correlation between echocardiography, angiographic, and hemodynamic findings. Ann. Radiol. (Paris), 20:419, 1977.

44. Henry, W.L., Clark, C.E., Glancy, D.L., and Epstein, S.E.: Echocardiographic measurement of the left ventricular outflow gradient in idiopathic hypertrophic subaortic stenosis. N. Engl. J. Med., 288:989, 1973.

45. Feizi, O. and Emanuel, R.: Echocardiographic

spectrum of hypertrophic cardiomyopathy. Br. Heart J., 37:1286, 1975.

46. King, J.F., DeMaria, A.N., Miller, R.R., Hilliard, G.K., Zelis, R., and Mason, D.T.: Markedly abnormal mitral valve motion without simultaneous intraventricular pressure gradient due to uneven mitral-septal contact in idiopathic hypertrophic subaortic stenosis. Am. J. Cardiol., 34:360, 1974.

47. Bolton, M.R., Jr., King, J.F., Polumbo, R.A., Mason, D., Pugh, D.M., Reis, R.L., and Dunn, M.I.: The effects of operation on the echocardiographic features of idiopathic hypertrophic subaortic stenosis. Circulation, 50:897, 1974.

48. Hardarson, T. and Curiel, R.: Study of clinical pharmacology of hypertrophic obstructive cardiomyopathy by noninvasive diagnostic investigations. Br. Heart J. 35:865, 1973.

49. Shah, P.M., Gramiak, R., Adelman, A.G., and Wigle, E.D.: Echocardiographic assessment of the effects of surgery and propranolol on the dynamics of outflow obstruction and hyperpranolol on the dynamics of outflow obstruction and hypertrophic subaortic stenosis. Circulation, 45:516, 1972.

50. Angoff, G.H., Wistran, D., Sloss, L.J., Markis, J.E., Come, P.C., Zoll, P.M., and Cohn, P.F.: Value of a noninvasively induced ventricular extrasystole during echocardiographic and phonocardiographic assessment of patients with idiopathic hypertrophic subaortic stenosis. Am. J. Cardiol., 42:919, , 1978.

51. Tajik, A.J., Gau, G.T., and Schattenberg, T.T.: Echocardiographic pseudo IHSS pattern in atrial septal defect. Chest, 62:324, 1972.

52. Greenwald, J., Yap, J.F., Franklin, M., and Lichtman, A.M.: Echocardiographic mitral systolic motion in left ventricular aneurysm. Br. Heart J., 37:684, 1975.

53. Maron, B.J., Gottidiener, J.S., Roberts, W.C., Henry, W.L., Savage, D.D., and Epstein, S.E.: Left ventricular outflow tract obstruction due to systolic anterior motion of the anterior mitral leaflet in patients with concentric left ventricular hypertrophy. Circulation, 57:527, 1978.

54. Levisman, J.A.: Systolic anterior motion of the mitral valve due to hypovolemia and anemia. Chest, 70:687, 1976.

55. Buckley, B.H. and Fortuin, N.J.: Systolic anterior motion of the mitral valve without asymmetric septal hypertrophy. Chest, 69:694, 1976.

56. Kronzon, I. and Glassman, E.: Mitral ring calcification in idiopathic hypertrophic subaortic stenosis. Am. J. Cardiol., 42:60, 1978.

57. Crawford, M.H., Groves, B.M., and Horwitz, L.D.: Dynamic left ventricular outflow tract obstruction and systolic anterior motion of the mitral valve in the absence of asymmetric septal hypertrophy. Am. J. Med., 65:703, 1978.

58. Mintz, G.S., Kotler, M.N., Segal, B.L., and Parry, W.R.: Systolic anterior motion of the mitral valve in the absence of asymmetric septal hypertrophy. Circulation, 57:256, 1978.

59. Boughner, D.R., Rakowski, H., and Wigle, E.D.: Mitral valve systolic anterior motion in the absence of hypertrophic cardiomyopathy. Circulation, 58:916, 1978.

59a. Drobinsky, G., Botreau-Roussel, P., and Grosgogeat, Y.: An echocardiographic trap: protosystolic advance of the mitral valve in normal subjects. Nouv. Presse Med., 5:1914, 1976.

60. Gardin, J.M., Stephanides, L.M., Kordecki, S., and Talano, J.V.: Systolic anterior motion in the absence of asymmetrical septal hypertrophy: a buckling phenomenon of the chordae tendinae. Circulation (Suppl. II), 58:121, 1978. (Abstract)

60a. Thompson, R., Ahmed, M., Pridie, R., and Yacoub, M.: Hypertrophic cardiomyopathy after aortic valve replacement. Am. J. Cardiol., 45:33, 1980.

61. Wei, J.Y., Weiss, J.L., and Bulkley, B.H.: Nonspecificity of the echocardiographic diagnosis of idiopathic hypertrophic subaortic stenosis: a clinicopathologic study. Circulation (Suppl. II), 58:237, 1978. (Abstract)

62. Harrison, E.E., Sbar, S.S., Martin, H., and Pupello, D.F.: Coexisting right and left hypertrophic subvalvular stenosis and fixed left ventricular outflow obstruction due to aortic valve stenosis. Am. J. Cardiol., 40:133, 1977.

63. Bloom, K.R., Meyer, R.A., Bove, K.E., and Kaplan, S.: The association of fixed and dynamic left ventricular outflow obstruction. Am. Heart J., 89:586, 1975.

64. Krueger, S.K., Hofschire, P.J., and Forker, A.D.: Echocardiographic features of combined hypertrophic and membranous subvalvular aortic stenosis: a case report. J. Clin. Ultrasound, 4:31, 1976.

64a. Hanrath, P., von Essen, R., Bleifeld, W., and Effert, S.: Idiopathic hypertrophic subaortic stenosis in aortic valve disease—diagnosis using echocardiography. Z. Kardiol., 65:964, 1976.

65. Aziz, K.U., Paul, M.H., Idriss, F.S., Wilson, A.D., and Muster, A.J.: Clinical manifestations of dynamic left ventricular outflow tract stenosis in infants with d-transposition of the great arteries with intact ventricular septum. Am. J. Cardiol., 44:290, 1979.

66. DiSessa, T.G., Childs, W., Ti, C., and Friedman, W.F.: Systolic anterior motion of the mitral valve in a one day old infant with d-transposition of the great vessels. J. Clin. Ultrasound, 6:186, 1978.

67. Yokota, Y., Kawanishi, H., Ohmori, K., Oda, A., Inoh, T., and Fukuzaki, H.: Studies on systolic anterior motion (SAM) pattern in idiopathic mitral valve prolapse by echocardiography. J. Cardiogr., 9:259, 1979.

68. Come, P.C., Bulkley, B.H., Goodman, Z.D., Hutchins, G.M., Pitt, B., and Fortuin, N.J.: Hypercontractile cardiac states simulating hypertrophic cardiomyopathy. Circulation, 55:901, 1977.

68a. Gutgesell, H.P., Mullins, C.E., Gillette, P.C., et al.: Transient hypertrophic subaortic stenosis in infants of diabetic mothers. J. Pediatr., 89:120, 1976.

69. Jinnouchi, J., Yoshioka, H., Koga, Y., and Toshima, H.: Mechanism of outflow obstruction in hypertrophic cardiomyopathy with asymmetric septal hypertrophy: two-dimensional echocardiographic study. J. Cardiogr., 7:23, 1977.

70. Kanaya, H., Genda, A., Funazu, T., Ishise, S., Kawasaki, S., Saiki, S., Mori, K., Oiwake, H., Nakayama, A., Hamada, M., and Takeda, R.: Clinical studies of patients showing so-called "SAM" (systolic anterior movement) by echocardiography. J. Cardiogr., 6:603, 1976.

71. Rodger, J.C.: Motion of mitral apparatus in hypertrophic cardiomyopathy with obstruction. Br. Heart J., 38:732, 1976.

72. Feigenbaum, H.: Clinical applications of echocardiography. Prog. Cardiovasc. Dis., 14:531, 1972.

73. Gramiak, R. and Shah, P.M.: Cardiac ultrasonog-

raphy: a review of current applications. Radiol. Clin. North Am., 9:469, 1971.

74. Chahine, R.A., Raizner, A.E., Nelson, J., Winters, W.L., Miller, R.R., and Luchi, R.J.: Midsystolic closure of aortic valve in hypertrophic cardiomyopathy: echocardiographic and angiographic correlation. Am. J. Cardiol., 43:17, 1979.

75. Joyner, C.R., Jr., Harrison, F.S., Jr., and Gruber, J.W.: Diagnosis of hypertrophic subaortic stenosis with a Doppler velocity flow detector. Ann. Intern. Med., 74:692, 1971.

76. Kinoshita, N., Nimura, Y., Miyatake, K., Nagata, S., Sakakibara, H., Hayashi, T., Asao, M., Terao, Y., and Matsuo, H.: Studies on flow patterns in the aortic arch in cases with hypertrophic cardiomyopathy using pulsed ultrasonic Doppler technique. J. Cardiogr., 8:325, 1978.

77. Boughner, D.R., Rakowski, H., and Wigle, E.D.: Idiopathic hypertrophic subaortic stenosis: combined Doppler and echocardiographic assessment. Circulation (Suppl. II), 54:191, 1976. (Abstract)

78. Cardiel, E.A., Alonso, M., Delcan, J.L., and Menarguez, L.: Echocardiographic sign of right-sided hypertrophic obstructive cardiomyopathy. Br. Heart J., 40:1321, 1978.

79. Brik, H., Meller, J., Bahler, A.S., Herman, M.V., and Teichholz, L.E.: Systolic anterior motion of the tricuspid valve in idiopathic hypertrophic subaortic stenosis. J. Clin. Ultrasound, 6:121, 1978.

80. Corya, B.C., Feigenbaum, H., Rasmussen, S., and Black, M.J.: Echocardiographic features of congestive cardiomyopathy compared with normal subjects and patients with coronary artery disease. Circulation, 49:1153, 1974.

81. Fujino, T., Ito, M., Kanaya, S., Imanishi, S., Fujino, M., Yamada, K., Hamanaka, Y., Kinoshita, R., Oya, I., and Mashiba, H.: Echocardiographic comparison of acute myocarditis with congestive cardiomyopathy. J. Cardiogr., 7:39, 1977.

82. Ghafour, A.S. and Gutgesell, H.P.: Echocardiographic evaluation of left ventricular function in children with congestive cardiomyopathy. Am. J. Cardiol., 44:1332, 1979.

83. Levisman, J.A.: Echocardiographic diagnosis of mitral regurgitation in congestive cardiomyopathy. Am. Heart J., 93:33, 1977.

84. Fortuin, N.J. and Pawsey, C.G.K.: The evaluation of left ventricular function by echocardiography. Am. J. Med., 63:1, 1977.

84a. Godley, R.W. et al.: Relation of incomplete mitral leaflet closure to the site of dyssynergy in patients with papillary muscle dysfunction. Circulation (Suppl. II), 60:204, 1979. (Abstract)

85. Child, J.S., Krivokapich, J., and Abbasi, A.S.: Increased right ventricular wall thickness on echocardiography in amyloid infiltrative cardiomyopathy. Am. J. Cardiol., 44:1391, 1979.

86. Rakowski, H., Boughner, D.R., Sole, M.J., and Wigle, E.D.: The echocardiographic diagnosis of amyloid cardiomyopathy. Circulation (Suppl. II), 54:84, 1976. (Abstract)

87. Giles, T.D., Le'on-Galindo, J., and Burch, G.E.: Echocardiographic findings in amyloid cardiomyopathy. South Med. J., 71:1393, 1978.

88. Child, J.S., Levisman, J.A., Abbasi, A.S., and MacAlpin, R.N.: Echocardiographic manifestations of infiltrative cardiomyopathy: a report of seven cases due to amyloid. Chest, 70:726, 1976.

88a. Chiaramida, S.A., Goldman, M.A., Zema, M.J., Pizzarello, R.A., and Goldberg, H.M.: Real-time cross-sectional echocardiographic diagnosis of infiltrative cardiomyopathy due to amyloid. J. Clin. Ultrasound, 8:58, 1980.

89. Borer, J.S., Henry, W.J., and Epstein, S.E.: Echocardiographic observations in patients with systemic infiltrative disease involving the heart. Am. J. Cardiol., 39:184, 1977.

90. Eggebrecht, R.F. and Kleiger, R.E.: Echocardiographic patterns in scleroderma. Chest, 71:47, 1977.

91. Smith, J.W., Clements, P.J., Levisman, J., Furst, D., and Ross, M.: Echocardiographic features of progressive systemic sclerosis (PSS): correlation with hemodynamic and postmortem studies. Am. J. Med., 66:28, 1979.

92. Gottdiener, J.S., Moutsopoulos, H.M., and Decker, J.L.: Echocardiographic identification of cardiac abnormality in scleroderma and related disorders. Am. J. Med., 66:391, 1979.

93. Noda, H., Nakamura, K., Komatsu, Y., Nagai, Y., Shimizu, K., Adachi, F., Kikuchi, N., Kondo, M., and Hirosawa, K.: Echocardiogram of five cases with secondary cardiomyopathy. J. Cardiogr., 8:191, 1978.

94. Henry, W.L., Nienhuis, A.W., Wiener, M., Miller, D.R., Canale, V.C., and Piomelli, S.: Echocardiographic abnormalities in patients with transfusion-dependent anemia and secondary myocardial iron deposition. Am. J. Med., 64:547, 1978.

95. Mir, M.A.: Evidence for non-infiltrative cardiomyopathy in acute leukaemia and lymphoma: a clinical and echocardiographic study. Br. Heart J., 40:725, 1978.

96. Lorell, B., Alderman, E.L., and Mason, J.W.: Cardiac sarcoidosis. Am. J. Cardiol., 42:143, 1978.

97. Rees, A., Elbl, F., Minhas, K., and Solinger, R.: Echocardiographic evidence of outflow tract obstruction in Pompe's disease (glycogen storage disease of the heart). Am. J. Cardiol., 37:1103, 1976.

98. Mather, H.M., Boyd, M.J., and Jenkins, J.S.: Heart size and function in acromegaly. Br. Heart J., 41:697, 1979.

99. Smallridge, R.C., Rajfer, S., Davia, J., and Schaaf, M.: Acromegaly and the heart: an echocardiographic study. Am. J. Med., 66:22, 1979.

100. Shimada, H., Inoue, M., Tamura, T., Ishihara, T., Kanemitsu, H., and Ishikawa, K.: Echocardiograms in progressive muscle dystrophy. J. Cardiogr., 8:689, 1978.

101. Van der Hausaert, L.G. and Dumoulin, M.: Hypertrophic cardiomyopathy in Friedreich's ataxia. Br. Heart J., 38:1291, 1976.

102. Hess, O.M., Turina, M., Senning, A., Goebel, N.H., Scholer, Y., and Krayenbuehl, H.P.: Pre- and postoperative findings in patients with endomyocardial fibrosis. Br. Heart J., 40:406, 1978.

103. Chew, C.Y.C., Ziady, G.M., Raphael, M.J., Nellen, M., and Oakley, C.M.: Primary restrictive cardiomyopathy: non-trophical endomyocardial fibrosis and hypereosinophilic heart disease. Br. Heart J., 39:399, 1977.

104. Eterovic, I., Angelini, P., Leachman, R., and Cooley, D.A.: Obliterative restrictive endomyocardial fibrosis: a surgical approach. Cardiovasc. Dis., 6:66, 1979.

CHAPTER 10

Pericardial Disease

PERICARDIAL EFFUSION

Detection of Pericardial Fluid

The technique that probably provided much of the impetus for the development of echocardiography in the United States was the detection of pericardial effusion.[1,2] Because a harmless, bedside examination for pericardial effusion has obvious clinical advantages, this technique has become one of the most popular applications of diagnostic ultrasound. [3-13,13a] The theory behind the echocardiographic technique for the detection of pericardial effusion is simple. Normally, the pericardial sac is only a potential space, and the heart is in direct contact with the surrounding structures. Echocardiographically, the anterior right ventricular wall is in direct contact with the stationary chest wall echoes, and the posterior left ventricular wall is in contact with the posterior pericardium and pleura. In the presence of pericardial effusion, this potential space fills with relatively echo-free fluid, and echocardiographic separation occurs between the anterior right ventricular wall and the chest wall[14] and between the posterior left ventricular wall and the posterior pericardium.[1]

Figure 10-1 shows a typical M-mode echocardiogram of a patient with pericardial effusion. The ultrasonic beam is directed through the left ventricular cavity at the same level at which left ventricular and right ventricular dimensions are made. The relatively echo-free space from the pericardial fluid (PE) can be seen between the chest wall and the anterior right ventricular wall

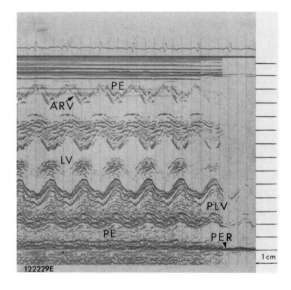

Fig. 10-1. M-mode echocardiogram of a patient with pericardial effusion. The pericardial effusion (PE) can be seen above the anterior right ventricular wall (ARV) and behind the posterior left ventricular wall (PLV). LV = left ventricle; PER = pericardium.

(ARV) and between the posterior left ventricular wall (PLV) and the pericardium (PER).

Although the fact that the echo-free space posterior to the left ventricular wall represents pericardial fluid has been accepted for many years, there has been relatively little direct proof. Figure 10-2 demonstrates a contrast echocardiographic study in a patient undergoing a therapeutic pericardiocentesis. A saline solution was injected through a needle in the pericardial sac, and contrast

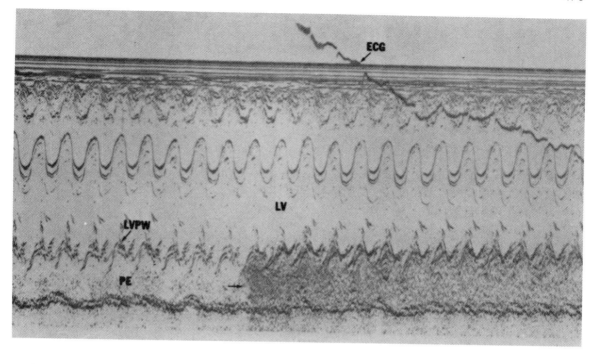

Fig. 10–2. Echocardiogram taken during a pericardiocentesis at which time contrast was injected into the pericardial sac. The echo-producing contrast *(arrow)* can be seen in the space occupied by the pericardial effusion (PE). LV = left ventricle; LVPW = left ventricular posterior wall. (From Chandraratna, P.A.N., et al.: Echocardiographic contrast studies during pericardiocentesis. Ann. Intern. Med., 87:199, 1977.)

echoes (arrow) were seen originating within the pericardial space.[15] This technique may be occasionally useful in pericardiocentesis to help identify the location of the needle. Occasionally, with a grossly bloody pericardial effusion it is difficult to determine whether one is in the pericardial space or within the cardiac chamber. Contrast echocardiography may assist in determining this differential point.

When the ultrasonic technique for detecting posterior pericardial effusion was first described, much attention was given to the fact that the posterior pericardial echo loses its normal cardiac motion in the presence of pericardial effusion.[1,2,5,16] This criterion was particularly important when few echoes were recorded from the posterior left ventricular wall. This observation is still valid with our newer techniques. The pericardial fluid acts as a buffer between the heart and the posterior pericardium, and the normal motion exhibited by the pericardium is damped and in most cases eliminated. However, in patients with small effusions or with vigorously beating hearts, the pericardial echo may still exhibit some motion.

The term relatively echo-free must be used to describe the pericardial fluid. Figure 10–1 shows that the pericardial fluid does produce echoes if the gain is sufficiently high. This echocardiogram demonstrates why proper controls are critical in the echocardiographic examination for pericardial effusion. As the gain is reduced, the echo-free space from the pericardial fluid (on the right of the tracing) is more obvious. As the gain is increased (left of the recording) the echoes may actually fill in the pericardial space, and the fluid may not be as obvious. Thus alterations in the gain or damping is a common technique for the detection of pericardial effusion. The "switch gain" modification has been advocated for this particular application.[17]

As with all M-mode echocardiographic examinations, there is a significant advantage to moving the transducer and obtaining an M-mode scan when examining for pericardial effusion.[18] Figure 10–3 shows an M-mode scan of the same patient in Figure 10–1. As one moves the transducer, the posterior echo-free space uniformly decreases as the ultrasonic beam traverses the base of the heart and the left atrium (LA). Usually the echo-free space is totally obliterated as the beam traverses the junction between the left ventricle and the left atrium (Fig. 10–4). However, occasionally one records fluid behind the left atrium even at the level of the aortic valve.[19-21] Figure 10–5 is another echocardiogram of the same patient in Figures 10–1 and 10–3. The ultrasonic beam is now directed at the aorta and left atrium, and one can detect an echo-free space from the pericardial fluid behind the left atrium.

One can detect pericardial effusion with the transducer in the subcostal area as well as along the left sternal border. Figure 10–6 shows an M-mode echocardiogram taken with the transducer along the left sternal

border in a patient with a large pericardial effusion. Although the echo from the posterior pericardium is barely visible in this photograph, the large echo-free spaces anterior and posterior to the pericardial effusion (PE) can be readily appreciated. Figure 10–7 shows a similar examination of the same patient with the transducer in the subcostal position. Again, a large echo-free space between the chest wall and anterior right ventricular wall (ARV) can be seen. The echo-free space behind the posterior left ventricular wall (PLV) is also demonstrated. The posterior pericardium is faintly visible at the posterior edge of the photograph.

Although the echocardiographic technique for the detection of pericardial effusion is time-proven as one of the basic uses of this examination, many technical details as well as potential pitfalls must be recognized. The effect of varying the gain has been mentioned. In addition, the direction and location of the transducer can also influence the

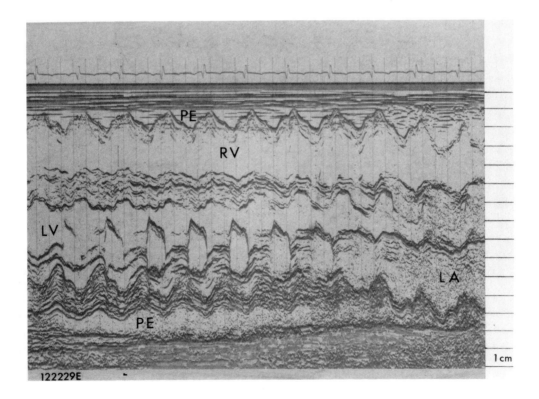

Fig. 10–3. M-mode scan of a patient with pericardial effusion. The pericardial effusion (PE) behind the left ventricle (LV) decreases as the ultrasonic beam is directed toward the left atrium (LA). RV = right ventricle.

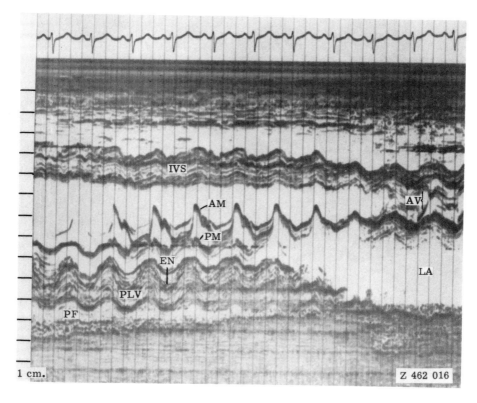

Fig. 10–4.   M-mode scan of a patient with pericardial effusion demonstrating how the pericardial fluid (PF) behind the posterior left ventricular wall (PLV) disappears as the ultrasonic beam is directed toward the left atrium (LA). IVS = interventricular septum: AV = aortic valve; AM = anterior mitral leaflet; PM = posterior mitral leaflet; EN = posterior left ventricular endocardium.

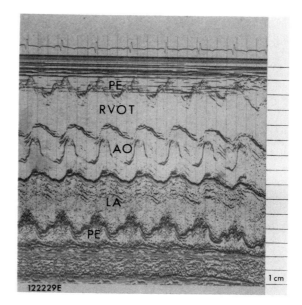

Fig. 10–5.   M-mode echocardiogram through the aorta (AO) and left atrium in a patient with pericardial effusion. The pericardial effusion (PE) is anterior to the right ventricular outflow tract (RVOT) and also posterior to the left atrium (LA).

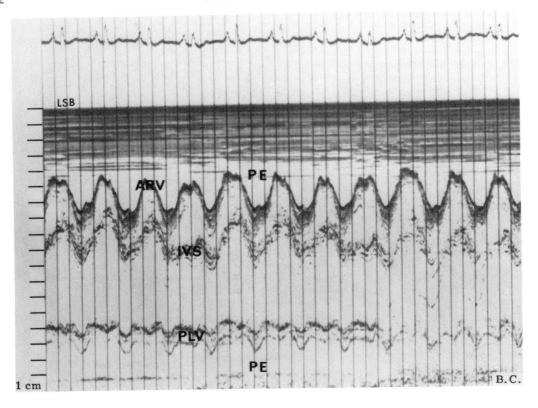

Fig. 10–6.   Echocardiogram taken with the transducer along the left sternal border (LSB) in a patient with a large pericardial effusion. The posterior pericardial echo is not recorded on this tracing. PE = pericardial effusion; ARV = anterior right ventricular wall; IVS = interventricular septum; PLV = posterior left ventricular wall.

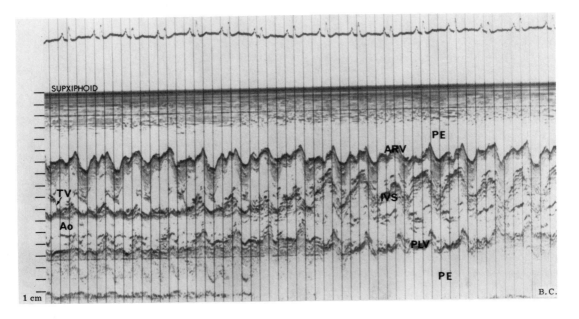

Fig. 10–7.   Another echocardiogram from the patient in Figure 10–6 with the transducer now in the subcostal or subxiphoid position. The large anterior pericardial effusion (PE) can again be seen. There is also a large echo-free space from the pericardial effusion behind the posterior left ventricular wall (PLV). ARV = anterior right ventricular wall; IVS = interventricular septum; TV = tricuspid valve; AO = aorta.

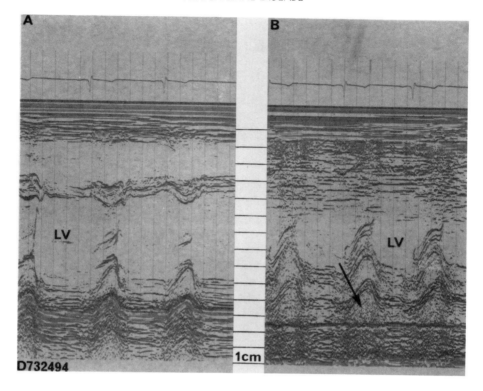

Fig. 10–8.   M-mode echocardiograms demonstrating how a relatively echo-free space can be seen behind the posterior left ventricular wall when the transducer is pointed medially. *A,* The correct examination reveals the left ventricle (LV) with no echo-free space posterior to it. *B,* With medial angulation of the transducer, however, a relatively echo-free space *(arrow)* is visible behind the left ventricle.

echocardiographic diagnosis. A common error is for the echocardiographer to direct the ultrasonic beam too medially.[2,16] Figure 10–8 illustrates how one can artifactually produce a relatively echo-free space behind echoes originating from the posterior left ventricular wall. The proper echocardiographic examination is noted in Figure 10–8A. There is no evidence of pericardial effusion. However, when the transducer is purposefully directed medially (Fig. 10–8B), the artifactual pericardial effusion can be noted (arrow). The etiology of this technical false positive has never been adequately studied, although, judging from our experience with two-dimensional echocardiography, the space behind the left ventricular echoes could be originating from a portion of the right ventricle as the beam traverses the posterior-medial interventricular septum. The space could also be originating from the coronary sinus.

One must be careful about the diagnosis of pericardial effusion with only an echo-free space between the chest wall and the anterior right ventricular wall. Figure 10–9 shows a patient with an echo-free space between the anterior right ventricular wall (ARV) and the chest wall. The patient had no evidence of pericardial effusion. This false effusion may be due to an epicardial fat pad. In addition, the heart is not adherent to the chest wall and some separation in systole is probably usual. Because of this problem we have been reluctant to call the presence of pericardial effusion solely on the basis of an anterior echo-free space. Some evidence of posterior effusion should also be present.

Another potentially confusing echocardiogram is one that reveals a relatively echo-free space from the descending aorta. This structure passes posterior to the heart in the vicinity of the junction between the left atrium and left ventricle. The echocardio-

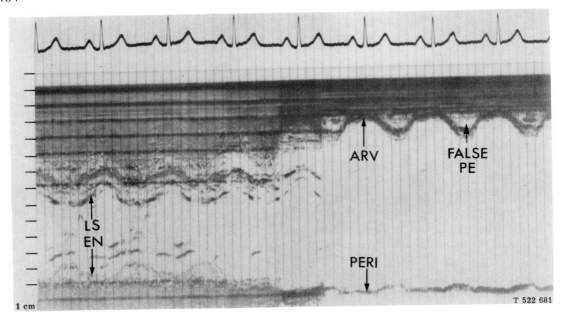

Fig. 10–9. Echocardiogram of a patient with no evidence of pericardial effusion who demonstrates a relatively echo-free space between the anterior right ventricular wall (ARV) and the chest wall. False PE = false pericardial effusion; LS = left side of septum; EN = posterior left ventricular endocardium; PERI = pericardium.

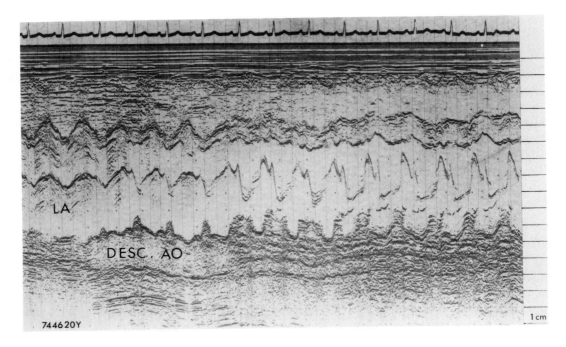

Fig. 10–10. M-mode scan demonstrating the relatively echo-free space originating in the descending aorta (DESC AO) behind the left atrium (LA).

graphic appearance of this vessel has been recently identified primarily with the assistance of two-dimensional echocardiography. Figure 10–10 shows an M-mode recording whereby the echo-free space from the descending aorta is evident. One can easily see how such a tracing might be confused with pericardial effusion. A two-dimensional study should readily identify the descending aorta (Fig. 10–11) and hence avoid any confusion.

Most false-positive and false-negative echocardiograms for pericardial effusion are due to faulty technique. However, a few false positives and false negatives in the lit-

erature warrant special consideration. The first reported false negative was in a patient with a loculated effusion on the right side of the heart.[16] In another patient with loculated effusion due to adhesions, the proper diagnosis was only obtained with an M-mode scan.[18] Another reported false negative was apparently in a patient with acute hemopericardium and a clot-filled pericardial sac.[22] The nature of the disease was apparently not revealed on the echocardiogram. In one reported patient with a false-positive effusion, there was a giant left atrium.[23] This massive chamber, visible behind the left ventricle, gave the appearance of an echo-free space posterior to the left ventricle. Another false-positive effusion was reported secondary to a foramen of Morgagni hiatus hernia. In this patient there was an echo-free space anterior to the right ventricle.[24]

A number of articles have noted confusing echocardiograms of patients with extracardiac tumors or masses.[25–28] Many of these echocardiograms gave superficial appearances of pericardial effusion. However, on close examination none showed classic signs of pericardial fluid.

Although two-dimensional echocardiography is not essential for the qualitative diagnosis of pericardial effusion, this technique can be particularly helpful in some of the confusing situations. This spatially oriented technique can frequently obviate the false positives and false negatives reported in the literature that are due to tumors or loculation.[29,30] Figure 10–12 shows a long-axis and short-axis two-dimensional echocardiogram of a patient with a large pericardial effusion. The effusion (PE) is primarily visible posteriorly in the long-axis study and both posteriorly and laterally in the short-axis examination. The short-axis study is particularly helpful in showing how the fluid tends to collect posteriorly in the posterior cul-de-sac. The amount of fluid anterior and medial to the heart is significantly less.

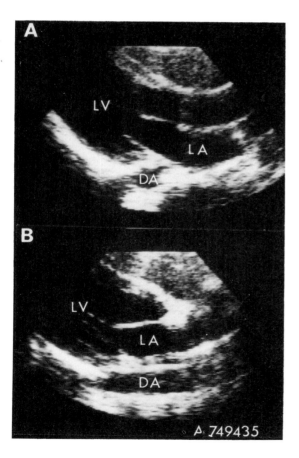

Fig. 10–11. Two-dimensional echocardiograms demonstrating the descending aorta. A, The echo-free space from the descending aorta (DA) is posterior to the junction between the left ventricle (LV) and the left atrium (LA) in the parasternal long-axis view. B, By changing the plane of the examination to render it parallel to the descending aorta, one can appreciate the length of the descending aorta.

Differentiation Between Pericardial Effusion and Pleural Effusion

Fortunately, left pleural effusion is not a frequent problem in the echocardiographic

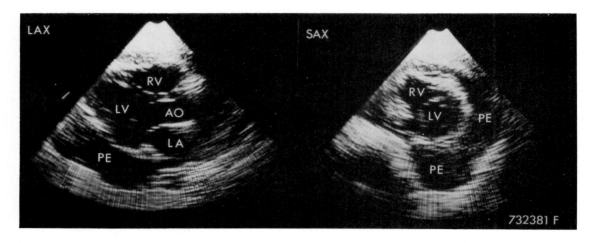

Fig. 10–12.   Long-axis (LAX) and short-axis (SAX) two-dimensional echocardiograms of a patient with a large pericardial effusion. The pericardial effusion (PE) can be seen accumulating posteriorly and laterally. RV = right ventricle; LV = left ventricle; AO = aorta; LA = left atrium.

diagnosis of pericardial effusion, because it usually accumulates along the pleural surface rather than in the retrocardiac space. However, retrocardiac pleural effusions can occur (Fig. 10–13). This patient has a large relatively echo-free space posterior to the left ventricular wall and one might interpret this space as indicative of pericardial effusion. Several features in this echocardiogram should exclude the possibility of pericardial effusion. First, the posterior echo-free space is large and thus represents an unusually large pericardial effusion. Such a large posterior effusion occurring without some evidence of anterior pericardial effusion would be rare. There is no echo-free area anterior to the right ventricle.

M-mode scanning can help distinguish pleural effusion from pericardial effusion. Figure 10–14 demonstrates an M-mode scan in the patient with a large pleural effusion. The echo-free space behind the left ventricular wall is again noted. As the ultrasonic beam is directed toward the left atrium, there is a rather sudden cessation of the echo-free space behind the heart. This type of scan should be easily distinguished from one in which there is a gradual decrease in the echo-free space owing to pericardial effusion (Figs. 10–3, 10–4).

Pericardial and pleural effusion can occasionally occur together. Figure 10–15 shows

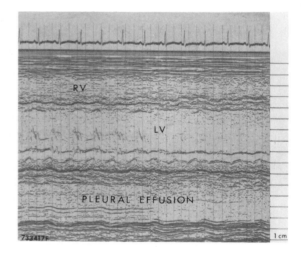

Fig. 10–13.   M-mode echocardiogram of a patient with a large pleural effusion. RV = right ventricle; LV = left ventricle.

a patient in such a situation. The key to the diagnosis of both pericardial effusion and pleural fluid is to find an echo between the two echo-free spaces that arises from the pericardium. As the ultrasonic beam is directed toward the base of the heart, the pericardial echo blends into the posterior left atrial wall (PLA), whereas the pleural space persists awhile. The pleural fluid seems to end abruptly, and the pleural echo

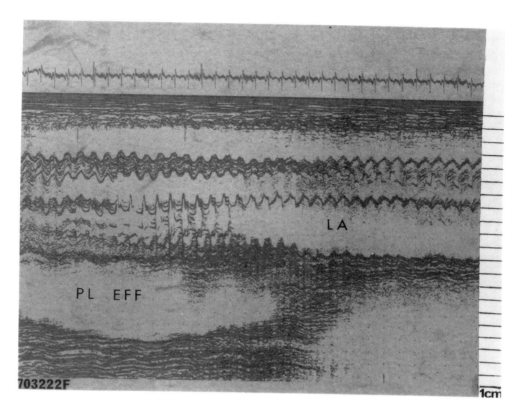

Fig. 10–14. M-mode scan of a patient with a large pleural effusion. The echo-free space from the pleural effusion (PL EFF) ends rather abruptly as the ultrasonic beam is directed toward the left atrium (LA).

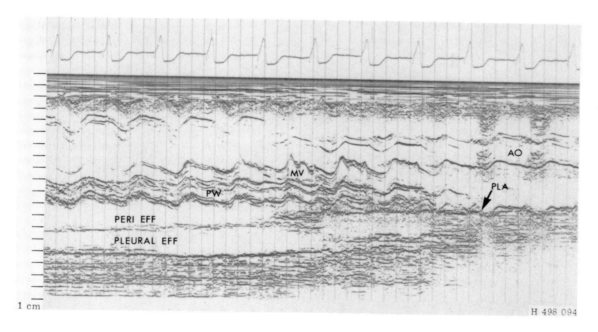

Fig. 10–15. M-mode scan of a patient with pericardial and pleural effusions. The large echo-free space behind the posterior left ventricular wall (PW) is divided by an echo thought to originate from the pericardium. The pericardial space virtually disappears at the posterior left atrial wall (PLA). The pleural space persists a while longer but ends rather abruptly at the junction of the left ventricle and left atrium. AO = aorta; MV = mitral valve. (From Chang, S.: M-mode Echocardiographic Techniques and Pattern Recognition. Philadelphia, Lea & Febiger, 1976.)

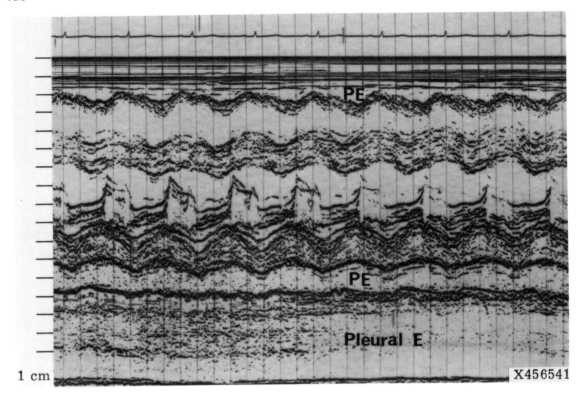

Fig. 10–16.   M-mode echocardiogram of a patient with pericardial and pleural effusions (E). In this patient the pericardial effusion (PE) can be seen both anteriorly and posteriorly.

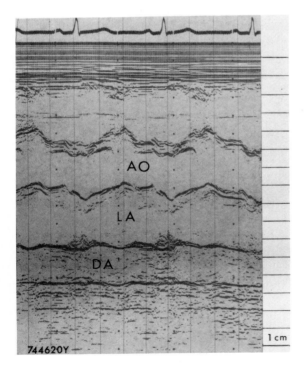

Fig. 10–17.   M-mode echocardiogram through the aorta (AO) and left atrium demonstrating the echo-free space of the descending aorta (DA) behind the left atrium (LA).

does not gradually meet the left atrial wall. Figure 10–16 shows yet another patient with pleural and pericardial effusion. The pericardial fluid (PE) can be seen anteriorly and posteriorly, and a large pleural effusion appears behind the posterior pericardial effusion. The echo from the pleura is barely visible at the edge of the photograph.

Two-dimensional echocardiography may also be helpful in differentiating pleural from pericardial effusion. It has been noted that pericardial effusion separates the descending aorta from the posterior cardiac structures.[30a] The separation can be appreciated in the short-axis or long-axis examinations. Pleural effusion does not produce any separation between the descending aorta and the posterior left ventricular wall.

Both pleural and pericardial effusion can be confused with the descending aorta. Figure 10–17 demonstrates an M-mode echocardiogram in which the descending aorta is recorded behind the left atrium. One might suspect a collection of fluid posterior to the left atrium. Figure 10–10 is the M-mode scan of the same patient and shows that the echo-free space is limited to the junction between the left atrium and the left ventricle. The two-dimensional echocardiogram (Fig. 10–11) could eliminate possible confusion.

Quantitation of Pericardial Fluid

There have been several efforts to use M-mode echocardiography to quantitate pericardial effusion.[10,31] Such efforts are difficult for the following reasons. First, the separation between the posterior pericardium and the posterior left ventricular epicardium varies according to the direction of the transducer. Figure 10–18 shows an M-mode scan of a patient with a large pericardial effusion. This scan shows that the amount of posterior echo-free space produced by the pericardial fluid increases as the ultrasonic beam moves toward the cardiac apex. If the ultrasonic beam is directed toward the apex, one assumes the presence of a larger effusion than when the beam is directed through the body of the left ventricle. In addition, the M-mode echocardiographic examination provides no information about the amount of pericardial fluid laterally or at the apex. Thus any attempt to quantitate pericardial fluid by way of M-mode echocardiography must consider potential error. Despite this limitation, one might still confidently predict that the patient in Figure 10–3 has a moderate pericardial effusion, as judged by the fact that the posterior left ventricular wall is never in contact with the pericardium and that even in the vicinity of the mitral valve echoes, there

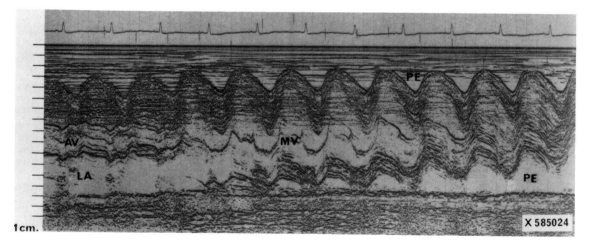

Fig. 10–18. M-mode scan of a patient with a large pericardial effusion. Note how the posterior echo-free space increases as the ultrasonic beam approaches the cardiac apex. The entire heart is moving vigorously, distorting the motion of all cardiac echoes. PE = pericardial effusion; MV = mitral valve; AV = aortic valve; LA = left atrium. (From Bonner, A.J., et al.: An unusual precordial pulse and sound associated with large pericardial effusion. Chest, 68:829, 1975.)

is a centimeter's separation between the posterior ventricular wall and the pericardium.[31] Figure 10–18 shows a considerably larger separation between the posterior and left ventricular wall and the pericardium as well as a large anterior pericardial effusion. One would thus anticipate a larger pericardial effusion. In contrast, the echocardiogram in Figure 10–19 shows a minor separation between the posterior left ventricular wall (EP) and the pericardium (PER) and another small separation anteriorly. Anything other than a relatively small pericardial effusion would be a surprise in this patient.

The patient in Figure 10–19 had renal failure, long-standing hypertension, and concentric left ventricular hypertrophy. Pericardial effusion is a fairly common finding in patients with long-standing renal disease[32] and in patients with heart failure.[33] The echocardiographic technique is so sensitive in detecting small effusions that it is sometimes difficult to distinguish a small effusion from the normal amount of pericardial fluid.[33]

A formula for quantitating the degree of pericardial effusion by way of M-mode echocardiography has been proposed.[31] This for-

mula requires a uniform distribution of the pericardial fluid and is based on quantitating the volume of the pericardial sac and subtracting the volume of the total heart. As previously noted, there are many limitations to quantitating pericardial effusion with M-mode echocardiography, and attempts to put a number on such an estimation would have considerable scatter.

Two-dimensional echocardiography is probably a more rational approach to quantitating pericardial effusion. Although M-mode echocardiography has better axial resolution and thus is superior in the qualitative diagnosis (especially in patients with small effusions), the spatial orientation inherent in two-dimensional echocardiography permits a better estimation of the distribution and amount of fluid. Figure 10–12 demonstrates the two-dimensional findings in a patient with a large pericardial effusion. The fluid is not evenly distributed around the heart. There is an accumulation of fluid posteriorly in the cul-de-sac and much less fluid is seen anteriorly. This type of recording demonstrates the difficulty in quantitating the pericardial fluid with M-mode echocardiography alone. Figure 10–20 shows

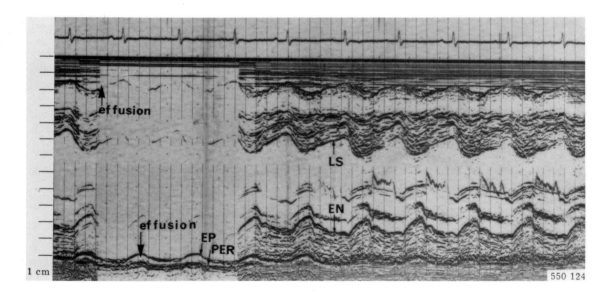

Fig. 10–19.   Echocardiogram of a patient with left ventricular hypertrophy and a small pericardial effusion. The small echo-free space can be seen both anteriorly and posteriorly. LS = left septum; EN = posterior ventricular endocardium; EP = posterior left ventricular epicardium; PER = pericardium. (From Chang, S.: M-mode Echocardiographic Techniques and Pattern Recognition. Philadelphia, Lea & Febiger, 1976.)

long- and short-axis two-dimensional echo-cardiograms of a patient with a small pericardial effusion. The pericardial space (PE) can be seen only posteriorly behind the left ventricle. Both long-axis and short-axis views show this location to be the only area of fluid collection. This recording is fairly comparable to an M-mode study and shows why M-mode echocardiography is quite accurate, especially in the case of small effusions.

In general, it is possible to quantitate or semiquantitate the amount of pericardial fluid by way of echocardiography. If the M-mode technique is used alone, then an M-mode scan should certainly be an important part of the examination.[34] Two-dimensional echocardiography probably

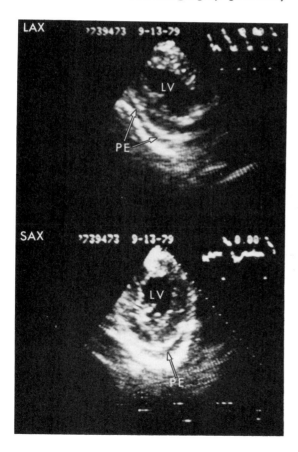

Fig. 10–20. Long-axis (LAX) and short-axis (SAX) two-dimensional echocardiograms of a patient with a small pericardial effusion. The small echo-free space from the pericardial effusion (PE) is visible posterior to the left ventricle (LV).

provides a better idea as to the quantitation of fluid, especially if it is large or loculated. No formula has been derived thus far for using two-dimensional echocardiography to quantitate the amount of pericardial fluid.

Cardiac Motion in Patients With Pericardial Effusion

Early use of echocardiography to detect pericardial effusion revealed that cardiac motion may be significantly altered in patients with large effusions.[35,35a] Figure 10–18 illustrates the excessive cardiac displacement that can occur with a large pericardial effusion. The most striking finding is wide excursion of the anterior right ventricular wall. In this echocardiogram, the amplitude of motion of the anterior right ventricular wall is approximately 2 cm. In addition, during most of the cardiac cycle the anterior and posterior cardiac walls are moving in similar directions. Thus the entire heart is being displaced within the massive pericardial fluid.

Occasionally, the cardiac motion may be so distorted that one may have difficulty making the proper diagnosis. Figure 10–21 shows a patient with a massive pericardial effusion that is principally anterior. The amount of cardiac motion distorts the pattern of all cardiac echoes. It is difficult to identify the various echoes. The fact that no intracardiac structures are recorded in this figure is partially because of this excessive cardiac motion and because much of the ultrasonic energy is reflected by the anterior wall of the heart. The echocardiogram with massive effusion and "swinging heart" can be confusing at times; if the echocardiographer is not alert to this possibility, the diagnosis can be missed. The person performing this examination is usually impressed with the excessive cardiac motion exhibited by the anterior cardiac wall.

If one analyzes the pattern of motion in Figure 10–21, it is noted that the motion of the cardiac echoes usually corresponds to two cardiac cycles. As a result, in most areas the QRS complex changes slightly as the position of the heart is altered by excessive motion.[35,36] Figure 10–22A shows another example of massive pericardial effusion whereby the entire heart is moving so that with every other depolarization it is in another position. The height of the electrocardiographic R wave clearly alternates. With the removal of a small amount of pericardial fluid (Fig. 10–22B), the alternating cardiac motion stops and the electrocardiographic alternation, or electrical alternans, also ceases. This echocardiographic finding in patients with pericardial effusion was instrumental in establishing the mechanism for the electrical alternation found in patients with pericardial effusion.[35–38]

Most of these patients, at least the adults, who exhibit this marked cardiac motion on the echocardiogram have a pericardial effusion due to a malignancy. Another cause could be chronic tuberculosis pericarditis, although this etiologic factor is not as common. A possible explanation why these conditions produce such excessive cardiac motion is because a "swinging heart" requires a large, chronically accumulated pericardial effusion and a minimum of adhesions. The bloody fluid with its possibly increased lubricity may permit the heart to move more freely. In children, swinging of the heart with pericardial effusion may be seen with benign viral pericarditis as well as with malignancies.

The excessive cardiac motion that occurs with pericardial effusion obviously distorts the echocardiogram.[39] Figure 10–23 shows an M-mode echocardiogram of a large pericardial effusion and excessive cardiac motion. With ventricular systole the entire heart moves posteriorly. Thus it is not surprising that the mitral valve also moves posteriorly. Some authors have indicated that such cardiac motion may distort the mitral valve motion to the point that a false-positive mitral valve prolapse can be produced (Fig. 10–23, arrow).[39–41] Even aortic valve and pulmonary valve motion have been distorted with large pericardial effusion.[40] The apparent paradoxical motion of the posterior left ventricular wall noted in Figure 10–23 could also be misinterpreted as ventricular dys-

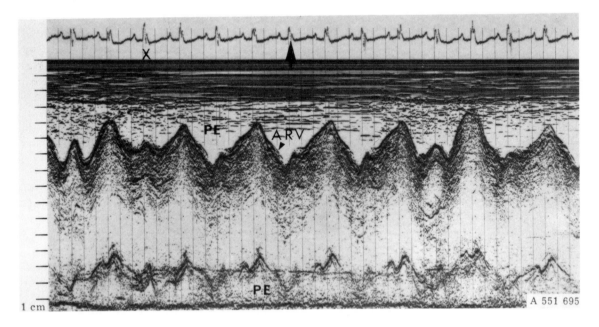

Fig. 10–21. M-mode echocardiogram of a patient with a massive pericardial effusion (PE). The anterior pericardial space is unusually large, and the echoes from the anterior right ventricular wall (ARV) are very echo-producing. The entire tracing is distorted because of excessive motion, and identification of the cardiac echoes can be confusing. The motion of the cardiac echoes is out of sequence to the electrocardiogram, which is distorted because of positional changes of the heart. The QRS marked X is different from that marked by an arrow. (From Chang, S.: M-mode Echocardiographic Techniques and Pattern Recognition. Philadelphia, Lea & Febiger, 1976.)

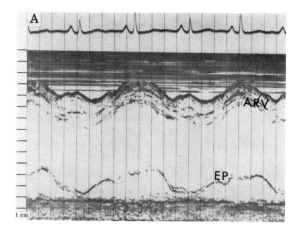

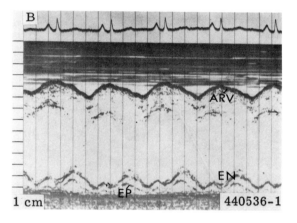

Fig. 10–22. Echocardiogram of a patient with massive pericardial effusion. *A*, The anterior right ventricular echo (ARV) and the posterior left ventricular epicardial echo (EP) move essentially in similar directions. The position of the heart is slightly different with each cardiac cycle. The corresponding electrocardiogram shows classic electrical alternation. *B*, Following removal of some of the pericardial effusion, the cardiac excursions are synchronous with each electrical depolarization. Electrical alternation is no longer present. EN = posterior left ventricular endocardium.

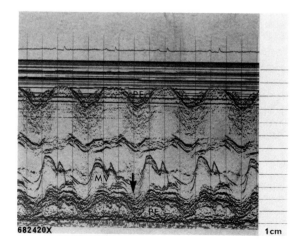

Fig. 10–23. Echocardiogram of a patient with a large pericardial effusion and excessive cardiac motion. The pericardial effusion (PE) can be seen anteriorly and posteriorly. During systole the entire heart, including the mitral valve (MV), moves posteriorly, producing a false impression of mitral valve prolapse *(arrow)*.

kinesis. The important point to remember is that the presence of a large pericardial effusion and excessive cardiac motion markedly limits any M-mode echocardiographic diagnosis that is based on the pattern of cardiac motion.

Excessive displacement of the heart with massive pericardial effusion can also be appreciated in real-time two-dimensional echocardiography. Figure 10–24 demonstrates two frames of a patient with a massive effusion and a marked change in the position of the heart. In one two-dimensional study, the authors were impressed by a counterclockwise rotation of the heart with systole, with massive pericardial effusion.[42]

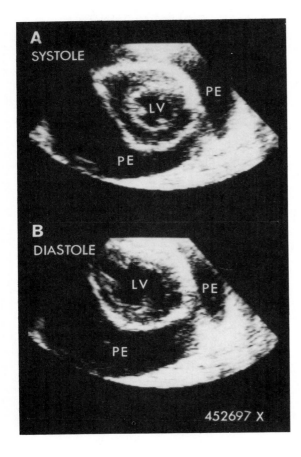

Fig. 10–24.   Short-axis two-dimensional echocardiogram of a patient with a large pericardial effusion, demonstrating the shift in cardiac position from systole to diastole. PE = pericardial effusion; LV = left ventricle.

Cardiac Tamponade

Several reports in the literature have demonstrated the echocardiographic findings in patients with cardiac tamponade due to pericardial effusion.[43–47,47a] Probably the first echocardiographically reported case of cardiac tamponade was in a patient with acute pericardial effusion secondary to perforation of the heart at cardiac catheterization.[2] In this case the patient's cardiac motion decreased markedly with reduced total amplitude of the left ventricular posterior wall excursion.

In one study, the investigators emphasized the cyclical respiratory changes in the right ventricular dimension and the mitral diastolic slope in patients with pericardial effusion and tamponade.[43] With inspiration there was an abrupt and dramatic increase in the right ventricular dimension at the expense of the left ventricle (Fig. 10–25). It should be remembered that this finding is only an exaggeration of the normal situation. A clear distinction between normal and abnormal has not been established yet. The investigators also noted a decrease in mitral diastolic slope with inspiration. In Figure 10–25 the area of the mitral valve is decreased, suggesting a decreased mitral valve flow and left ventricular stroke volume with inspiration. Other investigators have also emphasized the change in right ventricular dimension with cardiac tamponade.[44,45] One group believed that a right ventricular end-diastolic dimension at the end of expiration, which was 2 mm or less, was indicative of tamponade.[44] Figure 10–26 is another M-mode echocardiogram of a patient with pericardial effusion and cardiac tamponade. The right ventricular dimension at end-diastole (RV_E) at expiration is quite small. Figure 10–27 shows the post-pericardiocentesis M-mode echocardiogram of the same patient. The right ventricular dimension is much larger, and the respiratory variation noted in Figure 10–26 is no longer present.

Figure 10–26 also demonstrates a recently described finding in cardiac tamponade: posterior motion of the anterior right ventricular wall during diastole (large arrow).[47a] The abnormal right ventricular diastolic motion is not present in Figure 10–27 following

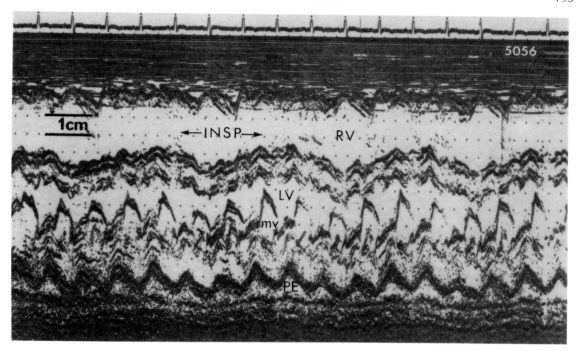

Fig. 10–25. M-mode echocardiogram of a patient with cardiac tamponade. With inspiration (INSP), the size of the right ventricle (RV) suddenly increases, and the size of the left ventricle (LV) decreases as the interventricular septum moves posteriorly. The total amplitude and opening of the mitral valve (mv) also decreases with inspiration. PE = pericardial effusion.

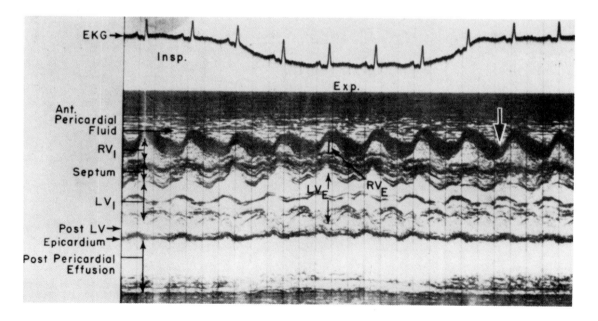

Fig. 10–26. M-mode echocardiogram of a patient with pericardial effusion and cardiac tamponade. The right ventricle during expiration (RV_E) is markedly diminished. There is also posterior motion of the right ventricular wall in diastole *(large arrow.)* INSP = inspiration; EXP = expiration; LV_E = left ventricle with expiration. (From Settle, H.P., et al.: Echocardiographic study of cardiac tamponade. Circulation, 56:951, 1977. By permission of the American Heart Association, Inc.)

pericardiocentesis and relief of the tamponade. Figure 10–25 also shows diastolic posterior motion of the right ventricular wall with inspiration. The mechanism is not totally understood, but the observation is intriguing and could be a reliable sign for the presence of tamponade.

Despite these reports there is still considerable skepticism among echocardiographers as to the reliability of echocardiography in the diagnosis of cardiac tamponade. Both false positives and false negatives have been observed, and the role of echocardiography in cardiac tamponade must await further confirmation. Serial changes in right ventricular dimensions and respiratory variations are probably more reliable than trying to use these criteria to determine the presence of tamponade from a single echocardiogram.[47]

The possible role of two-dimensional echocardiography in patients with tamponade is uncertain. In one patient a change in the shape of the anterior right ventricular wall was noted in the presence of tamponade.[44] Another study demonstrated that two-dimensional echocardiography was superior to the M-mode technique in detecting a large effusion and a relatively small left ventricle in a patient who developed tamponade following cardiac surgery.[46]

PERICARDITIS

Thickened Pericardium

The echocardiographic findings in cases of a thickened pericardium have been described.[49–50,50a,b] Occasionally, one may find what appears to be a significantly thickened pericardium in the presence of pericardial

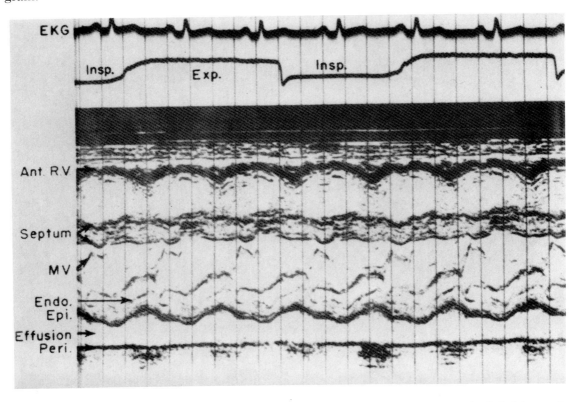

Fig. 10–27.   Echocardiogram of the patient in Figure 10–26 after pericardiocentesis and relief of the cardiac tamponade. With removal of the pericardial fluid, the size of the right ventricle increases, the respiratory variation decreases, and the amount of posterior pericardial effusion decreases. The abnormal diastolic motion of the right ventricular wall seen in Figure 10–26 is no longer present. RV = right ventricle; MV = mitral valve; ENDO = endocardium; EPI = epicardium; PERI = pericardium; INSP = inspiration; EXP = expiration. (From Settle, H.P., et al.: Echocardiographic study of cardiac tamponade. Circulation, 56:951, 1977. By permission of the American Heart Association, Inc.)

effusion. Figure 10–28 shows an example of a patient with pericardial effusion (PE) who has a double echo (arrow) next to the left ventricular epicardium. This finding is highly suggestive of a thickened visceral pericardium. It is not uncommon to find a band of echoes along the parietal pericardium with pericardial effusion. Figure 10–4 shows a band of relatively fuzzy echoes along the posterior border of the pericardial fluid. In this type of situation, it is frequently difficult to determine exactly where the pericardial echo is. Whether this band of echoes represents a thickened parietal pericardium or an accumulation of particular matter within the pericardial fluid, which is layered against the parietal pericardium, has not been established. Unless the thickened pericardium is recorded as relatively dense echoes, such as in Figure 10–28 (arrow), a thickened pericardium is not usually diagnosed echocardiographically. It is probably best detected when serial echocardiograms show the evolution of pericardial fluid into a thickened mass of echoes behind the posterior left ventricular wall.[51]

Two-dimensional echocardiography can frequently demonstrate band-like intrapericardial echoes in patients with pericardial effusion.[51a] These fibrinous structures may be seen undulating freely within the pericardial fluid, or they may be attached to either the visceral or parietal pericardium. These findings may be suspicious for an effusive-constrictive type of pericarditis.[51a]

One can occasionally be confident of a thickened pericardium even without pericardial effusion. Figure 10–29 shows such an example. The thickened pericardium is identified as a band of dense echoes (PER) behind the relatively echo-free posterior left ventricular myocardium (PLV). Pericardial thickening can be distinguished from pericardial effusion by the fact that the pericardial echoes move with exactly the same amplitude of motion as the left ventricular epicardium. One cannot be absolutely certain that the thickened pericardium does not represent pericardial effusion with adhesions; however, it does not represent an uncomplicated pericardial effusion. In addition, the intensity of the pericardial echoes

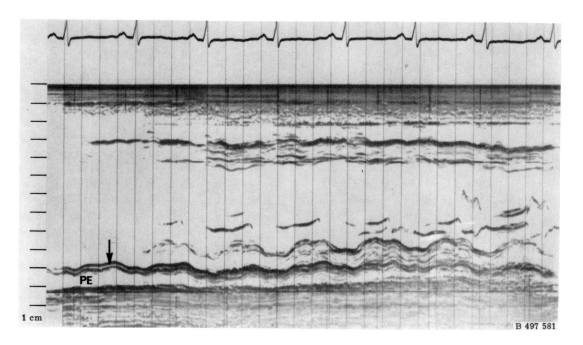

Fig. 10–28.   Echocardiogram of a patient with pericardial effusion (PE) who also demonstrates a double echo *(arrow)* in the vicinity of the left ventricular epicardium. Such a recording makes one suspect thickening of the visceral pericardium.

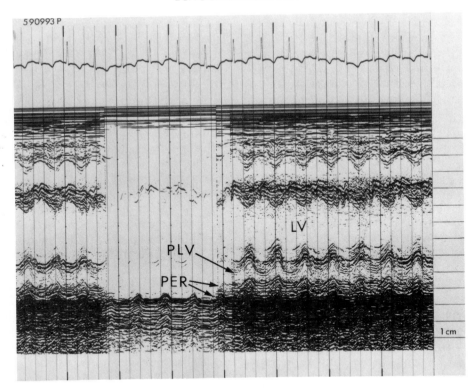

Fig. 10–29.   M-mode echocardiogram of a patient with a thickened pericardium. A band of dense echoes originating from the pericardium (PER) can be seen posterior to the relatively echo-free space of the posterior left ventricular myocardium (PLV). All pericardial echoes move synchronously and exhibit the same amplitude of motion as the epicardium of the posterior left ventricular wall. LV = left ventricle.

certainly suggests that there is something other than relatively homogeneous pericardial fluid.

Figure 10–30 represents another cause for a thickened pericardium. In this patient the distance between the epicardial (EPI) and pericardial (PER) echoes is actually greater than the thickness of the posterior left ventricular wall. The epicardial and pericardial echoes move equally and indicate a thickened pericardium rather than a pericardial effusion. This patient did not, however, have pericarditis; he had a metastatic tumor involving the pericardium.

Although there are reports that echocardiography is helpful in the diagnosis of pericardial thickening,[48,50] the echocardiographic diagnosis of thickened pericardium is not one of the more established applications of this diagnostic technique. Questions over the reliability and reproducibility of this examination are still unsettled, despite the considerable interest in this area for many years. The echocardiographic signs for a thickened pericardium are not pathognomonic. Multiple echoes from the vicinity of the posterior left ventricular epicardium and pericardium, possibly the result of reverberations, are not unusual.[50] In one study to determine the accuracy of echocardiography in detecting a thickened pericardium, 76 percent of the patients who had the echocardiographic diagnosis of a thickened pericardium actually had a thickened pericardium at surgery or autopsy.[50]

Constrictive Pericarditis

Many echocardiographic signs indicative of constrictive pericarditis have been introduced into the literature.[49,50,50b,52–57] One of the first and probably the most reliable signs of constriction is a flattening of the mid- and late diastolic motion of the left ventricular wall. Figure 10–31 demonstrates an echo-

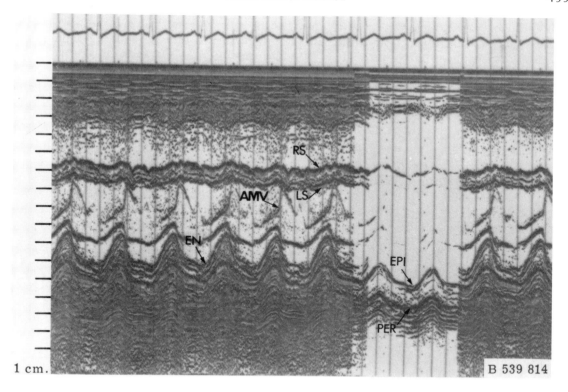

Fig. 10–30. Echocardiogram of the left ventricle and pericardium in a patient with tumor invading the pericardium. At surgery the pericardium behind the heart was markedly thickened by tumor and is represented in this echocardiogram by the space between the posterior left ventricular epicardium (EPI) and the pericardium (PER). LS = left septum; RS = right septum; AMV = anterior mitral valve; EN = posterior left ventricular endocardium.

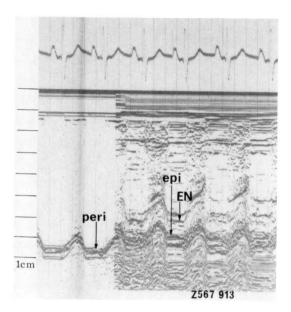

Fig. 10–31. Echocardiogram of a patient with constrictive pericarditis. Filling abruptly ceases in early diastole with virtually flat endocardial (EN), epicardial (ep), and pericardial (peri) echoes during the latter two-thirds of diastole. The distance between the epicardial and pericardial echoes is thought to represent the thickness of the pericardium.

cardiogram of a patient with constrictive pericarditis. The systolic and early diastolic motion of the posterior left ventricular wall and pericardium are normal; however, following early ventricular filling the left ventricular wall motion abruptly stops and becomes flat. There is no gradual downward motion with mid-diastole and atrial systole. This finding is probably the most consistent in patients with constrictive pericarditis.[49,54–56,58] In fact, one group of authors indicated that if the left ventricular endocardial echo is not at least more than 1 mm more posterior than it was at the onset of mid-diastole, then one should consider the possibility of constrictive pericarditis.[58]

A rapid early diastolic, or E to F, slope of the mitral valve has also been noted in patients with constrictive pericarditis.[50,55,56] Figure 10–32 illustrates two mitral valve

recordings from the same patient whose tracing appears in Figure 10–31. At times there seems to be duplication of the mitral valve that may merely be a function of the angulation of the leaflet. There is rapid and early closure of the mitral valve (Fig. 10–32B). At other times a more normal mitral valve can be appreciated (Fig. 10–32A).

Interventricular septal motion may also be abnormal in patients with constrictive pericarditis.[52,55,59] Figure 10–33 shows an example of abnormal septal motion in a patient with constrictive pericarditis. The principal finding is an exaggerated anterior motion of the septum with atrial filling. Since the posterior free wall of the left ventricle is unable to expand properly, an increase in left ventricular volume with atrial systole produces a marked displacement of the septum. The anterior motion of the left septum (LS)

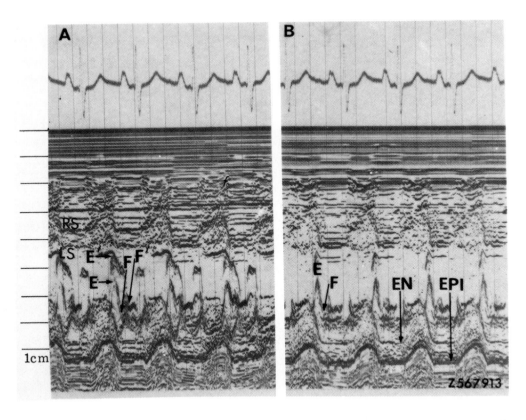

Fig. 10–32. Mitral valve and left ventricular echocardiograms of the patient in Figure 10–31. There are several echoes from the mitral valve, one of which closes rapidly with a steep diastolic closing slope (E–F). Another mitral valve echo shows a slightly slower slope (E'–F'). The echocardiograms again show flat motion of the left ventricular echoes during diastole. RS = right side of septum; LS = left side of septum. EN = posterior left ventricular endocardium; EPI = posterior left ventricular epicardium.

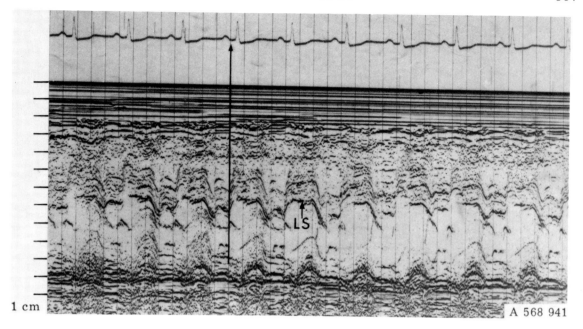

Fig. 10–33.   Echocardiogram of the interventricular septum of a patient with constrictive pericarditis. During atrial systole and before ventricular depolarization *(arrows)*, there is a brisk anterior motion of the septum (LS) that remains anterior throughout ventricular ejection. The septum then moves downward or posteriorly with ventricular relaxation.

occurs at the end of the electrocardiographic P wave (arrow). This timing should be distinguished from that which occurs with right ventricular volume overload. In the latter situation the brisk anterior septal motion occurs after the onset of ventricular depolarization.

Yet another echocardiographic finding with constrictive pericarditis is premature opening of the pulmonary valve.[57,60,60a] Figure 10–34 demonstrates a pre- and postoperative pulmonary valve echocardiogram in a patient with constriction. Prior to surgical removal of the thickened pericardium, there is a brisk, downward, opening motion of the pulmonary valve (arrow) before the electrocardiographic P wave. The explanation for this opening is that it is presumably a result of the marked increase in right ventricular diastolic pressure in mid-diastole. The right ventricular pressure rises abruptly and transiently exceeds the pulmonary artery pressure, permitting opening of the pulmonary valve. Following relief of the constriction (Fig. 10–34B) the premature

opening is no longer seen in the pulmonary valve.[57,60] This echocardiographic finding is not that common and probably indicates a marked elevation in right ventricular diastolic pressure.

Thus the echocardiographer has a constellation of signs available for the diagnosis of constrictive pericarditis. Unfortunately, no one sign is totally reliable. The flat diastolic motion of the posterior left ventricular wall is probably the most frequent sign. However, it is not pathognomonic for constriction. Cardiac dilatation, especially when relatively acute, may cause a normal pericardium to be relatively restrictive and mid- and late diastolic filling may be reduced. The echocardiographic diagnosis of constrictive pericarditis is probably best made if one can find two or more signs indicative of constriction.

ABSENT PERICARDIUM

The normal pericardium exerts considerable influence on cardiac motion. It is well recognized that besides providing some stability to the location of the heart within the

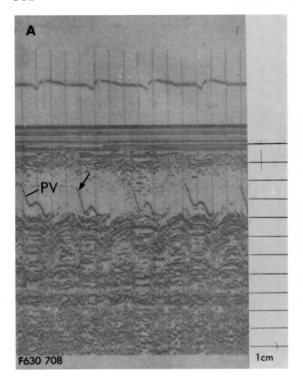
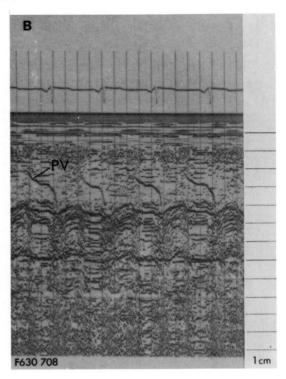

Fig. 10–34. Pulmonary valve echocardiogram of a patient with constrictive pericarditis before and after surgical removal of the pericardium. A, Preoperatively, there is a rapid downward motion *(arrow)* of the pulmonary valve (PV) prior to atrial systole. B, Postoperatively, there is only the normal gradual posterior motion of the pulmonary valve during diastole.

chest, the pericardium also limits the degree of dilatation of the heart. Following surgical removal of the pericardium, the heart frequently expands. The posterior left ventricular wall motion may become exaggerated. Patients who have congenital absence of the left pericardium also exhibit excessive motion of the posterior left ventricular wall.[61,61a] One of the consequences is that excessive cardiac motion can influence the pattern of motion of the entire heart. The heart also shifts to the left, often leaving more of the right ventricle visible than is usual on a routine left parasternal echocardiogram. The resultant excessive cardiac motion distorts the cardiac echoes, especially the interventricular septum. With ventricular systole the exaggerated posterior left ventricular wall motion produces anterior displacement of the interventricular septum. Thus, with congenital absence of left pericardium, one notes dilatation of the right ventricle, exces-

sive posterior left ventricular wall motion, and paradoxical motion of the interventricular septum. These findings are almost indistinguishable from those of a right ventricular volume overload.[61] Fortunately, many other clinical signs help in the differential diagnosis, such as marked shift of the cardiac silhouette to the left on the chest roentgenogram. Although the two-dimensional echocardiographic findings with absence of left pericardium have not been reported, it is hoped that this technique is also able to differentiate between right ventricular volume overload and absence of the left pericardium.

REFERENCES

1. Feigenbaum, H., Waldhausen, J.A., and Hyde, L.P.: Ultrasound diagnosis of pericardial effusion. J.A.M.A., *191*:107, 1965.
2. Feigenbaum, H., Zaky, A., and Waldhausen, J.A.: Use of ultrasound in the diagnosis of pericardial effusion. Ann. Intern. Med., 65:443, 1966.

3. Anonymous: Ultrasound in the diagnosis of pericardial effusion. Chin. Med. J., 7:411, 1973.

4. Bilek, J., Lukas, D., and Hula, J.: Echocardiography in pericardial effusion: case report. Vnitr. Lek., 16:428, 1970.

5. Feigenbaum, H.: Echocardiographic diagnosis of pericardial effusion. Am. J. Cardiol., 26:475, 1970.

6. Follath, F. and Heierli, B.: Echocardiography in pericardial effusion. Schweiz. Med. Wochenschr., 104:1572, 1974.

7. Goldberg, B.B., Ostrum, B.J., and Isard, J.J.: Ultrasonic determination of pericardial effusion. J.A.M.A., 202:103, 1967.

8. Klein, J.J. and Segal, B.L.: Pericardial effusion diagnosed by reflected ultrasound. Am. J. Cardiol., 22:57, 1968.

9. Moss, A. and Bruhn, F.: The echocardiogram: an ultrasound technic for the detection of pericardial effusion. N. Engl. J. Med., 274:380, 1966.

10. Pate, J.W., Gardner, H.C., and Norman R.S.: Diagnosis of pericardial effusion by echocardiography. Ann. Surg., 165:826, 1967.

11. Rothman, J., Chase, N.E., Kricheff, I.I., Mayoral, R., and Beranbaum, E.R.: Ultrasonic diagnosis of pericardial effusion. Circulation, 35:358, 1967.

12. Soulen, R.L., Lapayowker, M.D., Tyson, R.R., et al.: Angiography ultrasound and thermography in the study of peripheral vascular disease. Radiology, 105:115, 1972.

13. Werning, C.: Ultrasound diagnostics of pericardial effusion. Dtsch. Med. Wochenschr., 97:816, 1972.

13a. Riba, A.L. and Morganroth, J.: Unsuspected substantial pericardial effusions detected by echocardiography. J.A.M.A., 236:2623, 1976.

14. Edler, I.: Diagnostic use of ultrasound in heart disease. Acta Med. Scand., 308:32, 1955.

15. Chandraratna, P.A.N., First, J., Langevin, E., and O'Dell, R.: Echocardiographic contrast studies during pericardiocentesis. Ann. Intern. Med., 87:199, 1977.

16. Feigenbaum, H., Zaky, A., and Waldhausen, J.A.: Use of reflected ultrasound in detecting pericardial effusion. Am. J. Cardiol., 19:84, 1967.

17. Griffith, J.M. and Henry, H.L.: Switched gain: a technique for simplifying ultrasonic measurement of cardiac wall thickness. I.E.E.E. Trans. Biomed. Eng., 22:337, 1975.

18. Abbasi, A.S., Ellis, N., and Flynn, J.U.: Echocardiographic M-scan technique in the diagnosis of pericardial effusion. J. Clin. Ultrasound, 1:300, 1973.

19. Lemire, F., Tajik, A.J., Giuliani, E.R., Gau, G.T., and Schattenberg, T.T.: Further echocardiographic observations in pericardial effusion. Mayo Clin. Proc., 51:13, 1976.

20. Greene, D.A., Kleid, J.J., and Naidu, S.: Unusual echocardiographic manifestation of pericardial effusion. Am. J. Cardiol., 39:112, 1977.

21. Tajik, A.J.: Echocardiography in pericardial effusion. Am. J. Med., 63:29, 1977.

22. Kerber, R.E. and Payvandi, M.N.: Echocardiography in acute hemopericardium: production of false-negative echocardiograms by pericardial clots. Circulation (Suppl. III), 56:24, 1977. (Abstract)

23. Ratshin, R.A., Smith, M.K., and Hood, W.P., Jr.: Possible false-positive diagnosis of pericardial effusion by echocardiography in presence of large left atrium. Chest, 65:112, 1974.

24. Popp, R.L. and Harrison, D.C.: Echocardiography. In Noninvasive Cardiology. Edited by A.M. Weissler. New York, Grune & Stratton, 1974.

25. Foote, W.C., Jefferson, C.M., and Price, H.L.: False-positive echocardiographic diagnosis of pericardial effusion: result of tumor encasement of the heart simulating constrictive pericarditis. Chest, 71:546, 1977.

26. Lin, T.K., Stech, J.M., Eckert, W.G., Lin, J.J., Farha, S.J., and Hagan, C.T.: Pericardial angiosarcoma simulating pericardial effusion by echocardiography. Chest, 73:881, 1978.

27. Chandraratna, P.A.N., Littman, B.B., Serafini, A., Whayne, T., and Robinson, H.: Echocardiographic evaluation of extracardiac masses. Br. Heart J., 40:741, 1978.

28. Millman, A., Meller, J., Motro, M., Blank, H.S., Horowitz, I., Herman, M.V., and Teichholz, L.E.: Pericardial tumor or fibrosis mimicking pericardial effusion by echocardiography. Ann. Intern. Med., 86:434, 1977.

29. Martin, R.P., Rakowski, H., French, J., and Popp, R.L.: Localization of pericardial effusion with wide angle phased array echocardiography. Am. J. Cardiol., 42:904, 1978.

30. Friedman, M.J., Sahn, D.J., and Haber, K.: Two-dimensional echocardiography and B-mode ultrasonography for the diagnosis of loculated pericardial effusion. Circulation, 60:1644, 1979.

30a. Haaz, W.S., Mintz, G.S., Kotler, M.N., and Parry, W.R.: Two-dimensional echocardiographic recognition of the descending thoracic aorta: value in differentiating pericardial from pleural effusions. Am. J. Cardiol., 45:401, 1980. (Abstract)

31. Horowitz, M.S., Schultz, C.S., Stinson, E.B., Harrison, D.C., and Popp, R.L.: Sensitivity and specificity of echocardiographic diagnosis of pericardial effusion. Circulation, 50:239, 1974.

32. Kleiman, J.H., Motta, J., London, E., Pennell, J.P., and Popp, R.L.: Pericardial effusions in patients with end-stage renal disease. Br. Heart J., 40:190, 1978.

33. Berger, M., Bobak, L., Jelveh, M., and Goldberg, E.: Pericardial effusion diagnosed by echocardiography: clinical and electrocardiographic findings in 171 patients. Chest, 74:174, 1978.

34. D'Cruz, I., Prabhu, R., Cohen, H.C., and Glick, G.: Potential pitfalls in quantification of pericardial effusions by echocardiography. Br. Heart J., 39:529, 1977.

35. Feigenbaum, H., Zaky, A., and Grabhorn, L.: Cardiac motion in patients with pericardial effusion: a study using ultrasound cardiography. Circulation, 34:611, 1966.

35a. Krueger, S.K., Zucker, R.P., Dzindzio, B.S., and Forker, A.D.: Swinging heart syndrome with predominant anterior pericardial effusion. J. Clin. Ultrasound, 4:113, 1976.

36. Gabor, G.E., Winsberg, F., and Bloom, H.S.: Electrical and mechanical alternation in pericardial effusion. Chest, 59:341, 1971.

37. Yuste, P., Torres, Carballada, M.A., and Miguel Alonso, J.L.: Mechanism of electric alternans in pericardial effusion: study with ultrasonics. Arch. Inst. Cardiol. Mex., 45:197, 1975.

38. Rinkenberger, R.L., Polumbo, R.A., Bolton, M.R., and Dunn, M.: Mechanism of electrical alternans in patients with pericardial effusion. Cathet. Cardiovasc. Diagn., 4:63, 1978.

39. Levisman, J.A. and Abbasi, A.A.: Abnormal motion of the mitral valve with pericardial effusion: pseudo-prolapse of the mitral valve. Am. Heart J., 91:18, 1976.

40. Nanda, N.C., Gramiak, R., and Gross, C.M.: Echocardiography of cardiac valves in pericardial effusion. Circulation, 54:500, 1976.

41. Vignola, P.A., Pohost, G.M., Curfman, G.D., and Myers, G.S.: Correlation of echocardiographic and clinical findings in patients with pericardial effusion. Am. J. Cardiol., 37:701, 1976.

42. Matsuo, H., Matsumoto, M., Hamanaka, Y., Ohara, T., Senda, S., Inoue, M., and Abe, H.: Rotational excursion of heart in massive pericardial effusion studied by phased-array echocardiography. Br. Heart J., 41:513, 1979.

43. D'Cruz, I.A., Cohen, H.C., Prabhu, R., and Glick, G.: Diagnosis of cardiac tamponade by echocardiography: changes in mitral valve motion and ventricular dimensions, with special reference to paradoxical pulse. Circulation, 52:460, 1975.

44. Schiller, N.B. and Botvinick, E.H.: Right ventricular compression as a sign of cardiac tamponade: an analysis of echocardiographic ventricular dimensions and their clinical implications. Circulation, 56:774, 1977.

45. Settle, H.P., Adolph, R.J., Fowler, N.O., Engel, P., Agruss, N.S., and Levenson, N.I.: Echocardiographic study of cardiac tamponade. Circulation, 56:951, 1977.

46. Hochberg, M.S., Merrill, W.H., Bruber, M., McIntosh, C.L., Henry, W.L., and Morrow, A.G.: Delayed cardiac tamponade associated with prophylactic anticoagulation in patients undergoing coronary bypass grafting: early diagnosis with two-dimensional echocardiography. J. Thorac. Cardiovasc. Surg., 75:777, 1978.

47. Martins, J.B. and Kerber, R.E.: Can cardiac tamponade be diagnosed by echocardiography? Circulation, 60:737, 1979.

47a. Shina, S., Yaginuma, T., Kondo, K., Kawai, N., and Hosoda, S.: Echocardiographic evaluation of impending cardiac tamponade. J. Cardiogr., 9:555, 1979.

48. Horowitz, M.S., Rossen, R.M., Harrison, D.C., and Popp, R.L.: Ultrasonic evaluation of constrictive pericardial disease. Circulation (Suppl. II), 50:87, 1974. (Abstract)

49. Cohen, M.V., and Greenberg, M.A.: Constrictive pericarditis: early and late complication of cardiac surgery. Am. J. Cardiol., 43:657, 1979.

50. Schnittger, I., Bowden, R.E., Abrams, J., and Popp, R.L.: Echocardiography: pericardial thickening and constrictive pericarditis. Am. J. Cardiol., 42:388, 1978.

50a. Chandraratna, P.A.N. and Imaizumi, T.: Echocardiographic diagnosis of thickened pericardium. Cardiovasc. Med., 3:1279, 1978.

50b. Elkayam, U., Kotler, M.N., Segal, B., and Parry, W.: Echocardiographic findings in constrictive pericarditis: a case report. Isr. J. Med. Sci., 12:1308, 1976.

51. Allen, J.W., Harrison, E.C., Camp, J.C., Borsari, A., Turnier, E., and Lau, F.Y.K.: The role of serial echocardiography in the evaluation and differential diagnosis of pericardial disease. Am. Heart J., 93:560, 1977.

51a. Martin, R.P., Bowden, R., Filly, K., and Popp, R.L.: Intrapericardial abnormalities in patients with pericardial effusion: findings by two-dimensional echocardiography. Circulation, 61:568, 1980.

52. Pool, P.E., Seagren, S.C., Abbasi, A.S., Charuzi, Y., and Kraus, R.: Echocardiographic manifestations of constrictive pericarditis: abnormal septal motion. Chest, 68:684, 1975.

53. Candell-Riera, J., DelCastillo, G., Permanyer-Miralda, G., and Soler-Soler, J.: Echocardiographic features of the interventricular septum in chronic constrictive pericarditis. Circulation, 57:1154, 1978.

54. D'Cruz, I.A., Levinsky, R., Anagnostopoulos, C., and Cohen, H.C.: Echocardiographic diagnosis of partial pericardial constriction of the left ventricle. Radiology, 127:755, 1978.

55. Yamamoto, T., Makihata, S., Yasutomi, N., Tanimoto, M., Ando, H., Iwasaki, T., Yorifuji, S., Shimizu, Y., and Miyamoto, T.: Echocardiographic and impedance cardiographic manifestations of constrictive pericarditis. J. Cardiogr., 8:719, 1978.

56. Matsuo, H., Kitabatake, A., Matsumoto, M., Hamanaka, Y., Beppu, S., Nagata, S., Tamai, M., Ohara, T., Senda, S., and Nimura, Y.: Echocardiographic manifestation of constrictive pericarditis and pericarditis with effusion. Cardiovasc. Sound Bull., 5:173, 1975.

57. Nishimoto, M., Tanaka, C., Oku, H., Ikuno, Y., Kawai, S., Furukawa, K., Takeuchi, K., and Shiota, K.: Presystolic pulmonary valve opening in constrictive pericarditis. J. Cardiogr., 7:55, 1977.

58. Voelkel, A.G., Pietro, D.A., Folland, E.D., Fisher, M.L., and Parisi, A.F.: Echocardiographic features of constrictive pericarditis. Circulation, 58:871, 1978.

59. Gibson, T.C., Grossman, W., McLaurin, L.P., Moos, S., and Craige, E.: An echocardiographic study of the interventricular system in constrictive pericarditis. Br. Heart J., 38:738, 1976.

60. Wann, L.S., Weyman, A.E., Dillon, J.C., and Feigenbaum, H.: Premature pulmonary valve opening. Circulation, 55:128, 1977.

60a. Hada, Y., Sakamoto, T., Hayashi, T., Ichiyasu, H., and Amano, K.: Echocardiogram of normal pulmonary valve: physiological data and effect of atrial contraction on the valve motion. Jpn. Heart J., 18:421, 1977.

61. Payvandi, M.N. and Kerber, R.E.: Echocardiography in congenital and acquired absence of pericardium. Circulation, 53:86, 1976.

61a. Hermann, H., Raizner, A.E., Chahine, R.A., et al.: Congenital absence of the left pericardium: an unusual palpation finding and echocardiographic demonstration of the defect. South. Med. J., 69:1222, 1976.

Cardiac Masses

Echocardiography is possibly becoming the diagnostic procedure of choice for the detection of cardiac masses. There are an increasing number of reports of using echocardiography to detect a wide variety of intra- and extracardiac masses. Two-dimensional echocardiography has markedly improved the diagnostic ability of this ultrasonic examination. It is becoming apparent that echocardiography may have greater sensitivity and reliability in the diagnosis of cardiac masses than any other cardiologic test.

One type of cardiac mass—vegetations—was discussed in Chapter 6. This chapter primarily discusses tumors and thrombi.

INTRACARDIAC TUMORS

Left Atrial Tumors

The most common cardiac tumor is the left atrial myxoma. It is usually pedunculated and arises by way of a stalk from the interatrial septum. Since the tumor is usually mobile, it moves with the flow of blood. Thus the tumor drops through the mitral orifice with ventricular diastole. Since the tumor may impede the flow of blood from the left atrium to the left ventricle, the condition frequently mimics mitral stenosis.[1] The clinical symptoms and signs may be identical with those of mitral stenosis. In addition, the tumor causes many systemic manifestations, including fever and anemia, and may be confused with such diseases as bacterial endocarditis, cerebral vascular accident,[2,3] rheumatic fever, or even cardiomyopathy.[4] Thus, although the clinical diagnosis of left

atrial myxoma may be difficult,[1] it is extremely important because a tumor is potentially lethal owing to heart failure, systemic emboli, or sudden death. If correctly diagnosed, the condition is curable since the tumor is easily excised surgically and is rarely malignant.[5]

Probably one of the most exciting and rewarding echocardiographic diagnoses is the detection of a left atrial myxoma.[6–13,13a] More than a dozen left atrial tumors have been detected echocardiographically at the Indiana University Medical Center echocardiographic laboratories. In more than half of the cases, the initial diagnosis was made by the echocardiographic technician performing the examination. Figure 11–1 shows the

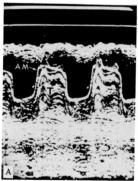
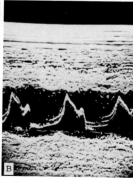

Fig. 11–1. Echocardiograms of a patient with a pedunculated, highly mobile left atrial tumor. A, Preoperative echocardiogram shows multiple echoes from the tumor (T) moving about behind the anterior mitral leaflet (AM). B, Postoperative echocardiogram shows absence of these echoes. (From Nasser, W.K., et al.: Atrial myxoma. Part II. Phonocardiographic, echocardiographic, hemodynamic, and angiographic features of nine cases. Am. Heart J., 83:810, 1972.)

preoperative and postoperative M-mode echocardiogram of one of our earlier patients who had a left atrial myxoma. In the preoperative echocardiogram (A), the echo from the anterior leaflet of the mitral valve (AM) superficially resembles mitral stenosis because the diastolic slope is reduced. In fact, this patient was originally examined echocardiographically at another hospital, and the echocardiographic diagnosis was mitral stenosis. Careful examination reveals, however, that the anterior leaflet is not thickened and that the echocardiogram should not have been misinterpreted as mitral stenosis. More important, the mitral valve is filled with a mass of echoes that are posterior to the anterior leaflet during diastole. The tumor was highly mobile and some of the echoes from the tumor even appear anterior to the mitral valve leaflet. At surgery the tumor was relatively small and on a long stalk. The postoperative echocardiogram (B) is basically normal.

Figure 11–2 actually shows a better echocardiographic way of detecting a left atrial tumor. The technique utilizes an M-mode scan from the vicinity of the mitral valve into the left atrium. One again sees a cloud of tumor echoes (T) behind the anterior leaflet of the mitral valve (MV). In this patient, the echo-producing mass almost completely fills the mitral valve throughout diastole. By directing the ultrasonic beam into the left atrium, one can follow the echo-producing mass (T) into the left atrium and can see how it practically fills the entire left atrial cavity. There is only a small posterior echo-free space that is not filled with tumor. The aortic valve, which shows signs of increased blood flow, is seen anterior to the tumor-filled left atrium. An M-mode scan is more informative than an isolated examination of the mitral valve (such as in Figure 11–1), although both echocardiograms clearly show the atrial myxoma. As might be expected from the tracing in Figure 11–2, the tumor was massive and caused severe hemodynamic impairment. The patient was extremely ill, and immediately following the tracing of this echocardiogram, the tumor was surgically removed. Angiographic confirmation was not obtained. The postoperative echocardiogram that appears in Figure 11–3 shows a dramatic difference. Aside from residual di-

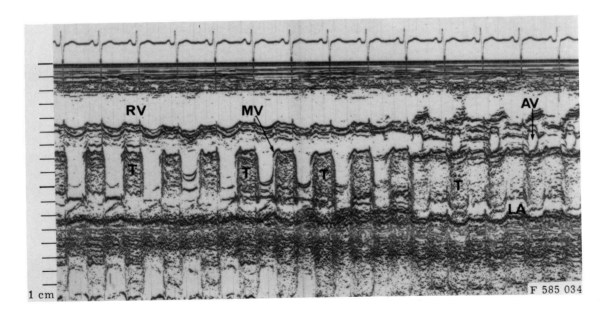

Fig. 11–2.   M-mode scan of a patient with a left atrial myxoma. The tumor echoes (T) are visible behind the anterior leaflet of the mitral valve (MV) during diastole and almost completely fill the left atrium (LA) during ventricular systole. RV = right ventricle; AV = aortic valve. (From Chang, S.: M-mode Echocardiographic Techniques and Pattern Recognition. Philadelphia, Lea & Febiger, 1976.)

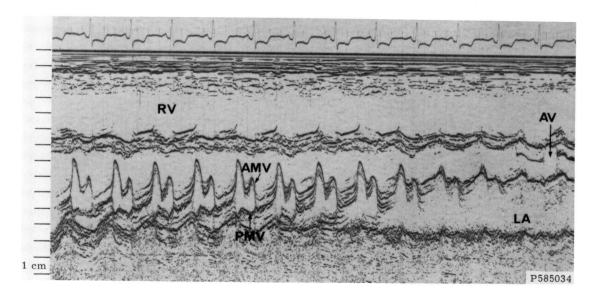

Fig. 11–3.   Postoperative echocardiogram of the patient in Figure 11–2. The echoes from the atrial myxoma are completely gone. RV = right ventricle; AMV = anterior mitral valve leaflet; PMV = posterior mitral valve leaflet; AV = aortic valve; LA = left atrium. (From Chang, S.: M-mode Echocardiographic Techniques and Pattern Recognition. Philadelphia, Lea & Febiger, 1976.)

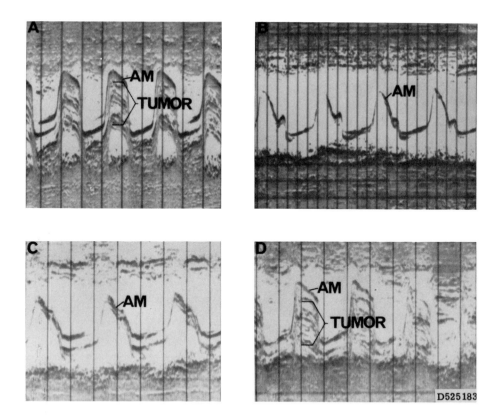

Fig. 11–4.   Serial mitral valve echocardiograms of a patient with a malignant left atrial myxoma. A, Preoperative echocardiogram shows a tumor behind the anterior mitral leaflet (AM). B, Postoperative tracing shows disappearance of tumor echoes. C, A later echocardiogram again reveals the heart as free of tumor echoes. D, Nine months later, however, tumor echoes can again be recorded behind the anterior mitral leaflet. The patient eventually died of malignancy.

latation of the right ventricle and left atrium, the echocardiogram is normal.

One of the obvious advantages of echocardiography is its ability to obtain serial examinations. The preoperative and postoperative echocardiograms shown in Figures 11–1, 11–2, and 11–3 strikingly demonstrate the effectiveness of surgery. On rare occasion a left atrial tumor may be malignant[13b] and may recur. Figure 11–4 illustrates serial mitral valve echocardiograms of a malignant left atrial tumor. The preoperative mitral valve echocardiogram (A) shows the tumor behind the mitral valve. The postoperative echocardiogram (B) shows a normal anterior mitral leaflet. Figure 11–4C is an echocardiogram taken several months later; the mitral valve still does not show any evidence of a tumor. However, approximately nine months following surgery the echocardiogram again showed an echoproducing mass behind the anterior mitral leaflet before the onset of any symptoms; the tumor indeed recurred (Fig. 11–4D).[14] The patient ultimately succumbed to the malignancy.

Although the echocardiographic diagnosis of a left atrial myxoma is dramatic and frequently obvious, like all other aspects of echocardiography it is not always simple. The M-mode recordings may not always exactly resemble those in Figures 11–1 and 11–2.[15] Figure 11–5 is an M-mode scan of a patient with a large atrial myxoma. The scan does not superficially resemble Figure 11–2 because of the lack of echoes within the left atrial cavity. Admittedly, there is an extra echo (T) within the left atrium and behind the aorta, but the band of echoes customarily seen in the left atrium is not apparent. One cannot appreciate the size of this tumor by this echocardiogram. Figure 11–6 is another examination of the same patient, only this time the transducer is directed a little more medially when recording the left atrium. Part of the tricuspid valve is recorded. In this location, the more characteristic band-like echoes from the tumor are visible within the body of the left atrium, as are the multiple echoes behind the mitral valve that are basically no different from those seen in Figure 11–5. Thus the direction of the transducer

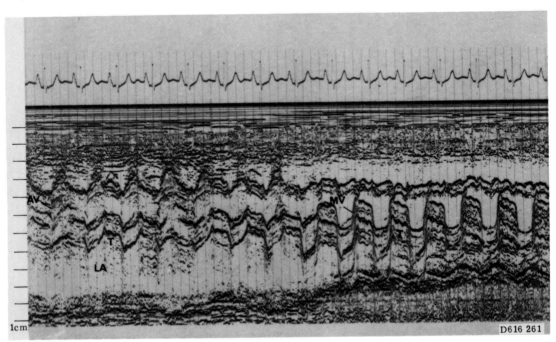

Fig. 11–5. M-mode echocardiogram of a patient with an atrial myxoma that was not markedly echo producing. Only the leading edge of the tumor (T) was visible within the left atrium (LA). The tumor echoes were visible behind the mitral valve (MV) during diastole. AV = aortic valve.

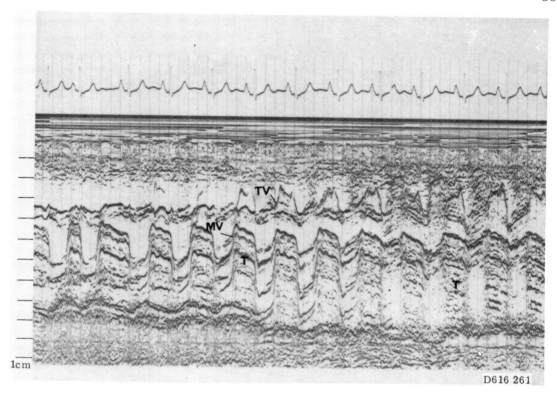

Fig. 11–6.   Another echocardiogram of the patient in Figure 11–5. When the transducer is pointed medially within the left atrium, the tumor echoes (T) are better recorded. The tumor echoes are recorded primarily during diastole and are located at the junction of the left atrium and the mitral valve. TV = tricuspid valve; MV = mitral valve.

may require occasional alteration to fully appreciate the atrial portion of the tumor echoes. Since the exact location of left atrial tumor varies from patient to patient, the echocardiograms may differ.

The literature reports many confusing echocardiograms with respect to the diagnosis of left atrial myxoma. Examples of dense, relatively homogeneous myxomas have been reported whereby only the leading edge of the myxoma is seen with relatively few echoes from the body of the tumor.[15,16] Possibly the most difficult left atrial myxoma to detect with M-mode echocardiography is the immobile left atrial tumor.[17] Figure 11–7 is an M-mode mitral valve echocardiogram of a patient with a left atrial myxoma. No evidence on this tracing even suggests the possibility of a left atrial myxoma. Mitral valve motion certainly does not suggest any obstruction to filling of the

left ventricle. Figure 11–8 demonstrates another M-mode recording of the same patient with the ultrasonic beam directed toward the aorta and left atrium. One now sees a band of echoes apparently attached to the posterior wall of the aorta, which is also the anterior wall of the left atrium. The mass of echoes proved to originate from an immobile tumor within the left atrium. Unfortunately, one may see a similar band of echoes behind the posterior wall of the aorta in patients who do not have a left atrial myxoma. One can only suggest the diagnosis for Figure 11–8; a definitive diagnosis is difficult.

There are M-mode echocardiographic examinations that may simulate left atrial tumors. For example, Figure 11–9 shows a situation in which a left atrial myxoma might conceivably be suspected. On the right side of the tracing, one records an anterior mitral leaflet that appears moderately stenotic; a

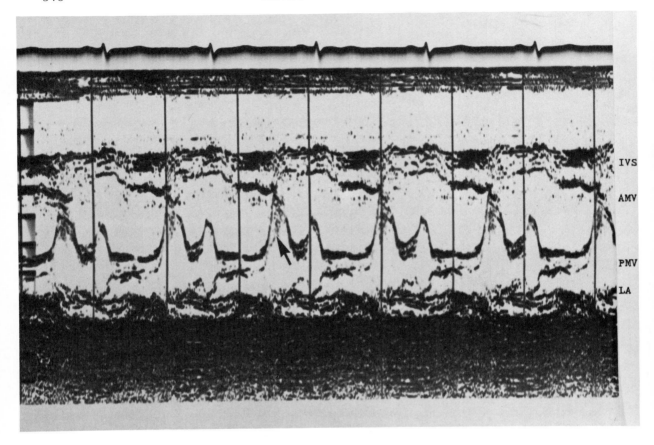

Fig. 11–7.   M-mode mitral valve echocardiogram of a patient with a left atrial myxoma. Aside from a few echoes *(arrow)* behind the mitral valve in diastole, this recording reveals no signs of a tumor. IVS = interventricular septum; AMV = anterior mitral valve; PMV = posterior mitral leaflet; LA = left atrium.

thick echo-producing band that most likely represents a fibrotic posterior mitral valve leaflet appears posteriorly. However, if only an isolated view of this mitral valve is obtained, this tracing might superficially resemble an atrial tumor. Fortunately, an M-mode scan was obtained, and as the ultrasonic beam is directed toward the left atrium, the posterior mitral leaflet disappears and the apparent tumor is no longer present. As noted in Figure 11–2, when a left atrial myxoma is present, the tumor continues to be recorded within the left atrial cavity.

Another confusing situation can occur with mitral valve prolapse. With a redundant, prolapsing mitral valve, one may obtain a recording that superficially resembles an atrial myxoma (Fig. 11–10). The posterior leaflet during diastole may assume a peculiar

orientation so that the ultrasonic beam cuts across the frequently redundant, wavy posterior leaflet in such a way that it appears as a mass of echoes (false tumor) behind the anterior leaflet. During systole, the prolapsing nature of the valve (p) is evident. This confusing band of echoes commonly occurs at the junction between the left ventricle and the left atrium and disappears as the ultrasonic beam is directed into the cavity of the left atrium.

Probably one of the most confusing echocardiograms is seen in Figure 11–11. This tracing demonstrates an echo-producing mass (arrow) attached to the mitral valve that persists throughout the recording. Part of the mass seems to be within the anterior portion of the left atrium and is still present deep into the left ventricle. This mass clearly does not

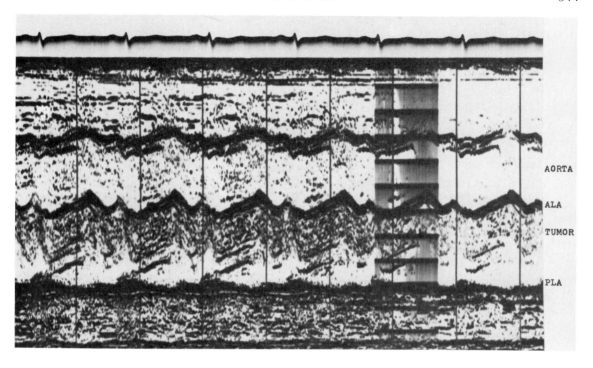

Fig. 11–8.   Another M-mode echocardiogram of the patient in Figure 11–7. With the ultrasonic beam directed toward the left atrium and aorta, the echo-producing tumor is seen attached to the anterior left atrial wall (ALA). PLA = posterior left atrial wall.

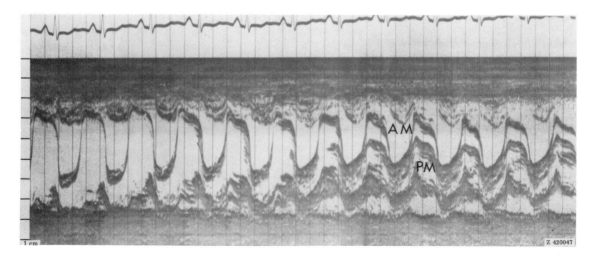

Fig. 11–9.   M-mode scan of the heart of a patient with mitral stenosis. One might confuse the fibrotic posterior mitral valve leaflet (PM) with a left atrial tumor. To differentiate between the two, the ultrasonic beam is directed toward the left atrium (left side of tracing). True tumor echoes should increase, whereas posterior mitral leaflet echoes disappear. AM = anterior mitral valve leaflet.

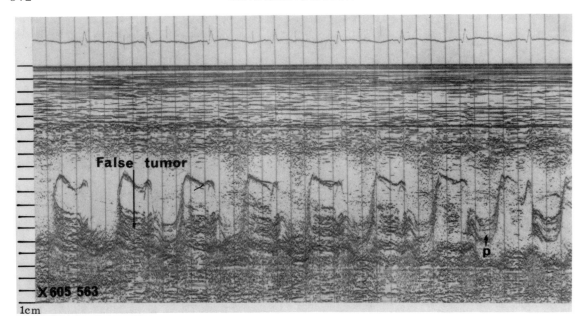

Fig. 11–10. Echocardiogram of a patient with marked mitral valve prolapse (p). During diastole the posterior leaflet assumes an almost vertical position and produces a mass of echoes behind the anterior leaflet that can simulate an atrial myxoma. (From Chang, S.: M-mode Echocardiographic Techniques and Pattern Recognition. Philadelphia, Lea & Febiger, 1976.)

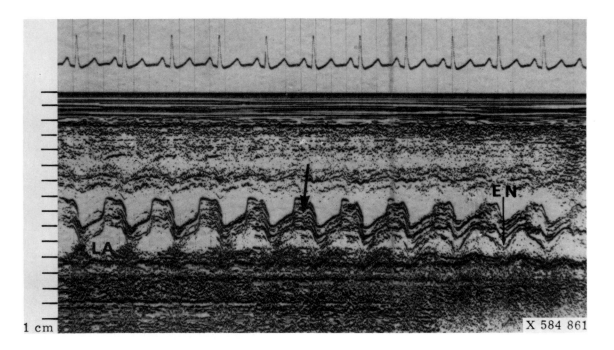

Fig. 11–11. Mitral valve echocardiogram of a patient with a nonbacterial thrombotic mass *(arrow)* involving the mitral valve. LA = left atrium; EN = posterior left ventricular endocardium.

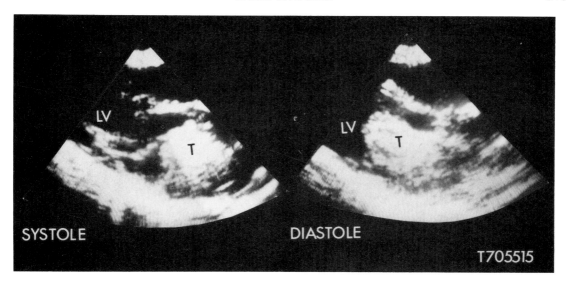

Fig. 11–12.   Long-axis two-dimensional echocardiogram of a patient with a left atrial myxoma. The tumor (T) is visible in the left atrium during systole and in the left ventricle (LV) during diastole.

represent the typical left atrial myxoma, which is pedunculated and moves in and out of the left atrium. However, some echo-producing mass was directly attached to the mitral valve itself. This patient proved to have a nonbacterial thrombotic involvement of the mitral valve and required surgical replacement of that valve. There is no way the echocardiogram could distinguish this mass from a neoplasm. Many similar confusing echocardiograms have been reported in the literature.[18–20] In addition, there has been a report of a fibrolipoma attached to the mitral valve that closely resembled Figure 11–11.[21]

Two-dimensional echocardiography can obviate some of the confusing situations involved in left atrial tumors.[17,22–27] A real-time two-dimensional examination can produce a spectacular recording of a mobile tumor.[24] Figure 11–12 shows a long-axis view of a large left atrial myxoma. The movement of the tumor (T) from systole to diastole is appreciable in these two still frames. The real-time examination was obviously more spectacular. Although the two–dimensional echocardiogram of a mobile left atrial myxoma is dramatic and can be helpful in convincing surgeons that a mass is present and requires removal, it is unusual for the two-dimensional technique to detect a mobile

tumor that could not be adequately diagnosed with M-mode echocardiography. The biggest advantage in two-dimensional echocardiography is detecting left atrial tumors that are not mobile.[17] Figure 11–13 is a long-axis two-dimensional echocardiogram of a

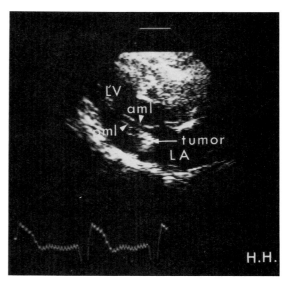

Fig. 11–13.   Long-axis two-dimensional echocardiogram of a patient with a small immobile tumor in the left atrium next to the mitral valve. aml = anterior mitral leaflet; pml = posterior mitral leaflet; LV = left ventricle; LA = left atrium.

patient with a small, immobile tumor at the junction between the left atrium and left ventricle. The tumor was actually on the atrial side of the mitral valve, immediately adjacent to the posterior mitral leaflet (pml). The M-mode echocardiogram of this patient was almost identical to Figure 11–10, except there was no evidence of mitral valve prolapse. The nature of this mass was not readily apparent on the M-mode echocardiogram. The two-dimensional study, however, clearly demonstrated that the echoes were from a tumor at the junction of the left atrium and left ventricle and not merely a peculiar mitral valve. A two-dimensional study would have probably also avoided the confusion in the patient whose echocardiograms were shown in Figures 11–7 and 11–8. Thus, if one suspects an immobile left atrial tumor, two-dimensional echocardiography is probably the examination of choice.

Right Atrial Tumors

Right atrial myxomas are less common than the left atrial variety, although several such tumors have been detected echocardi-

ographically.[13,28–32,32a] Figure 11–14 is an example of a patient with a right atrial myxoma. The tumor is represented by a mass of echoes filling the right ventricle during diastole; these echoes are not visualized during systole. There is an acoustic shadow caused by the tumor, making the septal echoes (IVS) difficult to record during diastole. The postoperative echocardiogram is shown in Figure 11–14B. The echo-producing mass within the right ventricle is no longer present.

A few cases of biatrial myxomas have been reported.[33,34,34a] Figure 11–15 demonstrates an M-mode scan from a patient with biatrial myxomas. The left atrial tumor shows the classic M-mode findings with a mass of echoes posterior to the anterior mitral leaflet (AM). Note the small echo-free gap between the valve leaflet and the tumor mass at the onset of diastole. This small echo-free gap is useful in differentiating a mobile tumor that follows the movement of blood from a mass of echoes that is attached to the valve itself. The echoes from the right tumor (R) appear within the right ventricle in diastole.

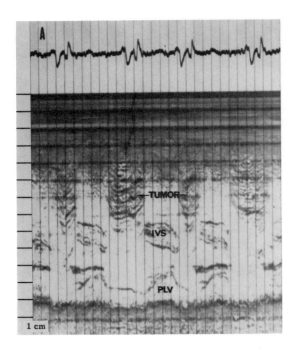 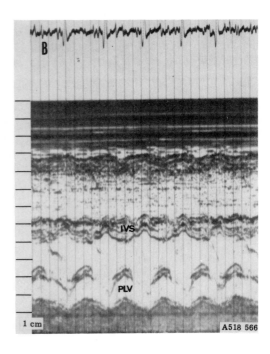

Fig. 11–14. Pre- and postoperative echocardiograms of a patient with a right atrial myxoma. A, During diastole, the tumor produces a band of echoes in the right ventricle. B, Following removal of the tumor, these echoes are absent. IVS = interventricular septum; PLV = posterior left ventricular wall.

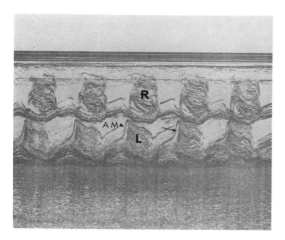

Fig. 11–15. M-mode echocardiogram of a patient with biatrial myxomas. The right tumor (R) appears in the right ventricle during diastole. The left tumor (L) is posterior to the anterior mitral leaflet (AM) in diastole. There is a small echo-free gap *(arrow)* between the mitral leaflet and the left atrial tumor in early diastole.

Although the M-mode echocardiogram in Figure 11–15 is quite diagnostic, a two-dimensional study can provide additional information. Figure 11–16 shows the two-dimensional echocardiogram of the patient in Figure 11–15. The long-axis examination is fairly identical to the M-mode study. The right and left tumors are again seen on either side of the interventricular septum. The four-chamber view is probably more informative since it shows that the right tumor is considerably larger than the left. The right ventricular chamber was grossly dilated, and the tumor practically filled the entire right ventricle in diastole. The real-time examination can frequently demonstrate the attachment of the tumors.

Although almost all echocardiographically detected right atrial tumors reported in the literature are myxomas, there are reports of secondary tumors invading the right atrium.[35,36] We have seen a tumor extend into the right atrium via the inferior vena cava. These tumors are frequently immobile and thus are best detected with two-dimensional echocardiography.

A large vegetation on a tricuspid valve can be difficult to distinguish echocardiographically from a right atrial tumor at times.[37,38] Two-dimensional echocardiography is better than the M-mode technique in making the differential diagnosis.

Occasionally, a prominent eustachian valve can produce prominent echoes within the right atrium. This structure must be identified to eliminate possible confusion with a right atrial mass.[39] There is also a report of a neonate who had a persistent right sinus venosus valve that produced an echocardiogram similar to one showing a right atrial

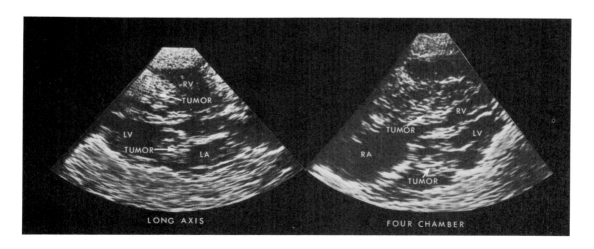

Fig. 11–16. Long-axis and four-chamber two-dimensional echocardiograms of the patient whose M-mode tracing appears in Figure 11–15. The findings in the long-axis view are similar to those in the M-mode recording and again demonstrate the left and right tumors. The four-chamber examination reveals that the right tumor is larger and almost fills the dilated right ventricle (RV). LV = left ventricle; LA = left atrium; RA = right atrium.

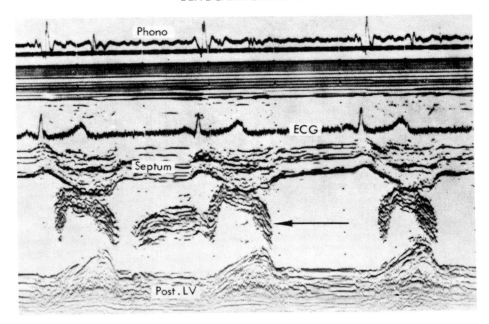

Fig. 11–17.   Left ventricular echocardiogram of a patient with a pedunculated tumor *(arrow)* within the left ventricle (LV). (From Levisman, J.A., et al.: Echocardiographic diagnosis of a mobile, pedunculated tumor in the left ventricular cavity. Am. J. Cardiol., 36:957, 1975.)

tumor.[40] A thrombus of the inferior vena cava may occasionally resemble a right atrial tumor.[40a]

Left Ventricular Tumors

A variety of left ventricular tumors have been detected echocardiographically.[41-49,49a] These include left ventricular myxoma,[41,43,44,49] fibroma,[46] rhabdomyosarcoma,[42] and organized thrombus. The tumors may be mobile or immobile. Figure 11–17 shows an M-mode echocardiogram of a mobile left ventricular tumor that proved to be an organized thrombus. The echoes from the mass (arrow) move anteriorly against the septum with ventricular systole. Such tumors frequently appear within the left ventricular outflow tract in systole.

Immobile left ventricular masses are more difficult to detect with M-mode echocardiography. Figure 11–18 shows an M-mode scan of a patient with a left ventricular tumor involving the apical half of the ventricle. As one scans toward the apex, the mass of echoes from the neoplasm (T) becomes evident. This echocardiogram, however, is not absolutely diagnostic for a ventricular mass.

One can obtain similar types of tracings by merely directing the beam so that it no longer passes through the center of the cavity. One cannot confidently say that the echoes in the apical half of this tracing were

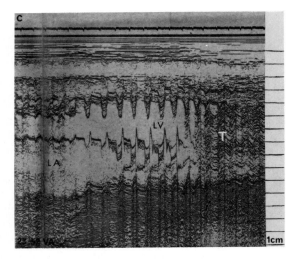

Fig. 11–18.   M-mode scan of a patient with a left ventricular tumor involving the apical half of the left ventricle. The echoes from the tumor (T) can be noted as the ultrasonic beam moves toward the apex. LV = left ventricle; LA = left atrium.

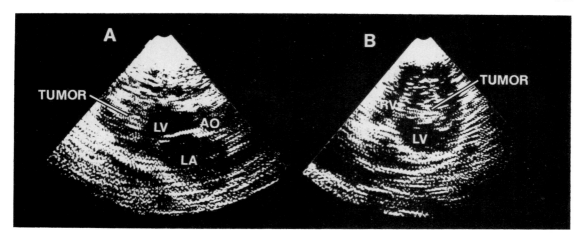

Fig. 11–19. Long-axis, A, and short-axis, B, two-dimensional echocardiograms of a patient with a left ventricular tumor whose M-mode recording appears in Figure 11–18. LV = left ventricle; AO = aorta; La = left atrium; RV = right ventricle. (From Feigenbaum, H.: Echocardiography. In Heart Disease. Edited by E. Braunwald. Philadelphia, W.B. Saunders, 1980.)

clearly abnormal. Figure 11–19 is the two-dimensional echocardiogram from that patient. Long-axis (A) and short-axis (B) views demonstrate the tumor mass within the left ventricular cavity. The correct diagnosis is more convincing on the two-dimensional study. One can appreciate the size and configuration of the tumor by way of this spatially oriented technique. This example again demonstrates why immobile tumors

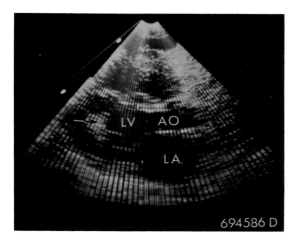

Fig. 11–20. Long-axis two-dimensional echocardiogram of a patient with an echo-producing mass of fibrous tissue (arrow) occupying the apical half of the left ventricle (LV). The patient had a form of endomyocardial fibrosis. AO = aorta; LA = left atrium.

are best detected with two-dimensional rather than M-mode echocardiography.

Occasionally, a tumor is not within the cavity of the left ventricle but primarily involves the interventricular septum.[50,51] The echocardiogram would reveal a wide interventricular septum. When the tumor is cystic, the mass is relatively echo free.[51]

Not all left ventricular masses are neoplastic. The tumors can be secondary to clot as in Figure 11–17. In addition, Figure 11–20 shows a two-dimensional echocardiogram similar to that in Figure 11–19. The apical half of the ventricular cavity was obliterated by an echo-producing mass. At surgery the obstructing tissue was a form of endomyocardial fibrosis, not neoplasm.[52]

Right Ventricular Tumors

Right ventricular tumors have also been detected echocardiographically.[53–58] Most tumors reported in the literature have been myxomas. One case of metastatic melanoma has been described.[53] The tumors are usually, but not always, mobile. A pedunculated myxoma may produce right ventricular outflow tract obstruction and simulate pulmonic stenosis.[56,57] Pedunculated, mobile, right ventricular myxomas appear similar to a right atrial myxoma, such as in Figures 11–14, 11–15, and 11–16. Figure 11–21 shows an

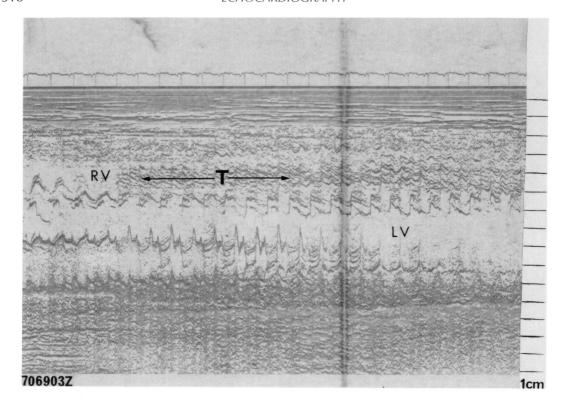

Fig. 11–21.   M-mode scan of a patient with an immobile right ventricular tumor. The tumor echoes (T) can be seen occupying the right ventricular cavity (RV). LV = left ventricle.

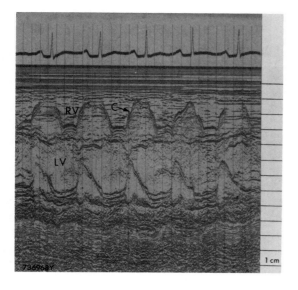

Fig. 11–22.   M-mode echocardiogram of a patient with a Swan-Ganz catheter (C) within the right ventricle (RV). LV = left ventricle.

M-mode echocardiogram of an immobile right ventricular mass appearing in the right ventricular outflow tract. An M-mode scan is necessary to ensure that the mass of echoes within the right ventricle is not artifactual.

One must be aware of iatrogenic echoes within the right ventricle and right ventricular outflow tract. A common cause for such echoes is a Swan-Ganz catheter traversing the right ventricle.[58a,58b] Figure 11–22 demonstrates an M-mode echocardiogram with an echo from a Swan-Ganz catheter in the right ventricular outflow tract (C). Such an echo may simulate a tricuspid valve or occasionally may resemble a mobile right ventricular tumor.

EXTRACARDIAC TUMORS

A variety of extracardiac tumors have been detected by echocardiography.[59–65] The pathology includes mediastinal cyst,[59]

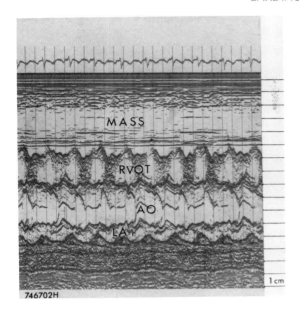

Fig. 11–23. Echocardiogram of a patient with a large mediastinal mass that displaces the heart posteriorly and markedly decreases the size of the left atrium (LA). AO = aorta. RVOT = right ventricular outflow tract.

thymoma,[61] and a variety of pericardial tumors.[62,64,65] Basically, the extracardiac tumors appear either anterior or posterior to the heart. Figure 11–23 demonstrates a large mediastinal mass anterior to the heart. There is a large, relatively echo-free space from the cystic mass that lies between the chest wall and the heart. Such masses can obviously distort the echocardiogram. For example, the left atrium is markedly reduced in Figure 11–23 because of the compression by the mediastinal mass.

Figure 11–24 illustrates a posterior extracardiac mass. This echocardiogram shows a tumor that invaded the posterior pericardium. The echocardiogram demonstrates what appears to be a thick pericardium. Its size, however, suggests more than mere thickening. Of course, posterior tumors may be even larger than that shown in Figure 11–24 and can distort the echocardiogram significantly. In one report, the extracardiac tumor was compressing the left atrium with

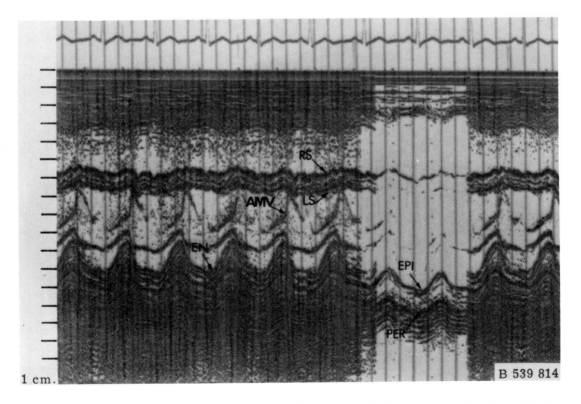

Fig. 11–24. M-mode echocardiogram of a patient with tumor invading the posterior pericardium. The tumor appears between the posterior left ventricular epicardium (EPI) and the posterior pericardium (PER). RS = right septum; LS = left septum; AMV = anterior mitral valve leaflet; EN = posterior left ventricular endocardium.

extension of the tumor into the left atrial cavity.[63] Two-dimensional echocardiography has been reported as particularly helpful in some of these extracardiac tumors.[63] In addition, some investigators have recommended examining the heart from the right sternal border when the heart is displaced by a mediastinal mass.[59,65]

INTRACARDIAC THROMBI

Left Atrial Thrombi

The left atrium is a frequent site for thrombi. Unfortunately, most of these clots are small and occur in the vicinity of the left atrial appendage, an area only recently recognized by way of two-dimensional echocardiography. Occasionally, a large left atrial clot may be seen along the posterior left atrial wall.[66-71] Figure 11–25 shows a large clot that produced a band of linear echoes within the left atrium. In the preoperative left atrial echocardiogram (A), one might have difficulty identifying the posterior left atrial wall. An M-mode scan into the left ventricle may or may not have been helpful in identifying the true left atrial wall. At surgery a large clot was indeed lying against the poste-

rior wall of the left atrium and was removed. The postoperative echocardiogram (B) is distinctly different. The extra linear echoes labeled clot in the preoperative tracing are no longer present.

Unfortunately, extra echoes within the left atrium are commonly seen. Left atrial echocardiograms quite similar to that in Figure 11–25A have been reported in patients in whom no atrial clot was found during surgery or at autopsy. These echoes could be originating from reverberations, the interatrial septum, or even pulmonary veins. Thus the echocardiograms seen in Figure 11–25 are compatible with but by no means diagnostic of a left atrial thrombus.

We had the opportunity to examine one patient with a mobile clot within the left atrium (Fig. 11–26). This thrombus was not attached to the walls and was floating freely within the left atrial cavity. Echoes from this clot can be seen within the left atrium and form a randomly appearing series of echoes moving extensively within the body of the left atrium. Although mobile left atrial clots are much easier to detect with M-mode echocardiography, such thrombi are extremely rare.

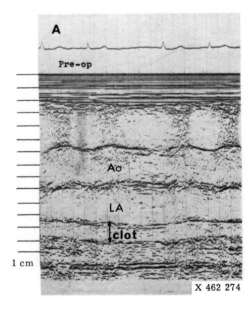
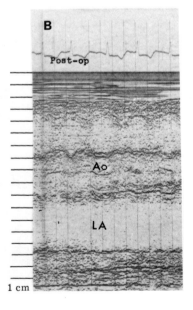

Fig. 11–25. Echocardiograms of a patient with mitral valve disease and clot within the left atrium. A, Prior to surgery, multiple linear echoes were present within the left atrial cavity (LA). B, Following surgical removal of the thrombus, these echoes disappeared. Thus they were thought to originate from the clot. (From Chang, S.: M-mode Echocardiographic Techniques and Pattern Recognition. Philadelphia, Lea & Febiger, 1976.)

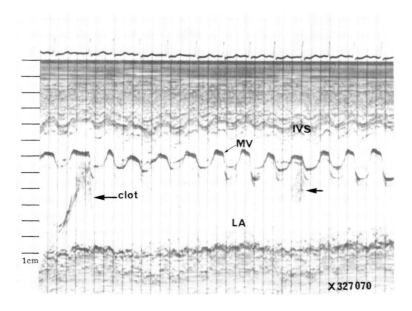

Fig. 11–26. Left atrial echocardiogram of a patient with a mobile clot that was floating freely within the cavity of the left atrium. IVS = interventricular septum; MV = mitral valve; LA = left atrium. (From Chang, S.: M-mode Echocardiographic Techniques and Pattern Recognition. Philadelphia, Lea & Febiger, 1976.)

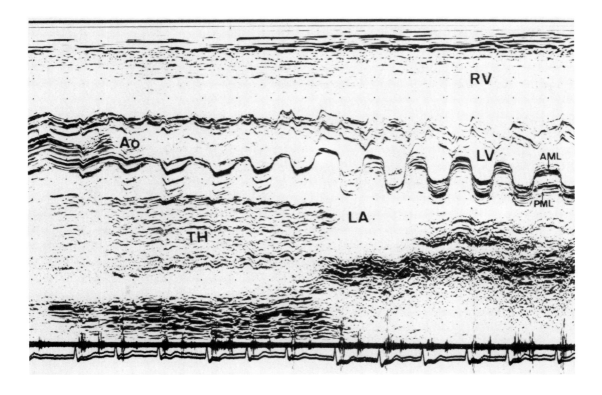

Fig. 11–27. M-mode scan of a patient with mitral stenosis and a large thrombus (TH) within the left atrium (LA). AO = aorta; RV = right ventricle; LV = left ventricle; AML = anterior mitral leaflet; PML = posterior mitral leaflet. (From Machii, K.: Atlas of Cross-sectional Echocardiography. Tokyo, Toshiba Corporation, 1978.)

Figure 11–27 is a more striking and probably more convincing M-mode echocardiogram of a large atrial thrombus. The echoes from the large thrombus (TH) are centrally located in the left atrial cavity in this patient with mitral stenosis. One again cannot be absolutely certain of the diagnosis of a thrombus. However, the echocardiogram here is far more suspicious than in Figure 11–25A.

Figure 11–28 is a long-axis two-dimensional echocardiogram of the patient in Figure 11–27. A large, spherical, echo-producing mass within the left atrium is even more convincing with this two-dimensional study. The thrombus (TH) almost completely fills the dilated left atrium. Although there are relatively few reports of using two-dimensional echocardiography for the diagnosis of left atrial thrombi,[72,73] one certainly expects the two-dimensional technique to be better than M-mode. It is hoped that if we can improve our technique for examining the left atrial appendage (Fig. 11–29), then we may be able to see some of the more common left atrial thrombi.

Left Ventricular Thrombi

Although occasional left ventricular thrombi have been detected with M-mode echocardiography,[74–77] this examination is relatively insensitive for finding such clots. A large percentage of these clots occur in or near the left ventricular apex, and this area is not examined well with M-mode echocardiography. On the other hand, two-dimensional echocardiography is proving successful in detecting thrombi, especially those near the apex.[77–80] These clots most often occur in acute myocardial infarction or cardiomyopathy. Figure 11–30 demonstrates the most commonly used examination for detecting left ventricular thrombi. This apical four-chamber view shows a large clot (CL) at the apex in this patient with coronary artery disease. These thrombi usually are stationary, although they may show considerable motion at times. When a large mobile clot is found within the left ventricular cavity, the question of whether surgical intervention is indicated frequently arises.

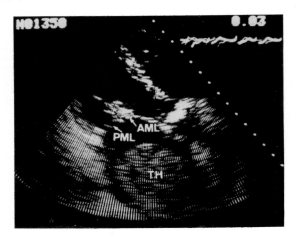

Fig. 11–28. Two-dimensional long-axis echocardiogram of a patient with a left atrial thrombus whose M-mode echocardiogram is shown in Figure 11–27. The large spherical thrombus (TH) is visible within the dilated left atrium. AML = anterior mitral leaflet; PML = posterior mitral leaflet. (From Machii, K.: Atlas of Cross-sectional Echocardiography. Tokyo, Toshiba Corporation, 1978.)

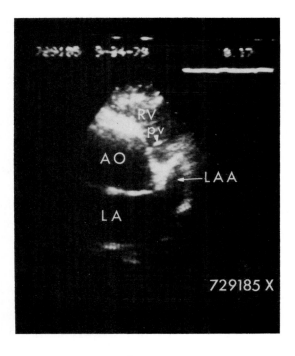

Fig. 11–29. Short-axis two-dimensional echocardiogram of the left atrium demonstrating the location of the left atrial appendage (LAA). RV = right ventricle; AO = aorta; LA = left atrium; pv = pulmonary valve.

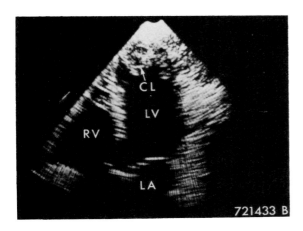

Fig. 11–30. Apical, four-chamber two-dimensional echocardiogram demonstrating a clot (CL) in the apex of the left ventricle (LV). RV = right ventricle; LA = left atrium.

Although the apical four- and two-chamber views are most commonly used for the detection of ventricular thrombi, the standard long- and short-axis views may also be helpful in the diagnosis. Figure 11–31 shows a long-axis (LAX) and short-axis (SAX) examination of a patient with a large clot that virtually fills the entire apex of the left ventricle. The short-axis examination demonstrates a rim of cavity that is not completely filled with clot. Figure 11–32 illustrates similar long- and short-axis examinations in a

patient with a smaller clot (CL) within a dyskinetic apex. This patient actually had two clots, one smaller than the other. The multiple views help to better assess the size and shape of the thrombi.

Thus two-dimensional echocardiography is proving a good method for the detection of left ventricular thrombi. The sensitivity and reliability appear satisfactory. This technique still misses small thrombi; however, it is unlikely that a clot as small as that seen in Figure 11–32 would be detected by any other technique, including angiography. Thus it is possible that echocardiography may be the most sensitive clinical tool available for the diagnosis of ventricular clots.

One must recognize potential false positives in the detection of mural thrombi. One should not misdiagnose a papillary muscle for a thrombus. Figure 11–33 shows a short-axis two-dimensional echocardiogram of a normal left ventricle at the level of the papillary muscle. The examination records only one papillary muscle (pm), which superficially might resemble a mural clot. With further searching, the other papillary muscle can be seen, and the potential misdiagnosis of thrombus can be avoided. An even more confusing echocardiogram appears in Figure 11–34. In diastole (A), one sees a mass of echoes (arrow) within the left ventricular cavity. These echoes have fine oscillations in

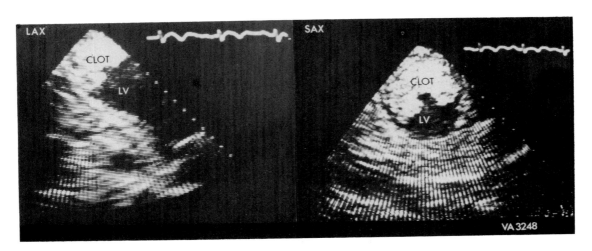

Fig. 11–31. Long-axis (LAX) and short-axis (SAX) two-dimensional echocardiograms of a patient with a large clot in the apex of the left ventricle (LV).

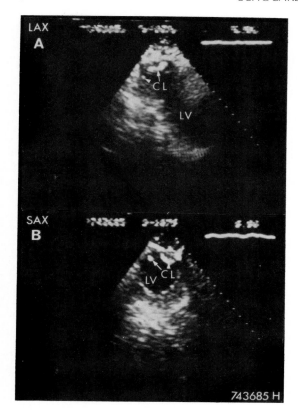

Fig. 11–32. Long-axis (LAX) and short-axis (SAX) two-dimensional echocardiograms of a patient with a small clot (CL) in an apical aneurysm of the left ventricle (LV).

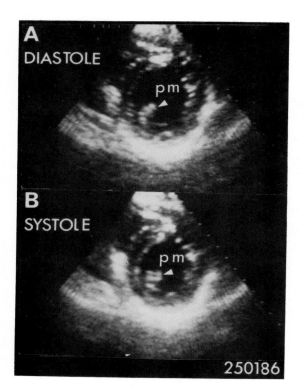

Fig. 11–33. Short-axis two-dimensional echocardiogram of a normal left ventricle at the level of the papillary muscles. Only one papillary muscle (pm) is recorded and may superficially resemble a mural thrombus.

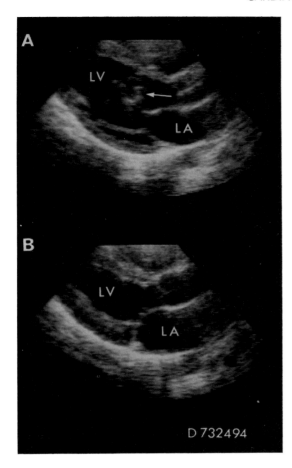

Fig. 11-34. Parasternal long-axis two-dimensional echocardiograms of a normal individual in diastole and systole. A, In diastole, a mass of echoes (arrow) are seen within the left ventricular cavity (LV). These echoes are artifacts due to reverberations and simulate a left ventricular mass. B, In systole, the echoes are absent. LA = left atrium.

the real-time examination and superficially resemble a mass within the cavity of the left ventricle. During ventricular systole (B), these echoes disappear. The abnormal echoes in Figure 11-34 are totally artifactual as the result of reverberations. The exact source of the reverberations is not totally understood. The reverberations are a function of the repetition rate of the echographic system and can be eliminated by changing the repetition rate. Thus, although echocardiography, especially two-dimensional echocardiography, is proving to be extremely important in the diagnosis of intracardiac masses,

one must be aware of potential false positives.

REFERENCES

1. Nasser, W.K., et al.: Atrial myxoma. I. Clinical and pathologic features in nine cases. Am. Heart J., 83:694, 1972.
2. Lortscher, R.H., Toews, W.H., Nora, J.J., Wolfe, R.R., and Spangler, R.D.: Left atrial myxoma presenting as rheumatic fever. Chest, 66:302, 1974.
3. Steimetz, E.F., Calanchini, P.R., and Anguilar, M.J.: Left atrial myxoma as a neurological problem: a case report and review. Stroke, 4:451, 1973.
4. Popp, R.L., and Levine, R.: Left atrial mass simulating cardiomyopathy. J. Clin. Ultrasound, 1:96, 1973.
5. Edmands, R.E., Linback, R.E., Mercho, J.P., Roushdi, H.A., and Wunsch, C.M.: Atrial myxoma: a curable disorder—a case report. J. Ind. State Med., 67:903, 1974.
6. Bass, N.M. and Sharratt, G.P.: Left atrial myxoma diagnosed by echocardiography with observations on tumour movement. Br. Heart J., 35:1332, 1973.
7. Effert, S. and Domanig, E.: The diagnosis of intraatrial tumor and thrombi by the ultrasonic echo method. German Med. Mth. 4:1, 1959.
8. Finegan, R.E. and Harrison, D.C.: Diagnosis of left atrial myxoma by echocardiography. N. Engl. J. Med., 282:1022, 1970.
9. Gustafson, A., Edler, I., Dahlback, O., Kaude, J., and Persson, S.: Left atrial myxoma diagnosed by ultrasound cardiography. Angiology, 24:554, 1973.
10. Kostis, J.B., and Moghadam, A.N.: Echocardiographic diagnosis of left atrial myxoma. Chest, 58:550, 1970.
11. Popp, R.L., and Harrison, D.C.: Ultrasound in the diagnosis of atrial tumor. Ann. Intern. Med., 71:785, 1969.
12. Schattenberg, T.T.: Echocardiographic diagnosis of left atrial myxoma. Mayo Clin. Proc., 43:620, 1968.
13. Wolfe, S.B., Popp, R.L., and Feigenbaum, H.: Diagnosis of atrial tumors by ultrasound. Circulation, 39:615, 1969.
13a. Abdulla, A.M., Stefadouros, M.A., Mucha, E., Moore, H.V., and O'Malley, G.A.: Left atrial myxoma: echocardiographic diagnosis and determination of size. J.A.M.A., 238:510, 1977.
13b. Winer, H.E., Kronzon, I., Fox, A., Hines, G., Trehan, N., Antapol, S., and Reed, G.: Primary cardiac chondromyxosarcoma—clinical and echocardiographic manifestations: a case report. J. Thorac. Surg., 74:567, 1977.
14. Zackia, A.H., Weber, D.J., Ramsey, C., and Wong, B.: Recurrence of left atrial myxoma. J. Cardiovasc. Surg. (Torino), 25:467, 1974.
15. Giuliani, E.R., Lemire, F., and Schattenberg, T.T.: Unusual echocardiographic findings in a patient with left atrial myxoma. Mayo Clin. Proc., 53:469, 1978.
16. Nasser, W.K., et al.: Atrial myxoma. II. Phonocardiographic, echocardiographic, hemodynamic, and angiographic features in nine cases. Am. Heart J., 83:810, 1972.
17. Chadda, K.D., Pochaczevsky, R., Gupta, P.K., Lichstein, E., and Schwartz, I.S.: Nonprolapsing atrial myxoma: clinical echocardiographic and angiographic correlations. Angiology, 29:179, 1978.
18. Weymann, A.E., Rankin, R., and King, H.: Leoffler's

endocarditis presenting as mitral and tricuspid stenosis. Am. J. Cardiol., 40:438, 1977.

19. Pasternak, R.C., Cannom, D.S., and Cohen, L.S.: Echocardiographic diagnosis of large fungal verruca attached to mitral valve. Br. Heart Jr., 38:1209, 1976.

20. Fitchett, D.H. and Oakley, C.M.: Granulomatous mitral valve obstruction. Br. Heart J., 38:112, 1976.

21. Barberger-Gateau, P., Paquet, M., Desaulniers, D., and Chenard, J.: Fibrolipoma of the mitral valve in a child. Circulation, 58:955, 1978.

22. Kerber, R.E., Kelly, D.H., Jr., and Gutenkauf, C.H.: Left atrial myxoma demonstrated by stop-action cardiac ultrasonography. Am. J. Cardiol., 34:838, 1974.

23. Matsumoto, M., Matsuo, H., Nagata, S., Oyama, S., Nimura, Y., Asoh, M., Miyazaki, H., Hamaji, M., Nakata, T., Kobayashi, Y., and Shimada, H.: Left atrial myxoma detected by ultrasound cardiogram. Med. Ultrasonics, 10:9, 1972.

24. Rogers, E.W., Weyman, A.E., Noble, R.J., and Bruins, S.C.: Left atrial myxoma infected with Histoplasma capsulatum. Am. J. Med., 64:683, 1978.

25. Lappe, D.L., Bulkley, B.H., and Weiss, J.L.: Two-dimensional echocardiographic diagnosis of left atrial myxoma. Chest, 74:55, 1978.

26. Seward, J.B., Gura, G.M., Hagler, D.J., and Tajik, S.J.: Evaluation of M-mode echocardiography and wide-angle two-dimensional sector echocardiography in the diagnosis of intracardiac masses. Circulation (Suppl. II), 58:234, 1978. (Abstract)

27. Hibi, N., Gukui, Y., Nishimura, K., Miwa, A., and Kambe, T.: Real time observation of left atrial myxoma with high speed B mode echocardiography. J. Clin. Ultrasound, 7:34, 1979.

28. Harbold, N.B., Jr. and Gau, G.T.: Echocardiographic diagnosis of right atrial myxoma. Mayo Clin. Proc., 48:284, 1973.

29. Farooki, Z.Q., Green, E.W., and Arciniegas, E.: Echocardiographic pattern of right atrial tumour motion. Br. Heart J., 38:580, 1976.

30. Pernod, J., Piwnica, A., and Duret, J.C.: Right atrial myxoma: an echocardiographic study. Br. Heart J., 40:201, 1978.

31. Meyers, S.N., Shapiro, S.E., Barresi, V., et al.:Right atrial myxoma with right to left shunting and mitral valve prolapse. Am. J. Med., 62:308, 1977.

32. Frishman, W., Factor, S., Jordon, A., Hellman, C., Elkayam, U., LeJemtel, T., Strom, J., Unschuld, H., and Becker, R.: Right atrial myxoma: unusual clinical presentation and atypical glandular histology. Circulation, 59:1070, 1979. (Case report)

32a.Atsuchi, Y., Nagai, Y., Nakamura, K., et al.: Echocardiographic diagnosis of prolapsing right atrial myxoma. Jpn. Heart J., 17:798, 1976.

33. Fitterer, J.D., Spicer, M.J., and Nelson, W.P.: Echocardiographic demonstration of bilateral atrial myxomas. Chest, 70:282, 1976.

34. Nicholson, K.G., Prior, A.L., Norman, A.G., Naik, D.R., and Kennedy, A.: Bilateral atrial myxomas diagnosed preoperatively and successfully removed. Br. Med. J., 2(6084):440, 1977.

34a.Gustafson, A.G., Edler, I.G., and Dahlback, O.K.: Bilateral atrial myxomas diagnosed by echocardiography. Acta Med. Scand., 201:391, 1977.

35. Horgan, J.H., Beachley, M.C., Kemp, V.E., Greenfield, L.J., Behm, F.G., Centor, R.M., and Goodman, A.C.: Primary and secondary right atrial

tumors detected by echocardiography. J. Clin. Ultrasound, 5:92, 1977.

36. Farooki, Z.Q., Henry, J.G., and Green, E.W.: Echocardiographic diagnosis of right atrial extension of Wilms' tumor. Am. J. Cardiol., 36:363, 1975.

37. Chandraratna, P.A.N. and Aronow, W.S.: Spectrum of echocardiographic findings in tricuspid valve endocarditis. Br. Heart J., 42:528, 1979.

38. Come, P.C., Kurland, G.S., and Vine, H.S.: Two dimensional echocardiography in differentiating right atrial and tricuspid valve mass lesions. Am. J. Cardiol., 44:1207, 1979.

39. Bommer, W.J., Kwan, O.L., Mason, D.T., and De-Maria, A.N.: Identification of prominent eustachian valves by M-mode and two-dimensional echocardiography: differentiation from right atrial masses. Am. J. Cardiol., 45:402, 1980. (Abstract)

40. Battle-Diaz, J., Stanley, P., Kratz, C., Fouron, J-C., Guerin, R., and Davignon, A.: Echocardiographic manifestations of persistence of the right sinus venosus valve. Am. J. Cardiol., 43:850, 1979.

40a.Broadbent, J.C., Tajik, A.J., and Wallace, R.B.: Thrombus of inferior vena cava presenting as right atrial tumor: roentgenographic, phonoechocardiographic, angiographic, and surgical findings. J. Thorac. Cardiovasc. Surg., 72:722, 1976.

41. Levisman, J.A., MacAlpin, R.N., Abbasi, A.S., Ellis, N., and Eber, L.M.: Echocardiographic diagnosis of a mobile, pedunculated tumor in the left ventricular cavity. Am. J. Cardiol., 36:957, 1975.

42. Farooki, Z.Q., Henry, J.G., Arciniegas, E., and Green, EX.W.: Ultrasonic pattern of ventricular rhabdomyoma in two infants. Am. J. Cardiol., 34:842, 1974.

43. Meller, J., Teichholz, L.E., Pichard, A.O., Matta, R., Litwak, R., Herman, M.V., and Massie, K.F.: Left ventricular myxoma: echocardiographic diagnosis and review of the literature. Am. J. Med., 63:816, 1977.

44. Morgan, D.L., Palazola, J., Reed, W., Bell, H.H., Kindred, L.H., and Beauchamp, G.D.: Left heart myxomas. Am. J. Cardiol., 40:611, 1977.

45. Orsmond, G.S., Knight L., Dehner, L.P., Nicoloff, D.M., Nesbitt, M., and Bessinger, F.B.: Alveolar rhabdomyosarcoma involving the heart: an echocardiographic, angiographic, and pathologic study. Circulation, 54:834, 1976. (Case report)

46. Oliva, P.B., Breckinridge, J.C., Johnson, M.L., Brantigan, C.O., and O'Meara, O.P.: Left ventricular outflow obstruction produced by a pedunculated fibroma in a newborn. Chest, 74:590, 1978.

47. Rees, A.H., Elbl, F.E., Minhas, K.V., and Solinger, R.E.: Echocardiographic evidence of left ventricular tumor in a neonate. Chest, 73:433, 1978.

48. Ports, T.A., Cogan, J., Schiller, N.B., and Rapaport, E.: Echocardiography of left ventricular masses. Circulation, 58:528, 1978.

49. Sabot, G., Fauvel, J.M., and Bounhoure, J.P.: Echocardiographic diagnosis of mobile left ventricular tumour. Br. Heart J., 42:113, 1979.

49a.Tomoike, H., Kawaguchi, K., Takeshita, A., et al.: Echocardiographic recognition of the cardiac mural tumor. Jpn. Heart J., 17:106, 1976.

50. Horgan, J.H., O'M Shiel, F., and Goodman, A.C.: Tumor invasion of the interventricular septum detected by conventional echocardiography. J. Clin. Ultrasound, 4:133, 1976.

51. Farooki, Z.Q., Adelman, S., and Green, E.W.:

Echocardiographic differentiation of a cystic and a solid tumor of the heart. Am. J. Cardiol., 39:107, 1977.

52. Eterovic, I., Angelini, P., Leachman, R., and Cooley, D.A.: Obliterative restrictive endomyocardial fibrosis: a surgical approach. Cardiovasc. Dis., 6:66, 1979.

53. Ports, T.A., Schiller, N.B., and Strunk, B.L.: Echocardiography of right ventricular tumors. Circulation, 56:439, 1977.

54. Nanda, N.C., Barold, S.S., Gramiak, R., Ong, L.S., and Heinle, R.A.: Echocardiographic features of right ventricular outflow tumor prolapsing into the pulmonary artery. Am. J. Cardiol., 40:272, 1977.

55. Asayama, J., Kunishige, H., Katsume, H., Watanabe, T., Matsukubo, H., Endo, N. Matsuura, T., Ijichi, H., Onouchi, Z., Tomizawa, M., Goto, M., and Nakata, K.: The ultrasound cardiographic findings of myxoma in the right ventricular wall. Cardiovasc. Sound Bull., 5:129, 1975.

56. Jaffe, C.C., Kelley, M.J., and Taunt, K.A.: Two-dimensional echocardiographic identification of a right ventricle tumor. Radiology, 129:471, 1978.

57. Chandraratna, P.A.N., Pedro, S., Elkins, R.C., and Grantham, N.: Echocardiographic, angiocardiographic, and surgical correlations in right ventricular myxoma simulating valvar pulmonic stenosis. Circulation, 55:619, 1977.

58. Roelandt, J., Bletter, W.B., Leuftink, E.W., van-Dorp, W.G., tenCate, F., and Nauta, J.: Ultrasonic demonstration of right ventricular myxoma. J. Clin. Ultrasound, 5:191, 1977.

58a. Charuzi, Y., Kraus, R., and Swan, H.J.C.: Echocardiographic interpretation in the presence of Swan-Ganz intracardiac catheters. Am. J. Cardiol., 40:989, 1977.

58b. Kirkman, P.M., Reeves, W.C., and Zelis, R.: Echocardiographic diagnostic pitfalls induced by indwelling Swan-Ganz catheters. Practical Cardiol., November, 1978.

59. Koch, P.C., Kronzon, I., Winer, H.E., Adams, P., and Trubek, M.: Displacement of the heart by a giant mediastinal cyst. Am. J. Cardiol., 40:445, 1977.

60. Tingelstad, J.B., McWilliams, N.B., and Thomas, C.E.: Confirmation of a retrosternal mass by echocardiogram. J. Clin. Ultrasound, 4:129, 1976.

61. Canedo, M.I., Otken, L., and Stefadouros, M.A.: Echocardiographic features of cardiac compression by a thymoma simulating cardiac tamponade and obstruction of the superior vena cava. Br. Heart J., 39:1038, 1977.

62. Farooki, Z.Q., Hakimi, N., Arciniegas, E., and Green, E.W.: Echocardiographic features in a case of intrapericardial teratoma. J. Clin. Ultrasound, 6:108, 1978.

63. Yoshikawa, J., Sabah, I., Yanagihara, K., Owaki, T., Kato, H., and Tanemoto, K.: Cross-sectional echocardiographic diagnosis of large left atrial tumor and extracardiac tumor compressing the left atrium. Am. J. Cardiol., 42:853, 1978.

64. Lin, T.K., Stech, J.M., Eckert, W.G., Lin, J.J., Farha, S.J., and Hagan, C.T.: Pericardial angiosarcoma simulating pericardial effusion by echocardiography. Chest, 73:881, 1978.

65. Chandraratna, P.A.N., Littman, B.B., Serafini, A., Whayne, T., and Robinson, H.: Echocardiographic evaluation of extracardiac masses. Br. Heart J., 40:741, 1978.

66. Klepacki, Z., Surlowica-Sidun, B., and Zarebska, L.: Intra-atrial thrombus detected by ultrasonocardiography. Kardiol. Pol., 17:83, 1974.

67. Phillips, B.J., Friedeward, V.E., Jr., Kinard, S.A., and Diethrich, E.B.: Calcified intra-atrial mass detected by M-mode echocardiography and multihead transducer scanning: a case report. J. Clin. Ultrasound, 2:245, 1974. (Abstract)

68. Poehlmann, H.W., Basta, L.L., and Brown, R.E.: Left atrial thrombus detected by ultrasound: a case report. J. Clin. Ultrasound, 3:65, 1975.

69. Spangler, R.D. and Okin, J.T.: Illustrative echocardiogram: echocardiographic demonstration of a left atrial thrombus. Chest, 67:716, 1975.

70. Graboys, T.B., Sloss, L.J., and Ockene, I.A.: Echocardiographic diagnosis of left atrial thrombus—a case report. J. Clin. Ultrasound, 5:284, 1977.

71. Spangler, R.D. and Okin, J.T.: Illustrative echocardiogram: echocardiographic demonstration of a left atrial thrombus. Chest, 67:716, 1975.

72. Mikell, F.L., Asinger, R.W., Rourke, T., Hodges, M., Sharma, B., and Francis, G.S.: Two-dimensional echocardiographic demonstration of left atrial thrombi in patients with prosthetic mitral valves. Circulation, 60:1183, 1979. (Case report)

73. Denbow, C.E., Tajik, A.J., Seward, J.B., and Pluth, J.R.: Massive thrombus in body of left atrium: clinical profile and surgical experience. Circulation (Suppl. II), 68:232, 1978. (Abstract)

74. Horgan, J.H., O'M Shiel, F., and Goodman, A.C.: Demonstration of left ventricular thrombus by conventional echocardiography. J. Clin. Ultrasound, 4:287, 1976.

75. Kramer, N.E., Rathod, R., Chawla, K.K., Patel, R., and Towne, W.D.: Echocardiographic diagnosis of left ventricular mural thrombi occurring in cardiomyopathy. Am. Heart J., 96:381, 1978.

76. Dejoseph, R.L., Shiroff, F.A., Levenson, L.W., Martin, C.E., and Zelis, R.F.: Echocardiographic diagnosis of intraventricular clot. Chest, 71:417, 1977.

77. van den Bos, A.A., Bletter, W.B., and Hagemeijer, F.: Progressive development of a left ventricular thrombus. Detection and evolution studied with echocardiographic techniques. Chest, 74:307, 1978.

78. DeMaria, A.N., Bommer, W., Neumann, A. Grehl, T., Weinart, L., DeNardo, S., Amsterdam, E.A., and Mason, D.T.: Left ventricular thrombi identified by cross-sectional echocardiography. Ann. Intern. Med., 90:14, 1979.

79. Meltzer, R.S., Guthaner, D., Rakowski, H., Popp, R.L., and Martin, R.P.: Diagnosis of left ventricular thrombi by two-dimensional echocardiography. Br. Heart J., 42:261, 1979.

80. Mikell, F., Asinger, R., Rourke, T., Hodges, M., Sharma, B., and Francis, G.: Detection of intracardiac thrombi by two-dimensional echocardiography (2DE). Circulation (Suppl. II), 58:43, 1978. (Abstract)

Diseases of the Aorta

ECHOCARDIOGRAPHIC EXAMINATION OF THE AORTA

Although the echocardiographic examination of the aorta has been recognized for many years,[1] interest in this structure has been renewed in recent years. Figure 12–1 shows an M-mode scan from the left ventricle into the base of the heart and the aorta (AO). The anterior wall of the aorta is continuous with the echoes from the interventricular septum (LS), and the posterior wall of the aorta is continuous with the anterior mitral valve leaflet. Within the aorta are the characteristic box-like echoes from the aortic valve. A larger recording of a normal aortic root is illustrated in Figure 12–2. The characteristic features that identify the aorta are the two dominant parallel echoes that move upward or anteriorly with systole and posteriorly with diastole. The walls of the aorta are

very echo producing; these echoes are usually the easiest to record. Although the motion of the two walls is similar, the amplitude of motion of the anterior wall is somewhat more, so that the distance between the two walls is slightly greater in systole than in diastole.

Although aortic root measurements can be obtained at any time in the cardiac cycle, the measurement is usually obtained in diastole, as indicated in Figure 12–2. The measurement may be taken from the trailing edge or posterior edge of the anterior wall echo to the leading edge of the posterior wall echo, as in Figure 12–2. However, according to the American Society of Echocardiography, the measurement should be taken from the leading edge of the anterior wall of the aorta to the leading edge of the posterior wall of the aorta.

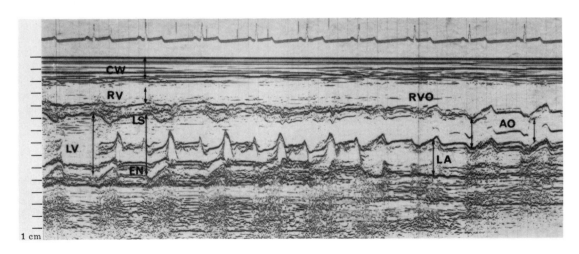

Fig. 12–1.   M-mode scan from the left ventricle (LV) to the aorta (AO) and left atrium (LA). CW = chest wall; RV = right ventricle; LS = left septum; EN = posterior left ventricular endocardium; RVO = right ventricular outflow tract.

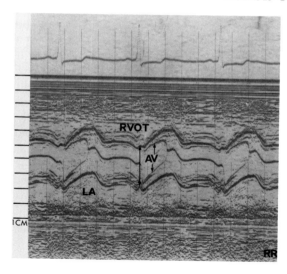

Fig. 12–2. Echocardiogram of the aortic root bounded anteriorly by the right ventricular outflow tract (RVOT) and posteriorly by the left atrium (LA). The aortic valve leaflets (AV) lie within the aortic wall echoes. (From Chang, S.: M-mode Echocardiographic Techniques and Pattern Recognition. Philadelphia, Lea & Febiger, 1976.)

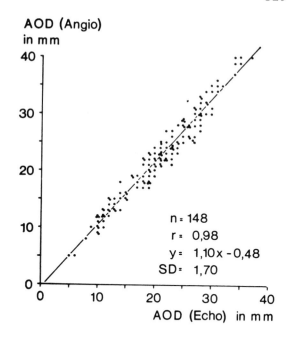

Fig. 12–3. Correlation between the aortic root diameter measured angiographically (Angio) and echocardiographically (Echo). (From Lundstrom, N.R. and Mortensson, W.: Clinical applications of echocardiography in infants and children. II. Estimation of aortic root diameter and left atrial size. A comparison between echocardiography and angiocardiography. Acta Paediatr. Scand. 63:33, 1974.)

Several investigators have correlated the echocardiographic measurement of aortic root diameter with similar angiographic measurements.[2,3] The graph in Figure 12–3 shows the results of such a study in infants and children. This study demonstrated an excellent relationship between the M-mode echocardiographic and angiographic measurements.

There is increasing interest in the motion of the aortic root. Many investigators have used the pattern of motion of the posterior aortic wall as an indicator of changes in left atrial volume (see Chapter 4). Several hemodynamic measurements have utilized the amplitude of motion of the aorta in judging cardiac output, stroke volume, or overall cardiac performance.

Much of the renewed interest in using echocardiography to examine the aorta is due to the advent of two-dimensional echocardiography. It has been demonstrated that with the two-dimensional technique virtually the entire aorta is now available for ultrasonic examination. Figure 12–4 demonstrates a long-axis view of the root of the aorta. As in the case of its M-mode counter-

part, the anterior wall is continuous with the interventricular septum and the posterior wall connects with the anterior leaflet of the mitral valve. The two aortic walls run parallel to each other. In diastole, the slight bulging of sinuses of Valsalva can be noted (arrows). The short-axis two-dimensional examination of the aorta demonstrates the circular configuration of this great vessel (Fig. 12–5). The aortic valve is visible within the root of the aorta.

There is a limit to how much ascending aorta can be visualized echocardiographically. Two-dimensional echocardiography has some advantage over M-mode echocardiography in appreciating more of the ascending aorta. However, much of the artery lies directly below the sternum, making ultrasonic examination difficult.

Suprasternal echocardiography has made the arch of the aorta accessible to echocardiographic examination. Although M-mode

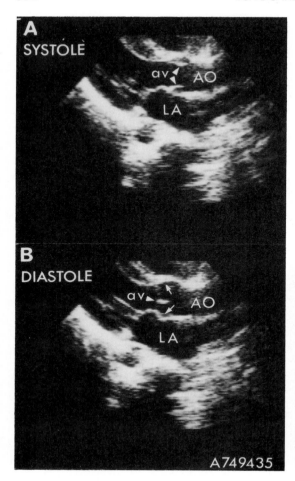

Fig. 12–4. Long-axis two-dimensional echocardiograms of the aorta (AO) in systole, *A*, and diastole, *B*. In diastole the sinuses of Valsalva *(arrows)* are prominent. av = aortic valve; LA = left atrium.

The most recent development in the echocardiographic examination of the aorta is the realization that the descending aorta can be seen with the transducer in the parasternal position.[7,8] Figure 12–8A demonstrates a long-axis parasternal two-dimensional echocardiogram with a circular echo-free space behind the junction of the left ventricle and left atrium. This area has frequently been confused with a dilated coronary sinus. By altering the plane of the examination so that it runs parallel to the long axis of the aorta (Fig. 12–8B), one can visualize the length of the aorta (DA). In fact, with further adjust-

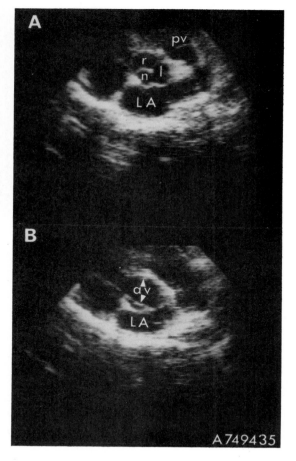

Fig. 12–5. Short-axis two-dimensional echocardiograms of the aorta in diastole and systole. *A*, In diastole, the closed aortic leaflets are seen within the aorta. *B*, In systole, the open leaflets (av) can be recorded. r = right coronary cusp; n = noncoronary cusp; l = left coronary cusp; pv = pulmonary valve; LA = left atrium.

echocardiography has been used to examine the arch of the aorta,[4,5] the two-dimensional technique is superior.[6] Figure 12–6 demonstrates a two-dimensional echocardiogram of the aortic arch obtained from the suprasternal notch. One can see the curve of the aortic arch, the descending aorta, and several branches coming off of the aorta. An examination perpendicular to the arch of the aorta can also be obtained by turning the transducer 90°. Figure 12–7 demonstrates such a study. The arch of the aorta is now relatively circular, and the more linear right pulmonary artery is visible below the arch.

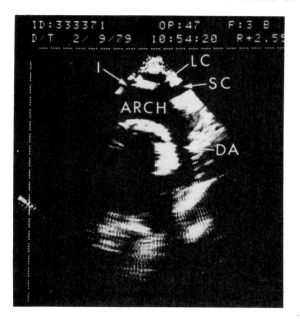

Fig. 12–6. Suprasternal two-dimensional echocardiogram of the arch of the aorta and the descending aorta (DA). I = innominate artery; LC = left common carotid artery; SC = subclavian artery.

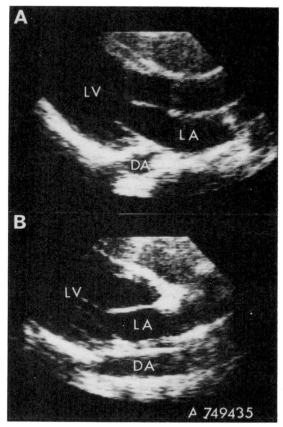

Fig. 12–8. Parasternal two-dimensional echocardiograms of the descending aorta (DA). A, The standard long-axis view shows the descending aorta as a circular, echo-free space posterior to the junction of the left ventricle (LV) and the left atrium (LA). B, By making the examining plane parallel to the descending aorta, the length of the descending aorta can be visualized.

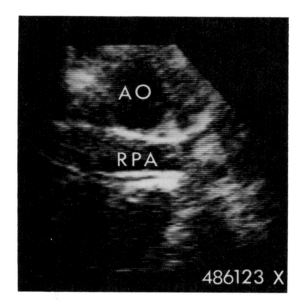

Fig. 12–7. Suprasternal two-dimensional echocardiogram perpendicular to the arch of the aorta. The arch of the aorta (AO) is seen as a relatively circular, echo-free space. The right pulmonary artery (RPA) is seen in its long dimension.

ment of the angulation of the transducer, one can see the descending aorta curve upward toward the arch (Fig. 12–9). The descending aorta need not always appear below the junction of the left atrium and left ventricle. Figure 12–10 shows a long-axis two-dimensional echocardiogram in which the descending aorta (DA) is posterior to the left atrium. This figure also shows that the size of the aorta may vary somewhat from diastole to systole.

The descending aorta can also be clearly seen with M-mode echocardiography.[7] Figure 12–11 shows an M-mode scan in which the descending aorta is recorded posterior to

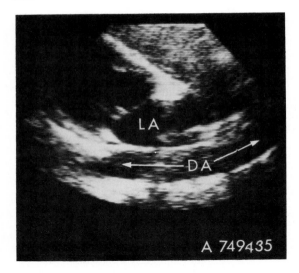

Fig. 12–9. Two-dimensional echocardiogram showing the curved descending aorta (DA) behind the left atrium (LA).

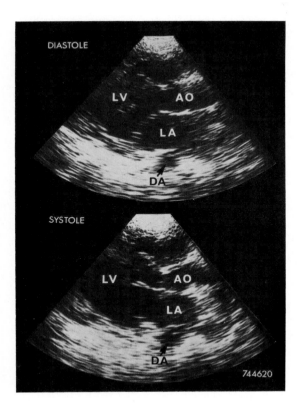

Fig. 12–10. Parasternal two-dimensional echocardiograms showing the descending aorta (DA) behind the left atrium (LA). The descending aorta is slightly larger in systole than in diastole. LV = left ventricle; AO = aorta.

the left atrial wall. This echo-free space has offered some difficulty in the diagnosis of pericardial effusion, pleural effusion, or even intra-atrial structures. Figure 12–12 is another M-mode recording of the patient in Figure 12–11 and illustrates how confusion can arise from the descending aorta echocardiogram. This recording is not totally dissimilar from that seen with a left atrial membrane, cor triatriatum, left atrial clot, or fluid behind the left atrium. Fortunately, the confusion can be eliminated by M-mode scanning, such as in Figure 12–11 or with the two-dimensional examination.

The abdominal aorta can also be examined ultrasonically. This examination is done primarily by way of a contact B-mode abdominal ultrasonograph. With increased use of real-time two-dimensional systems, interest in using such devices for examining the abdominal aorta is also increasing . The echocardiographic literature offers relatively little information concerning the abdominal aorta, although this is a routine examination in abdominal ultrasound.[8a–c]

DILATATION OF THE AORTA AND ANEURYSMS

If the root of the aorta can be examined and measured quantitatively, then this examination should be useful in detecting aortic aneurysms or dilated aortas.[9–14,14a] Figure 12–13 shows a dilated aorta. The upper limits of normal for the aortic dimension is less than 4 cm (see Appendix). In this patient the aortic root measures almost 5 cm. The exact location of the ultrasonic measurement is assisted by the identification of the aortic valve (AV).

Figure 12–14 shows a patient with an aortic aneurysm located immediately beyond the aortic valve (AV). The root of the aorta at the level of the aortic valve is also dilated; the distance between the walls is more than 4 cm. Just beyond the aortic valve is a striking increase in aortic size as the ultrasonic beam scans superiorly. Normally, the aortic walls move in a parallel fashion upward or anteriorly with systole. In this patient the anterior wall at the level of the aortic valve is flat, and the posterior wall exhibits posterior systolic expansion. The systolic expansion is

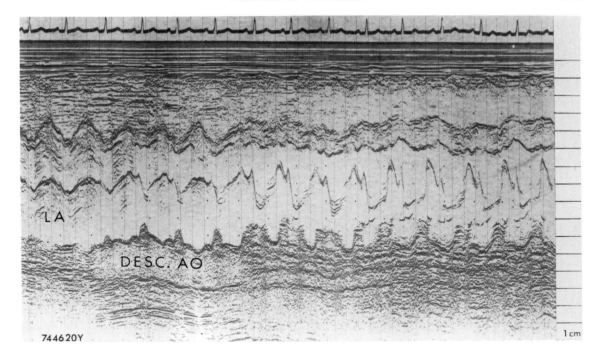

Fig. 12–11.   M-mode scan demonstrating the echo-free space of the descending aorta (DESC AO). LA = left atrium.

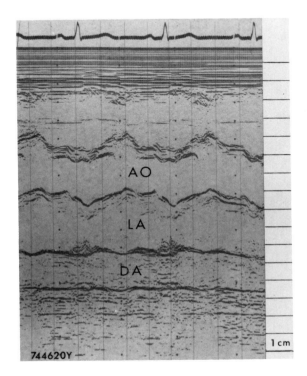

Fig. 12–12.   M-mode echocardiogram of the aorta (AO), left atrium (LA), and descending aorta (DA).

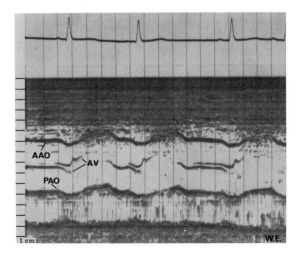

Fig. 12–13.   Echocardiogram of a patient with a dilated aorta. AAO = anterior aortic wall; PAO = posterior aortic wall; AV = aortic valve.

more apparent in the aneurysmal portion of the aorta.

Figure 12–15 shows an M-mode echocardiogram of the aorta in which systolic expansion occurs at the aortic valve level (arrow). The left atrium, posterior to the aorta, is so distorted by the dilated aorta that hardly any cavity is seen.

Another echocardiogram of a dilated aorta appears in Figure 12–16. The aortic valve demonstrates a feature not uncommon in aortic root dilatation.[11,13] There is early systolic closure (arrow) somewhat similar to that seen with subaortic stenosis or mitral regurgitation. A possible explanation for this early systolic closure is that the dilated root produces eddy currents beyond the aortic annulus that partially close the valve in early systole. A similar type of phenomenon has

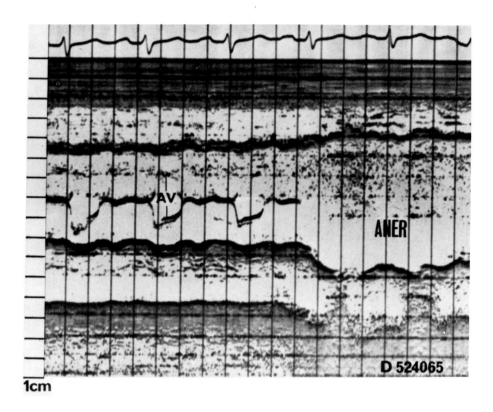

Fig. 12–14.   M-mode scan of a patient with an aortic aneurysm. There are marked changes in the size of the aorta at the level of the aortic valve (AV) and immediately beyond the aortic valve where the aneurysmal dilatation (ANER) occurs. Systolic expansion of the aorta also exists.

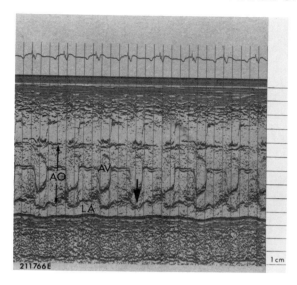

Fig. 12–15. M-mode echocardiogram of a dilated aorta (AO) at the level of the aortic valve (AV). Note systolic expansion *(arrow)* of the posterior aortic wall and the markedly diminished size of the left atrium (LA).

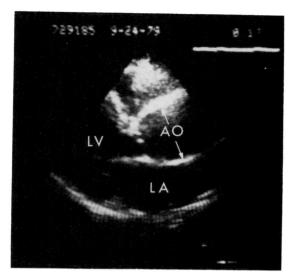

Fig. 12–17. Long-axis two-dimensional echocardiogram of a patient with a dilated aorta (AO). LV = left ventricle; LA = left atrium.

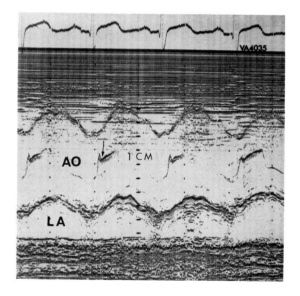

Fig. 12–16. M-mode echocardiogram of a patient with a markedly dilated aorta (AO). Note early systolic closure *(arrow)* of the aortic valve. LA = left atrium.

been noted with dilatation of the pulmonary artery.

Figure 12–17 demonstrates a long-axis parasternal two-dimensional examination of a patient with a dilated aorta. A generalized increase in the aorta is evident as the vessel gradually increases in size from its origin. Figure 12–18 shows marked dilatation or actual aneurysm of the root of the aorta in a young patient with Marfan's syndrome.[12–14] The aorta markedly increases at the attachment of the aortic valve leaflets (AV).

Two-dimensional echocardiography permits the recording of a variety of unusual aneurysms, especially in the arch of the aorta. Figure 12–19 shows a two-dimensional study of the arch of the aorta of a child and demonstrates a massive aneurysm between the arch and descending aorta that was presumably congenital in origin. Another interesting aneurysm is demonstrated in Figure 12–20. This echocardiogram reveals a small aneurysm, arising from the arch of the aorta, that was believed to be traumatic in origin.

Some investigators have suggested that a dilated aorta is best examined from the right sternal position.[10] They were able to measure the size of the aorta in eight patients with dilated aortas but could adequately re-

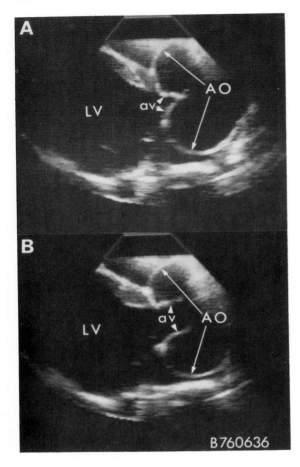

Fig. 12–18.   Diastolic, *A*, and systolic, *B*, long-axis, parasternal two-dimensional echocardiograms of a patient with Marfan's syndrome. The aorta (AO) is markedly dilated. Note the marked discrepancy between the aortic valve (av) opening and the size of the aorta. LV = left ventricle.

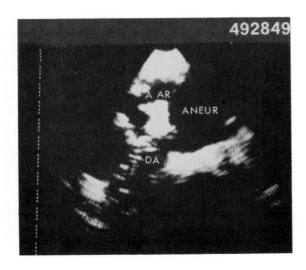

Fig. 12–19.   Suprasternal two-dimensional echocardiogram demonstrating a massive aneurysm (ANEUR) between the arch of the aorta (A AR) and the descending aorta (DA) of a child. The aneurysm was presumably congenital.

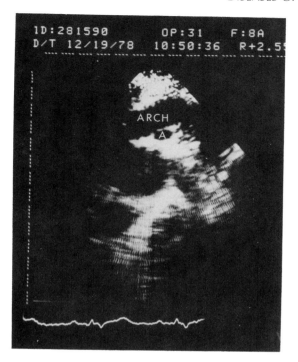

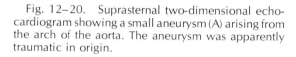

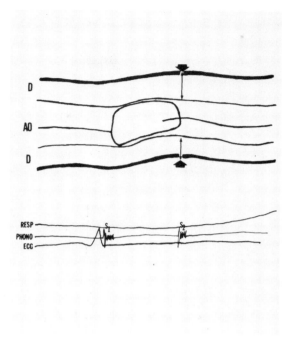

Fig. 12–20.   Suprasternal two-dimensional echocardiogram showing a small aneurysm (A) arising from the arch of the aorta. The aneurysm was apparently traumatic in origin.

Fig. 12–21.   Diagram demonstrating the principle for echocardiographic diagnosis of aortic dissection. The aortic walls are indicated by heavy arrows. The thinner arrows denote echoes originating from the false lumen of the dissection. D = dissection; AO = aorta. (From Nanda, N.C., Gramiak, R., and Shah, P.M.: Diagnosis of aortic root dissection by echocardiography. Circulation, 48:506, 1973.)

cord only five of the eight from the usual left parasternal transducer position.

DISSECTING ANEURYSM

There has been much interest in the echocardiographic diagnosis of dissecting aortic aneurysms.[15-26] The diagram in Figure 12–21 shows the theory behind the M-mode echocardiographic diagnosis of a dissecting aneurysm. In such a condition, there is duplication of the aortic root echoes whereby the extra echoes represent the false lumen. Whether double echoes occur anteriorly *and* posteriorly depends on the extent of the dissection. One might only have an anterior or posterior dissection. If the dissection is circumscribed, then double echoes are found along both walls of the aorta. The aortic valve echoes are within the two inner echoes, which usually are less echo producing than the outer wall echoes, which represent the true walls of the aorta. In addition to finding the double echoes from the aortic walls, the

other criterion necessary for the diagnosis of dissecting aortic aneurysm is that the root of the aorta must be dilated and more than 4 cm.[17] Figure 12–22 is an echocardiogram of a patient with a dissecting aneurysm. The aortic valve echocardiogram is faintly visible following the second cardiac complex. A strong echo from the posterior aortic wall is also readily apparent. The anterior aortic wall is comprised of a thick band of parallel running echoes that apparently originate from the blood within the false lumen of the dissection (D). There is also a faint echo between the aortic valve leaflets and the posterior aortic wall. The space between the faint echo and the posterior aorta is the lumen of the posterior dissection (D). The true lumen of the aorta (AO) lies between the fainter echoes. Figure 12–23 shows preoperative (a) and postoperative (b) echocardiograms of another patient with a dissecting aneurysm.

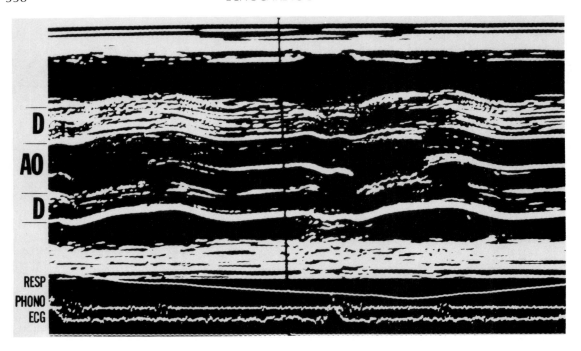

Fig. 12–22.   Echocardiogram of a patient with dissection of the aorta. The false lumen from the dissection (D) lies between the aortic wall and the echoes from the aortic valve. AO = aortic lumen. (From Nanda, N.C., Gramiak, R., and Shah, P.M.: Diagnosis of aortic root dissection by echocardiography. Circulation, 48:506, 1973.)

The anterior false lumen is fairly apparent, although the posterior false lumen is not quite as obvious because the posterior endothelial echo is faint. In the postoperative echocardiogram, both false lumens are obliterated.

Although several independent investigators have confirmed the echocardiographic findings in dissecting aortic aneurysms,[15–17,27–30,30a] one must beware of false positives, which can be created depending on how the ultrasonic beam transects the root of the aorta. Several false positives have been noted.[20,26,27,31,32] Among the conditions that can produce echocardiograms similar to those seen in dissection are abscess in the interventricular septum, dilatation in the sinus of Valsalva, and even sclerosis in and around the aortic root. These conditions can all produce duplication of aortic wall echoes, leading to possible confusion. An intramural aortic abscess may also produce an echocardiogram similar to that seen with a dissecting aneurysm.[32a] Figure 12–24 shows a fairly common aortic valve echocardiogram in which duplication of echoes can be seen along both aortic walls. Although this echocardiogram might be superficially confused with dissection, it does not reveal a major criterion for dissection, that is, aortic dilatation. The total diameter of the aorta is well within normal limits, and one really should not entertain the possibility of dissection in this patient. A more confusing echocardiogram is Figure 12–25. This M-mode scan begins in the aorta, and the ultrasonic beam is then directed toward the left ventricle. When the aorta is examined, the echoes duplicate in the vicinity of the posterior aortic wall. If one uses the more posterior of the echoes for the aortic wall measurement, then dilatation is present and one can envision a false lumen involving the posterior aortic wall. This patient did not have a dissection, and the duplication of echoes was merely a function of a prominent sinus of Valsalva. The more anterior of the two posterior aortic echoes came from the

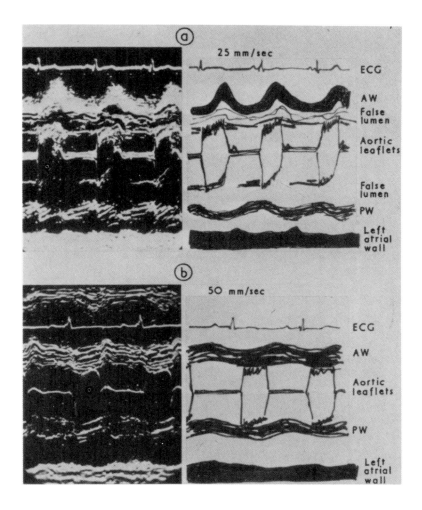

Fig. 12–23.   Echocardiograms of a patient with aortic dissection before, *a*, and after, *b*, surgical repair of the dissection. A false lumen is visible between the anterior aortic wall and the aortic valve leaflets in the preoperative tracing. The false lumen is no longer present in the postoperative tracing. PW = posterior wall of the aorta. AW = anterior wall of the aorta. (From Nanda, N.C., Gramiak, R., and Shah, P.M.: Diagnosis of aortic root dissection by echocardiography. Circulation, *48*:506, 1973.)

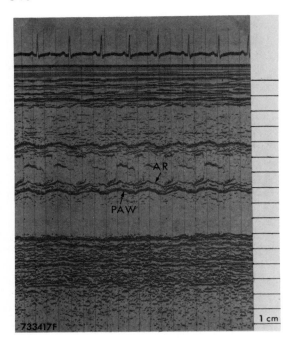

Fig. 12–24. M-mode echocardiogram of an aorta that demonstrates double echoes in the vicinity of the posterior aortic wall (PAW). The more anterior echo (AR) probably originates from the aortic root. The aorta is not dilated, and this patient does not have a dissection.

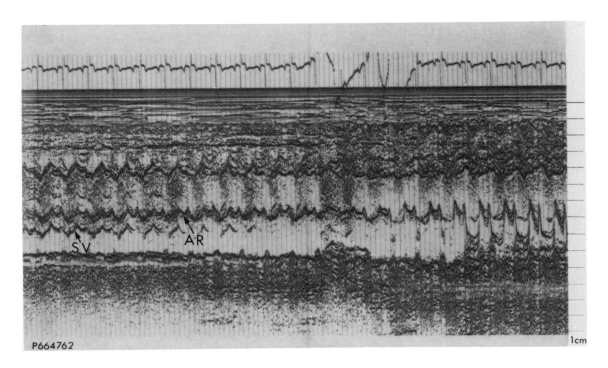

Fig. 12–25. M-mode scan demonstrating a common cause of duplication of echoes in the vicinity of the posterior aortic wall. The more posterior double echo (SV) originates from a prominent sinus of Valsalva. The more anterior posterior echo (AR) originates from the aortic root. This patient does not have a dissection.

aortic annulus, the more posterior from the sinus. At a certain point in the scan, the two echoes appeared simultaneously and gave the false impression of a possible dissection.

An interesting finding in one patient with a dissecting aortic aneurysm is an oscillation of the intimal flap.[21] Figure 12–26 is an illustration taken from that paper and shows a moving echo believed to originate from the oscillating flap within the false lumen of the dissection. Another report notes a similar type of M-shaped intimal flap in the arch of the aorta detected by way of the suprasternal examination.[18] A torn intimal flap was also recorded echocardiographically in a patient who apparently had cystic medial necrosis of the aorta.[22] The false lumen was actually not recorded.

The two-dimensional examination of dissecting aneurysms has been described.[7,24,25,25a] Both ascending and descending aortic dissections have been noted with the two-dimensional technique. Figure 12–27 shows a two-dimensional echocardiogram and

diagram of a patient with dissection of the descending aorta. The greatly enlarged descending aorta can be seen posterior to the left atrium. In addition, the intimal tear is noted in the lumen of the echo-free space behind the left atrium.

Despite the many reports of using echocardiography for the diagnosis of dissecting aortic aneurysm, there is still a large number of confusing situations with false positives and false negatives. Thus one should be cautious when using echocardiography for this diagnosis. There are secondary signs of dissection, such as pericardial effusion or aortic insufficiency, which can be detected echocardiographically and may be helpful in making the proper diagnosis.

SINUS OF VALSALVA ANEURYSM

There are many reports in the literature describing the echocardiographic findings for sinus of Valsalva aneurysm.[25,33–42] The echocardiographic appearance can vary markedly, depending on the location of the

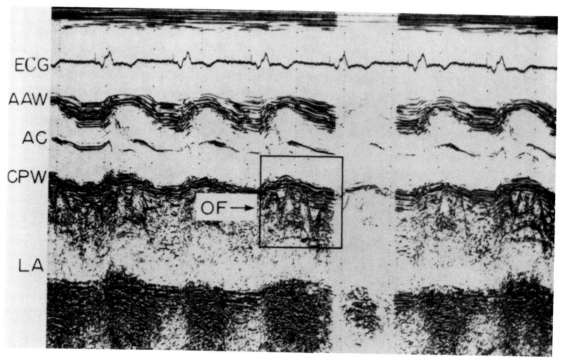

Fig. 12–26. M-mode echocardiogram of a patient with dissection of the aorta. Note the undulating echo from an oscillating flap (OF) within the dissection. AAW = anterior aortic wall; AC = aortic cusp; CPW = component of posterior aortic wall; LA = left atrium. (From Nicholson, W.J. and Cobbs, B.W., Jr.: Echocardiographic oscillating flap in aortic root dissecting aneurysm. Chest, 70:305, 1976.)

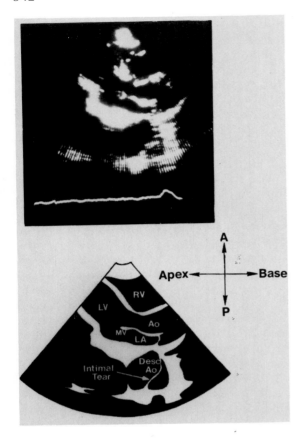

Fig. 12–27.   Parasternal long-axis two-dimensional echocardiogram and diagram of a patient with an aortic aneurysm and dissection of the descending aorta. The large echo-free space of the descending aorta (DescAo) can be seen posterior to the left atrium (LA). Within the descending aorta is a wavy echo from the intimal tear. RV = right ventricle; LV = left ventricle; AO = aorta; MV = mitral valve; A = anterior; P = posterior. (From Mintz, G.S., et al.: Two-dimensional echocardiographic recognition of the descending thoracic aorta. Am. J. Cardiol., 44:232, 1979.)

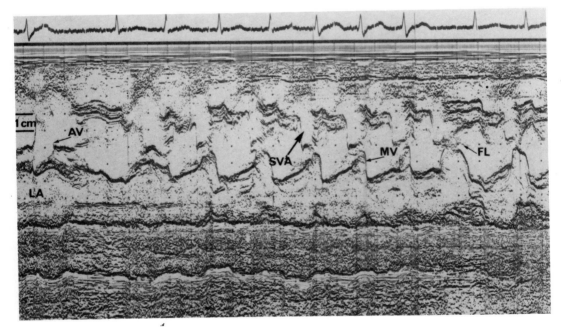

Fig. 12–28.   M-mode scan of a patient with a sinus of Valsalva aneurysm. The echoes from the aneurysm (SVA) are seen in the left ventricular outflow tract in diastole. Fine fluttering of the mitral valve apparatus (FL) is present. MV = mitral valve; AV = aortic valve; LA = left atrium.

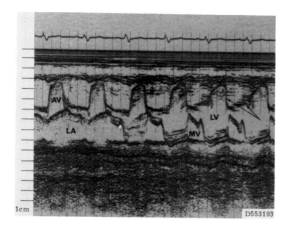

Fig. 12–29. Echocardiogram of a patient with a sinus of Valsalva aneurysm that ruptured into the interventricular septum. The markedly abnormal echoes *(arrows)* represent the aneurysm and the dissected interventricular septum. With diastole the aneurysm and the dissected septum fill with blood and expand into the left ventricular outflow tract. AV = distorted aortic valve; LA = left atrium; LV = left ventricle; MV = mitral valve. (From Rothbaum, D.A., et al.: Echocardiographic manifestations of right sinus of Valsalva aneurysm. Circulation, *49*:768, 1974.)

aneurysm, whether or not it ruptures, and if so, into which part of the heart it ruptures. Figure 12–28 is an M-mode scan of a patient with a sinus of Valsalva aneurysm. The abnormality produces a peculiar pattern of echoes in the left ventricular outflow tract. In early diastole the aneurysm fills with blood and herniates into the outflow tract. As noted in Figure 12–4, even the normal sinuses of Valsalva are more prominent in diastole. With systole the aneurysm moves back into the aorta and out of the outflow tract. Thus one is left with what appears to be a downward motion of the septal portion of the outflow tract toward the mitral valve. Actually, the abnormal motion is in the superior-inferior direction rather than the anterior-posterior direction. The aneurysm was also leaking into the left ventricle, producing aortic regurgitation. There is some fine fluttering (FL) noted just above the mitral valve.

Another sinus of Valsalva aneurysm is depicted in Figure 12–29. Here the aneurysm ruptured into the interventricular septum.

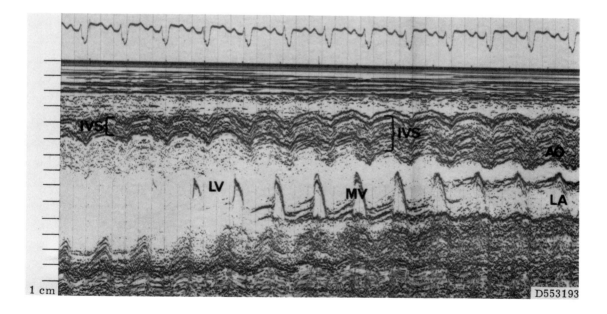

Fig. 12–30. Postoperative M-mode echocardiogram of the patient in Figure 12–29. A patch was placed over the ruptured sinus of Valsalva aneurysm, and the interventricular septal echoes no longer expand with diastole. The interventricular septum at the outflow tract is thickened and probably contains organizing clot. AO = aorta; LA = left atrium; LV = left ventricle; MV = mitral valve; IVS = interventricular septum. (From Rothbaum, D.A., et al.: Echocardiographic manifestations of right sinus of Valsalva aneurysm. Circulation, *49*:768, 1974.)

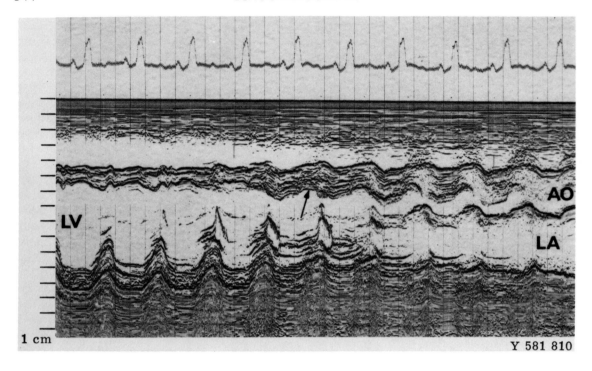

Fig. 12–31.   M-mode echocardiogram of a patient with an infected sinus of Valsalva aneurysm. The striking finding was thickening of the interventricular septum at the level of the left ventricular outflow tract *(arrow)*. Some extra echoes were also present between the aortic valve and the anterior wall of the aorta. Fine fluttering of the mitral valve is barely visible in this patient who also had aortic regurgitation. LV = left ventricle; LA = left atrium; AO = aorta.

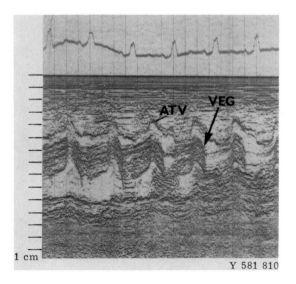

Fig. 12–32.   Another echocardiogram of the patient in Figure 12–31. The sinus of Valsalva aneurysm communicated with the right side of the heart with a vegetation (VEG) recorded immediately posterior to the anterior tricuspid valve (ATV). (From Chang, S.: M-mode Echocardiographic Techniques and Pattern Recognition. Philadelphia, Lea & Febiger, 1976.)

One again sees an apparent abrupt downward motion of the interventricular septum into the left ventricular outflow tract. This structure appears to be continuous with the aortic valve (AV), which is distorted. The unusual echoes (arrows) are actually the aneurysm and the left side of the dissected interventricular septum, both of which fill with blood in diastole and empty during systole. The postoperative echocardiogram, following patching of the communication between the sinus of Valsalva and the interventricular septum, is seen in Figure 12–30. Note that the large band of echoes from the interventricular septum, which is probably filled with blood and clot, is no longer in communication with the aorta and does not exhibit the dramatic expansile motion seen in Figure 12–29.

Sinus of Valsalva aneurysms can dissect into a variety of places. In addition to the interventricular septum, such aneurysms may dissect into the left ventricle and mimic aortic regurgitation (Fig. 12–28). A common location for aneurysms to dissect is the right heart near the junction between the right ventricle and right atrium. When such a dissection occurs, there frequently is systolic fluttering of the tricuspid valve.

The echocardiogram in Figure 12–31 shows a patient with an infected sinus of Valsalva aneurysm. One again finds excessive echoes in the vicinity of the left ventricular outflow tract (arrow). With further examination one also sees an echo-producing mass immediately posterior to the tricuspid valve that corresponds to the infected vegetation extending from the sinus of Valsalva aneurysm (Fig. 12–32). This patient also had free communication between the aorta and the right ventricle that produced a high right ventricular diastolic pressure with premature opening of the pulmonary valve.[43]

Two-dimensional echocardiography has been used for the detection of sinus of Valsalva aneurysms.[25,39,40,44] Figure 12–33 demonstrates a parasternal long-axis two-dimensional echocardiogram and diagram of a patient with a sinus of Valsalva aneurysm. Aneurysmal protrusion of the posterior aortic wall can be seen in the area of the posterior coronary sinus. In another report the two-dimensional technique could detect the ruptured sinus of Valsalva aneurysm (Fig. 12–34). In diastole (Fig. 12–34a), a direct communication between the right ventricular outflow tract and the aorta can be seen (arrow). During systole (Fig. 12–34b), the

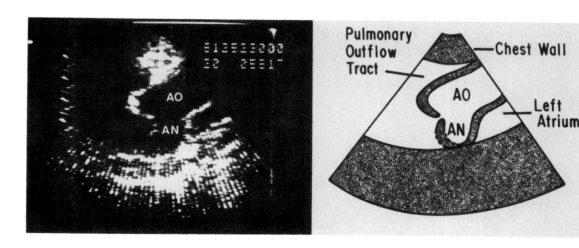

Fig. 12–33. Long-axis two-dimensional echocardiogram and diagram demonstrating a sinus of Valsalva aneurysm. Aneurysmal protrusion of the posterior aortic wall (AN) is visible in the area of the posterior coronary sinus. AO = aorta. (From DeMaria, A.N., et al.: Identification and localization of aneurysms of the ascending aorta by cross-sectional echocardiography. Circulation, 59:755, 1979. By permission of the American Heart Association, Inc.)

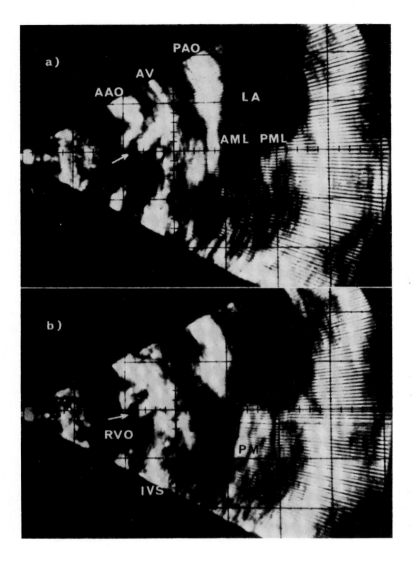

Fig. 12–34.   Long-axis two-dimensional echocardiograms of a patient with a ruptured sinus of Valsalva aneurysm. (Echographic orientation has superior at the top, inferior at the bottom, anterior on the left, posterior on the right.) During diastole, *a*, communication is visible between the aorta and the right ventricle *(arrow)*. In systole, *b*, communication is not apparent, and the aneurysm of the right sinus of Valsalva is visible with an opening into the right ventricular outflow tract *(arrow)*. AAO = anterior aortic wall; AV = aortic valve; PAO = posterior aortic wall; LA = left atrium; AML = anterior mitral leaflet; PML = posterior mitral leaflet; RVO = right ventricular outflow tract; IVS = interventricular septum; PM = papillary muscle. (From Nishimura, K., et al.: High-speed ultrasonocardiotomography: echocardiographic manifestation of right sinus of Valsalva aneurysm ruptured into the right ventricle. J. Cardiogr., 6:149, 1976.)

communication with the aorta is not as evident, although the aneurysm involving the right coronary sinus can be seen opening into the right ventricular outflow tract (arrow).

REFERENCES

1. Gramiak, R. and Shah, P.M.: Echocardiography of the aortic root. Invest. Radiol., 3:356, 1968.
2. Francis, G.S., Hagan, A.D., Oury, J., and O'Rourke, R.A.: Accuracy of echocardiography for assessing aortic root diameter. Br. Heart J., 37:376, 1975.
3. Lundstrom, N.R. and Martensson, W.: Clinical applications of echocardiography in infants and children. II. Estimation of aortic root diameter and left atrial size: a comparison between echocardiography and angiocardiography. Acta Paediatr. Scand., 63:33, 1974.
4. Goldberg, B.B.: Suprasternal ultrasonography. J.A.M.A., 215:245, 1971.
5. Goldberg, S.J., Allen, H.D., and Sahn, D.J.: *In* Pediatric and Adolescent Echocardiography. Chicago, Year Book Medical Publishers, Inc., 1975.
6. Sahn, D.J., Goldberg, S.J., McDonald, G., and Allen, H.D.: Suprasternal notch real-time cross-sectional echocardiography for imaging the pulmonary artery, aortic arch, and descending aorta. Am. J. Cardiol., 39:266, 1977. (Abstract)
7. Mintz, G.S., Kotler, M.N., Segal, B.L., and Parry, W.R.: Two dimensional echocardiographic recognition of the descending thoracic aorta. Am. J. Cardiol., 44:232, 1979.
8. Seward, J.B. and Tajik, A.J.: Noninvasive visualization of the entire thoracic aorta: a new application of wide-angle two-dimensional sector echocardiographic technique. Am. J. Cardiol., 43:387, 1979. (Abstract)
8a. Leopold, G.R., Goldberger, L.E., and Bernstein, E.F.: Ultrasonic detection and evaluation of abdominal aortic aneurysms. Surgery, 72:939, 1972.
8b. Goldberg, B.B.: Aortosonography. Int. Surg., 62:294, 1977.
8c. Maloney, J.D., Pairolero, P.C., Smith, B.F., Hattery, R.R., Brakke, D.M., and Spittell, J.A.: Ultrasound evaluation of abdominal aortic aneurysms. Cardiovasc. Surg. (Suppl. II), 56:80, 1977.
9. Kronzon, I., Weisinger, B., and Glassman, E.: Illustrative echocardiogram: cystic medial necrosis with severe aortic root dilatation. Chest, 66:79, 1974.
10. D'Cruz, I.A., Jain, D.P., Hirsch, L., Levinsky, R., Cohen, H.C., and Glick, G.: Echocardiographic diagnosis of dilatation of the ascending aorta using right parasternal scanning. Radiology, 129:465, 1978.
11. Atsuchi, Y., Nagai, Y., Komatsu, Y., Nakamura, K., Shibuya, M., and Hirosawa, K.: Echocardiographic manifestations of annulo-aortic ectasia: its "paradoxical" motion of the aorta and premature systolic closure of the aortic valve. Am. Heart J., 93:428, 1977.
12. Tanaka, K., Yoshikawa, J., Kato, H., Owaki, T., Ishihara, K., Kuroda, A., Okumachi, F., Takagi, Y., Uchihira, F., Baba, K., Tomita, Y., Syomura, T., Chikusa, H., Hirashima, N., Inoue, K., Nakamura, T., Watanabe, S., and Yoshizumi, M.: Echocardiographic assessment of cardiac abnormalities in Marfan's syndrome. Cardiovasc. Sound Bull., 5:437, 1975.
13. Atsuchi, Y., Nagai, Y., Komatsu, Y., Nakamura, K., Kondo, M., Shibuya, M., and Hirosawa, K.: Echocardiographic manifestations of annulo-aortic ectasia. Cardiovasc. Sound Bull., 5:653, 1975.
14. Koiwaya, Y., Tomoike, H., Tanaka, S., Takeshita, A., Kuroiwa, A., Nakamura, M., Shibuya, H., Tokunaga, K., and Hirata, T.: UCG findings in annulo-aortic ectasia: comparison with operative findings in two cases. Cardiovasc. Sound Bull., 5:667, 1975.
14a. Alter, B.R., Treasure, R.L., Humphrey, S.H., Murgo, J.P., and McGranahan, G.M., Jr.: Echocardiographic detection of a subannular aortic aneurysm. Am. Heart J., 96:525, 1978.
15. Millward, D.K., Robinson, N.J., and Craige, E.: Dissecting aortic aneurysm diagnosed by echocardiography in a patient with rupture of the aneurysm into the right atrium. Am. J. Cardiol., 30:427, 1972.
16. Moothart, R.W., Spangler, R.D., and Blout, S.G., Jr.: Echocardiography in aortic root dissection and dilatation. Am. J. Cardiol., 36:11, 1975.
17. Nanda, N.C., Gramiak, R., and Shah, P.M.: Diagnosis of aortic root dissection by echocardiography. Circulation, 48:506, 1973.
18. Kasper, W., Meinertz, T., Kersting, F., Lang, K., and Just, H.: Diagnosis of dissecting aortic aneurysm with suprasternal echocardiography. Am. J. Cardiol., 42:291, 1978.
19. Clark, P.I. and Glasser, S.P.: Problem: vague chest symptoms and new aortic regurgitation. Cardiovasc. Med., 4:805, 1979.
20. Nanda, N.C., Ong, L.S., and Barold, S.S.: Aortic root dissection: unusual echocardiographic motion pattern. Ann. Intern. Med., 85:79, 1976.
21. Nicholson, W.J. and Cobbs, B.W., Jr.: Echocardiographic oscillating flap in aortic root dissecting aneurysm. Chest, 70:305, 1976.
22. Krueger, S.K., Wilson, C.S., Weaver, W.F., Reese, H.E., Caudill, C.C., and Rourke, T.: Aortic root dissection: echocardiographic demonstration of torn intimal flap. J. Clin. Ultrasound, 4:35, 1976.
23. Nanda, N., Lever, H., Gramiak, R., Ross, A., Reeves, W., Hess, P., Zesk, J., and Combs, R.: Reliability of echocardiography in the diagnosis of aortic root dissection. Circulation (Suppl. III), 56:68, 1977. (Abstract)
24. Matsumoto, M., Matsuo, H., Ohara, T., and Abe, H.: Use of kymo-two-dimensional echoaortocardiography for the diagnosis of aortic root dissection and mycotic aneurysm of the aortic root. Ultrasound Med. Biol., 3:153, 1977.
25. DeMaria, A.N., Bommer, W., Neumann, A., Weinert, L., Bogren, H., and Mason, D.T.: Identification and localization of aneurysms of the ascending aorta by cross-sectional echocardiography. Circulation, 59:755, 1979.
25a. Matsumoto, M., Matsuo, H., Ohara, T., Yoshioka, Y., and Abe, H.: A two-dimensional echoaortocardiographic approach to dissecting aneurysms of the aorta to prevent false-positive diagnoses. Radiology, 127:491, 1978.
26. Krueger, S.K., Starke, H., Forker, A.D., and Eliot, R.S.: Echocardiographic mimics of aortic root dissection. Chest, 67:441, 1975.
27. Brown, O.R., Popp, R.L., and Kloster, F.E.: Echocardiographic criteria for aortic root dissection. Am. J. Cardiol., 36:17, 1975.
28. Kronzon, I. and Mehta, S.S.: Illustrative echocardiogram: aortic root dissection. Chest, 65:88, 1974.
29. Weill, F., Kraehenbuhl, J., Jr., Ricatee, J.P., Aucant, D., Gillet, M., and Makridis, D.: Ultrasonic diag-

nosis of aortic dissections and aneurysmal fissurations. Ann. Radiol. (Paris), *17*:49, 1974.

30. Yuste, P., Aza, V., Minguez, I., Cerezo, L., and Martinez-Bardiu, C.: Dissecting aortic aneurysm diagnosed by echocardiography. Br. Heart J., *36*:111, 1974.

30a. Di Luzio, V., Purcaro, A., Boccanelli, A., et al.: Echocardiographic diagnosis of the dissection of the thoracic aorta. G. Ital. Cardiol., *6*:677, 1976.

31. Krueger, S.K., Starke, H., Forker, A.D., and Eliot, R.S.: Echocardiographic mimics of aortic root dissection. Chest, *67*:441, 1975.

32. Hirschfeld, D.S., Rodriguez, H.J., and Schiller, N.B.: Duplication of aortic wall seen by echocardiography. Br. Heart J., *38*:943, 1976.

32a. Fox, S., Kotler, M.N., Segal, B.L., and Parry, W.: Echocardiographic diagnosis of acute aortic valve endocarditis and its complications. Arch. Intern. Med., *137*:85, 1977.

33. Rothbaum, D.A., Dillon, J.C., Chang, S., and Feigenbaum, H.: Echocardiographic manifestation of right sinus of Valsalva aneurysm. Circulation, *49*:768, 1974.

34. Cooperberg, P., Mercer, E.N., Mulder, D.S., and Winsberg, F.: Rupture of a sinus of Valsalva aneurysm: report of a case diagnosed preoperatively by echocardiography. Radiology, *113*:171, 1974.

35. Matsumoto, M., Matsuo, H., Beppu, S., Yoshioka, Y., Kawashima, Y., Nimura, Y., and Abe, H.: Echocardiographic diagnosis of ruptured aneurysm of sinus of Valsalva: report of two cases. Circulation, *53*:382, 1976.

36. Warren, S.G., Waugh, R.A., Kisslo, J., and Johnson, M.L.: Echocardiographic abnormalities in ruptured right coronary sinus of Valsalva aneurysm. Circulation (Suppl. III), *50*:249, 1974. (Abstract)

37. Haraoka, S., Ueda, M., Saito, D., Ogino, Y., Yoshida, H., and Kusuhara, S.: Echocardiographic findings of a case of sinus of Valsalva aneurysm ruptured into left ventricle: abnormal echoes in the left ventricular outflow tract. J. Cardiogr., *8*:293, 1978.

38. DeSa'Neto, A., Padnick, M.B., Desser, K.B., and Steinhoff, N.C.: Right sinus of Valsalva-right atrial fistula secondary to nonpenetrating chest trauma: a case report with description of noninvasive diagnostic features. Circulation, *60*:205, 1979.

39. Nishimura, K., Hibi, N., Kato, T., Fukui, Y., Arakawa, T., Tatematsu, H., Miwa, A., Tada, H., Kambe, T., and Sakamoto, N.: Real-time observation of ruptured right sinus of Valsalva aneurysm by high speed ultrasonocardiotomography: report of a case. Circulation, *53*:732, 1976.

40. Nishimura, K., Hibi, N., Kato, T., Fukui, Y., Arakawa, T., Tatematsu, H., Miwa, A., Tada, H., and Kambe, T.: High-speed ultrasonocardiotomography: echographic manifestation of right sinus of Valsalva aneurysm ruptured into the right ventricle. J. Cardiogr., *6*:149, 1976.

41. Matsumoto, M., Matsuo, H., Beppu, S., Yoshioka, Y., Kawashima, Y., Nimura, Y., and Abe, H.: Echocardiographic diagnosis of ruptured aneurysm of sinus of Valsalva: report of two cases. Circulation, *53*:382, 1976.

42. Wong, B.Y.S., Bogart, D.B., and Dunn, M.I.: Echocardiographic features of an aneurysm of the left sinus of Valsalva. Chest, *73*:105, 1978.

43. Weyman, A.E., Dillon, J.C., Feigenbaum, H., and Chang, S.: Premature pulmonic valve opening following sinus of Valsalva aneurysm rupture into the right atrium. Circulation, *51*:556, 1975.

44. Mintz, G.S., Kotler, M.N., Segal, B.L., and Parry, W.R.: Comparison of two-dimensional and M-mode echocardiography in the evaluation of patients with infective endocarditis. Am. J. Cardiol., *43*:738, 1979.

Appendix:
Echocardiographic Measurements and Normal Values

Appendices A through D provide normal values for M-mode echocardiographic measurements. The four sets of values were derived at different institutions at different times during the course of the development of echocardiography.

APPENDIX A: TRADITIONAL NORMAL ECHOCARDIOGRAPHIC VALUES

Appendix A presents data obtained in 1972 that represent the oldest normal values. These measurements do not utilize current American Society of Echocardiography recommendations. Most measurements are from trailing edge to leading edge.

Definition of Echocardiographic Measurements. *Right ventricular dimension (RVD)* represents the distance between the trailing echoes of the anterior right ventricular wall and the leading echo of the right side of the interventricular septum at the R wave of the electrocardiogram. *Left ventricular internal dimension (LVID)* is measured from the trailing edge of the left side of the septum to the leading edge of the posterior endocardium at the R wave of the electrocardiogram. *Posterior left ventricular wall thickness* represents the distance between the leading edge of the posterior left ventricular endocardium and the leading edge of the

epicardium at the R wave of the electrocardiogram. *Posterior left ventricular wall amplitude* is the maxium amplitude of the posterior left ventricular endocardial echo. *Interventricular septal (IVS) wall thickness* is the distance between the leading edge of the left septal echo and the trailing edge of the right septal echo at the R wave of the electrocardiogram. *Midinterventricular septal (IVS) amplitude* is the amplitude of motion of the left septal echo with the ultrasonic beam traversing the midportion of the left ventricle. *Apical interventricular septal (IVS) amplitude* is the systolic amplitude of motion of the left septal echo with the ultrasonic beam directed toward the apex in the vicinity of the papillary muscles. *Left atrial dimension (LAD)* represents the distance between the trailing edge of the posterior aortic wall echo and the leading edge of the posterior left atrial wall echo at the level of the aortic valve at end-systole. *Aortic root dimension* is the distance between the leading edge of the anterior aortic wall and the leading edge of the posterior aortic wall at the R wave of the electrocardiogram. *Aortic cusp separation* represents the distance between the trailing edge of the anterior aortic valve leaflet and the leading edge of the posterior aortic valve leaflet in early systole.

TABLE A–1. Adult Normal Values

	Range (cm.)	Mean (cm.)	Number
Age (years)	13 –54	26	134
Body Surface Area (M²)	1.45– 2.22	1.8	130
RVD-flat	0.7 – 2.3	1.5	84
RVD-left lateral	0.9 – 2.6	1.7	83
LVID-flat	3.7 – 5.6	4.7	82
LVID-left lateral	3.5 – 5.7	4.7	81
Post. LV wall thickness	0.6 – 1.1	0.9	137
Post. LV wall amplitude	0.9 – 1.4	1.2	48
IVS wall thickness	0.6 – 1.1	0.9	137
Mid IVS amplitude	0.3 – 0.8	0.5	10
Apical IVS amplitude	0.5 – 1.2	0.7	38
Left atrial dimension	1.9 – 4.0	2.9	133
Aortic root dimension	2.0 – 3.7	2.7	121
Aortic cusps separation	1.5 – 2.6	1.9	93
Mean rate of circumferential shortening (Vcf)	1.02– 1.94 circ./sec.	1.3 circ./sec.	38

TABLE A–2. Adult Normal Values, Corrected for Body Surface Area

	Range (cm.)	Mean (cm.)	Number
RVD/M²—flat	0.4–1.4	0.9	76
RVD/M²—left lateral	0.4–1.4	0.9	79
LVID/M²—flat	2.1–3.2	2.6	77
LVID/M²—left lateral	1.9–3.2	2.6	81
LAD/M²	1.2–2.2	1.6	127
Aortic root/M²	1.2–2.2	1.5	115

TABLE A–3. Normal Values for Children Arranged by Weight

	Weight (lbs.)	Mean (cm.)	Range (cm.)	Number of Subjects
RVD	0– 25	.9	.3–1.5	26
	26– 50	1.0	.4–1.5	26
	51– 75	1.1	.7–1.8	20
	76–100	1.2	.7–1.6	15
	101–125	1.3	.8–1.7	11
	126–200	1.3	1.2–1.7	5
LVID	0– 25	2.4	1.3–3.2	26
	26– 50	3.4	2.4–3.8	26
	51– 75	3.8	3.3–4.5	20
	76–100	4.1	3.5–4.7	15
	101–125	4.3	3.7–4.9	11
	126–200	4.9	4.4–5.2	5
LV and IV septal wall thickness	0– 25	.5	.4– .6	26
	26– 50	.6	.5– .7	26
	51– 75	.7	.6– .7	20
	76–100	.7	.7– .8	15
	101–125	.7	.7– .8	11
	126–200	.8	.7– .8	5
LA dimension	0– 25	1.7	.7–2.3	26
	26– 50	2.2	1.7–2.7	26
	51– 75	2.3	1.9–2.8	20
	76–100	2.4	2.0–3.0	15
	101–125	2.7	2.1–3.0	11
	126–200	2.8	2.1–3.7	5
Aortic root	0– 25	1.3	.7–1.7	26
	26– 50	1.7	1.3–2.2	26
	51– 75	2.0	1.7–2.3	20
	76–100	2.2	1.9–2.7	15
	101–125	2.3	1.7–2.7	11
	126–200	2.4	2.2–2.8	5
Aortic valve opening	0– 25	.9	.5–1.2	26
	26– 50	1.2	.9–1.6	26
	51– 75	1.4	1.2–1.7	20
	76–100	1.6	1.3–1.9	15
	101–125	1.7	1.4–2.0	11
	126–200	1.8	1.6–2.0	5

TABLE A–4.   Normal Values for Children Arranged by Body Surface Area

	BSA (M.²)	Mean (cm.)	Range (cm.)	Number of Subjects
RVD	.5 or less	.8	.3–1.3	24
	.6 to 1.0	1.0	.4–1.8	39
	1.1 to 1.5	1.2	.7–1.7	29
	over 1.5	1.3	.8–1.7	11
LVID	.5 or less	2.4	1.3–3.2	24
	.6 to 1.0	3.4	2.4–4.2	39
	1.1 to 1.5	4.0	3.3–4.7	29
	over 1.5	4.7	4.2–5.2	11
LV and IV septal wall thickness	.5 or less	.5	.4– .6	24
	.6 to 1.0	.6	.5– .7	39
	1.1 to 1.5	.7	.6– .8	29
	over 1.5	.8	.7– .8	11
LA dimension	.5 or less	1.7	.7–2.4	24
	.6 to 1.0	2.1	1.8–2.8	39
	1.1 to 1.5	2.4	2.0–3.0	29
	over 1.5	2.8	2.1–3.7	11
Aortic root	.5 or less	1.2	.7–1.5	24
	.6 to 1.0	1.8	1.4–2.2	39
	1.1 to 1.5	2.2	1.7–2.7	29
	over 1.5	2.4	2.0–2.8	11
Aortic valve opening	.5 or less	.8	.5–1.0	24
	.6 to 1.0	1.3	.9–1.6	39
	1.1 to 1.5	1.6	1.3–1.9	29
	over 1.5	1.8	1.5–2.0	11

Fig. B–1.   Methods of measurement.

Abbreviations:

LVD (D)–(A.S.E.)*	Left ventricular internal dimension at end-diastole measured at onset of QRS complex
LVD (D)–(MAX)	Maxium left ventricular internal dimension at end-diastole
LVD (S)–(A.S.E.* and MIN)	Left ventricular internal dimension at end-systole measured at peak posterior motion of ventricular septum (also corresponds to minimum internal dimension)
ST (D)–(A.S.E.)*	Ventricular septal thickness at end-diastole measured at onset of QRS complex
ST (D)	Ventricular septal thickness in late diastole measured immediately before atrial systole
ST (S)	Ventricular septal thickness at end-systole measured at maximum thickness
PWT (D) (A.S.E.)*	Left ventricular posterobasal free wall thickness at end-diastole measured at onset of QRS complex
PWT (D)	Left ventricular posterobasal free wall thickness in late diastole measured immediately before atrial systole
PWT (S)	Left ventricular posterobasal free wall thickness at end-systole measured at maximum thickness
AO–(A.S.E.)*	Aortic root dimension at end-diastole measured at onset of QRS complex from leading edge of anterior wall of aorta to leading edge of posterior wall of aorta
LA–(A.S.E.)*	Left atrial dimension at end-systole measured at the maximum dimension from the leading edge of the posterior wall of aorta to the dominant line representing the posterior wall of the left atrium (identified by the switched-gain circuit or by manual damping)

* Measurement obtained by way of standards recommended by the American Society of Echocardiography

APPENDIX B: NORMAL ECHOCARDIOGRAPHIC MEASUREMENTS FROM INFANCY TO OLD AGE

Appendix B is provided by Henry et al.[1,2] He and his associates developed new normal measurements in 1978 that account for changes in age and are based on the American Society of Echocardiography's recommendations.

Methods of measurement are shown in Figure B–1. The method for using the normal data graphs is exemplified in Figure B–2A and B.

The 387 subjects initially screened were between 21 and 97 years of age. Subjects were excluded if they had (1) history of heart disease or hypertension, (2) abnormal EKG or chest roentgenogram, (3) obesity, (4) ab-

METHODS OF MEASUREMENT

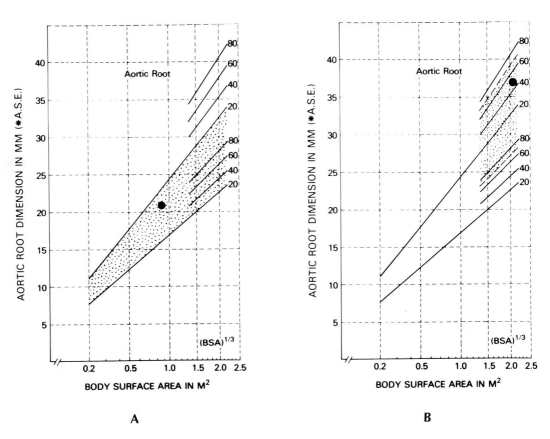

Fig. B–2.   Method for using normal data graphs.

A, An example of a normal data graph for subjects aged one month to 20 years. The graph was prepared for an 8-year-old child with a body surface area of 0.9 m² and an aortic root dimension of 21 mm. Since the child is less than 20 years of age, the two lines that extend from 0.2 to 2.2 m² (labeled 20) are used as the upper and lower limits of normal. In this example, an aortic root dimension of 21 mm is within the 95% prediction limits of normal for an 8-year-old child with a body surface area of 0.9 m².

B, An example of a normal graph for subjects more than 20 years of age. This graph was prepared for a 70-year-old man with a body surface area of 2.2 m² and an aortic root dimension of 37 mm. For this subject, the upper limit of normal is determined by extrapolating a line midway between the upper limits for ages 60 and 80 (labeled 60 and 80). The lower limit of normal is extrapolated in the same way. In this example, an aortic root dimension of 37 mm is within the 95% prediction limits of normal for a 70-year-old patient with a body surface area of 2.2 m².

normal physical examination of the heart, or (5) abnormal or otherwise unsatisfactory echocardiograms. Of the 387 subjects initially screened, 251 were excluded. The remaining 136 subjects were included in the study (Table B–1).

TABLE B–1.   Newer Normal Data

Age	Males	Females	Total
1–5 days	7	6	13
1 month–20 years	45	47	92
21–30 years	15	10	25
31–40 years	9	15	24
41–50 years	16	13	29
51–60 years	19	10	29
61–70 years	9	8	17
71–97 years	10	2	12
Total	130	111	241

Echocardiographic parameters related to age and body surface area are (1) left ventricular internal dimensions (Figs. B–3 and B–4), (2) ventricular septal thickness (Fig. B–5), (3) left ventricular free wall thickness (Fig. B–6), (4) estimated left ventricular mass (Fig. B–7), (5) aortic root dimension (Fig. B–8), (6) left atrial dimension (Fig. B–9), and (7) mitral valve E–F slope (Fig. B–10). Except for mitral valve E–F slope, all parameters were derived from measurements that were obtained by way of standards recommended by the American Society of Echocardiography.

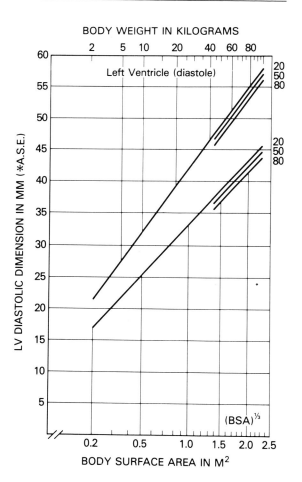

Fig. B–3.

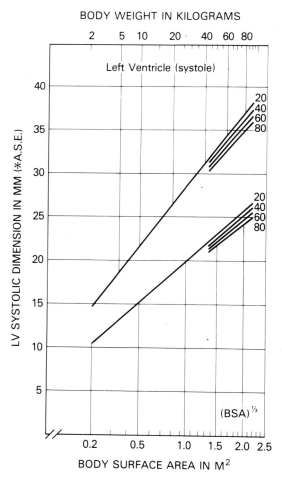

Fig. B–4.

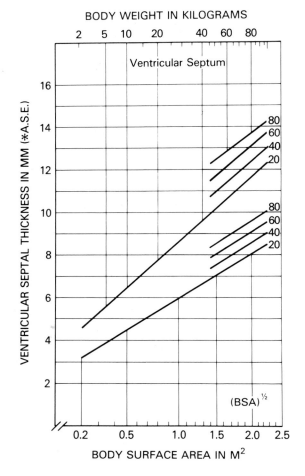

Fig. B–5.

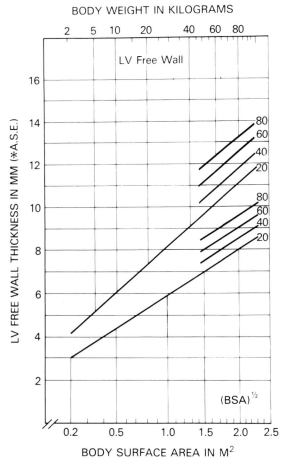

Fig. B–6.

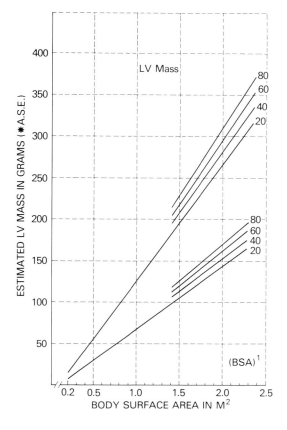

Fig. B–7.

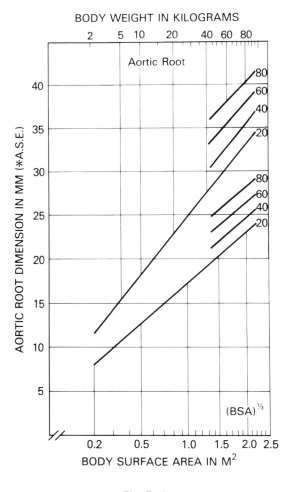

Fig. B–8.

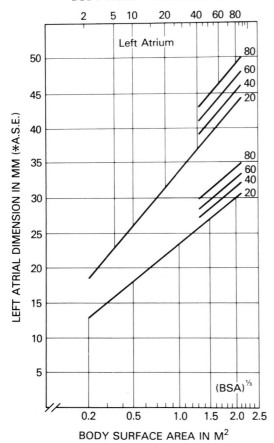

Fig. B–9.

Fig. B–10.

Normal echocardiographic parameters unrelated to age and body surface area are as follows:

1. Left ventricular fractional shortening
   Mean: 36%   95% prediction limits: 28–44%*
   (Mean: 37%   95% prediction limits: 29–45%†

2. Left ventricular ejection fraction (cubed)
   Mean: 74%   95% prediction limits: 64–83%*
   (Mean: 75%   95% prediction limits: 65–84%†

3. Ventricular septal thickening (younger normal data)
   Mean: 35%   95% prediction limits: 18–53%*

4. Left ventricular free wall thickening (younger normal data)
   Mean: 60%   95% prediction limits: 39–82%*

---

* Derived from measurements that were obtained by way of standards recommended by the American Society of Echocardiography
† Derived from measurement of left ventricular internal dimension at end-diastole at point of maximum dimension

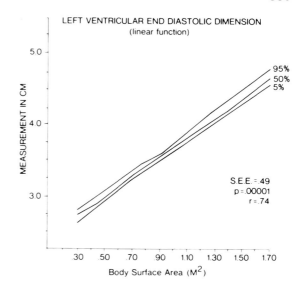

Fig. C–1.

APPENDIX C: ECHOCARDIOGRAPHIC MEASUREMENTS PLOTTED AGAINST BODY SURFACE AREA IN CHILDREN

Appendix C presents graphs that plot echocardiographic measurements against body surface area in a series of children (Figs. C–1 through C–10). The data are obtained from research performed by Goldberg, Allen, and Sahn.[3]

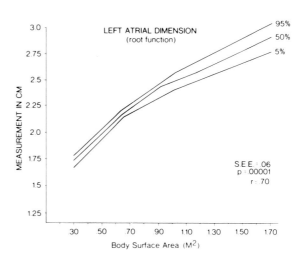

Fig. C–2.

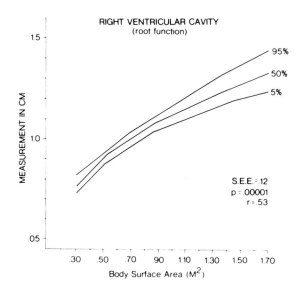

Fig. C–3.

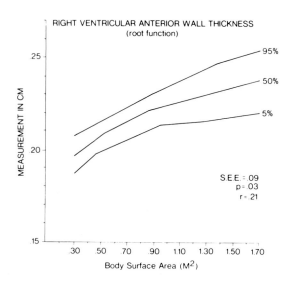

Fig. C–5.

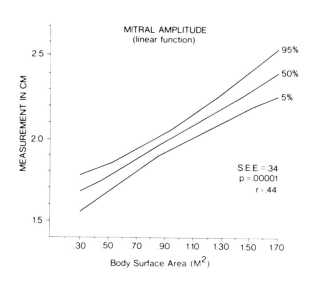

Fig. C–4.

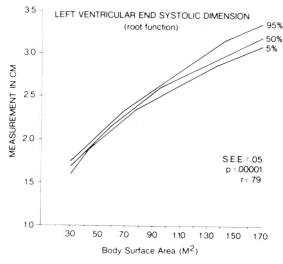

Fig. C–6.

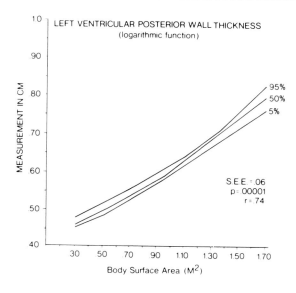

Fig. C–7.

SEPTAL THICKNESS
(root function)

Fig. C–9.

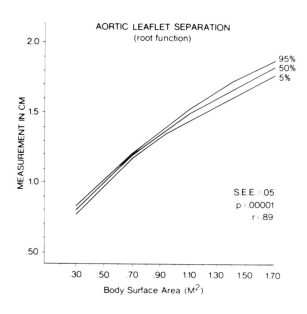

Fig. C–8.

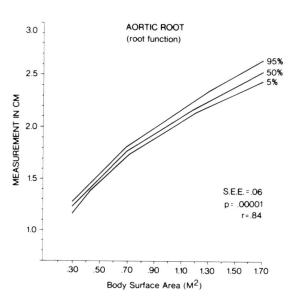

Fig. C–10.

TABLE D–1.　Normal Echocardiographic Values in Newborns

Reference	Hagan, et al.[5]	Meyer, Kaplan[6]	Solinger, et al.[7]	Godman, et al.[8]	Lundstrom[9]	Winsberg[10]	Sahn, et al.[11]	All Cases
Age of Patient	10–72 hr	1½–192 hr	6 hr–4 wk	1 wk–1 mo	1 wk–1 mo	12–120 hr	12–120 hr	1½ hr–1 mo
Weight	2.7–4.5 kg	2.3–4.9 kg	2.2–4.5 kg	1.9–4.3 kg	?	2.8–4.5 kg	2.7–4.5 kg	1.9–4.9 kg
No. of Cases	(200)	(50)	(240)	(50)	(10)	(11)	(72)	(633)
MVD	....	31–47	22–32	....	....	....	....	22–47 mm. (290)
MVTE	....	....	8.5–13.1	6.5–12.4	10–14	....	....	6.5–1.4 mm. (300)
MVDE	6–12	6–12	....	....	7– 9	....	....	6–12 mm. (210)
MVVS	60–130	36–80	....	....	....	....	....	36–130 mm./sec. (250)
TVD	....	24–32	13–19	8–13	12	....	....	13–32 mm. (290)
TVTE	7–14	8–14	8.8–14.2	....	....	....	....	8–14.2 mm. (300)
TVDE	....	....	....	....	....	....	....	7–14 mm. (200)
TVVS	60–116	34–56	....	....	....	....	....	34–11 mm./sec. (250)
ARD	8.1–12	7–12(S)	9.3–13.6(S)	8–11 (S)	....	....	....	7–13.6 mm. (540)
AVO	....	....	4–6.8	....	....	....	....	4–6.8 mm. (240)
PRD	9.4–13	....	10.7–15.8(S)	....	....	....	....	9.2–15.8 mm. (490)
PVO	....	....	5.8–9.9	....	....	....	....	5.8–9.9 mm. (240)
LAD	5–10	6–13(S)	6.8–13.5(S)	4–10.5(S)	....	....	....	4–13.5 mm. (540)
IST	1.8–4	....	2.1–4.5 (D)	....	....	....	....	1.8–4.5 mm. (440)
LVPW(S)	2.5–6	....	....	....	....	6	....	2.5–6 mm. (200)
LVPW(D)	1.6–3.7	....	2–4.6	....	....	....	....	1.6–4.6 mm. (440)
LVD(S)	8–18.6	....	....	....	....	8–12	....	8–18.6 mm. (211)
LVD(D)	12.23–3	12–20	16.1–24.1	12–20.4	....	16–20	....	12–24.1 mm. (351)
RVAW(S)	3.3–7.3	....	....	....	....	....	....	3.3–7.3 mm. (200)
RVAW(D)	2–4.7	....	1.1–4.1	....	....	....	....	1.1–4.7 mm. (440)
RVD(S)	5.5–11.4	....	....	....	....	....	....	5.5–11.4 mm. (200)
RVD(D)	6.1–15	10–17	10.4–17.7	10–17.5	....	....	....	6.1–17.7 mm. (540)
MVCF	....	....	....	....	....	....	0.92–2.2	0.92–2.2 circ./sec. (72)

MDV　= mitral valve depth
MVTE = mitral valve total excursion
MVDE = mitral valve diastolic excursion
MVVS = mitral valve velocity slope
TVD　= triscupid valve depth
TVTE = triscupid valve total excursion
TVDE = triscupid valve diastolic excursion
TVVS = triscupid valve velocity slope

ARD　= aortic root diameter
AVO　= aortic valve opening
PRD　= pulmonary root diameter
PVO　= pulmonary valve opening
LAD　= leit atrial dimension
IST　= interventricular septal thickness
LVPW = leit ventricular posterior wall
LVD　= left ventricular dimension

RVAW = right ventricular anterior wall
RVD　= right ventricular dimension
MVCF = mean velocity circumferential fiber shortening
(S)　= systole
(D)　= diastole

APPENDIX D: NORMAL ECHOCARDIOGRAPHIC VALUES IN NEWBORNS

Table D–1, reprinted from an article by Moss et al.,[4] lists from the literature some normal echocardiographic values for newborns.

REFERENCES

1. Henry, W.L., Ware, J., Gardin, J.M., Hepner, S.I., McKay, J., and Weiner, M.: Echocardiographic measurements in normal subjects: growth-related changes that occur between infancy and early adulthood. Circulation, 57:278, 1978.
2. Gardin, J.M., Henry, W.L., Savage, D.D., Ware, J.H., Burn, C., and Borer, J.S.: Echocardiographic measurements in normal subjects: evaluation of an adult population without clinically apparent heart disease. J. Clin. Ultrasound, 7:439, 1979.
3. Goldberg, S.J., Allen, H.D., and Sahn, D.J.: Pediatric and Adolescent Echocardiography. Chicago, Yearbook Medical Publishers, 1975.
4. Moss, A.J., Gussoni, C.C., and Isabel-Jones, J.: Echocardiography in congenital heart disease. West. J. Med., 124:102, 1976.
5. Hagan, A.D., Deely, W.J., Sahn, D.J., Karliner, J., Friedman, W.F., and O'Rourke, R.: Ultrasound evaluation of systolic anterior septal motion in patients with and without right ventricular volume overload. Circulation, 50:1221, 1973.
6. Meyer, R.A. and Kaplan, S.: Echocardiography in the diagnosis of hypoplasia of the left or right ventricle in the neonate. Circulation, 46:55, 1972.
7. Solinger, R., Elbl, F., and Minhas, K.: Echocardiography in the normal neonate. Circulation, 47:108, 1973.
8. Godman, M.J., Tham, P., and Kidd, B.S.L.: Echocardiography in the evaluation of the cyanotic newborn infant. Br. Heart J., 36:154, 1974.
9. Lundstrom, N.R. and Elder, I.: Ultrasoundcardiography in infants and children. Acta Paediatr. Scand., 60:117, 1971.
10. Winsberg, F.: Echocardiography of the fetal and newborn heart. Invest. Radiol., 7:152, 1972.
11. Sahn, D.J., Deely, W.J., Hagan, A.D., and Friedman, W.F.: Echocardiographic assessment of left ventricular performance in normal newborns. Circulation, 49:232, 1974.

Index

Page numbers in *italics* refer to illustrations; page numbers followed by t refer to tables.